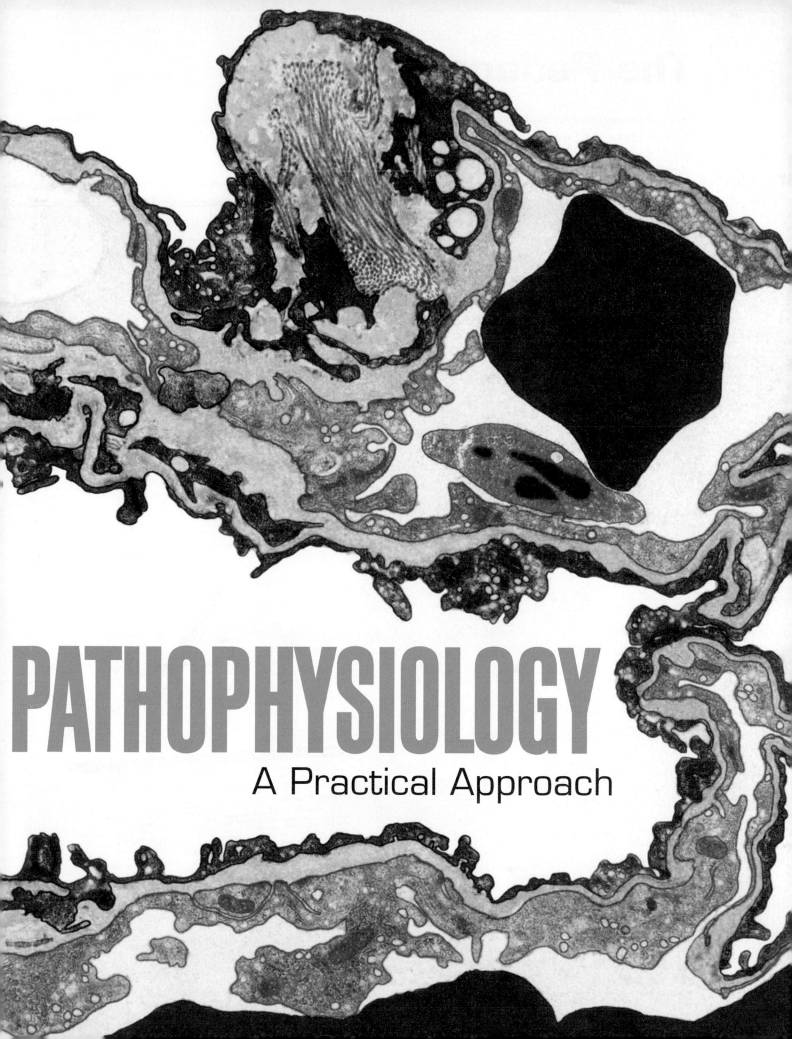

PATHOPHYSIOLOGY

A Practical Approach

The Pedagogy

Pathophysiology: A Practical Approach focuses on driving comprehension through a variety of strategies that meet the learning needs of students while generating enthusiasm about the topic. This interactive approach addresses different learning styles, making this the ideal text to ensure mastery of key concepts. The pedagogical aids that appear in most chapters include the following:

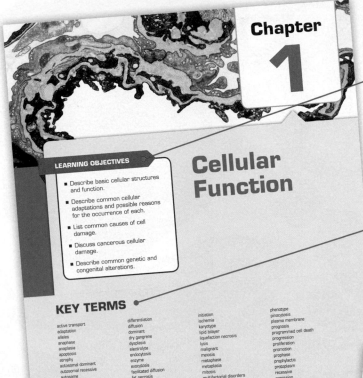

Chapter Objectives These objectives provide instructors and students with a snapshot of the key information they will encounter in each chapter. They can serve as a checklist to help guide and focus study.

Key Terms Found in a list at the beginning of each chapter and in bold within the chapter, these terms will create an expanded vocabulary in evidence-based practice. Visit **http://go.jblearning.com/story** to see these terms in an interactive glossary and use flashcards and word puzzles to nail the definitions.

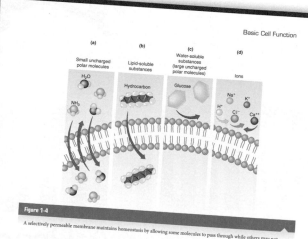

Figure 1-4

A selectively permeable membrane maintains homeostasis by allowing some molecules to pass through while others may not.

Exchanging Material

Cellular permeability is the ability of the cell to allow passage of some substances through the membrane while not permitting others. To accomplish this process, cells have gates that may be opened or closed by proteins, chemical signals, or electrical charges. Being selectively permeable allows the cell to maintain internal balance, or homeostasis. Some substances have free passage in and out of the cells, including enzymes, glucose, and electrolytes. Enzymes are proteins that facilitate chemical reactions in cells, while glucose is a sugar molecule that provides energy. Electrolytes are chemicals that are charged conductors when dissolved in water. Passage across the cell membrane is accomplished through several mechanisms, including diffusion, osmosis, facilitated diffusion, active transport, endocytosis, and exocytosis.

Diffusion is the movement of solutes, particles dissolved in a solvent, from an area of higher concentration to lower concentration (Figure 1-5). The degree of diffusion depends on the permeability of the membrane and the concentration gradient, which is the difference in concentrations of substances on either side of the membrane. Smaller particles diffuse more easily than

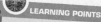

LEARNING POINTS

To illustrate diffusion, consider an elevator filled beyond capacity with people. When the door opens, the people near the door naturally fall out—moving from an area of high concentration to an area with less concentration with no effort. In the body, gases are exchanged in the lungs by diffusion. Unoxygenated blood enters the pulmonary capillaries where it picks up oxygen from the inhaled air of the alveoli, while dropping off carbon dioxide to the alveoli to be exhaled.

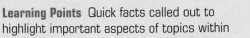

Learning Points Quick facts called out to highlight important aspects of topics within each chapter.

Myth Busters Common myths and misconceptions highlighted and debunked.

Clinical Cases Found in select chapters, these vignettes provide critical-thinking challenges for students and are accompanied by follow up discussion questions and answers.

Chapter Summary Summaries are included at the end of each chapter to provide a concise review of material covered in each chapter.

Learning Aids Features within the text meant to enhance the student's learning experience. Includes bolded key terms for easy identification, web resources for additional reading and information, and full-color illustrations and photos for enhanced visual understanding.

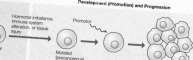

Conversion (or Initiation)   Development (Promotion) and Progression

DNA-reactive carcinogen
Inherited mutation
Epigenetic carcinogen   Normal cell
Hormonal imbalance, immune system alteration, or tissue injury   Promotor   Mutated (precancerous) cell   Malignant cells (cancer)

Mutation   Oncogenes activated and expressed
Normal DNA   Mutated DNA   Mutated DNA

Figure 1-20

Carcinogenesis: the stages leading to cancer.

complex interactions between carcinogen exposure and genetic mutations. Numerous genes have been identified as causing cancers. Oncogenes activate cell division and influence embryonic development. Some of these cancer-producing genes can remain harmless until altered by a genetic or acquired mutation. Common causes of acquired genetic mutations include viruses, radiation, environmental and dietary carcinogens, and hormones. Other factors that can increase a person's likelihood of developing cancer include age, nutritional status, hormonal balance, and stress response. As we age, statistically there is a higher

likelihood of a DNA transcription error occurring, as well as more carcinogen exposure. Examples of how changes in nutritional status increase the likelihood of cancer can be seen in free radical damage. Some cancers almost feed off of hormones, meaning they grow faster in the presence of particular hormones. Finally, the immune system is impaired during stress states, which can impair its ability to find and respond to carcinogenesis.

The loss of differentiation that occurs with cancer is referred to as anaplasia. Anaplasia occurs in varying

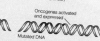

MYTH BUSTERS

MYTH 1: Standing in front of a microwave oven while it is cooking can increase your risk for cancer.

This is a common myth that may have some truth in it. Cancer risk has been linked to increased levels of ionizing radiation (e.g., X-rays) because they detach electrons from atoms. Microwaves use non-ionizing microwave radiation to heat food. Early microwave ovens emitted higher levels of this radiation, which may have increased cancer risk slightly. Research has never been able to determine whether cancer risk increased with non-ionizing radiation exposure. Currently, Food and Drug Administration guidelines limit the amount of the non-ionizing radiation microwave ovens can emit, further decreasing the cancer risk.

MYTH 2: Using cell phones can increase your risk of cancer.

This is another common myth. Cell phones use the same non-ionizing microwave radiation as microwave ovens to emit a signal. Even with the close proximity to your head while in use, evidence does not support that there is an increase in brain cancer risk. Using a cell phone for an extended period at one time will indeed heat your ear for the same reason that the microwave heats your food. But no clear evidence suggests that this extended use increases cancer risk.

CASE STUDY

HISTORY

Mrs. Turner is a 47-year-old Caucasian female who has been admitted to the general surgical floor with a lump in her right breast. She generally has enjoyed good health up to this admission. Mrs. Turner neither smokes nor drinks and follows a daily exercise regimen. Approximately 2 months ago, Mrs. Turner's husband noticed a small lump in her right breast. She gave this finding little attention, assuming that the lump was like the many others she tended to experience around her menses. The lump, however, failed to resolve after her menses, and Mrs. Turner became concerned when it seemed to grow bigger.

Mrs. Turner is the mother of 2 children, 8 and 6 years old. Mrs. Turner took birth control pills for 5 years after the birth of her second child. Last year she chose to discontinue birth control pill use and turned to an alternative method of birth control. Mrs. Turner is the only child born to her parents late in their life. Her father is alive and well, but her mother died of breast cancer 5 years ago. A family history revealed a strong history of both heart disease and cancer on both sides of Mrs. Turner's family.

CURRENT STATUS

On exam, a 2–3-cm mass was palpated in the upper quadrant of her right breast. This mass felt firm, was fixed to the chest wall, and was tender to the touch. The remaining breast skin was normal in appearance with no discoloration or retraction of the skin. One node, approximately the size of a pea, was palpated under the right axilla. Palpation of the left breast revealed two 1–2-cm soft, movable masses. Mrs. Turner said that she noticed these lumps in her left breast 2 weeks ago but stated that the lumps in her left breast became palpable and bothersome about 12 days from the start of menses. A reproductive history disclosed that the onset of menses occurred at the age of 10. There is no history of dysmenorrhea associated with her periods, though she states that her breasts become tender and lumpy a week or two before her menses. She has had no pregnancies that were delivered by cesarean section. Her one and only Papanicolaou (Pap) smear was done 2 years ago and produced a normal result. The remaining exam findings were unremarkable. Mammography confirmed the presence of a 3-cm mass in the upper quadrant of the right breast and three 1.5-cm masses in the left breast. The result of a bone scan and other diagnostic procedures were negative.

1. Mrs. Turner is considered to be at increased risk for developing breast cancer. Which of the following factors is most positively related to this high-risk profile?

    A. History of breast cancer in family members

    B. History of cystic breast disease

    C. Early onset of menarche

    D. Trauma related to birth of her children

2. Which of the following best explains the existence of an enlarged right axillary lymph node in Mrs. Turner?

    A. The lymph node is the result of an inflammatory reaction that normally occurs with the onset of her current menses.

    B. The existence of the node is the result of an increased strain on the lymphatic system as a result of cellular degeneration.

    C. The lymph node exists to provide nutrients to the rapidly growing cancer cells.

    D. The lymph node is the result of cancer cells spreading to different tissues within the body.

Mrs. Turner was taken to surgery 3 days later, and a modified radical mastectomy was performed. A histological exam was used to classify the tumor using the TNM staging system. An estrogen receptor assay performed on the removed tissue confirmed that Mrs. Turner's tumor was estrogen dependent. She returned to her room with a drain in place. Her dressing was dry and intact. She was able to turn, cough, and breathe deeply on her own. Her temperature remained within normal limits after surgery. Progesterone therapy was initiated daily. Ambulation was started on the 2nd postoperative day.

3. Mrs. Turner's tumor was staged at stage III using the TNM staging system. Pathological exam of the surgically removed tissue sample placed Mrs. Turner's tumor in category type II. The need to state and classify tumors is important for which of the following reasons?

    A. Treatment is based on the knowledge of tumor size, extent, and tissue type.

    B. Tumor staging is useful for studying a number of researchable factors, from survival to treatment response.

    C. A consistent classification system provides a way to catalogue individuals with breast tumors for statistical analysis.

    D. All of the above.

4. Which activities by Mrs. Turner increase her likelihood for a good prognosis?

5. What was the rationale for hormone therapy with Mrs. Turner?

Chapter Summary

Cells are the basic units of life, and they face many challenges in order to survive. These challenges include hypoxia, nutritional changes, infection, inflammation, and chemicals. Cells adapt to the challenges in an attempt to prevent or limit damage as well as death. This adaptation may be reversible or permanent.

Neoplasms arise from abnormal cellular proliferation or differentiation. These neoplasms can be benign or malignant. Benign tumors are more differentiated; therefore, they are more like the parent cells. Benign tumors are less likely to cause problems in the host or metastasize except in terms of location. On the other hand, malignant tumors are less differentiated; therefore, they are more like the parent cells. Malignant tumors are more likely to cause problems in the host and metastasize.

Genetic and congenital disorders can develop from factors that disrupt normal fetal development or interact with defective genes. These factors, or teratogens, can include radiation, infections, or chemicals. Genetic and congenital disorders may be present at birth or may not appear until later in life. Exploring these basic cellular and genetic concepts and issues will lay the foundation for understanding where disease begins.

Case Study Answers

1. A
2. D
3. D
4. Not smoking or drinking; routine exercise; overall good health
5. Because the tumor is hormone dependent, hormone therapy with more progesterone-like drugs will strangulate the supply of estrogen to the cancer. The tumor will shrink or growth will slow

References

Chiras, D. (2008). *Human biology* (6th ed.). Sudbury, MA: Jones and Bartlett.

Elling, B., Elling, K., & Rothenberg, M. (2004). *Anatomy and physiology.* Sudbury, MA: Jones and Bartlett.

Lewin, B., Cassimeris, L., Lingappa, V., & Plopper, G. (Eds.). (2007). *Cells.* Sudbury, MA: Jones and Bartlett.

Mosby's medical, nursing, & allied health dictionary (7th ed.). (2005). St. Louis, MO: Mosby.

Porth, C. (2006). *Essentials of pathophysiology* (6th ed.). Philadelphia, PA: Lippincott Williams & Wilkins.

Professional guide to pathophysiology (2nd ed.). (2007). Philadelphia, PA: Lippincott Williams & Wilkins.

Resources

www.cellsalive.com
www.cancer.org
www.cdc.gov
www.medlineplus.gov
www.nih.gov
www.rarediseases.org

go.jblearning.com/story

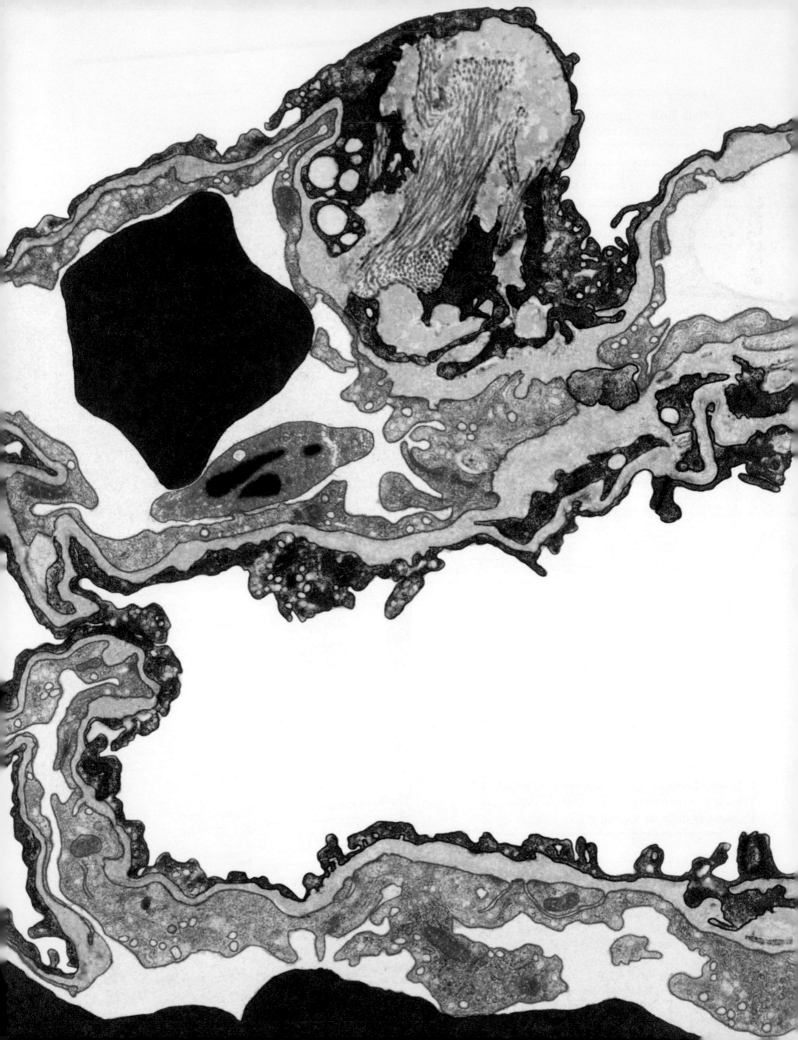

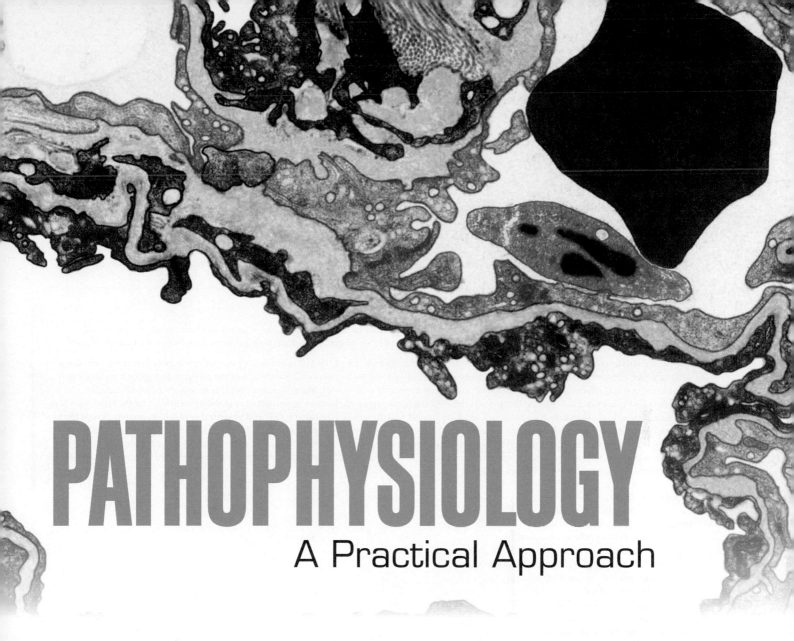

PATHOPHYSIOLOGY
A Practical Approach

Lachel Story, PhD, RN

Assistant Professor
School of Nursing
University of Southern Mississippi
Hattiesburg, Mississippi

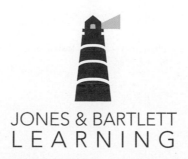

JONES & BARTLETT
LEARNING

World Headquarters
Jones & Bartlett Learning
40 Tall Pine Drive
Sudbury, MA 01776
978-443-5000
info@jblearning.com
www.jblearning.com

Jones & Bartlett Learning Canada
6339 Ormindale Way
Mississauga, Ontario L5V 1J2
Canada

Jones & Bartlett Learning International
Barb House, Barb Mews
London W6 7PA
United Kingdom

Jones & Bartlett Learning books and products are available through most bookstores and online booksellers. To contact Jones & Bartlett Learning directly, call 800-832-0034, fax 978-443-8000, or visit our website, www.jblearning.com.

Substantial discounts on bulk quantities of Jones & Bartlett Learning publications are available to corporations, professional associations, and other qualified organizations. For details and specific discount information, contact the special sales department at Jones & Bartlett Learning via the above contact information or send an email to specialsales@jblearning.com.

The author, editor, and publisher have made every effort to provide accurate information. However, they are not responsible for errors, omissions, or for any outcomes related to the use of the contents of this book and take no responsibility for the use of the products and procedures described. Treatments and side effects described in this book may not be applicable to all people; likewise, some people may require a dose or experience a side effect that is not described herein. Drugs and medical devices are discussed that may have limited availability controlled by the Food and Drug Administration (FDA) for use only in a research study or clinical trial. Research, clinical practice, and government regulations often change the accepted standard in this field. When consideration is being given to use of any drug in the clinical setting, the health care provider or reader is responsible for determining FDA status of the drug, reading the package insert, and reviewing prescribing information for the most up-to-date recommendations on dose, precautions, and contraindications, and determining the appropriate usage for the product. This is especially important in the case of drugs that are new or seldom used.

Production Credits
Chief Executive Officer: Ty Field
President: James Homer
SVP, Chief Operating Officer: Don Jones, Jr.
SVP, Chief Technology Officer: Dean Fossella
SVP, Chief Marketing Officer: Alison M. Pendergast
SVP, Chief Financial Officer: Ruth Siporin
Publisher: Kevin Sullivan
Acquisitions Editor: Amy Sibley
Associate Editor: Patricia Donnelly
Editorial Assistant: Rachel Shuster
Production Manager: Carolyn F. Rogers
Associate Production Editor: Cindie Bryan
Marketing Manager: Meagan Norlund
V.P., Manufacturing and Inventory Control: Therese Connell
Composition: Publishers' Design & Production Services, Inc.
Cover and Text Design: Kristin E. Parker
Associate Artist and Photo Researcher: Carolyn Arcabascio
Cover and Title Page Image: © Science Photo Library/age fotostock
Printing and Binding: Courier Kendallville
Cover Printing: Courier Kendallville

To order this product, use ISBN: 978-1-4496-2408-8

Library of Congress Cataloging-in-Publication Data
Story, Lachel.
    Pathophysiology : a practical approach / Lachel Story.
            p. ; cm.
    Includes bibliographical references and index.
    ISBN 978-0-7637-7238-3
  1. Physiology, Pathological.   I. Title.
    [DNLM: 1.   Pathology—Nurses' Instruction. 2.   Physiology—Nurses' Instruction.   QZ 140 S887p 2011]
    RB113.S84 2011
    616.07--dc22
            2010023127

6048

Printed in the United States of America
15 14 13 12   10 9 8 7 6 5 4 3

Contents

Preface

Teaching pathophysiology for more than 6 years and nursing for more than 15 years, I noticed a lack of pathophysiology books that students could relate to, and high student frustration in learning the convoluted material. Pathophysiology—while being the foundation of much of nursing education from medical-surgical to pharmacology, it is often an insurmountable barrier for students. Often students are faced with a copious amount of complicated information to weed through that bogs them deep in a marsh. While some students are bogged down in an information marsh, other students are seeking more information in a skeleton book that has been cut to the bone. Nursing faculty join the students on this frustrating, Goldilocks journey by trying to make the available resources fit. Nursing students and faculty have pathophysiology books available that provide either way too much information or way too little. This book will provide the right fit with a practical guide to pathophysiology by providing information in a student-friendly, understandable way. This is a book where extraneous information is omitted, leaving only necessary information. The information in this book is presented in an more accessible manner by considering readability, providing colorful graphics, and giving the content context and meaning.

This ground-breaking book will provide a springboard for faculty and students to come together as co-learners to explore this fascinating content. As this co-learning is stimulated, pathophysiology is no longer just mindlessly deposited into the students in a stifling manner; rather, learning for the students and the faculty becomes an empowerment pedagogy. This book will provide students with an understandable and practical resource for learning pathophysiology. The faculty will have a resource that speaks to students and resources to engage students. Health professionals will also be able to refer the book to refresh their memory on concepts in a pragmatic way.

Acknowledgments

First, I would like to thank my husband, Tom, and children, Clayton and Mason, for their never-ending love and encouragement. I would also like to express my deepest gratitude to my mom, Carolyn, and dad, Tommy, because I would not be who I am today without them. I would also like to acknowledge all my students past, present, and future for constantly teaching me for more than I could ever teach them and for all their feedback—I heard it and I hope this is more what you had in mind. Finally, I would like to convey my appreciation to my colleagues for their gracious mentoring and support.

Reviewers

Tanya L. Rogers, APRN, BC, MSN, EdD
Associate Professor of Nursing
School of Nursing and Allied Health Administration
Fairmont State University
Fairmont, West Virginia

Jennifer K. Sofie, MSN, ANP, FNP
Adjunct Assistant Professor
College of Nursing
Montana State University
Bozeman, Montana

Joan Stokowski, MSN
Assistant Professor
Department of Health Careers
Illinois Central College
Peoria, Illinois

Brenda D. Tilton, RN, MSN, FNP-BC
Assistant Professor of Nursing
School of Nursing
Southern State Community College
Hillsboro, Ohio

Vickie Walker, DNP, RN
Assistant Professor of Nursing
School of Nursing
Gardner-Webb University
Boiling Springs, North Carolina

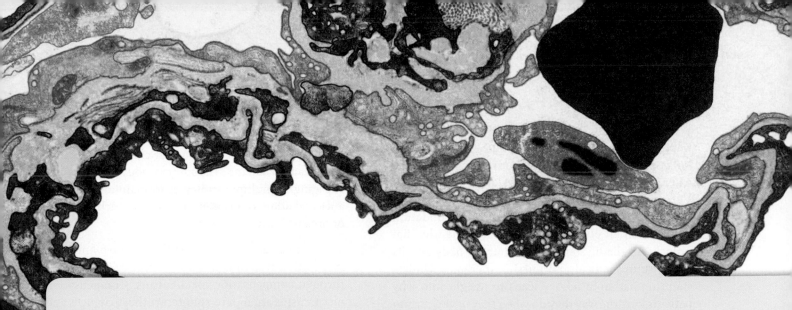

Introduction to Pathophysiology

LEARNING OBJECTIVES

- Define pathophysiology and identify its importance for clinical practice.

- Identify key health and disease concepts.

KEY TERMS

acute	epidemiology	idiopathic	pathophysiology
chronic	etiology	insidious	predisposing factor
complication	exacerbation	manifestation	prognosis
convalescence	health	negative feedback system	remission
disease	homeostasis	pandemic	syndrome
epidemic	iatrogenic	pathogenesis	

Pathophysiology Concepts

What is meant by pathophysiology? And why is it so important to understand, especially for nurses? Essentially, pathophysiology is the study of what happens when normal anatomy and physiology goes wrong. Veering off this normal path can cause diseases or abnormal states. Pathophysiology is the foundation upon which all of nursing is built. It is the why that unlocks all the mysteries of the human body and its response to medical and nursing therapies. Understanding pathophysiology leads to insight into why patients look the way they do when they have a certain disease, why the medicines we give them work, why the side effects of treatments occur, and why the complications transpire. Pathophysiology provides the rationale for evidence-based medicine. Now, it is important to ask, why are so many students mystified by pathophysiology? Students often get lost in the minute details and the complicated nuances of pathophysiology. Pathophysiology, when brought back to the basics and framed in a practical context, can bring meaning and understanding to the world of health and disease in which people live.

Health and Disease

To understand disease, first health is clarified. Health may be considered the absence of disease. Health can be expanded to include wellness of mind, body, and spirit. This normal state may vary due to genetic, age, and gender differences, and it becomes relative to the individual's baseline. Negative events in any one of these three areas can cause issues in the other—these areas coexist. Humans are complicated and do not exist in a vacuum. Just like the mind, body, and spirit are interrelated, humans are interrelated with their environment, including the physical ecology as well as social factors. These environmental factors play a significant role in an individual's health, whether negatively or positively.

On the flip side of health is disease. Disease is the state when a bodily function is no longer occurring normally. Diseases range from merely causing temporary stress to causing life-changing complications. Exploring concepts of homeostasis is a good place to start in understanding the origins of disease.

Homeostasis

Many words can be used to describe homeostasis, such as equilibrium, balance, consistency, and stability. Some examples of this relative consistency can be seen in things like blood pressure, pulse, and temperature. Every part of the human body, from cells to the organs, needs balance to maintain its bodily functions. In some cases, such as with pH, minimal changes can cause significant problems. The human body is constantly engaging in multiple strategies to maintain this balance and addressing external stressors such as injury or organism invasion.

Homeostasis is a self-regulating, give-and-take system that responds to minor changes in the body through compensation mechanisms. Compensation mechanisms attempt to counteract those changes and return the body to its normal state (**Figure I–1**). Several brain structures are instrumental in maintaining this balance, including the medulla oblongata, hypothalamus, reticular formation, and pituitary gland. The medulla oblongata is located in the brain stem and controls vital functions such as blood pressure, temperature, and pulse. The reticular formation is a network of nerve cells in the brain stem and the spinal cord that also controls vital functions. The reticular formation relays information to the hypothalamus. The hypothalamus controls homeostasis by communicating to the pituitary gland. The pituitary gland, or the

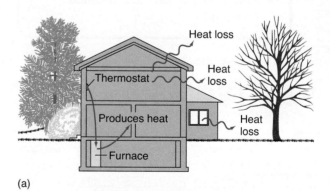

(a)

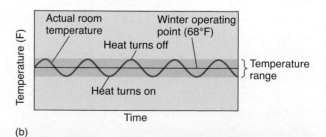

(b)

Figure I-1

Homeostasis is like a house. (a) Heat is maintained in a house by a furnace, which compensates for heat loss. (b) A hypothetical temperature graph.

master gland, regulates other glands that contribute to growth, maturation, and reproduction.

Two types of feedback systems exist to maintain homeostasis: negative and positive. The negative feedback system is the most common type and works to maintain a deficit in the system. Examples of negative feedback systems include temperature and glucose regulation. Positive feedback systems, though few in number, take the body away from homeostasis. An amplified response occurs in the same direction as the original stressor. Examples of positive feedback systems include childbirth, sneezing, and blood clots.

Disease Development

Etiology is the cause of a disease. Etiologic factors may include infectious agents, chemicals, or environmental factors, to name a few. Etiologic factors may also be unknown, or idiopathic. Additionally, diseases can be caused by an unintended, or iatrogenic, effect of a medical treatment. Predisposing factors are tendencies that put an individual at risk for developing certain diseases. Examples of predisposing factors are similar to etiology factors and may include dietary imbalances and carcinogen exposure. Identifying the etiology and predisposing factors of diseases can be instrumental in preventing the disease by distinguishing at-risk populations. The healthcare system is turning toward more disease prevention because of the long-term financial implications.

The development of a disease is called pathogenesis. Some diseases are self-limiting, while others are chronic and never resolve. Some diseases cause reversible changes while others cause irreparable damage. The body will attempt to limit the damage with compensatory mechanisms. When those mechanisms can no longer maintain relative consistency, disease occurs. The onset of the disease may be sudden or acute. Acute onset of a disease may include pain or vomiting, but a gradual, or insidious onset may have vague signs. Hypertension can occur in this subtle manner.

Disease duration is another important concept to consider. A disease may be short term, or acute, occurring and resolving quickly. Gastroenteritis and tonsillitis are examples of acute diseases. When an acute disease does not resolve after a short period, it may move into a chronic state. A chronic disease often has less notable signs and occurs over a longer period. Chronic diseases may not ever resolve but may become manageable. Diabetes mellitus and depression are examples of chronic diseases. Additionally, people with chronic diseases can experience an acute event of that disease, complicating care. An example of this phenomenon can be seen when an asthmatic patient has an acute asthma attack.

Recognition of a disease when it is encountered is important in diagnosis, or identification, of disease. Manifestations are the clinical effects or evidence of a disease. These may include both signs—what can be seen or measured—and symptoms—what the patient describes. Syndrome refers to a group of signs and symptoms that occurs together. Some diseases may include episodes of remission and exacerbation. Remission occurs when the manifestations subside, and exacerbation occurs when the manifestations increase again. Systemic lupus erythematosus is an example of a disease that experiences remission and exacerbation.

Recovering from a disease and limiting any residual effects are important aspects of disease. Convalescence is the stage of recovery following a disease that may last for days or months. Prognosis refers to an individual's likelihood of a full recovery or regaining normal functioning. Complications are new problems that arise because of a disease. For example, renal failure can be a complication of uncontrolled hypertension.

Understanding factors affecting the health and disease of populations is the cornerstone to understanding prevention and containment. Epidemiology refers to tracking patterns of diseases in a group of people. This tracking includes occurrence, incidence, prevalence, transmission, and distribution of the disease. Epidemics occur when there are increasing disease numbers in a group. When the epidemic expands to a larger population, it becomes a pandemic.

Summary

Pathophysiology is the basis for understanding the intricate world of the human body, its response to disease, and the rationale for treatment. Understanding pathophysiology can assist the nurse to better anticipate situations, correct issues, and provide appropriate care. The concepts of health and disease, although complex, need not cause stress to nursing students or patients. These concepts can open a world of wonder of which to be in awe.

Bibliography

Mosby's medical, nursing, & allied health dictionary. (2005). (7th ed.) St. Louis, MO: Mosby.

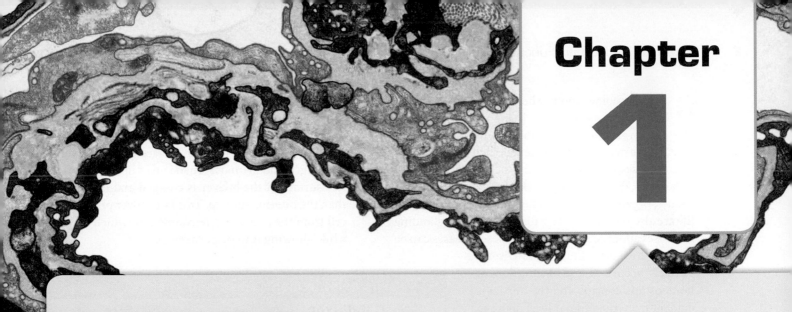

Cellular Function

- Describe basic cellular structures and function.

- Describe common cellular adaptations and possible reasons for the occurrence of each.

- List common causes of cell damage.

- Discuss cancerous cellular damage.

- Describe common genetic and congenital alterations.

KEY TERMS

active transport
adaptation
alleles
anaphase
anaplasia
apoptosis
atrophy
autosomal dominant
autosomal recessive
autosome
benign
cancer
carcinogenesis
caseous necrosis
cell membrane
chromosome
coagulative necrosis
congenital
crenation
curative
cytoplasm
deoxyribonucleic acid (DNA)

differentiation
diffusion
dominant
dry gangrene
dysplasia
electrolyte
endocytosis
enzyme
exocytosis
facilitated diffusion
fat necrosis
free radicals
gangrene
gas gangrene
genes
genetics
glucose
grading
heterozygous
homozygous
hyperplasia
hypertrophy

initiation
ischemia
karyotype
lipid bilayer
liquefaction necrosis
lysis
malignant
meiosis
metaphase
metaplasia
mitosis
multifactorial disorders
necrosis
neoplasm
nucleotide
nucleus
oncogene
organelle
osmosis
osmotic pressure
palliative
phagocytosis

phenotype
pinocytosis
plasma membrane
prognosis
programmed cell death
progression
proliferation
promotion
prophase
prophylactic
protoplasm
recessive
remission
selectively permeable
sex-linked
telophase
teratogens
TNM staging
tumor
wet gangrene

athophysiology inquiry begins with exploring the basic building blocks of living organisms. Cells give organisms their immense diversity. Organisms can be made up of a single cell, such as with bacteria or viruses, or billions of cells, such as with humans. In humans, these building blocks work together to form tissues, organs, and organ systems. These basic units of life are also the basic units of disease. As understanding increases about specific diseases, these diseases can be reduced to their cellular level. Diseases likely occur because of some loss of homeostatic control, and the impact is evident from the cellular level on up to the system level. Understanding cellular dysfunctions associated with diseases has led to improved prevention and treatment of those diseases. Therefore, understanding basic cellular function and dysfunction is essential to understanding pathophysiology.

Basic Cell Function

Cells are complex miniorganisms that are the result of millions of years of evolution. Cells can only arise from a pre-existing cell. Cells, while varying greatly in size and shape (**Figure 1-1**), have the remarkable ability to exchange materials with their immediate surroundings, obtain energy from organic nutrients, synthesize complex molecules, and replicate themselves.

The basic components of cells include the cytoplasm, the nucleus, and the cell membrane. The cytoplasm, or protoplasm, is a colorless, viscous liquid containing water, nutrients, ions, dissolved gases, and waste products where the cellular work takes place. The cytoplasm supports all the internal cellular structures called organelles (**Figure 1-2**). Organelles, or little organs, perform the work that maintains the cell's life (**Table 1-1**). The cytoplasm also surrounds the nucleus. The nucleus, or the control center, contains all the genetic information (DNA) for the cell and is surrounded by a double membrane (**Figure 1-3**). The nucleus regulates cell growth, metabolism, and reproduction. The cell membrane, or

plasma membrane, is the semipermeable boundary containing the cell and its components (**Figure 1-4**). A lipid bilayer, or fatty double covering, makes up the membrane. The interior surface of the bilayer is uncharged and primarily made up of lipids. The exterior surface of the bilayer is charged and is less fatty than the interior surface. This fatty cover protects the cell from the aqueous environment in which it exists while allowing it to be permeable.

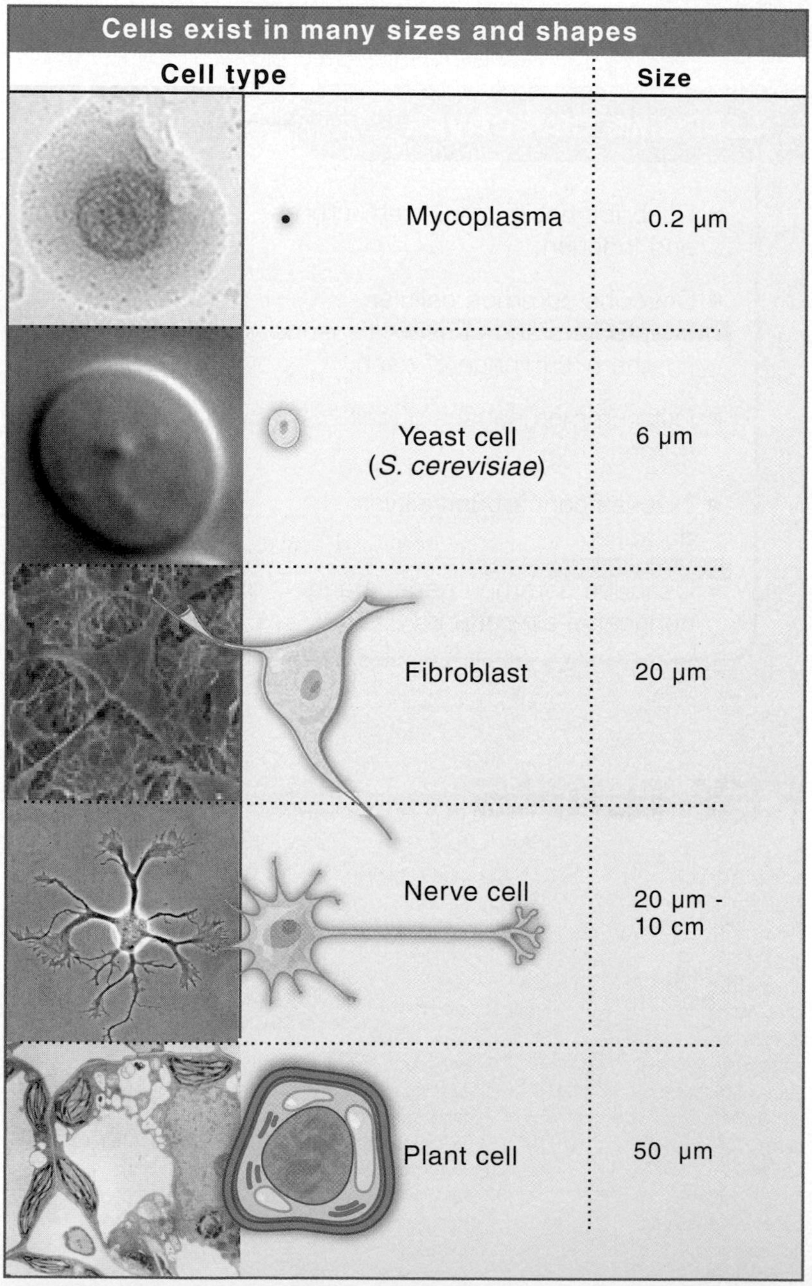

Cells exist in many sizes and shapes		
Cell type		**Size**
	Mycoplasma	0.2 μm
	Yeast cell (*S. cerevisiae*)	6 μm
	Fibroblast	20 μm
	Nerve cell	20 μm - 10 cm
	Plant cell	50 μm

Figure 1-1

Cells vary greatly in size and shape. Some cells are spherical, while others are long extensions.

Table 1-1 Overview of Cell Organelles

Organelle	Structure	Function
Nucleus	Round or oval body; surrounded by nuclear envelope	Contains the genetic information necessary for control of cell structure and function; DNA contains hereditary information
Nucleolus	Round or oval body in the nucleus consisting of DNA and RNA	Produces ribosomal RNA
Endoplasmic reticulum	Network of membranous tubules in the cytoplasm of the cell. Smooth endoplasmic reticulum contains no ribosomes. Rough endoplasmic reticulum is studded with ribosomes	Smooth endoplasmic reticulum (SER) is involved in the production of phospholipids and has many different functions in different cells; round endoplasmic reticulum (RER) is the site of the synthesis of lysosomal enzymes and proteins for extracellular use
Ribosomes	Small particles found in the cytoplasm; made of RNA and protein	Aid in the production of proteins on the RER and polysomes
Polysome	Molecule of mRNA bound to ribosomes	Site of protein synthesis
Golgi complex	Series of flattened sacs usually located near the nucleus	Sorts, chemically modifies, and packages proteins produced on the RER
Secretory vesicles	Membrane-bound vesicles containing proteins produced by the RER and repackaged by the Golgi complex; contain protein hormones or enzymes	Store protein hormones or enzymes in the cytoplasm awaiting a signal for release
Food vacuole	Membrane-bound vesicle containing material engulfed by the cell	Stores ingested material and combines with lysosome
Lysosome	Round, membrane-bound structure containing digestive enzymes	Combines with food vacuoles and digests materials engulfed by cells
Mitochondria	Round, oval, or elongated structures with a double membrane. The inner membrane is thrown into folds.	Complete the breakdown of glucose, producing nicotine adenine dinucleotide (NADH) and adenosine triphosphate (ATP)
Cytoskeleton	Network of microtubules and microfilaments in the cell	Gives the cell internal support, helps transport molecules and some organelles inside the cell, and binds to enzymes of metabolic pathways
Cilia	Small projections of the cell membrane containing microtubules; found on a limited number of cells	Propel materials along the surface of certain cells
Flagella	Large projections of the cell membrane containing microtubules; found in humans only on sperm cells	Provide motive force for sperm cells
Centrioles	Small cylindrical bodies composed of microtubules arranged in nine sets of triplets; found in animal cells, not plants	Help organize spindle apparatus necessary for cell division

Sources: Chiras, D. (2008). *Human biology* (6th ed.). Sudbury, MA: Jones & Bartlett Learning.

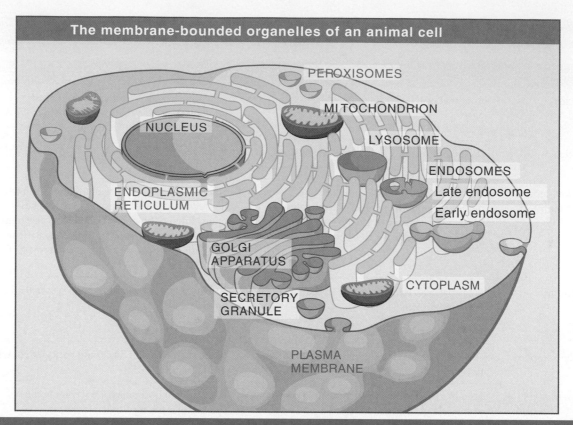

The membrane-bounded organelles of an animal cell

Figure 1-2

The cytoplasm contains several organelles.

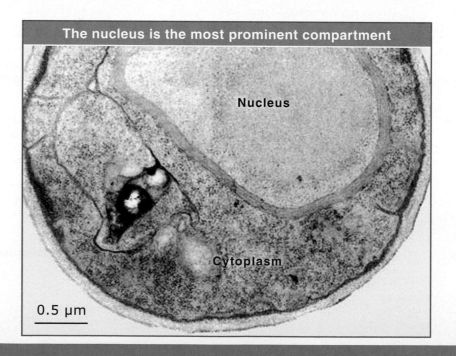

The nucleus is the most prominent compartment

Nucleus

Cytoplasm

0.5 μm

Figure 1-3

Although the proportion of the cell that is taken up by the nucleus varies according to cell type, the nucleus is usually the largest and most prominent cellular compartment.

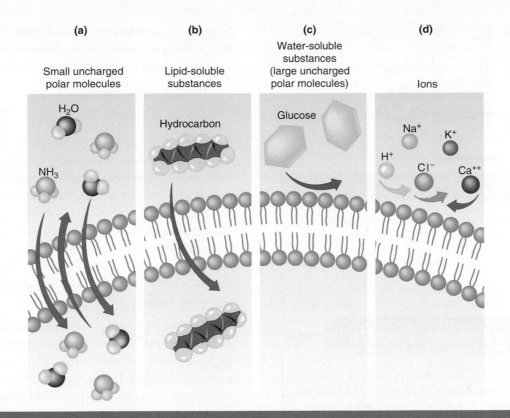

(a) Small uncharged polar molecules

(b) Lipid-soluble substances

(c) Water-soluble substances (large uncharged polar molecules)

(d) Ions

Figure 1-4

A selectively permeable membrane maintains homeostasis by allowing some molecules to pass through while others may not.

Exchanging Material

Cellular permeability is the ability of the cell to allow passage of some substances through the membrane while not permitting others. To accomplish this process, cells have gates that may be opened or closed by proteins, chemical signals, or electrical charges. Being selectively permeable allows the cell to maintain internal balance, or homeostasis. Some substances have free passage in and out of the cells, including enzymes, glucose, and electrolytes. Enzymes are proteins that facilitate chemical reactions in cells, while glucose is a sugar molecule that provides energy. Electrolytes are chemicals that are charged conductors when dissolved in water. Passage across the cell membrane is accomplished through several mechanisms, including diffusion, osmosis, facilitated diffusion, active transport, endocytosis, and exocytosis.

Diffusion is the movement of solutes, particles dissolved in a solvent, from an area of higher concentration to lower concentration (Figure 1-5). The degree of diffusion depends on the permeability of the membrane and the concentration gradient, which is the difference in concentrations of substances on either side of the membrane. Smaller particles diffuse more easily than

LEARNING POINTS

To illustrate diffusion, consider an elevator filled beyond capacity with people. When the door opens, the people near the door naturally fall out—moving from an area of high concentration to an area with less concentration with no effort. In the body, gases are exchanged in the lungs by diffusion. Unoxygenated blood enters the pulmonary capillaries where it picks up oxygen from the inhaled air of the alveoli, while dropping off carbon dioxide to the alveoli to be exhaled.

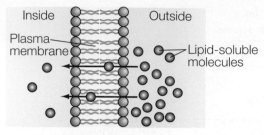

Simple diffusion

Figure 1-5

Lipid-soluble substances pass through the membrane directly via simple diffusion.

LEARNING POINTS

To understand osmosis, envision a plastic bag with holes in it that are only permeable to water and filled with water and sugar. If this bag is submerged in distilled water (contains no impurities), the bag will begin to swell because the water is attracted to the sugar. The water shifts to the higher concentrations of sugar in an attempt to dilute the sugar concentrations (**Figure 1-6**). In our bodies, osmosis allows the cells to remain hydrated.

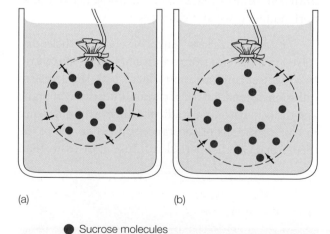

(a)　　　　　　　　　(b)

● Sucrose molecules

Figure 1-6

(a) When a bag of sugar water is immersed in a solution of pure water, (b) water will diffuse into the bag toward the lower concentrations of water, causing the bag to swell.

larger ones, and less viscous solutions diffuse more rapidly than thicker solutions. Many substances, such as oxygen, enter the cell through diffusion.

Osmosis is the movement of water or another solvent across the cellular membrane from an area of low solute concentration to an area of high solute concentration. The membrane is permeable to the solvent but not the solute. Movement usually continues until concentrations of the solute equalize on both sides of the membrane. Osmotic pressure refers to the tendency of water to move by osmosis. If too much water enters the cell membrane, the cell will swell and burst (lysis). If too much water moves out of the cell, the cell shrinks (crenation). Osmosis helps regulate fluid balance in the body, and examples can be found in the functioning of the kidneys.

Facilitated diffusion is the movement of substances from an area of lower concentration to an area of higher concentration with the assistance of a carrier molecule (**Figure 1-7**). Energy is not required, and the number of molecules that can transport is directly equivalent to the concentration of the carrier molecule. Glucose is transported into the cells by this method using insulin.

Active transport is the movement of a substance from an area of lower concentration to an area of higher concentration, against a concentration gradient (Figure 1-7). This movement will require a carrier molecule and energy because of the effort required to go against the gradient. This energy is usually in the form of adenosine triphosphate (ATP).

Endocytosis is bringing a substance into the cell (**Figure 1-8**). The membrane surrounds the particles, engulfing them. Phagocytosis, or cell eating, is when the process involves solid particles. Pinocytosis, or cell

LEARNING POINTS

To understand active transport, consider the overfilled elevator again. If the door opens and someone from outside the elevator attempts to get in, it will require much effort (energy) to enter the full elevator. The sodium-potassium pump is an example of active transport in the body. Energy is required to move sodium out of the cell where the concentrations are high and move potassium into the cell where the concentrations are high.

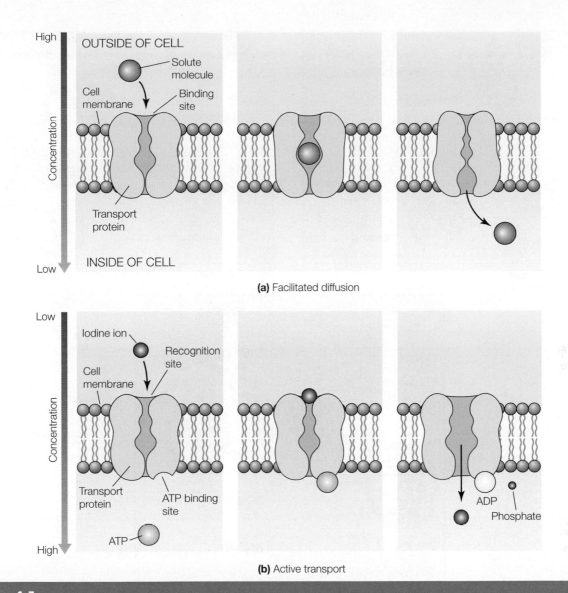

High

OUTSIDE OF CELL

Concentration

Solute
molecule

Cell
membrane

Binding
site

Transport
protein

Low   INSIDE OF CELL

(a) Facilitated diffusion

Low

Iodine ion

Recognition
site

Cell
membrane

Concentration

Transport
protein

ATP binding
site

ATP

ADP

Phosphate

High

(b) Active transport

Figure 1-7

Facilitated diffusion and active transport: (a) Water-soluble molecules can also diffuse through membranes with the assistance of proteins in facilitated diffusion. (b) Other proteins use energy from ATP to move against concentration gradients in a process called active transport.

drinking, is when the process involves a liquid. Components of the immune system use endocytosis, particularly phagocytosis, to consume and destroy bacteria and other foreign material. **Exocytosis** is the release of materials from the cell, usually with the assistance of a vesicle (a membrane-bound sac) (Figure 1-8). Often glands secrete hormones using exocytosis.

Energy Production

Energy can be a mystery to many of us. To understand energy, first we must understand that it comes

in many forms. Cells can obtain energy from two main sources—the breakdown of glucose (a type of carbohydrate) and the breakdown of triglycerides (a type of fat). Food enters the gastrointestinal tract, where it is broken down into sugars, amino acids, and fatty acids. These substances then are either converted to larger molecules (e.g., glucose to glycogen, amino acids to proteins, and fatty acids to triglycerides and fats), stored until needed, or metabolized to make ATP. When used to make ATP, all three sources of energy must first be converted to acetyl coenzyme A (acetyl CoA). Acetyl CoA enters the Kreb cycle, a high-electron-producing

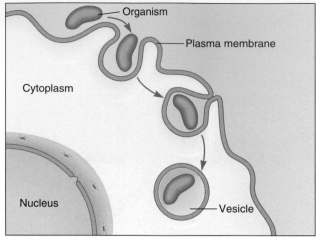

(a) ENDOCYTOSIS

PINOCYTOSIS

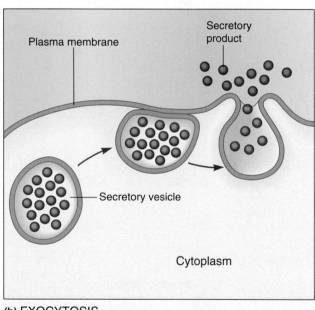

(b) EXOCYTOSIS

Figure 1-8

(a) Cells can engulf large particles, cell fragments, and even entire cells. (b) Cells can also get rid of large particles.

process, of the mitochondria. These molecules then go through a complex series of reactions, which result in the production of large amounts of ATP (**Figure 1-9**).

Replication and Differentiation

A cell's basic requirement for life is ensuring that it can reproduce. Many cells divide numerous times throughout the life span while others die and are replaced with new cells. **Proliferation** is the regulated process by which cells divide and reproduce. The most common form of cell division, where the cell divides into two

separate cells, is **mitosis** (**Figure 1-10**). In mitosis, the division of one cell results in two genetically identical and equal daughter cells. This process occurs in four phases—prophase, metaphase, anaphase, and telophase. In **prophase**, the chromosomes condense and the nuclear membrane disintegrates. In **metaphase**, the spindle fibers attach to centromeres and chromosomes align. Chromosomes separate and move to opposite poles in **anaphase**. Finally, chromosomes arrive at each pole, and new membranes are formed in **telophase**. **Meiosis** is a form of cell division that occurs only in mature sperm and ova (Figure 1-10). Normally, human

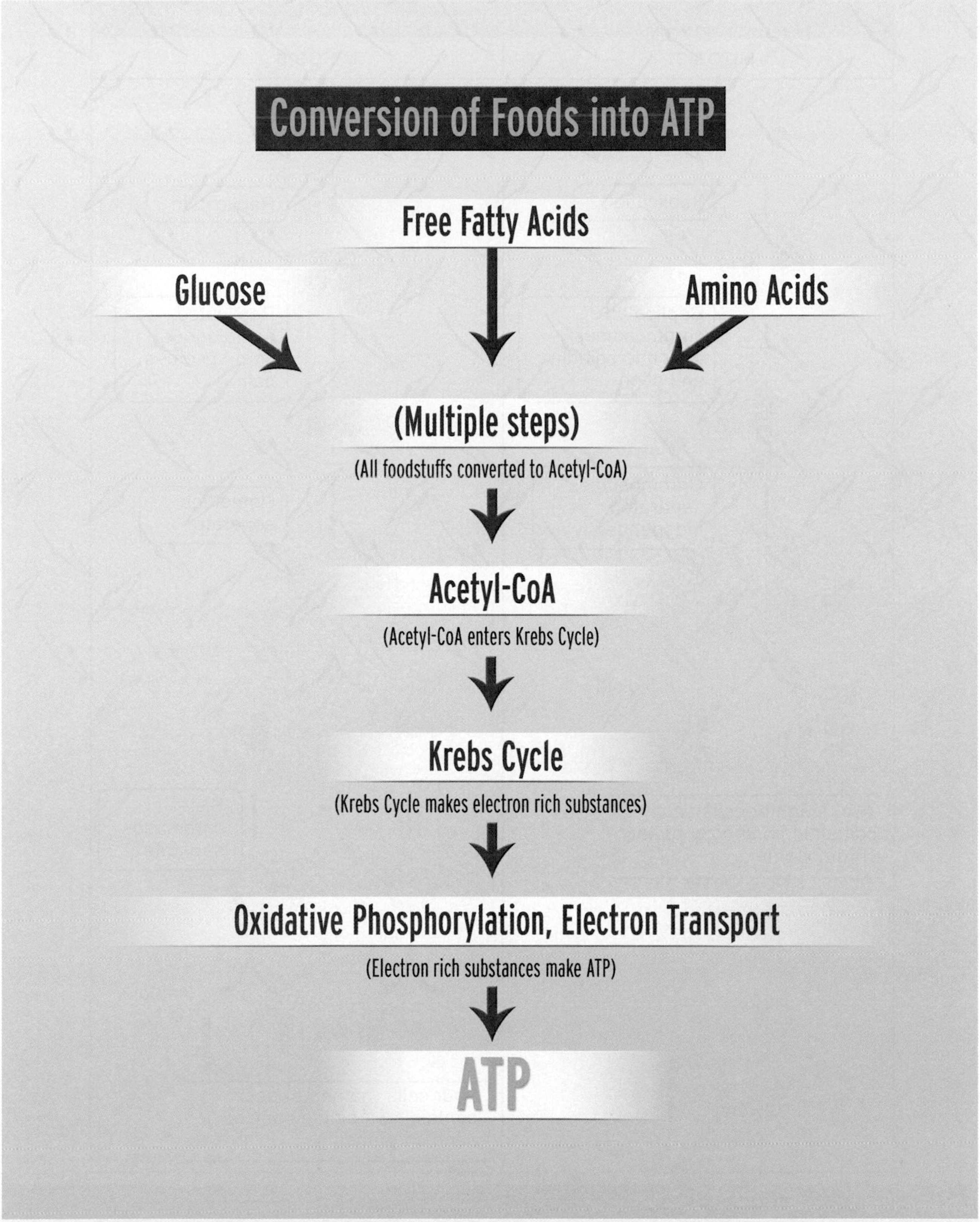

Conversion of Foods into ATP

Free Fatty Acids

Glucose

Amino Acids

(Multiple steps)

(All foodstuffs converted to Acetyl-CoA)

Acetyl-CoA

(Acetyl-CoA enters Krebs Cycle)

Krebs Cycle

(Krebs Cycle makes electron rich substances)

Oxidative Phosphorylation, Electron Transport

(Electron rich substances make ATP)

ATP

Figure 1-9

Conversion of foods into ATP.

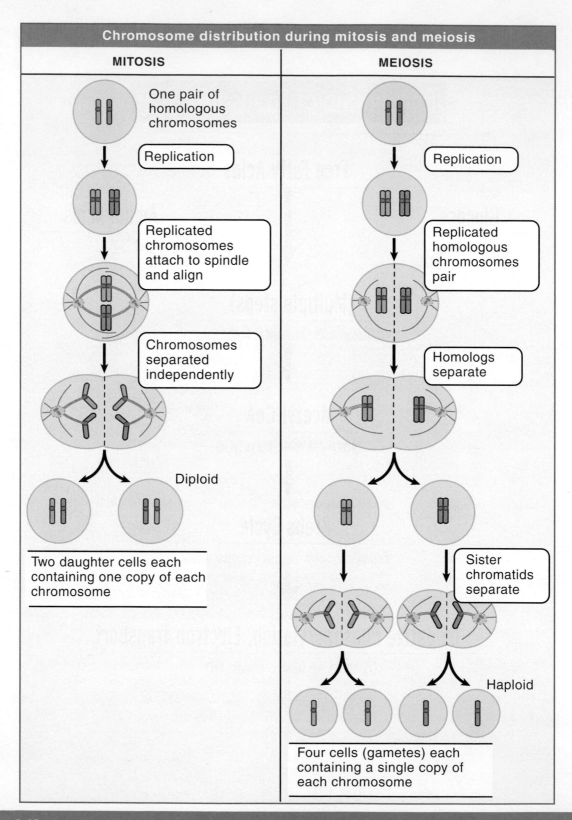

Chromosome distribution during mitosis and meiosis

MITOSIS	MEIOSIS

One pair of homologous chromosomes

Replication

Replicated chromosomes attach to spindle and align

Chromosomes separated independently

Diploid

Two daughter cells each containing one copy of each chromosome

Replication

Replicated homologous chromosomes pair

Homologs separate

Sister chromatids separate

Haploid

Four cells (gametes) each containing a single copy of each chromosome

Figure 1-10

Mitosis and meiosis.

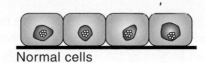

Normal cells

Hypertrophy

Atrophy

Hyperplasia

Dysplasia

Metaplasia

Neoplasia
(malignancy)

Figure 1-11

Cellular adaptation: abnormal cellular growth patterns.

cells contain 46 chromosomes, but sperm and ova contain 23 each. When the sperm and ova join, the resulting organism has 46 chromosomes.

Differentiation is a process by which cells become specialized in terms of cell type, function, structure, and cell cycle. This process does not begin until approximately 15–60 days after the sperm and ova unite. During this time, the embryo is the most susceptible to damage because of environmental influences. The differentiation is the process by which the primitive stem cells of the embryo develop into the highly specialized cells of the human (e.g., cardiac cells and nerve cells).

Cellular Adaptation and Damage

Cellular Adaptation

Cells are constantly exposed to a variety of environmental factors that can cause damage. Cells attempt to prevent their own death from environmental changes through adaptation. Cells may modify their size, numbers, or types in an attempt to manage these changes and maintain homeostasis. These changes may involve one or a combination of these modifications. These modifications may be normal or abnormal depending on whether they were mediated through standard pathways. These modifications may also be permanent or reversible, but regardless, once the stimulus is removed, the adaptation ceases. These adaptive changes include atrophy, hypertrophy, hyperplasia, metaplasia, and dysplasia (**Figure 1-11**).

Atrophy occurs because of decreased work demands on the cell. The body attempts to work as efficiently as possible to conserve energy and resources. When cellular work demands decrease, the cells decrease in size and number. These atrophied cells utilize less oxygen, and their organelles decrease in size and number. Causes of atrophy include disuse, denervation, endocrine hypofunction, inadequate nutrition, and ischemia. An example of disuse atrophy can be seen in the muscle shrinking of the extremity that has been in a cast for a long time. Denervation atrophy is closely associated to disuse and can be seen in the muscle shrinking of paralyzed extremities. Atrophy because of a loss of endocrine function can be seen as the reproductive organs of postmenopausal women shrink. With a lack of nutrition and blood flow, cells shrink because of a lack of necessary substances—much like when water and fertilizer are withheld from a plant.

The opposite of atrophy is **hypertrophy**. Hypertrophy occurs when cells increase in size in an attempt to meet increased work demand. This change may be a result of normal or abnormal changes. These changes are commonly seen in cardiac and skeletal muscle. To illustrate this process resulting from normal changes, consider what happens when a body builder diligently performs bicep curls with weights—the biceps get larger. An abnormal hypertrophic change can be seen with hypertension. Just as the bicep muscle grows larger from the increased work, the cardiac muscle will thicken and enlarge because of increased workload placed on it because of the hypertension. The bicep muscle increases in strength and function when its workload is increased; however, the heart loses the flexibility to fill with blood and pump the blood when the cardiac muscle increases in size. This abnormal hypertrophic change can lead to complications such as cardiomyopathy and heart failure (see Chapter 4).

Hyperplasia refers to an increase in the number of cells in an organ or tissue. This increase only occurs in cells that have the ability to perform mitotic division, such as epithelial cells. This process is usually a result of normal stimuli. Examples of hyperplasia include menstruation, liver regeneration, wound healing, and skin warts. Hyperplasia is different from hypertrophy, but they often occur together because of similar triggers.

The process of one adult cell being replaced by another cell type is **metaplasia**. This change is usually initiated by chronic irritation and inflammation providing a more virulent cell line. The cell types do not cross over the overarching cell type. For instance, epithelial cells may be converted to another type of epithelial cells, but they will not be replaced with nerve cells. Some examples of metaplastic changes can be seen in ciliary changes that occur in the respiratory tract because of chronic smoking or vitamin A deficiency. Metaplasia does not necessarily lead to cancerous changes; however, if the stimulus is not removed, cancerous changes will likely occur.

The final cellular adaption is dysplasia. In **dysplasia**, the cells mutate into cells of a different size, shape, and appearance. Although dysplasia is abnormal, it is potentially reversible by removing the trigger. Dysplastic changes are often implicated as precancerous cells. The reproductive and respiratory tracts are common sites for this type of adaptation because of increased exposure to carcinogens (e.g., cigarette smoke, human papillomavirus).

Cellular Death and Injury

Cellular injury can occur in many ways and is usually reversible up to a point. Whether the injury is reversible or irreversible usually depends on the severity of the injury and intrinsic factors (e.g., blood supply and nutritional status). Cell injury can occur because of (1) physical agents (e.g., mechanical forces and extreme temperature), (2) chemical injury (e.g., pollution, lead, and drugs), (3) radiation, (4) biologic agents (e.g., viruses, bacteria, and parasites), and (5) nutritional imbalances.

Death is a part of the human existence, and it is no different at the cellular level. When cellular injury becomes irreversible, it usually results in cell death. The process of eliminating unwanted cells is called **programmed cell death** and usually occurs through the **apoptosis** mechanism (**Figure 1-12**). Programmed cell death refers to cell death that occurs as a specific point in development. Apoptosis specifically occurs because of morphologic (structure or form) changes. This mechanism of cell death is not limited to developmental causes but may be a result of environmental triggers. Apoptosis is important in tissue development, immune defense, and cancer prevention. However, this mechanism can result in inappropriate destruction of cells if it is unregulated. This inappropriate activation of apoptosis can occur in degenerative neurologic diseases such as Alzheimer's disease (see Chapter 11).

It is important to note that not all cell death is apoptotic. Cell death can occur because of ischemia or necrosis (Figure 1-12). **Ischemia** refers to decreased blood flow to tissue or an organ. This lack of blood flow essentially strangles the tissue or organ by limiting necessary nutrients and oxygen. Ischemia can leave the cells damaged to the extent that they cannot survive, or **necrosis**. The difference between apoptosis and necrosis lies mostly in the cell's morphologic changes. In apoptosis, the cells condense or shrink, and in necrosis, the cells swell and burst.

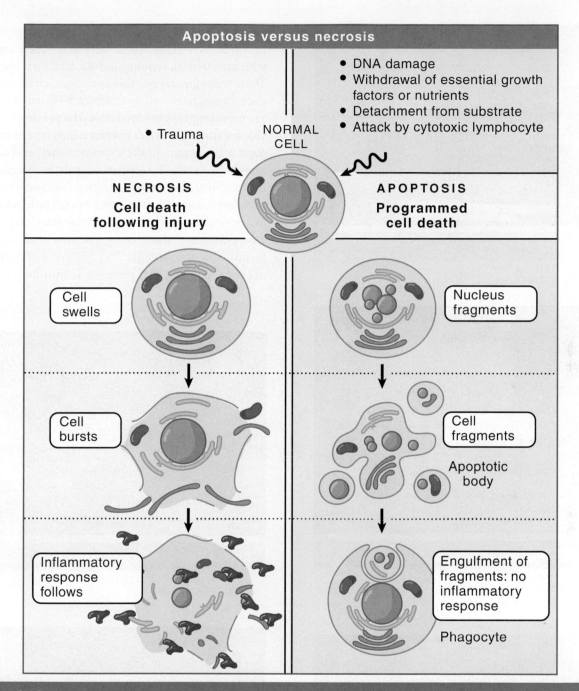

Apoptosis versus necrosis

- DNA damage
- Withdrawal of essential growth factors or nutrients
- Detachment from substrate
- Attack by cytotoxic lymphocyte

- Trauma

NORMAL CELL

NECROSIS
Cell death following injury

APOPTOSIS
Programmed cell death

Cell swells

Nucleus fragments

Cell bursts

Cell fragments

Apoptotic body

Inflammatory response follows

Engulfment of fragments: no inflammatory response

Phagocyte

Figure 1-12

Cellular damage can result in necrosis, which has a different appearance than apoptosis, as organelles swell and the plasma membrane ruptures.

Necrosis can take one of several pathways. Liquefaction necrosis (**Figure 1-13**) occurs when caustic enzymes dissolve and liquefy necrotic cells. The most common site of this type of necrosis is the brain because it contains a plentiful supply of these enzymes. Caseous necrosis (**Figure 1-14**) occurs when the necrotic cells disintegrate but the cellular debris remains for months or years. This type of necrosis has a cottage cheeselike appearance, and it is most common with pulmonary tuberculosis. Fat necrosis (**Figure 1-15**) occurs when

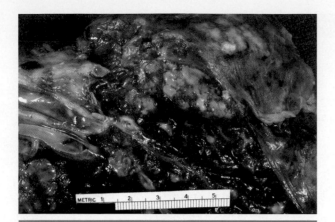

Figure 1-13

Liquefaction necrosis.

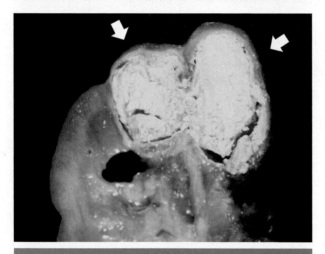

Figure 1-14

Caseous necrosis.

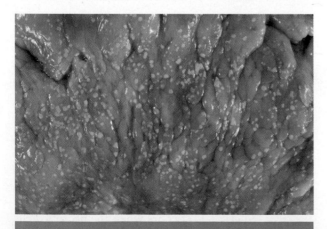

Figure 1-15

Fat necrosis.

lipase enzymes break down intracellular triglycerides into free fatty acids. These fatty acids then combine with magnesium, sodium, and calcium-forming soaps. These soaps give fat necrosis an opaque, chalky appearance. Coagulative necrosis (**Figure 1-16**) usually results as an interruption in blood flow. The pH drops (acidosis), denaturing the cell's enzymes. This type of necrosis most often occurs in the kidneys, heart, and adrenal glands. Gangrene is a form of coagulative necrosis that is a combination of impaired blood flow and a bacterial invasion. Gangrene usually occurs in the legs because of arteriosclerosis (hardening of the arteries) or in the gastrointestinal tract. Gangrene can occur in three forms—dry, wet, and gas. Dry gangrene (**Figure 1-17**) occurs when bacterial presence is minimal, and the

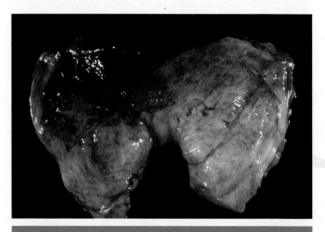

Figure 1-16

Coagulative necrosis.

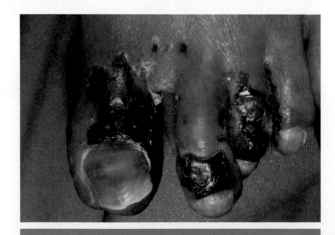

Figure 1-17

Dry gangrene.

skin has a dry, dark brown, or black appearance. **Wet gangrene** (**Figure 1-18**) occurs with liquefaction necrosis. Extensive damage from bacteria and white blood cells produce a liquid wound. Wet gangrene can occur in extremities and internal organs. **Gas gangrene** (**Figure 1-19**) develops because of *Clostridium*, an anaerobic bacterium. This type of gangrene is the most serious and has the most potential for being fatal. The bacterium releases toxins that kill surrounding cells, thus spreading rapidly. The release of gas bubbles from the tissue, often underneath the skin.

Another important mechanism of cellular injury to understand is free radicals. **Free radicals** are injurious, unstable agents that can cause cell death. This rapidly progressing pathway can cause a wide range of damage, and a single unbalanced atom initiates it. The atom has an unpaired electron, making it unstable. In an attempt to stabilize, the atom borrows an electron from a surrounding atom, usually rendering it unstable. This newly unstable atom will then borrow an electron from its neighbor, creating a domino effect that continues until the atom giving the electron is stable without it. The extent of damage that this process causes depends on how long this chain of events continues. The immune system is equipped with agents to protect or limit the damage (see Chapter 3) because of this process, and certain dietary components can aid in this fight (e.g., vitamins C, A, and E).

Neoplasm

When the process of proliferation or differentiation goes wrong, neoplasms can develop. A **neoplasm** or **tumor** is a cellular growth that is no longer responding to normal regulator processes usually because of a mutation. The disease state associated with this uncontrolled growth is **cancer**. Cancer's key features include rapid, uncontrolled proliferation and a loss of differentiation. Thus, cancer cells differ from normal cells in size, shape, number, differentiation, purpose, and function.

Carcinogenesis is the process by which cancer develops, and it occurs in three phases—initiation, promotion, and progression (**Figure 1-20**). **Initiation** involves the exposure of the cell to a substance or event (e.g., chemicals, viruses, or radiation), which causes DNA damage or mutation. Usually the body has enzymes that detect these events and repair the damage. If the event is overlooked, then the mutation can become permanent and is passed on to future cellular generations. **Promotion** involves the mutated cells' exposure to factors (e.g., hormones, nitrates, or nicotine) that promote growth. This phase may occur just after initiation or years later, and it can be reversible if the promoting factors are removed. In **progression**, the tumor invades, metastasizes (spreads), and becomes drug resistant. This final phase is permanent or irreversible.

A healthy body is equipped with the necessary defenses to shield against cancer (see Chapter 2). When those defenses fail, cancer prevails. Evidence suggests that these defenses fail because of a combination of

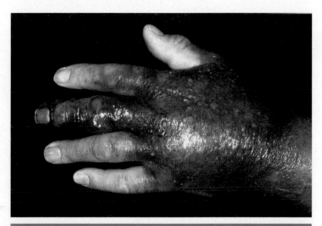

Figure 1-18

Wet gangrene.

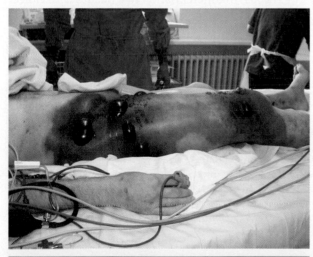

Figure 1-19

Gas gangrene.

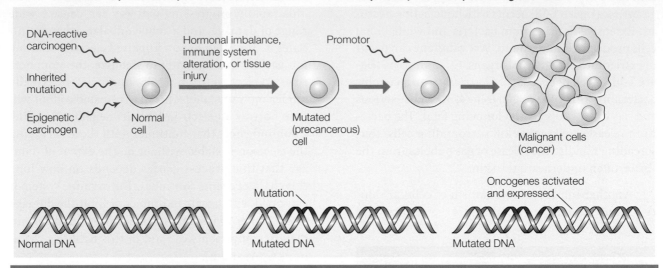

Conversion (or Initiation)   **Development (Promotion) and Progression**

Figure 1-20

Carcinogenesis: the stages leading to cancer.

complex interactions between carcinogen exposure and genetic mutations. Numerous genes have been identified as causing cancers. Oncogenes activate cell division and influence embryonic development. Some of these cancer-producing genes can remain harmless until altered by a genetic or acquired mutation. Common causes of acquired genetic mutations include viruses, radiation, environmental and dietary carcinogens, and hormones. Other factors that can increase a person's likelihood of developing cancer include age, nutritional status, hormonal balance, and stress response. As we age, statistically there is a higher

likelihood of a DNA transcription error occurring, as well as more carcinogen exposure. Examples of how changes in nutritional status increase the likelihood of cancer can be seen in free radical damage. Some cancers almost feed off of hormones, meaning they grow faster in the presence of particular hormones. Finally, the immune system is impaired during stress states, which can impair its ability to find and respond to carcinogenesis.

The loss of differentiation that occurs with cancer is referred to as anaplasia. Anaplasia occurs in varying

MYTH BUSTERS

MYTH 1: Standing in front of a microwave oven while it is cooking can increase your risk for cancer.

This is a common myth that may have some truth in it. Cancer risk has been linked to increased levels of ionizing radiation (e.g., X-rays) because they detach electrons from atoms. Microwaves use non-ionizing microwave radiation to heat food. Early microwave ovens emitted higher levels of this radiation, which *may* have increased cancer risk slightly. Research has never been able to determine whether cancer risk increased with non-ionizing radiation exposure. Currently, Food and Drug Administration guidelines limit the amount of the non-ionizing radiation microwave ovens can emit, further decreasing the cancer risk.

MYTH 2: Using cell phones can increase your risk of cancer.

This is another common myth. Cell phones use the same non-ionizing microwave radiation as microwave ovens to emit a signal. Even with the close proximity to your head while in use, evidence does not support that there is an increase in brain cancer risk. Using a cell phone for an extended period at one time will indeed heat your ear for the same reason that the microwave heats your food. But no clear evidence suggests that this extended use increases cancer risk.

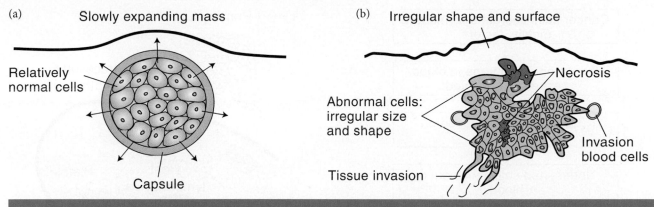

(a)

Slowly expanding mass

Relatively normal cells

Capsule

(b)

Irregular shape and surface

Necrosis

Abnormal cells: irregular size and shape

Invasion blood cells

Tissue invasion

Figure 1-21

Characteristics of (a) benign and (b) malignant tumors.

degrees. The less the cell resembles the original cell, the more anaplastic the cell. These anaplastic cells may begin functioning as completely different cells, often producing hormones or hormonelike substances.

Benign and Malignant Tumors

Two major types of neoplasm include benign and malignant (**Table 1-2; Figure 1-21**). Benign tumors usually consist of differentiated (less anaplastic) cells that are reproducing more than normal. Because of their differentiation, benign tumors are more like normal cells and cause fewer problems. Benign cells are usually encapsulated and are unable to metastasize. The tumor, however, can compress surrounding tissue as it grows. Benign tumors usually cause problems because of their

location due to that compression. Regardless of size, if the tumor is in sensitive areas such as the brain or spinal cord, it can cause devastating problems.

On the other hand, malignant tumors usually are undifferentiated (more anaplastic), nonfunctioning cells that are reproducing rapidly. Malignant tumors often penetrate surrounding tissue and spread to secondary sites. The tumor's ability to metastasize (**Figure 1-22; Figure 1-23**) is dependent on the ability to access and survive in the circulatory or the lymphatic system. Most commonly, the tumor metastasizes to tissue or organs near the primary site but can travel to distant sites (**Table 1-3**).

Regardless of the type of tumor, several factors are imperative for the tumor's progression and survival.

Table 1-2 Characteristics of Benign and Malignant Tumors		
	Benign Tumors	**Malignant Tumors**
Cells	Similar to normal cells Differentiated Mitosis fairly normal	Varied in size and shape Many undifferentiated Mitosis increased and atypical
Growth	Relatively slow Expanding mass Frequently encapsulated	Rapid growth Cells not adhesive, infiltrate tissue No capsule
Spread	Remains localized	Invades nearby tissue or metastasizes to distant sites through blood and lymph vessels
Systemic effects	Rare	Common
Life threatening	Only in certain locations (e.g., brain)	Yes, by tissue destruction and spread

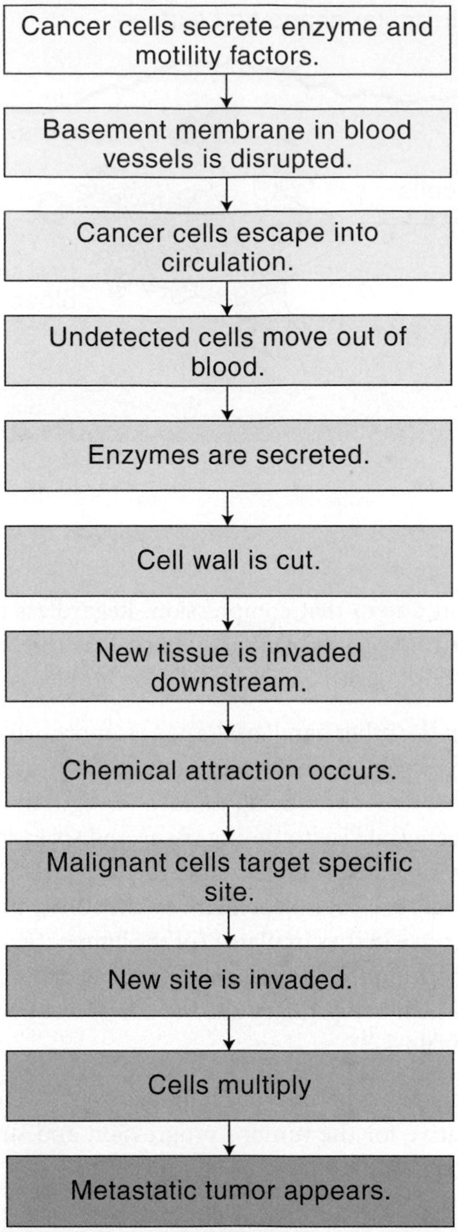
Cancer cells secrete enzyme and motility factors.
Basement membrane in blood vessels is disrupted.
Cancer cells escape into circulation.
Undetected cells move out of blood.
Enzymes are secreted.
Cell wall is cut.
New tissue is invaded downstream.
Chemical attraction occurs.
Malignant cells target specific site.
New site is invaded.
Cells multiply
Metastatic tumor appears.

Figure 1-22

How cancer metastasizes.

The tumor must have an adequate blood supply, and sometimes the tumor will divert the blood supply from surrounding tissue to meet its own needs. The tumor will only grow as large as what the blood supply will support. Location is imperative because it determines the cytology of the tumor as well as the tumor's ability to survive and metastasize. Host factors including age, gender, health status, and immune function will also affect the tumor. Alterations in some of these host factors can create a prime environment for the tumor to grow and prosper.

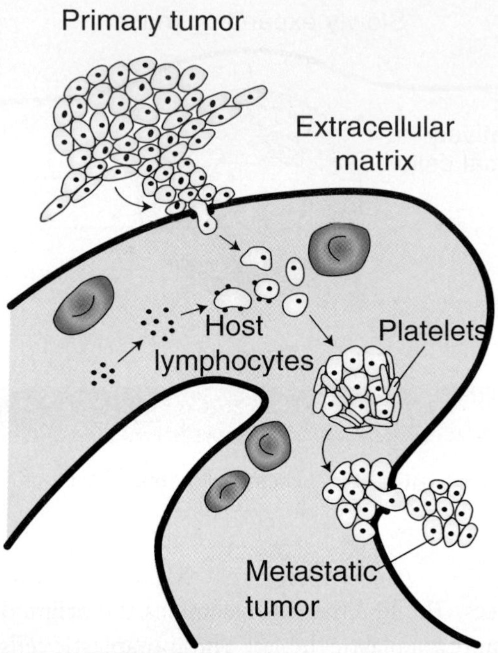
Primary tumor
Extracellular matrix
Host lymphocytes
Platelets
Metastatic tumor

Figure 1-23

Pathogenesis of metastasis.

Clinical Manifestations

In most cases, the prognosis improves the earlier the cancer is detected and treated. Many cases of cancer are first detected through the recognition of signs and symptoms by the healthcare provider, patient, or family. Heeding these warning signs is vital to initiating treatment early. The American Cancer Society (www.cancer.org) developed a list of warning signs it calls CAUTION signs (**Table 1-4**). Unfortunately, people

Table 1-3 Common Sites of Metastasis

Cancer Type	Sites for Metastasis
Breast	Axillary lymph nodes, lung, liver, bone, brain
Colorectal	Liver, lung, peritoneum
Lung	Liver, brain, bone
Ovarian	Peritoneum, diaphragm, liver, lung
Prostate	Bone
Testicular	Lungs, liver

Table 1-4 Cancer's Seven Warning Signs

C	hange in bowel or bladder habits
A	sore that doesn't heal
U	nusual bleeding or discharge
T	hickening or lump in the breast or elsewhere
I	ndigestion or difficulty swallowing
O	bvious change in a wart or mole
N	agging cough or hoarseness

Source: Adapted from the American Cancer Society (www.cancer.org).

often ignore or do not recognize the warning signs for a variety of reasons (e.g., denial and symptom ambiguity).

As the cancer progresses, the patient may present with signs and symptoms of advancing disease including anemia, cachexia, fatigue, infection, leukopenia, thrombocytopenia, and pain. Anemia, decreased red blood cells, can be a result of the bloodborne cancers (e.g., leukemias), chronic bleeding, malnutrition, chemotherapy, or radiation. Cachexia, a generalized wasting syndrome where the person appears emaciated, often occurs due to malnutrition. Fatigue, or feeling of weakness, is a result of the parasitic nature of a tumor, anemia, malnutrition, stress, anxiety, and chemotherapy. Factors that can increase the risk for infection include bone marrow depression, chemotherapy, and stress. Leukopenia (low leukocyte levels) and thrombocytopenia (low platelet levels) are common side effects of chemotherapy and radiation due to bone marrow depression. Pain is often associated with cancer due to tissue pressure, obstructions, tissue invasion, visceral stretching, tissue destruction, and inflammation.

Diagnosis

Diagnosis of cancer is complex and is specific to the type of cancer suspected. This chapter will provide a basic overview of cancer diagnostic procedures, and more specifics will be presented in future chapters as various cancers are discussed. A set of diagnostic procedures usually follows a thorough history and physical examination. These diagnostic procedures may vary depending on the type of cancer suspected. The intention of these diagnostic tests is to identify cancer cells, establish the cytology, and determine the primary site and any secondary sites; however, all these goals are not always accomplished. The healthcare provider will gather as much information as possible to paint the clearest, most complete picture possible of the patient in order to develop an appropriate treatment plan.

Some screening tests are used for early detection of cancer cells as well as staging the cancer (**Table 1-5**). These screening tests include X-rays, radioactive isotope scanning, computed tomography scans, endoscopies, ultrasonography, magnetic resonance imagining, positron emission tomography scanning, biopsies, and blood tests. Some of the blood tests may include tumor markers—substances secreted by the cancer cells—for specific cancers (**Table 1-6**). These tumor markers not only aid in cancer detection but also assist in tracking disease progression and treatment response.

Malignant cancer cells are classified in reference to the degree of differentiation (grading) and extent of disease (staging). The **grading** system determines the degree of differentiation on a scale of 1 to 4 in order of clinical severity. For instance, grade 1 cancers are well differentiated, meaning they are less likely to cause problems since they are more like the original tissue. On the other hand, grade 4 cancers are undifferentiated, meaning they are highly likely to cause problems because they do not resemble any characteristics of the original tissue. The **TNM staging** system evaluates the tumor size, nodal involvement, and metastatic progress (**Figure 1-24**).

Treatment

Cancer treatment usually includes a combination of chemotherapy, radiation, surgery, hormone therapy, and immunotherapy. Additionally, other strategies may include watchful waiting and alternative therapies (e.g., herbs, diet, and acupuncture). The goal of treatment is **curative** (eradicate the disease), **palliative** (treat symptoms to increase comfort), and **prophylactic** (preventative). With surgery, attempts are made to remove the tumor and surrounding tissue. Chemotherapy involves the administration of a wide range of medications that destroy replicating cells. Radiation includes the use of ionizing radiation to cause cancer cellular mutation and interrupt the tumor's blood supply. Radiation may be administered by external sources or with internal implanted sources. Hormone therapy involves administering specific hormones that

Table 1-5 Cancer Screening Guidelines

Screening Area	Recommendations
Breast	
Mammogram	• Every year age 40 and older
Clinical breast examination	• Every year age 40 and older; every 3 years for ages 20 to 39
Breast self-examination	• Suggested monthly for age 20 and older
Cervix	
Papanicolaou (Pap) test	• Every year beginning about 3 years after the onset of vaginal intercourse • Screen may stop for women age 70 and older who have had three consecutive normal Pap tests • Not necessary after a total hysterectomy unless done for treatment of cervical cancer
Endometrium	
Endometrial biopsy	• Yearly beginning at age of 35 for those women at risk for colon cancer
Prostate	
Prostate-specific antigen (PSA)	• Yearly beginning at age 50, unless at high risk, then beginning at age 40
Digital rectal examination	• Yearly beginning at age 50, unless at high risk, then beginning at age 40
Colon and Rectum	
Fecal occult blood test	• Yearly age 50 and older
Flexible sigmoidoscopy	• Every 5 years age 50 and older
Barium enema	• Every 5 years age 50 and older
Colonoscopy	• Every 10 years age 50 and older

Sources: Adapted from American Cancer Society (www.cancer.org) and National Cancer Institute (www.cancer.gov).

Table 1-6 Common Tumor Cell Markers

Marker	Malignant Condition	Nonmalignant Condition
Alpha-fetaprotein	• Liver cancer • Ovarian germ cell cancer • Testicular germ cell cancer	• Ataxia-telangiectasia • Cirrhosis • Hepatitis • Pregnancy
Carcinoembryonic antigen	• Bladder cancer • Breast cancer • Cervical cancer • Colorectal cancer • Kidney cancer • Liver cancer • Lung cancer • Lymphoma • Melanoma • Ovarian cancer • Pancreatic cancer • Stomach cancer • Thyroid cancer	• Inflammatory bowel disease • Liver disease • Pancreatitis • Tobacco use

Table 1-6 Common Tumor Cell Markers *(Continued)*

Marker	Malignant Condition	Nonmalignant Condition
CA 15-3	• Breast cancer • Lung cancer • Ovarian cancer • Prostate cancer	• Benign breast disease • Endometriosis • Hepatitis • Lactation • Benign ovarian disease • Pelvic inflammatory disease • Pregnancy
CA 19-9	• Bile duct cancer • Colorectal cancer • Pancreatic cancer • Stomach cancer	• Cholecystitis • Cirrhosis • Gallstones • Pancreatitis
CA 27-29	• Breast cancer • Colon cancer • Kidney cancer • Liver cancer • Lung cancer • Ovarian cancer • Pancreatic cancer • Stomach cancer • Uterine cancer	• Benign breast disease • Endometriosis • Kidney disease • Liver disease • Ovarian cysts • Pregnancy (first trimester)
CA 125	• Colorectal cancer • Gastric cancer • Ovarian cancer • Pancreatic cancer	• Endometriosis • Liver disease • Menstruation • Pancreatitis • Pelvic inflammatory disease • Peritonitis • Pregnancy
Human chorionic gonadotropin	• Choriocarcinoma • Embryonic cell carcinoma • Liver cancer • Lung cancer • Pancreatic cancer • Stomach cancer • Testicular cancer	• Marijuana use • Pregnancy
Lactate dyhydrogenase	• Almost all cancers • Ewing's sarcoma • Leukemia • Non-Hodgkin's lymphoma • Testicular cancer	• Anemia • Heart failure • Hypothyroidism • Liver disease • Lung disease
Neuron-specific enolase	• Kidney cancer • Melanoma • Neuroblastoma • Pancreatic cancer • Small-cell lung cancer • Testicular cancer • Thyroid cancer • Wilm's tumor	• Unknown
Prostatic acid phosphatase	• Prostate cancer	• Benign prostate conditions
Prostate-specific antigen	• Prostate cancer	• Benign prostatic hyperplasia • Prostatitis

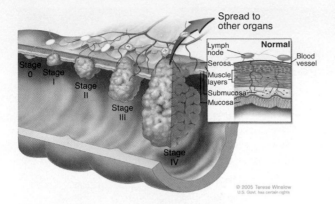

Spread to other organs

Stage 0
Stage I
Stage II
Stage III
Stage IV

Lymph node
Serosa
Muscle layers
Submucosa
Mucosa

Normal
Blood vessel

© 2005 Terese Winslow
U.S. Govt. has certain rights

Figure 1-24

TNM staging system. The example shown is staging of colorectal cancer.

inhibit the growth of certain cancers. Immunotherapy involves administering specific immune agents to alter the host's biological response to the cancer (e.g., interferons and interleukins).

Prognosis

A cure for cancer is usually defined as a 5-year survival without recurrence after diagnosis and treatment. Prognosis refers to the patient's likelihood for surviving the cancer. Prognosis is heavily dependent on the cancer's ability to metastasize. The more the cancer spreads to other sites by way of the circulation or lymph system, the worse the patient's prognosis. Early diagnosis and treatment usually improves the prognosis by treating the cancer before metastasis has occurred. Remission refers to when the cancer has responded to treatment and is under control. Remission may occur with some cancers, and generally, the patient does not exhibit any manifestations of cancer. Many cancers are preventable, so health-promoting education (e.g., smoking cessation, proper nutrition, and weight management) is vital to decreasing the prevalence and occurrences of all cancers. Though the likelihood of these cancers can be diminished with these strategies, it is noteworthy that cancer can develop in people with no risk factors. This unpredictable development contributes to the mystery and challenges surrounding cancer.

Genetic and Congenital Alterations

Genetic and congenital defects are important to understand because of the encompassing nature of these disorders. These diseases affect all levels of health care

and age groups by involving almost any tissue type and organs. Genetics is the study of heredity—the passage of physical, biochemical, and physiologic traits from biological parents to their children. Disorders and mutations that can result in serious disability or death can be transmitted through genetic material. Genetic disorders may or may not be present at birth. Congenital defects, often referred to as birth defects, usually develop during the prenatal phase of life and are apparent at birth or shortly thereafter.

Genetics

The cellular instructions and information are carried with our genes. A gene is a segment of deoxyribonucleic acid (DNA) and serves as a template of protein synthesis. DNA is a long double-stranded chain of nucleotides called chromosomes. The nucleotides consist of a five-carbon sugar (deoxyribose), a phosphate group, and one of four nitrogen bases (cytosine, thymine, guanine, or adenine). An estimated 3 billion nucleotides make up the human genome. Each gene can contain hundreds to thousands of these nucleotides. Of the 46 chromosomes, the 22 sets of paired chromosomes are called autosomes, and the remaining two make up the sex chromosomes (paired Xs for females and an X and a Y for males). A representation of a person's individual set of chromosomes is referred to as karyotype, and the physical expression of those genes is referred to as phenotype (e.g., blue eyes). Not all genes in the code are expressed.

Patterns of Inheritance

Each parent contributes one set of chromosomes. Some characteristics, or traits, are determined by one gene that may have many variants (alleles). A person who has identical alleles of each chromosome is homozygous for that gene; if the alleles are different, then they are said to be heterozygous for that gene. For unknown reasons, one allele on a chromosome may be more influential than the other in determining a specific trait. The more powerful, or dominant, allele is more likely to be expressed in the offspring than the less influential, or recessive, allele. Offspring will express the dominant allele in both homozygous and heterozygous allele pairs. On the other hand, offspring will only express the recessive allele in homozygous pairs.

The sex chromosomes (X and Y) can pass on genes when they are linked, or attached, to one of the sex chromosomes. For example, a male will transmit one copy of each X-linked gene to his daughter but none to

CASE STUDY

HISTORY

Mrs. Turner is a 47-year-old Caucasian female who has been admitted to the general surgical floor with a lump in her right breast. She generally has enjoyed good health up to this admission. Mrs. Turner neither smokes nor drinks and follows a daily exercise regimen. Approximately 2 months ago, Mrs. Turner's husband noticed a small lump in her right breast. She gave this finding little attention, assuming that the lump was like the many others she tended to experience around her menses. The lump, however, failed to resolve after her menses, and Mrs. Turner became concerned when it seemed to grow bigger.

Mrs. Turner is the mother of 2 children, 8 and 6 years old. Mrs. Turner took birth control pills for 5 years after the birth of her second child. Last year she chose to discontinue birth control pill use and turned to an alternative method of birth control. Mrs. Turner is the only child born to her parents late in their life. Her father is alive and well, but her mother died of breast cancer 5 years ago. A family history revealed a strong history of both heart disease and cancer on both sides of Mrs. Turner's family.

CURRENT STATUS

On exam, a 2–3-cm mass was palpated in the upper quadrant of her right breast. This mass felt firm, was fixed to the chest wall, and was tender to the touch. The remaining breast skin was normal in appearance with no discoloration or retraction of the skin. One node, approximately the size of a pea, was palpated under the right axilla. Palpation of the left breast revealed two 1–2-cm soft, movable masses. Mrs. Turner said that she noticed these lumps in her left breast 2 weeks ago but stated that the lumps in her left breast became palpable and bothersome about 12 days from the start of menses. A reproductive history disclosed that the onset of menses occurred at the age of 10. There is no history of dysmenorrhea associated with her periods, though she states that her breasts become tender and lumpy a week or two before her menses. She has had no pregnancies that were delivered by cesarean section. Her one and only Papanicolaou (Pap) smear was done 2 years ago and produced a normal result. The remaining exam findings were unremarkable. Mammography confirmed the presence of a 3-cm mass in the upper quadrant of the right breast and three 1.5-cm masses in the left breast. The result of a bone scan and other diagnostic procedures were negative.

1. Mrs. Turner is considered to be at increased risk for developing breast cancer. Which of the following factors is most positively related to this high-risk profile?

   A. History of breast cancer in family members

   B. History of cystic breast disease

   C. Early onset of menarche

   D. Trauma related to birth of her children

2. Which of the following best explains the existence of an enlarged right axillary lymph node in Mrs. Turner?

   A. The lymph node is the result of an inflammatory reaction that normally occurs with the onset of her current menses.

   B. The existence of the node is the result of an increased strain on the lymphatic system as a result of cellular degeneration.

   C. The lymph node exists to provide nutrients to the rapidly growing cancer cells.

   D. The lymph node is the result of cancer cells spreading to different tissues within the body.

Mrs. Turner was taken to surgery 3 days later, and a modified radical mastectomy was performed. A histological exam was used to classify the tumor using the TNM staging system. An estrogen receptor assay performed on the removed tissue confirmed that Mrs. Turner's tumor was estrogen dependent. She returned to her room with a drain in place. Her dressing was dry and intact. She was able to turn, cough, and breathe deeply on her own. Her temperature remained within normal limits after surgery. Progesterone therapy was initiated daily. Ambulation was started on the 2nd postoperative day.

3. Mrs. Turner's tumor was staged at stage III using the TNM staging system. Pathological exam of the surgically removed tissue sample placed Mrs. Turner's tumor in category type II. The need to state and classify tumors is important for which of the following reasons?

   A. Treatment is based on the knowledge of tumor size, extent, and tissue type.

   B. Tumor staging is useful for studying a number of researchable factors, from survival to treatment response.

   C. A consistent classification system provides a way to catalogue individuals with breast tumors for statistical analysis.

   D. All of the above.

4. Which activities by Mrs. Turner increase her likelihood for a good prognosis?

5. What was the rationale for hormone therapy with Mrs. Turner?

his son, whereas a female will transmit a copy to each offspring, male or female. An example of an X-linked disorder is Klinefelter's syndrome. Some traits require a combination of two or more genes and environmental factors, or multifactorial inheritance. Some examples of this type of inheritance include height, diabetes mellitus, and obesity.

Autosomal Dominant Disorders

Autosomal dominant disorders are single gene mutations that are passed from an affected parent to an offspring regardless of sex. Autosomal dominant disorders occur with homozygous and heterozygous allele pairs. In most cases, the offspring with the homozygous pair will have a more severe expression of the disorder as compared to the heterozygous pair. These disorders typically involve abnormalities with structural proteins. Examples of autosomal dominant disorders include Marfan syndrome and neurofibromatosis.

Marfan Syndrome

Marfan syndrome is a rare, degenerative, generalized disorder of the connective tissue (**Figure 1-25**). The condition results from a single gene mutation on chromosome 15 that leads to elastin and collagen defects. These defects produce varying ocular, skeletal, and cardiovascular disorders. Some clinical manifestations of Marfan syndrome include:

- Increased height
- Long extremities
- Arachnodactyly (long, spiderlike fingers)
- Sternum defects (e.g., funnel chest or pigeon breast)
- Chest asymmetry
- Scoliosis
- Kyphosis
- Nearsightedness
- Lens displacement (ocular hallmark)
- Valvular defects (e.g., redundancy of leaflets, stretching of the chordae tendineae, mitral valve prolapse, and aortic insufficiency)
- Coarctation of the aorta (most life threatening)

Multiple complications can occur with Marfan syndrome, including:

- Weak joints and ligaments that are prone to injury

- Cataracts
- Retinal detachment
- Severe mitral regurgitation
- Spontaneous pneumothorax
- Inguinal hernia

A thorough history and physical examination is vital in diagnosing Marfan syndrome. In most cases of Marfan syndrome, the family history is positive for the disease or the symptoms. A physical examination would reveal the presence of the hallmark lens displacement and other symptoms of the disease. Diagnostic procedures include a skin biopsy that would be positive for fibrillin, X-rays that would confirm the skeletal abnormalities, an echocardiogram that would reveal the cardiac abnormality, and a DNA analysis for the

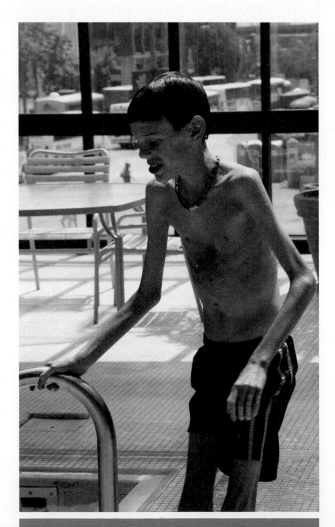

Figure 1-25

Marfan syndrome.

gene. Typical treatment focuses on relieving symptoms and may include:

- Surgical repair of aneurysms and valvular defects
- Surgical correction of ocular deformities
- Steroid and sex hormone therapy to aid in closure of long bones, thereby limiting height
- Beta-adrenergic blockers to limit complications from cardiac deformities
- Bracing and physical therapy for mild scoliosis and surgical correction for severe cases

Other strategies include avoiding contact sports, supportive care for both the patient and the family, and frequent checkups.

Neurofibromatosis

Neurofibromatosis is a condition that involves neurogenic (nervous system) tumors that arise from Schwann cells, which keep peripheral nerve fibers alive, and other similar cells. There are two main types. Type 1 (**Figure 1-26**) involves cutaneous lesions that may include raised lumps, café au lait spots (brown pigmented birthmarks), and freckling. Type 1 is caused by a mutation on chromosome 17. Type 2 involves bilateral acoustic (eighth cranial nerve) tumors that cause hearing loss. Type 2 is caused by a mutation on chromosome 22.

People with neurofibromatosis can be affected in many ways. An increased incidence of learning disabilities and seizure disorders are associated with neurofibromatosis. The appearance of the lesions may vary between individuals, but the lesions can be disfiguring in some cases. There is no cure for neurofibromatosis, but surgeries may be necessary to remove the lesions for palliative or safety reasons. A small risk that the type 1 lesions may develop into cancer exists. Other issues that may develop with type 1 include scoliosis and bone defects.

Autosomal Recessive Disorders

Autosomal recessive disorders are single gene mutations that are passed from an affected parent to an offspring regardless of sex, but they occur only in homozygous allele pairs. Those persons with heterozygous pairs are carriers only and exhibit no symptoms. The age of onset for these disorders is usually early in life, and they occur most commonly as deficiencies in enzymes and inborn errors in metabolism. Some

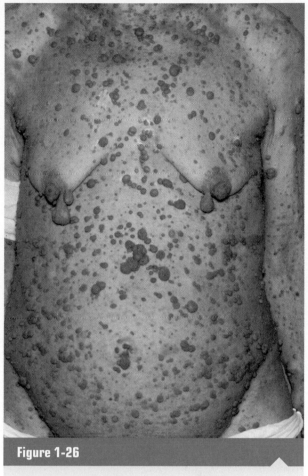

Figure 1-26

Neurofibromatosis type 1.

examples of autosomal recessive disorders include phenylketonuria (PKU) and Tay-Sachs disease.

Phenylketonuria

PKU is a deficiency of phenylalanine hydroxylase, the enzyme necessary for the conversion of phenylalanine to tyrosine, due to a mutation on chromosome 12. This deficiency leads to toxic levels of phenylalinine in the blood. If untreated, PKU leads to severe mental retardation. Symptoms develop slowly and can go undetected, and since untreated cases almost always lead to mental retardation, newborns are routinely screened for PKU shortly after birth by testing for high serum phenylalanine levels. If untreated, newborns can develop the following clinical manifestations:

- Failing to meet milestones
- Microcephaly
- Progressive neurological decline
- Seizures

- Hyperactivity
- Electrocardiograph (EKG) abnormalities
- Learning disability
- Mousy smelling urine, skin, hair, and sweat
- Eczema

Treatment for PKU involves a diet low in phenylalanine. Newborns may be breastfed, but the quantity has to be monitored. Special infant formulas are available for supplementation. Dietary restrictions include avoiding proteins and minimizing starches. Oral medications are available to lower phenylalanine (e.g., sapropterin [Kuvan]), and gene therapy has also demonstrated promise in treating PKU.

Tay-Sachs Disease

Tay-Sachs disease is a deficiency or absence of hexosaminidase A, which is necessary to metabolize certain lipids. These lipids accumulate and progressively destroy and demyelinate nerve cells. This destruction of nerve cells leads to a progressive mental and motor deterioration, often causing death by 5 years of age. Tay-Sachs almost exclusively affects individuals of Jewish descent. Clinical manifestations of Tay-Sachs include:

- Exaggerated Moro reflex (startle reflex) at birth
- Apathy to loud sounds by age 3–6 months
- Inability to sit up, lift head, or grasp objects
- Difficulty turning over
- Progressive vision loss
- Deafness and blindness
- Seizure activity
- Paralysis
- Spasticity
- Pneumonia

Tay-Sachs disease is diagnosed by a thorough history and physical examination as well as deficient serum and amniotic hexosaminidase A levels. Because of the devastating nature of this disease, genetic counseling is important for those of Jewish ancestry or with a positive family history. There is no known cure; most treatments are supportive. Those supportive approaches include parenteral nutrition (tube feedings), pulmonary hygiene (e.g., suctioning and postural drainage), skin care, laxatives, and psychological counseling.

Sex-Linked Disorders

Genes located on the sex chromosomes cause some genetic disorders. Most sex-linked disorders are X-linked. Females are frequently carriers because they have two X chromosomes while men with the defective X gene will be affected because they have only one X chromosome. X-linked disorders may be either recessive or dominant. Fragile X syndrome is an example of an X-linked disorder.

Fragile X Syndrome

Fragile X syndrome (**Figure 1-27**) is an X-linked dominant disorder associated with a single trinucleotide gene sequence on the X chromosome, which leads to a failure to express a protein necessary for neural tube development. Clinical manifestations of fragile X syndrome include:

- Mental retardation
- Behavioral and learning disabilities
- Prominent jaw and forehead
- Long, narrow face with long or large ears
- Connective tissue abnormalities
- Large testes
- Hyperactivity
- Seizures
- Speech difficulties
- Language delays
- Autistic-like behaviors

Diagnosis of fragile X syndrome involves the identification of clinical manifestations and a positive genetic test. There is no known cure for this condition. Treatment focuses on controlling individual symptoms. Genetic counseling is appropriate for persons with a positive family history. Behavioral and psychological support may be indicated for both parents and the affected child. Other supportive interventions include physical, speech, and occupational therapy.

Multifactorial Disorders

Most multifactorial disorders are a result of an interaction between genes and environmental factors. These disorders do not follow a clear-cut pattern of inheritance. Multifactorial disorders may be present at birth, as with cleft lip or palate, or they may be expressed later in life, as with hypertension. The environmental fac-

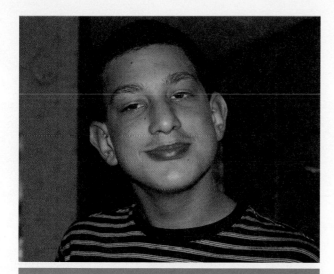

Figure 1-27

Fragile X syndrome.

tors may include any of a number of teratogens (birth defect–causing agents) such as infections, chemicals, or radiation.

Cleft Lip and Cleft Palate

Cleft lip and palate may occur together or separately. These conditions develop in the second month of pregnancy, when the facial structures do not fuse properly. The deformities may be unilateral or bilateral. Severity of the deformity varies from a mild notch to involving the lip, palate, and tongue (**Figure 1-28**). Feeding and nutritional issues may occur because of these structural problems. Clinical manifestations are obvious at

birth and can be detected with a prenatal ultrasound. A series of surgeries is performed to close the gap in the lip and palate. Speech therapy and feeding devices can minimize speech delays and nutritional deficits. Parental support is important to ensure the child's proper care and minimize caregiver stress.

Chromosomal Disorders

Chromosomal disorders are a major category of genetic disorders that result most often from alteration in chromosomal duplication or number. Oftentimes these disorders occur in utero because of some environmental influences (e.g., maternal age, drugs, and infections). The most vulnerable time for the fetus is at 15–60 days' gestation. This period immediately follows fertilization and implantation, when much of the cellular differentiation is occurring. More than 60 disorders fall in this category, many of which result in first trimester abortions. The more common examples of these disorders include trisomy 21, monosomy X, and polysomy X.

Trisomy 21

Trisomy 21, or Down syndrome, is a spontaneous chromosomal mutation that results in three copies of chromosome 21 (**Figure 1-29**). Risk increases with parental age and environmental teratogen exposure. Clinical manifestations can vary widely and are apparent at birth. These manifestations typically include:

- Hypotonia
- Distinctive facial features (e.g., low nasal bridge, epicanthic folds, protruding tongue, low-set ears, and small, open mouth)

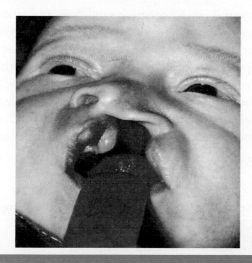

Figure 1-28

Cleft lip and palate.

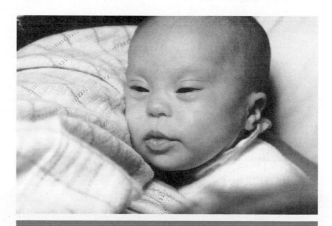

Figure 1-29

Down syndrome.

- Single crease on the palm (simian crease)
- White spots on the iris
- Mental retardation
- Congenital heart defects
- Strabismus and cataracts
- Poorly developed genitalia and delayed puberty

Early death can occur due to cardiac and pulmonary complications (e.g., hypertension, pneumonia). Persons with trisomy 21 are at increased susceptibility to leukemia and infections. Clinical presentation can be detected using four-dimensional ultrasounds. Other prenatal testing includes amniocentesis and serum hormone levels. There is no known cure for trisomy 21. Treatment strategies focus on symptom and complication management.

Monosomy X

Monosomy X, or Turner's syndrome, is a result of a deletion of part or all of an X chromosome (**Figure 1-30**). This condition only affects females who develop gonadal streaks instead of ovaries; therefore, these females will not menstruate. Other clinical manifestations may vary but often include:

- Short stature
- Lymphedema (swelling) of the hands and feet
- Broad chest with widely spaced nipples
- Low-set ears
- Small lower jaw
- Drooping eyelids
- Reproductive sterility
- Increased weight
- Small fingernails
- Webbing of the neck
- Coarctation of the aorta
- Horseshoe kidney
- Visual disturbances (e.g., glaucoma)
- Ear infections
- Hearing loss

Turner's syndrome is treated by administering female sex hormones to promote secondary sex characteristics and skeletal growth. Growth hormones may also be administered to further aid in skeletal growth. Diagnosis is often delayed until late childhood or early

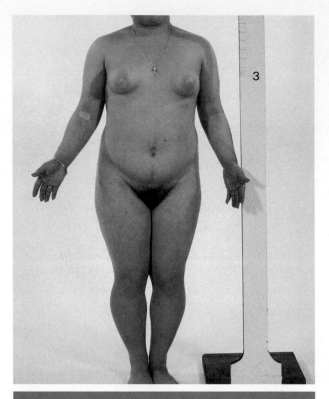

Figure 1-30

Turner's syndrome.

adolescence if the clinical presentation is more subtle, but chromosomal analysis can confirm diagnosis. Early treatment allows for early hormone replacement to minimize problems and detect complications.

Polysomy X

Polysomy X, or Klinefelter's syndrome, is a relatively common abnormality that results from an extra X chromosome—creating an XXY sex chromosome. Because of the presence of a Y chromosome, persons with this syndrome are male (**Figure 1-31**). The syndrome usually becomes apparent at puberty when testicles fail to mature, rendering affected boys infertile. Clinical manifestations of Klinefelter's syndrome include:

- Small penis, prostate gland, and testicles
- Sparse facial and body hair
- Sexual dysfunction (e.g., impotence, decreased libido)
- Gynecomastia (femalelike breasts)
- Long legs with a short, obese trunk
- Tall stature
- Behavioral problems

- Learning disabilities
- Increased incidence of pulmonary disease and varicose veins

Other problems that can develop include osteoporosis and breast cancer. Diagnostic procedures consist of history, physical examination, hormone levels, and chromosomal testing. Treatment includes male hormone replacement to promote secondary sex characteristics. A mastectomy may be performed in cases of gynecomastia and breast cancer. Psychological counseling and support may be beneficial to the patient and the parents.

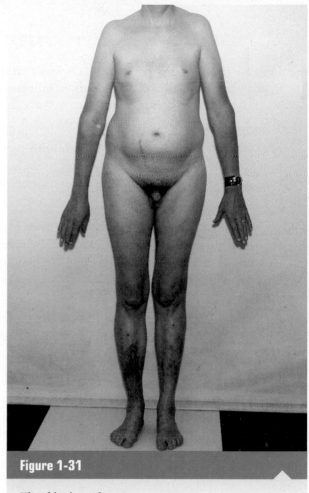

Figure 1-31

Klinefelter's syndrome.

Chapter Summary

Cells are the basic units of life, and they face many challenges in order to survive. These challenges include hypoxia, nutritional changes, infection, inflammation, and chemicals. Cells adapt to the challenges in an attempt to prevent or limit damage as well as death. This adaptation may be reversible or permanent.

Neoplasms arise from abnormal cellular proliferation or differentiation. These neoplasms can be benign or malignant. Benign neoplasms are more differentiated; therefore, they are more like the parent cells. Benign tumors are less likely to cause problems in the host or metastasize except in terms of location. On the other hand, malignant tumors are less differentiated; therefore, they are more like the parent cells. Malignant tumors are more likely to cause problems in the host and metastasize.

Genetic and congenital disorders can develop from factors that disrupt normal fetal development or interact with defective genes. These factors, or teratogens, can include radiation, infections, or chemicals. Genetic and congenital disorders may be present at birth or may not appear until later in life. Exploring these basic cellular and genetic concepts and issues will lay the foundation for understanding where disease begins.

Case Study Answers

1. A
2. D
3. D
4. Not smoking or drinking; routine exercise; overall good health

5. Because the tumor is hormone dependent, hormone therapy with more progesterone-like drugs will strangulate the supply of estrogen to the cancer. The tumor will shrink or growth will slow

References

Chiras, D. (2008). *Human biology* (6th ed.). Sudbury, MA: Jones and Bartlett.

Elling, B., Elling, K., & Rothenberg, M. (2004). *Anatomy and physiology.* Sudbury, MA: Jones and Bartlett.

Lewin, B., Cassimeris, L., Lingappa, V., & Plopper, G. (Eds.). (2007). *Cells.* Sudbury, MA: Jones and Bartlett.

Mosby's medical, nursing, & allied health dictionary (7th ed.). (2005). St. Louis, MO: Mosby.

Porth, C. (2006). *Essentials of pathophysiology* (6th ed.). Philadelphia, PA: Lippincott Williams & Wilkins.

Professional guide to pathophysiology (2nd ed.). (2007). Philadelphia, PA: Lippincott Williams & Wilkins.

Resources

www.cellsalive.com

www.cancer.org

www.cdc.gov

www.medlineplus.gov

www.nih.gov

www.rarediseases.org

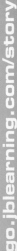

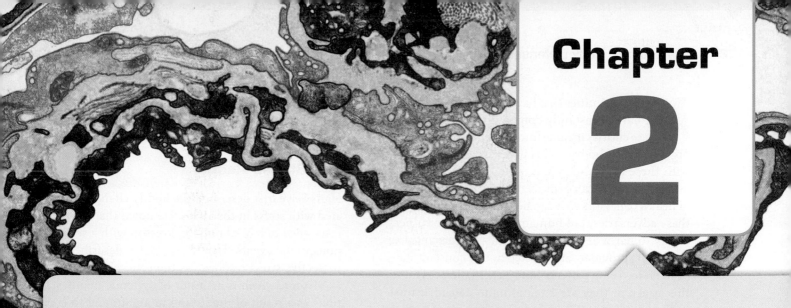

Body Defenses

KEY TERMS

acquired immunity
active acquired immunity
acute tissue rejection
alarm
allogenic
antibody-producing cell
antigen
autoimmune
autologous
B cell
chronic tissue rejection
cytotoxic cell

effector cell
exhaustion
first line of defense
general adaptation syndrome
graft-versus-host rejection
helper cell
host-versus-graft rejection
hyperacute tissue rejection
hypersensitivity
immunodeficiency
inflammatory response
interferon

killer cell
local adaptation syndrome
memory cell
opportunistic infections
passive acquired immunity
primary deficit
pyrogen
regulator cell
resistance
second line of defense
secondary immunodeficiency
suppressor cell

syngenic
systemic lupus erythematosus (SLE)
T cell
third line of defense
type I hypersensitivity
type II hypersensitivity
type III hypersensitivity
type IV hypersensitivity

variety of entities that have the potential of causing harm constantly bombard the human body. These entities include things such as stressors and organisms. The body's ability to resist damage and deal with these events will determine the effects of such events. Humans can arm themselves with an arsenal of health behaviors that can help them defend against these adversaries, but humans increase their vulnerability to harm as well. All patients we encounter as healthcare providers are affected by this constant state of warfare. These patients have either fallen victim to this attack or they are attempting to defend against it. Healthcare providers can identify those at risk or under attack and help those people take up arms to defeat these persistent adversaries.

Stress

Stress is a universal experience of human existence that can negatively affect the body's fragile homeostasis state (see Introduction). Stress can contribute directly to the development or exacerbation of disease. Stress can also contribute to negative behaviors such as smoking and drug abuse in an attempt to cope. Stress can arise from many events, even those that may be perceived as positive (e.g., weddings and vacations).

Understanding the nature of stress and the effects that it can have on the body is vital for healthcare providers in their interaction with the infirmed.

The Stress Response

Hans Selye first described the bodily changes associated with stress in the 1930s. He noted that the body responded to any stimuli, or stressor, with a series of nonspecific events (**Figure 2-1**). Selye described this protective stress response as the general adaptation syndrome, which is a cluster of systemic manifestations as a result of modifying in an attempt to cope with a stressor. Several factors can affect adaptation, including natural reserve, time, genetics, age, gender, health status, nutrition, sleep–wake cycles, hardiness, and psychosocial factors. The general adaptation syndrome includes three stages—alarm, resistance, and exhaustion (**Figure 2-2**). The alarm stage includes the generalized stimulation of the sympathetic nervous system resulting in the release of catecholamines and cortisol, or the fight-or-flight response. In the resistance stage, the body chooses the most effective and advantageous defense. Cortisol levels and the sympathetic nervous system return to normal, causing the fight-or-flight symptoms to disappear. The body will

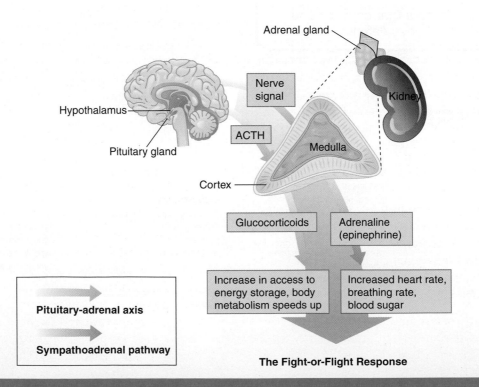

Figure 2-1

Physiological response to stress.

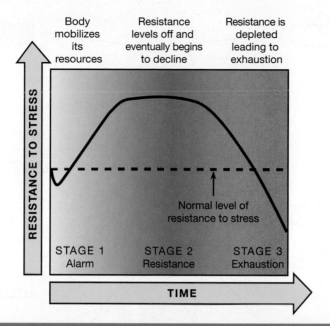

Body
mobilizes
its
resources

Resistance
levels off and
eventually begins
to decline

Resistance is
depleted
leading to
exhaustion

RESISTANCE TO STRESS

Normal level of
resistance to stress

STAGE 1
Alarm

STAGE 2
Resistance

STAGE 3
Exhaustion

TIME

Figure 2-2

General adaptation syndrome.

either adapt or alter in an attempt to limit problems or become desensitized to the stressor. Stress management techniques (e.g., meditation and relaxation) can assist in the desensitization process. If the stressor is prolonged or overwhelms the body, the exhaustion phase is initiated. During the exhaustion phase, the body becomes depleted and damage may appear as homeostasis can no longer be maintained. As the body's defenses are utilized, disease or death results. Diseases and ailments that have been attributed to stress include anxiety, depression, headaches, insomnia, infections, and cardiovascular disease (**Figure 2-3**).

The local adaptation syndrome is the localized version of general adaptation syndrome. In this syndrome, the body is attempting to limit the damage associated with the stressor by confining the stressor to one location. An example of this response can be seen in the local inflammatory reaction that results from tissue trauma. The inflammatory response will be discussed in an upcoming section.

Although there is some predictability to the stress response, there is some individual variability due to conditioning factors. These conditioning factors may include genetics, age, gender, life experiences, dietary status, and social support. The positive presence of these factors can limit and eliminate the likelihood of damage, disease, or death. The implementation of one or more coping strategies can also minimize

and eliminate negative stress effects. These strategies include lifestyle modifications such as physical activity, adequate sleep, and optimal dietary status. Other strategies include relaxation, distraction, and biofeedback. Unfortunately, maladaptive coping strategies may be used instead. These maladaptive strategies cause more problems than benefits and include activities such as smoking, consuming alcohol or drugs, and overeating. Healthcare professionals can assist patients to replace those negative strategies with more positive ones.

Immunity

The body is under constant assault by life-threatening microbes. Although the vast majority of microbes are harmless, occasionally they are not. The immune system is responsible for protecting the body against an array of microorganisms (e.g., bacteria, viruses, fungi, protozoans, and prions) as well as removing damaged cells and destroying cancer cells. Therefore, a functioning immune system is essential for survival. Fundamental to a properly functioning immune system is the ability to recognize and respond to a foreign agent, or antigen. Some immune cells circulate constantly, always on alert for an invasion, and others remain in tissue and organs, waiting to be activated (**Table 2-1**). Additionally, some of the body's structures serve as barriers, preventing invasion.

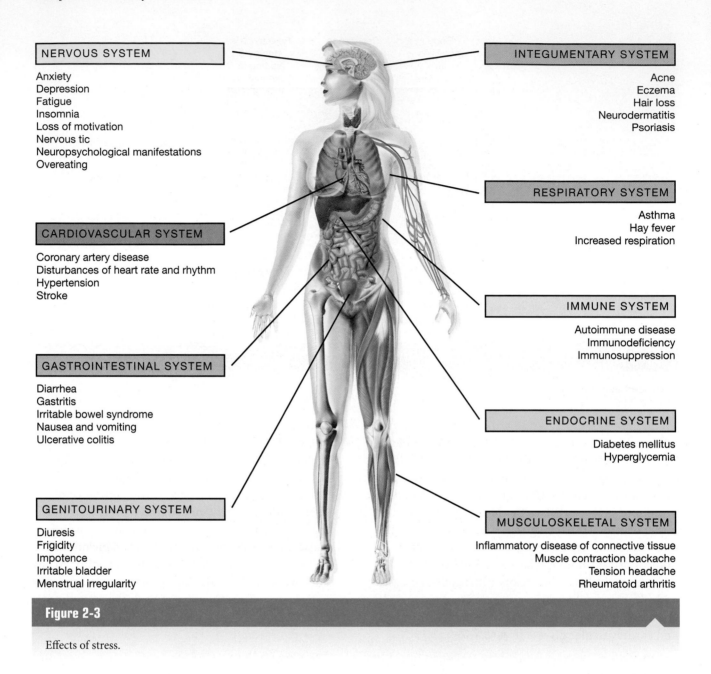

NERVOUS SYSTEM

Anxiety
Depression
Fatigue
Insomnia
Loss of motivation
Nervous tic
Neuropsychological manifestations
Overeating

CARDIOVASCULAR SYSTEM

Coronary artery disease
Disturbances of heart rate and rhythm
Hypertension
Stroke

GASTROINTESTINAL SYSTEM

Diarrhea
Gastritis
Irritable bowel syndrome
Nausea and vomiting
Ulcerative colitis

GENITOURINARY SYSTEM

Diuresis
Frigidity
Impotence
Irritable bladder
Menstrual irregularity

INTEGUMENTARY SYSTEM

Acne
Eczema
Hair loss
Neurodermatitis
Psoriasis

RESPIRATORY SYSTEM

Asthma
Hay fever
Increased respiration

IMMUNE SYSTEM

Autoimmune disease
Immunodeficiency
Immunosuppression

ENDOCRINE SYSTEM

Diabetes mellitus
Hyperglycemia

MUSCULOSKELETAL SYSTEM

Inflammatory disease of connective tissue
Muscle contraction backache
Tension headache
Rheumatoid arthritis

Figure 2-3

Effects of stress.

First Line of Defense

The immune system takes a multilayer approach to protection from antigens. The **first line of defense** includes physical and chemical barriers that indiscriminately protect against all invaders (nonspecific immunity). The most prominent barriers in this first line are the skin and mucous membranes. The skin is a thick, impermeable layer of epidermal cells overlying the rich vascular layer, or dermis. As newly produced skin cells push the dead ones outward, the dead cells produce a waterproof layer because of keratin contained in those dead cells. Although the skin does protect the human body from invasions, there are passageways that allow direct access to its interior (respiratory, digestive, and genitourinary tracts). These passageways are lined with a protective mucous membrane that is not as thick as skin, but these membranes do provide a moderate layer of protection. The first line also includes chemical barriers in conjunction with the physical barriers. The skin produces a slightly acidic substance that inhibits bacterial growth. Hydrochloric acid in the stomach destroys many ingested bacteria. Tears and saliva contain lysozyme, an enzyme that dissolves bacterial cell walls.

Table 2-1 Major Components of the Immune System

Antigen	A foreign agent that triggers the production of antibodies by the immune system.
Antibody	Proteins used by the immune system to identify and neutralize foreign agents, such as viruses and bacteria.
Autoantibody	An antibody made by the immune system that attacks an individual's own proteins.
Thymus	Located in the anterior superior mediastinum; functions are the development of T-lymphocytes and the production and secretion of thymosins.
Lymphatic tissue	Connective tissue containing many lymphocytes; transports immune cells, antigen-presenting cells, fatty acids, and fats; filters body fluids.
Bone marrow	Soft, fatty tissue found inside of bones. Contains stem cells and leukocytes.
Cells	
Neutrophils	An infection-fighting agent. Usually the first to arrive on the scene of an infection, neutrophils are attracted by various chemicals released by infected tissue. Neutrophils escape from the capillary wall and migrate to the site of infection. Once they get to the site, neutrophils phagocytize microorganisms, preventing the infection from spreading.
Basophils	White blood cells that bind IgE and release histamine in anaphylaxis.
Eosinophils	White blood cells involved in allergic reactions.
Monocytes	White blood cells that replenish macrophages and dendritic cells in normal states and respond to inflammation by migrating to infected tissue to become macrophages and dendritic cells, which elicits an immune response.
Macrophages	White blood cells within tissues, produced by differentiation of monocytes. Functions are phagocytosis and stimulating lymphocytes and other immune cells to respond to pathogens.
Mast cells	Connective tissue cells that contain histamine, heparin, hyaluronic acid, slow-reacting substance of anaphylaxis (SRS-A), and serotonin.
B cells (B lymphocytes)	B cells mature in the bone marrow where they differentiate into memory cells or immunoglobulin-secreting (antibody) cells. B cells eliminate bacteria, neutralize bacterial toxins, prevent viral reinfection, and produce immediate inflammatory response.
Plasma cells	White blood cells that develop from B cells and produce large volumes of specific antibodies.
T cells (T lymphocytes)	T cells are produced in the bone marrow and mature in the thymus, hence "T" cell. Two major types of T cells work to destroy antigens—regulator cells and effector cells.
Killer T cells	A type of T cell that destroys cells infected with viruses by releasing lymphokines that destroy cell walls. Also called cytotoxic cells and effector cells.
Memory B cells	Type of B cell that aids quick response to subsequent exposures to an antigen because memory cells recall the antigen as foreign, and antibody production is rapid.
Helper B cells	A type of regulator cell that activates, or calls up, B cells to produce antibodies.
NK lymphocytes	Natural killer cells that destroy cancer cells, foreign cells, and virus-infected cells.
Chemical Mediators	
Complement	A group of inactive proteins in the circulation that, when activated, stimulate the release of other chemical mediators, promoting inflammation, chemotaxis, and phagocytosis.
Histamine	Released by mast cells and basophils, especially during allergic reactions, triggering the inflammatory response. Increases the permeability of the capillaries to white blood cells and other proteins, in order to allow them to engage foreign invaders in the infected tissues.

(Continues)

Table 2-1 Major Components of the Immune System *(Continued)*

Kinins (e.g., bradykinin)	Induce vasodilation and contraction of smooth muscle.
Prostaglandins	A group of lipid compounds that have a variety of effects, including constriction or dilation in vascular smooth muscle cells, control of cell growth, and sensitizing spinal neurons to pain.
Leukotrienes	Fatty molecules of the immune system that contribute to contraction of bronchiolar smooth muscle.
Cytokines (messengers)	Small cell-signaling protein molecules that are extensively involved in intracellular communication. Includes interleukins, interferons, and lymphokines.
Tumor necrosis factor (TNF)	A group of cytokines that can cause cell death (apoptosis).
Chemotactic factors	Attract phagocytes to the area of inflammation.

Source: Adapted from Gould, B. (2010). *Pathophysiology for the health professions* (4th ed.). Philadelphia, PA: Elsevier.

Second Line of Defense

The first line of defense is not impenetrable. Tiny breaks in the skin or in the lining of the respiratory, digestive, or genitourinary tracts may permit an antigen invasion. The second line of defense is in place to respond to those antigens. The second line of defense involves a number of chemical and cellular agents. The second line includes four components: (1) inflammatory response, (2) pyrogens, (3) interferons, and (4) complement proteins.

Inflammatory Response

Damage or trauma to body tissue triggers a series of reactions referred to as the inflammatory response. The inflammatory reaction is characterized by erythema (redness), edema (swelling), heat, and pain at the site (**Figure 2-4**). The inflammatory response is triggered by a set of mediators, or mast cells, including histamine (stimulates vasodilatation) and prostaglandins (stimulates pain receptors in the area). Immediately after the injury, arterioles in the area briefly go into spasm and constrict to limit bleeding and the extent of injury. This vasoconstriction is immediately followed by vasodilatation, which increases blood flow to the injured area in an attempt to dilute toxins and provide essential immune cells (e.g., neutrophils, monocytes), nutrients, and oxygen. The vasodilatation increases capillary permeability, and as permeability increases, leukocytes line the vessel wall in preparation of immigration into the surrounding tissue. While the leukocytes are lining the vessel walls, endothelial cells in the vessel walls react to biochemical mediators that cause these vessels to retract. This retraction gives the leukocytes the space to migrate into the interstitial space to begin the cleanup process of phagocytosis, or the engulfing and digestion of foreign substances and cellular debris. In conjunction with phagocytosis, fibrinogen is transforming into fibrin. The fibrin will be used to wall off the injured area so that foreign substances are contained. A meshwork of new cells forms to use in the healing process. Blood clotting begins if blood vessels have been damaged.

Pyrogens

Pyrogens are molecules released by macrophages that have been exposed by bacteria. Pyrogens travel to the hypothalamus, the portion of the brain primarily responsible for controlling body temperature. These pyrogens turn the heat up on the bacteria, producing fever and creating an unpleasant environment for bacterial growth. Mild fevers cause the spleen and liver to remove iron from the blood, which is required by many bacteria to reproduce. Fever also increases metabolism, which facilitates healing and accelerates phagocytosis. However, severe fever (over 105° F) can be life threatening because it begins to denature vital proteins, especially enzymes needed for biochemical reactions.

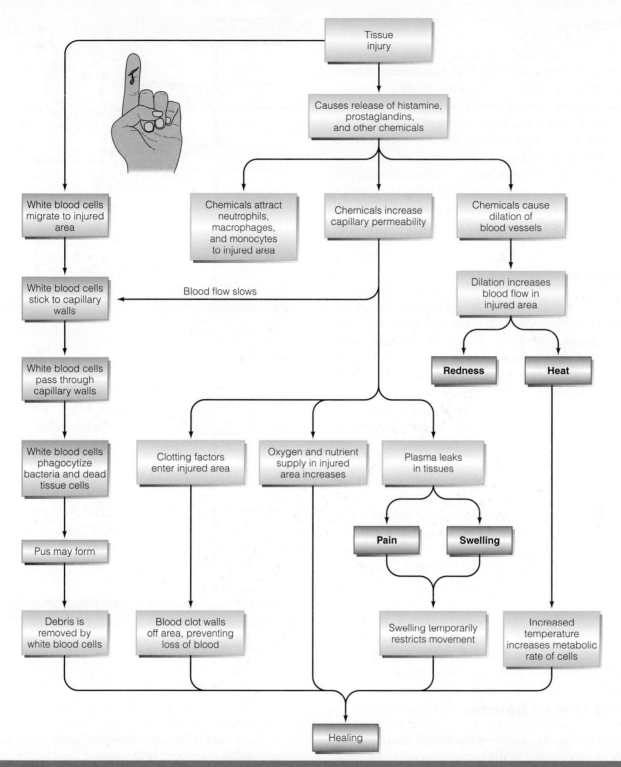

Figure 2-4

Inflammatory response.

Interferons

Interferons are small proteins released from cells infected by viruses (**Figure 2-5**). Interferons diffuse away from the site of invasion through the interstitial tissue and bind to receptors on the plasma membranes of noninfected cells. The binding of interferons to uninfected cells triggers the synthesis of enzymes that inhibit viral replication. Consequently, when viruses enter the previously uninfected cells, they cannot replicate and spread. Interferons do not protect cells already infected by a virus; they stop the spread. In essence, interferon production is the dying cells' attempt to protect other cells.

Complement Proteins

The complement system is a process that involves blood plasma proteins (~20) that enhances the action of antibodies. Complement proteins circulate in the blood in an inactive state. When foreign substances invade the body, the complement proteins are activated. We will briefly describe a few activities of this complex process. Five complement system proteins join together to form a large molecule, or membrane-attack complex. The membrane-attack complex embeds in the plasma membrane of bacteria, creating an opening into which water flows. The influx of water causes the bacterial cells to swell, burst, and die. Other complement proteins stimulate vasodilatation in an infected area as a part of the inflammatory response. Some complement proteins increase permeability of vessels, allowing white blood cells and plasma to pass quickly to the infected area. Additionally, other complement proteins serve as chemical attractants, drawing macrophages, monocytes, and neutrophils to the infected area where they phagocytize foreign cells. Finally, other complement proteins bind to microbes, forming a rough coat on the invader that promotes phagocytosis.

Third Line of Defense

The third line of defense is the body's own immune system. Key players in the recognition of the antigens that make it through the first two layers of immunity are T cells and B cells (**Figure 2-6**). T cells and B cells mingle with antigens as they circulate throughout the body's fluids and peripheral lymphoid tissue (e.g., tonsils, lymph nodes, spleen, and intestinal lymphoid tissue). There are two main reasons for this interaction: (1) to destroy the antigen (T cell function or cellular immunity), or (2) to produce antibodies against the antigen (B cell function or humoral immunity).

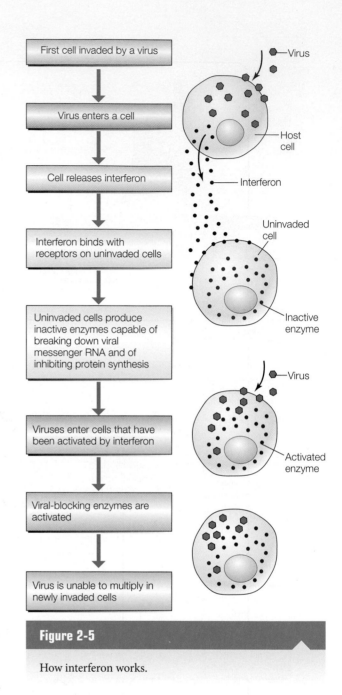

Figure 2-5

How interferon works.

T cells get their name from the place where they mature, the thymus. T cells are produced in the bone marrow, after which they enter the bloodstream and travel to the thymus for maturation. Two major types of T cells work to destroy antigens: (1) regulator cells, including helper T cells and suppressor T cells; and (2) effector cells, or killer cells. Helper cells activate, or call up, B cells to produce antibodies. Suppressor cells turn that antibody production off. Killer cells, or cytotoxic cells, destroy cells infected with viruses by releasing lymphokines that destroy cell walls. T cells

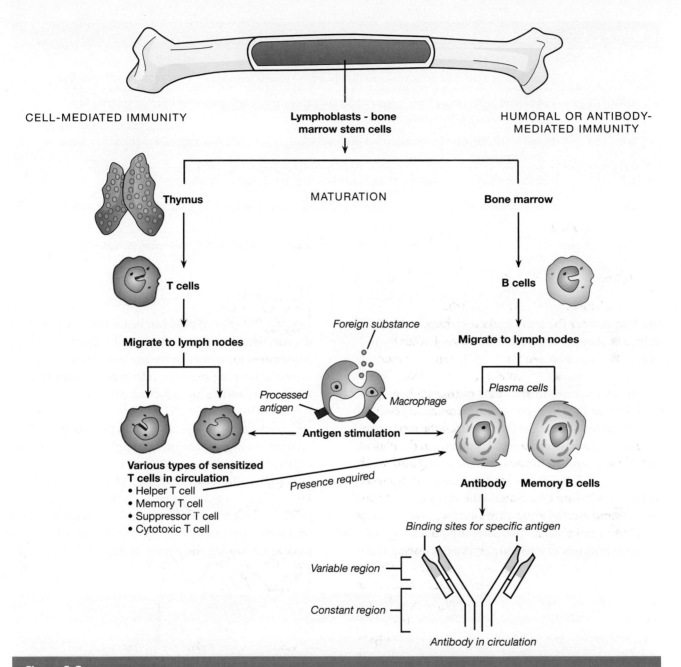

CELL-MEDIATED IMMUNITY   **Lymphoblasts - bone marrow stem cells**   HUMORAL OR ANTIBODY-MEDIATED IMMUNITY

Thymus   MATURATION   **Bone marrow**

T cells   **B cells**

Migrate to lymph nodes   *Foreign substance*   **Migrate to lymph nodes**

Processed antigen   *Macrophage*   *Plasma cells*

Antigen stimulation

Various types of sensitized T cells in circulation
• Helper T cell
• Memory T cell
• Suppressor T cell
• Cytotoxic T cell

Presence required   **Antibody   Memory B cells**

Binding sites for specific antigen

Variable region

Constant region

Antibody in circulation

Figure 2-6

Development of cellular and humoral immunity.

Table 2-2 Immunoglobulins and Their Functions

IgG	Main defense against bacteria; can cross the placenta to protect fetus against infections (passive immunity).
IgM	Fight blood infections and help trigger additional production of IgG; present in lymphocyte cells; first antibody made by a developing fetus.
IgA	Found in membranes of respiratory and gastrointestinal tract, tears, saliva, mucus, and colostrum; important in local immunity.
IgE	Protects the body in mucous membranes and skin; triggers allergic reactions.
IgD	Present in blood serum (in small amounts) and B cell surfaces; receptor for antigens; helps anchor cell membranes.

Source: Adapted from Gould, B. (2010). *Pathophysiology for the health professions* (4th ed.). Philadelphia, PA: Elsevier.

work to protect the body against viruses and cancer cells, and they are responsible for hypersensitivity and transplant rejection.

B cells mature in the bone marrow where they differentiate into memory cells or immunoglobulin-secreting (antibody) cells (**Table 2-2**). B cells eliminate bacteria, neutralize bacterial toxins, prevent viral reinfection, and produce immediate inflammatory response. Each B cell has receptor sites for a specific antigen, and when it encounters the antigen, the B cells activate and multiply into either antibody-producing cells or memory cells. The antibody-producing cells produce millions of antibody molecules during their 24-hour life span. B cells can begin this antigen production within 72 hours after initial antigen exposure. Subsequent exposures to the antigen produce a quick response because memory cells recall the antigen as foreign, and antibody production is rapid. This reaction is referred to as acquired immunity (**Table 2-3**). Active acquired immunity refers to this process gained by actively having the antigen through invasion or vaccination. In active immunity, the person makes his or her own antibodies, and protection is usually long term. Passive acquired immunity refers to the process gained by receiving antibodies made outside the body by another person, animal, or recombinant DNA. In passive immunity, the person is not actively produc-

Table 2-3 Types of Acquired Immunity

Type	Mechanism	Memory	Example
Natural active	Pathogens enter the body and cause illness; antibodies form	Yes	Person has rubella once
Artificial active	Vaccine (live or attenuated organisms) is injected into the body. No illness results, but antibodies form.	Yes	Person receives measles vaccine
Natural passive	Antibodies are passed directly from mother to child to provide temporary protection	No	Passage through placenta during pregnancy; consumption of breastmilk
Artificial passive	Antibodies are injected into the body (antiserum) to provide temporary protection or to minimize severity of an infection	No	Gammaglobulin injection to treat immunological disease, such as idiopathic thrombocytopenia purpura (ITP)

Source: Adapted from Gould, B. (2010). *Pathophysiology for the health professions* (4th ed.). Philadelphia, PA: Elsevier.

ing antibodies, and protection is short lived. Examples of passive immunity include mother-to-fetus transfer through placenta or breastfeeding transference.

Altered Immune Response

Malfunction at any point in any of the numerous and highly complex immune responses can create a pathologic state. Malfunctions may include exaggeration (hypersensitivity), misdirection (autoimmune), or diminution (immunodeficiency).

Hypersensitivity

Hypersensitivity is an inflated or inappropriate response to an antigen. The result is inflammation and destruction of healthy tissue. Hypersensitivity reactions may be immediate, occurring within minutes to hours of reexposure, or delayed, occurring several hours after reexposure. There are four types of hypersensitivity reactions: type I (IgE mediated), type II (tissue specific), type III (immune complex mediated), and type IV (cell mediated) (**Figure 2-7**).

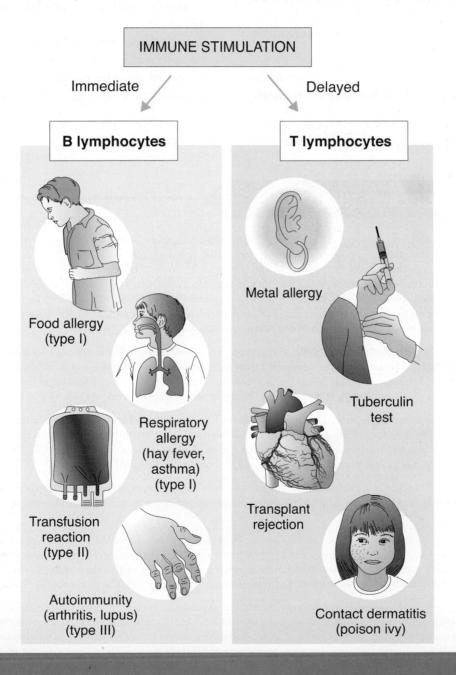

Figure 2-7

Classification of hypersensitivity reactions.

With type I hypersensitivity, allergens activate T cells, which bind to mast cells. Repeated exposure to relatively large doses of the allergens is usually necessary to cause this response. When enough IgE has been produced, the person is sensitized to the allergen. At the next exposure to the same antigen, the antigen binds with the surface IgE, releasing mediators (e.g., histamines, cytokines, and prostaglandins) and triggering the complement system. The effects of type I reactions include immediate inflammation and pruritus. Examples of type I reactions include hay fever, food allergies, and anaphylaxis. Treatment of type I reactions includes epinephrine, antihistamines, corticosteroids, and desensitizing injections.

Type II hypersensitivity generally involves the destruction of a target cell by an antibody-directed, cell-surface antigen. IgG or IgM reacts with an antigen on the cell, activating the complement system. The effects of type II reactions include cell lysis and phagocytosis. Examples of type II reactions include blood transfusion reactions and erythroblastosis fetalis. Treatment focuses on prevention and includes ensuring blood compatibility prior to transfusions and administering medication to prevent maternal antibody development (e.g., Rho[D] immune globulin [RhoGAM]).

In type III hypersensitivity, circulating antigen-antibody complexes accumulate and are deposited in the tissue. Common tissues include kidneys, joints, skin, and blood vessels. This accumulation triggers the complement system causing local inflammation and increased vascular permeability, so more complexes accumulate. Examples of type III reactions include

TRANSPLANT REACTIONS

The immune system's protective nature makes it challenging for patients receiving much-needed tissue and organ transplants and blood transfusion. Transplant success is closely tied to making the best possible tissue match. There are three types of tissue transplants—allogenic, syngenic, and autologous. Allogenic transplants are those in which tissue is used from the same species of similar tissue type, but it is not identical. Most transplants use allogenic tissue. Syngenic transplants use tissue from the identical twin of the host. With autologous transplants, the host and the donor are the same person. An example of this type of transplant is someone storing up his or her own blood prior to a scheduled surgery. Donors may be live or a cadaver, but regardless, making a close tissue match is fundamental to preventing rejection.

Rejection reactions are classified by timing. Hyperacute tissue rejections occur immediately to 3 days after the transplant. Hyperacute reactions occur due to a complement response in which the recipient has antibodies against the donor. This complement response triggers a systemic inflammatory reaction. The response is so quick that often the tissue has not had a chance to establish vascularization; as a result, the tissue becomes permanently necrotic.

Acute tissue rejections are the most common and treatable type of rejection. This type usually occurs between 4 days and 3 months following the transplant. Acute reactions are cell mediated and result in transplant cell destruction (lyses) or necrosis. The patient exhibits signs and symptoms of the inflammatory process including fever, redness, swelling, and tenderness at the graft site. Additionally, the patient may experience impaired functioning of the transplanted organ.

Chronic tissue rejection occurs from about 4 months to years after the transplant. This reaction is most likely due to an antibody-mediated immune response. Antibodies and complements deposit in the transplanted tissue vessel walls, resulting in decreased blood flow and ischemia.

Most rejection reactions are classified as host-versus-graft rejection; in other words, the host is fighting the graft. The graft fights the host in one type of reaction, or graft-versus-host rejection. This potentially life-threatening type of reaction occurs *only* with bone marrow transplants. The immunocompetent graft cells recognize the host cells as foreign and organize a cell-mediated attack. The host is usually immunocompromised and unable to fight the graft cells.

Identifying the rejection reaction is crucial to reversing it. Assessment including signs and symptoms of a healthy and unhealthy transplant organ is paramount. For example, if the kidneys are the transplanted organ, decreased urine output may indicate a failing transplant. Diagnostic procedures include laboratory tests to identify immune and inflammatory activity (e.g., white blood count) and specific tests to determine functioning of the transplanted organ. Treatment for transplant rejection usually begins with prevention. Prevention starts with ensuring a tissue match and initiating immunosuppressive therapy. The transplant patient will likely require immunosuppressive therapy for life. Once a rejection is suspected, immunosuppression therapy is intensified to reverse it.

SYSTEMIC LUPUS ERYTHEMATOSUS

Systemic lupus erythematosus (SLE) is a chronic inflammatory disorder that can affect any connective tissue. It is thought that B cells are activated for unknown reasons to produce autoantibodies and autoantigens that combine to form immune complexes. These immune complexes fight against the body's own tissues (e.g., nucleic acid, red blood cells, platelets, and lymphocytes). It is proposed that hyperactive helper T cells and subdued suppressor T cells create a prime environment for B cells to overproduce.

This unpredictable disorder most often harms the heart, joints, skin, lungs, blood vessels, liver, kidneys, and nervous system (**Table 2-4**). The disease occurs nine times more often in women than in men, especially between the ages of 15 and 50, and is more common in those of non-European descent.

Since patients with SLE can have a wide variety of symptoms and different combinations of organ involvement, no single test establishes the diagnosis of SLE. To improve the accuracy of the diagnosis of SLE, 11 criteria were established. Some patients suspected of having SLE may never develop enough criteria for a definite diagnosis. Other patients accumulate enough criteria only after months or years. When a person has four or more of these criteria, the diagnosis of SLE is strongly suggested. Nevertheless, the diagnosis of SLE may be made in some settings in patients with only a few of these classical criteria, and treatment may be instituted at this stage.

The 11 criteria used for diagnosing systemic lupus erythematosus include:

1. Butterfly rash over the cheeks of the face

2. Skin rash of patchy redness with hyperpigmentation and hypopigmentation that can cause scarring

3. Photosensitivity

4. Mucous membrane ulcers

5. Arthritis

6. Pleuritis or pericarditis (inflammation of the lining tissue around the heart or lungs)

7. Renal abnormalities (abnormal amounts of urine protein or clumps of cellular elements, called casts, detectable with a urinalysis)

8. Brain irritation (manifested by seizures and/or psychosis)

9. Blood abnormalities (low counts of white or red blood cells, or platelets)

10. Immunologic disorder (abnormal immune tests include anti-DNA)

11. Antinuclear antibody (positive antinuclear antibody testing)

In addition to the 11 criteria, other tests can be helpful in evaluating patients with SLE to determine the severity of organ involvement. These tests include routine testing of the blood to detect inflammation (e.g., erythrocyte sedimentation rate and C-reactive protein), blood-chemistry testing, direct analysis of internal body fluids, and tissue biopsies. Abnormalities in body fluids and tissue samples (kidney, skin, and nerve biopsies) can further support the diagnosis of SLE. The appropriate testing procedures are selected for the patient on an individual basis.

Treatment of SLE is directed at symptom management. General strategies include stress reduction, exercise, and sleep. Medical treatment includes nonsteriodal anti-inflammatory drugs to reduce pain and inflammation in joints, muscle, and other tissue. Corticosteroids may also be used to treat SLE. Corticosteroids are more potent than nonsteroidal anti-inflammatory drugs in reducing inflammation and restoring function when the disease is active, particularly when internal organs are affected, but they have multiple side effects (e.g., weight gain, risk for infection, hyperglycemia, high blood pressure) that must be considered. Antimalarial drugs can treat fatigue, joint pain, rashes, and pleural inflammation by suppressing the immune system. Immunosuppressants may be used for patients with kidney and nervous system involvement. Additionally, plasmapheresis can remove antibodies and other immune substances from the blood to suppress immunity.

autoimmune disorders (e.g., systemic lupus erythematosus and glomerulonephritis). Treatment for type III reactions is disease specific.

Type IV hypersensitivity involves a delayed processing of the antigen by the macrophages. Once processed, the antigen is presented to the T cells, resulting in the release of lymphokines that cause inflammation and antigen destruction. Examples of type IV reactions include tuberculin skin testing, transplant reactions, and contact dermatitis. Treatment for type IV reactions is disease specific.

Table 2-4 Common Manifestations of Systemic Lupus Erythematosus

Joints	Polyarthritis, with swollen, painful joints, without damage; arthralgia
Skin	Butterfly rash with erythema on cheeks and over nose or rash on body; photosensitivity—exacerbation with sun exposure; ulcerations in oral mucosa; hair loss
Kidneys	Glomerulonephritis with antigen-antibody deposit in glomerulus, causing inflammation with marked proteinuria and progressive renal damage
Lungs	Pleurisy—inflammation of the pleural membranes, causing chest pain
Heart	Carditis—inflammation of any layer of the heart, commonly pericarditis
Blood vessels	Raynaud's phenomenon—periodic vasospasms in fingers and toes, accompanied by pain
Central nervous system	Psychoses, depression, mood changes, seizures
Bone marrow	Anemia, leucopenia, thrombocytopenia

Autoimmune Disorders

In autoimmune reactions, the body's normal defenses become self-destructive—recognizing self as foreign. What causes this misdirected response is unclear. Some theories include etiologies that are viral, genetic, medicinal, hormonal, and environmental in nature. Autoimmune disorders affect women more often than men. Autoimmune disorders can affect any tissue or organ in the body, while some are systemic. These disorders are characterized by frequent, progressive periods of exacerbations (worsening of symptoms) and remissions (easing of symptoms). Physical and emotional stressors frequently trigger exacerbations. Examples of autoimmune disorders include systemic lupus erythematosus, rheumatoid arthritis, and Guillain-Barré syndrome. Because of the mysterious nature of autoimmune disorders, diagnostic procedures often begin with eliminating all other causes. Other laboratory tests used are specific to the suspected autoimmune disorder (e.g., rheumatoid factor for rheumatoid arthritis). Treatment for autoimmune disorders is disease specific but often includes coping and stress management strategies to prevent exacerbations.

Immunodeficiency

A diminished or absent immune response increases susceptibility to infections. Immunodeficiencies may be primary (reflecting a defect with the immune system) or secondary (reflecting an underlying disease or factor that is suppressing the immune system). The most common forms of immunodeficiency are caused by viral infections or are iatrogenic reactions to therapeutic drugs (e.g., corticosteroids and chemotherapy). The problem may be acute or chronic. Primary deficits involve basic developmental failures, many resulting from genetic or congenital abnormalities (e.g., hypogammaglobulinemia). Secondary or acquired immunodeficiency refers to a loss of immune function because of a specific cause. These causes may include infection, splenectomy, malnutrition, hepatic disease, drug therapy, or stress.

Immunodeficiency states predispose patients to opportunistic infections. Opportunistic infections are infections caused by pathogens that do not normally cause disease in healthy individuals (e.g., toxoplasmosis, Kaposi sarcoma, candidiasis infections). These infections often arise from a disruption of normal flora. Opportunistic infections can be difficult to treat successfully and can become life threatening. These infections need to be identified and treated early to improve the patient's prognosis.

Diagnosis of the immunodeficiency state includes the identification of recurrent or persistent infections. Diagnostic procedures consist of immunoglobulin levels, white blood cells, and T cell counts. Treatment for immunodeficiency states is individualized for the specific deficiency and may include gamma globulin, bone marrow transplants, or thymus transplants. Reverse isolation precautions (e.g., hand washing, limiting visitors, and avoiding fresh flowers) can limit the person's exposure to pathogens and thus decrease his or her risk for infection.

CLINICAL CASE

Mrs. Stubbs is a 24-year-old African American woman, living in a small rural town. Shortly after she gave birth to her second child, she suddenly began experiencing fatigue, anxiety, and heart palpitations. She contacted her healthcare provider, who believed the symptoms were related to the stress of having given birth in addition to caring for her toddler. The healthcare provider recommended that she rest and obtain some help caring for her two small children.

Mrs. Stubbs's symptoms worsened and then gradually resolved. Her family encouraged her to try to reduce the stress in her life. Approximately 1 year after the initial symptoms, she began experiencing abdominal pain. Her healthcare provider referred her to a gastroenterologist, who determined that due to her age and symptoms, her gallbladder was most likely causing the abdominal pain and prescribed a low-fat diet and increased physical activity.

Three years after the symptoms initially began, Mrs. Stubbs became pregnant with her third child. During the 6th month of her pregnancy, Mrs. Stubbs began to experience problems. She had premature contractions, increased fatigue, headaches, and swelling in her legs. Her healthcare provider prescribed bed rest due to overexertion. During the last 3 months of pregnancy, she remained on bed rest and the pregnancy was monitored with biweekly visits and ultrasounds. Her family played a central role in helping her with housekeeping and childcare for her two children. However, she was forced to take a leave of absence from her job due to the premature labor, but she delivered a healthy baby girl. Shortly after the birth of her third child, Mrs. Stubbs began experiencing new and puzzling symptoms. Her ankles and knees began to swell, and the edema was noted bilaterally. She also started to complain of joint pain in her ankles, knees, elbows, wrists, and fingers. She had difficulty climbing a flight of steps or dancing. Rest and over-the-counter pain medication relieved her symptoms, but it was difficult for her to find time for much rest due to the responsibilities of caring for a family and working full time. Her family was very concerned about her health and questioned why the healthcare provider was not able to find a cause for her problems.

Winters brought a new intolerance to low temperatures. While Mrs. Stubbs had never liked cold weather, suddenly she was having a problem with her hands and feet becoming painful and discolored when she was exposed to cold. Her extremities became painful, stiff, and altered in color when exposed to cold temperatures. She returned to her healthcare provider with this new development. The healthcare provider was perplexed and not sure what was causing the young woman's problems. The healthcare provider referred Mrs. Stubbs to a rheumatologist.

The rheumatologist examined Mrs. Stubbs and ran several blood tests. Mrs. Stubbs's antinuclear antibody test was positive at 1:640. Her anti-DNA antibody was elevated (normal is low or none). The rheumatoid arthritis factor was negative (normal is negative with < 60 U/mL), and her sedimentation rate was 62 mm/hr (normal is up to 20 mm/hr for females).

The rheumatologist told her that he could not be sure of her condition, but that he was considering the possibility that it could be lupus. He emphatically told her, however, that it was not a positive diagnosis, and he certainly did not want to label her with such a devastating disease unless he was certain. He prescribed an anti-inflammatory medication and told her to return home and rest. Mrs. Stubbs was frustrated—no one had been able to find an answer to why she felt so sick. She tried to talk to her family and friends, but they did not seem to understand what she was going through. Even the healthcare providers did not seem to hear what she was telling them.

While medication reduced the pain and swelling in her joints, she continued to experience fatigue, abdominal pain, and intolerance to cold weather. She was frustrated and felt as if no one were listening to her complaints. Her spouse, family, and friends did not understand why she felt so bad when she looked as if there were nothing wrong with her. To Mrs. Stubbs, it seemed as if she would never feel healthy again.

During the summer months, Mrs. Stubbs experienced a strange, red, raised rash with itching after having been out in the sun. She had always enjoyed the outdoors, and she had never had a rash after being in the sun. In addition, she began to develop small, raised sores on her legs and arms. The joint pain, swelling, and fatigue continued. Convinced that there must be something wrong with her, she began researching information on rheumatologic conditions. Based on her symptoms and the lab test results performed in the past, she began to suspect that she had lupus.

Mrs. Stubbs returned to the rheumatologist, who, after reexamining diagnosed her with systemic lupus erythematosus. She met 5 of the 11 American College of Rheumatology (ACR) criteria for diagnosis, including butterfly rash/facial erythema, nonerosive arthritis, hematologic or blood disorder (anemia), immunologic disorder (abnormal anti-DNA antibody test), and a positive antinuclear antibody titer. A 1-month course of a corticosteroid with tapered doses was prescribed. An anti-inflammatory agent was added to the regimen prior to the corticosteroid being weaned off. The rheumatologist reassured Mrs. Stubbs as she left his office that he would be available for her and would help her manage the disease.

As Mrs. Stubbs left the rheumatologist's office, her feelings were mixed. She was thankful to know she was not crazy and to have a diagnosis. She was also angry and bitter that it took so long to find a cause for her symptoms. She was relieved that she could finally tell her family and friends why she felt so sick. She was also very afraid because she was not certain what her future would hold once she had been diagnosed with the chronic disease lupus. Mrs. Stubbs journey is typical for those with SLE, full of frustrations and unknowns.

Source: NetCE (n.d.).

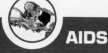

AIDS

AIDS is a deadly, sexually transmitted disease caused by the human immunodeficiency virus (HIV), a retrovirus. HIV attacks and weakens the immune system. There are two primary strains of the virus. The HIV-1 strain is the most prevalent strain in the United States, and the HIV-2 is the most prevalent strain in Africa. According to the Centers for Disease and Control and Prevention (CDC), HIV is the second leading cause of death in individuals 24 to 44 years of age in the United States. African Americans have the highest rate of new cases as compared to other ethnic groups. New cases among women have risen significantly in the last 30 years. Homosexual and bisexual men remain in the high-risk groups as well.

HIV is transmitted through direct contact with infected blood, blood products, or body fluids (e.g., human milk, vaginal secretions, semen, cerebrospinal fluid, and saliva). Even though saliva and tears can contain HIV, it is in low concentrations. The risk of acquiring HIV from an accidental needle stick is minimal (1 in 300), but the risk of transmission from sharing needles is significantly greater (1 in 150). There is a 13–40% chance of an infected mother transmitting it to her child, but administration of antiretroviral therapy can decrease the transmission risk by approximately 68%. The most common antiretroviral drug used to prevent maternal transmission is Retrovir (zidovudine), which has a high safety index. Cesarean delivery can further decrease the risk of HIV transmission to the fetus.

Being a retrovirus, the HIV requires a host to survive. Once the HIV gains access to the body, the virus invades the CD4 cells. Once inside the CD4 cells, the virus uses an enzyme, reverse transcriptase, to convert the viral RNA to DNA. The viral DNA is then integrated into the CD4's DNA. As the infected CD4 cell reproduces, it inadvertently produces viral copies. Meanwhile, the virus replicates inside the CD4 to the point that the cell membrane is compromised, releasing millions of viral copies into the bloodstream. Each viral copy then attaches to a new CD4 to start the process over again.

The HIV infectious process takes three forms—immunodeficiency, autoimmunity, and neurologic dysfunction (**Figure 2-8**). The immunodeficiency aspect includes opportunistic infections. The autoimmunity aspect includes lymphoid interstitial pneumonitis, arthritis, and hypergammaglobulinemia. Finally, the neurologic dysfunction aspect includes the AIDS dementia complex, HIV encephalopathy, and peripheral neuropathies. Once infected, the individual may not experience any symptoms other than a brief episode of flulike symptoms (e.g., fever, malaise, headache, and lymphopathy) referred to as the acute HIV infection. After this brief early infection episode, the individual may be asymptomatic for months to years while the virus is methodically infecting and destroying CD4 cells. As more and more CD4 cells are destroyed, the individual begins to have symptoms (e.g., lymphopathy, diarrhea, weight loss, fever, cough, shortness of breath). The individual becomes more symptomatic as more CD4 cells are destroyed. Over the next 10 years, serious clinical manifestations begin appearing as the individual moves into the late phase of infections. HIV in children may appear differently. Children who are HIV positive may experience the following:

- Difficulty gaining weight
- Difficulty growing normally
- Problems walking
- Delayed mental development
- Severe forms of common childhood illnesses such as ear infections (otitis media), pneumonia, and tonsillitis

Diagnosis is established through a set of laboratory tests as early as 1 month postexposure. In the past, the enzyme-linked immunosorbent assay, in combination with the Western blot was used to confirm diagnosis. Now, several rapid tests can give highly accurate information within as little as 20 minutes. These tests look for antibodies to the virus using blood or fluid samples collected on a treated pad that is rubbed on the upper and lower gums. The oral test is almost as sensitive as the blood test and eliminates the need for drawing blood. A positive reaction on a rapid test requires a confirming blood test. The tests are relatively new and were originally approved for use only in certified laboratories; they may not be widely available. The Food and Drug Administration has also approved one HIV test for home use. The Home Access HIV-1 test is as accurate as a clinical test. Unlike a home pregnancy test, the test is mailed in and then results are retrieved from a toll-free number in 3 to 7 business days, ensuring privacy and anonymity. All positive results are retested.

Once HIV/AIDS is confirmed, a test to predict the probable disease progression, or viral load, will be conducted. The plasma viral load, or number of viral particles per milliliter of blood, is an indication of clinical progression—the higher the viral load, the further the progression. The test for viral load is also known as the polymerase chain reaction. The polymerase chain reaction is the most appropriate test for infants because of the mother's circulating antibodies. The aim of antiretroviral therapy is to reduce the viral load to a point that the body's immune system can keep the virus in check. Viral load can also be an indicator of treatment success, along with other indicators (e.g., CD4 count and presence of opportunistic infections).

Viral diseases

1. HIV encephalopathy
2. Progressive multifocal leukoencephalopathy
3. Shingles, recurrent (zoster)
4. Cytomegalovirus retinitis
5. Recurrent herpes simplex lesions

Bacterial diseases

6. Persistent pneumonia
7. Tuberculosis
8. *Mycobacterium avium* complex
9. *Salmonella* septicemia

Fungal diseases

10. Cryptococcosis
11. Candidiasis
12. Histoplasmosis
13. Coccidioidomycosis
14. *Pneumocystis* pneumonia

Protozoal diseases

15. Toxoplasmosis
16. Chronic *Cryptosporidium* diarrhea

Cancers

17. Lymphomas of brain, lymphatic tissue
18. Kaposi sarcoma

Miscellaneous conditions

19. Persistent diarrhea
20. Persistent generalized lymphadenopathy
21. Wasting syndrome
22. Night sweats
23. Persistent fever

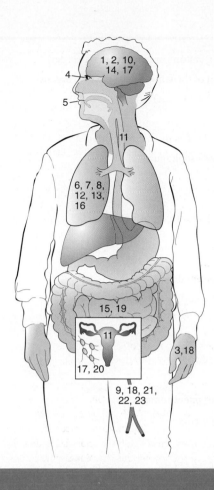

Figure 2-8

Effects of AIDS.

HIV infection progression is classified based on two systems: CD4 count and symptom presentation. CD4 classification includes the following categories:

- *Category 1:* CD4 cell count ≥ 500 cells/mm^3
- *Category 2:* CD4 cell count 200–499 cells/mm^3
- *Category 3:* CD4 cell count < 200 cells/mm^3

Classification based on clinical symptom presentation includes the following categories and their corresponding symptoms:

- *Category A:*
  - Asymptomatic HIV infection
  - Persistent, generalized lymph node enlargement
  - Acute HIV infection with accompanying illness or history of acute HIV infection
- *Category B:*
  - Bacillary angiomatosis (skin infection)
  - Oropharyngeal or vaginal candidiasis (yeast) infection
  - Fever or diarrhea lasting longer than a month

(Continues)

- Idiopathic thrombocytopenic purpura (autoimmune bleeding disorder)
- Pelvic inflammatory disease (infection of the female reproduction organs)
- Peripheral neuropathy (peripheral nerve damage)
  - *Category C:*
    - Bacterial pneumonia, recurrent (≥ 2 episodes in 12 months)
    - Candidiasis of the respiratory tract and esophagus
    - Invasive cervical cancer
    - Fungal infections
    - Parasitic and protozoan infections (> 1-month duration)
    - Cytomegalovirus disease
    - Encephalopathy
    - Herpes simplex: chronic ulcers (> 1-month duration)
    - Histoplasmosis
    - Kaposi sarcoma
    - Lymphoma
    - *Mycobacterium avium* complex
    - *Mycobacterium tuberculosis*
    - *Pneumocystis jiroveci* (formerly *carinii*) pneumonia
    - Progressive multifocal leukoencephalopathy
    - *Salmonella* septicemia
    - Toxoplasmosis of the brain
    - Wasting syndrome due to HIV (involuntary weight loss > 10% of baseline body weight) associated with either chronic diarrhea (≥ 2 loose stools per day ≥ 1 month) or chronic weakness and documented fever ≥ 1 month

Although there is no cure for AIDS, antiretroviral therapy is used to control the reproduction of HIV and slow the progression of the disease. Highly active antiretroviral therapy is the recommended approach and includes three or more antiretroviral medications from different classes. The five approved classes include nucleoside reverse transcriptase inhibitors, nucleoside reverse transcriptase inhibitors, protease inhibitors, nucletside reverse transcriptase inhibitors, and fusion inhibitors. Other treatment strategies may include medications to treat specific opportunistic infections as they arise. An HIV vaccine has been in development for years, but an effective and safe vaccine has yet to be developed.

Preventing HIV transmission is a worldwide public health priority. Prevention includes the following strategies:

- Avoiding contact with bodily fluids
- Avoiding activities that increase risk of exposure to those bodily secretions (e.g., drug use, multiple sexual partners)
- Education
- Using condoms with every sexual experience

Developing a Strong Immune System

The key to preventing infectious diseases is building a strong immune system. Many people assume that the best way to stay healthy is to avoid exposure. However, because the immune system is a memory system, the immune system needs to be exposed early to antigens to operate optimally. Exposure to microbes is limited today because of small family units, good sanitation, and widespread antibiotic use. Research suggests that avoiding oversanitizing our environment can increase exposure to microbes earlier and develop a stronger immune system.

At-risk individuals and states that specifically put individuals at risk for an impaired immune system include:

- The very young and the very old
- Poor nutrition
- Impaired skin integrity
- Circulatory issues
- Alterations in normal flora due to antibiotic therapy

- Chronic diseases especially diabetes mellitus
- Corticosteroid therapy
- Chemotherapy
- Smoking
- Alcohol consumption
- Immunodeficiency states

Strategies to build a healthy immune system include:

- Increasing fluid intake
- Eating a well-balanced diet
- Increasing antioxidants and protein intake
- Getting adequate sleep
- Avoiding caffeine and refined sugar
- Spending time outdoors
- Reducing stress

Chapter Summary

Humans are in a constant state of warfare with often unseen enemies. The body takes a multilevel approach to prevent attacks and eliminate invaders. Problems can occur at these levels that can lead to overreactions, underreactions, and inappropriate reactions. These altered reactions can lead to disease states that can negatively affect the body. Multiple conditions can impair the body's ability to battle, but when armed with the appropriate weapons, the body becomes a fighting machine that can withstand many a fierce invader.

References

Chiras, D. (2008). *Human biology* (6th ed.). Sudbury, MA: Jones and Bartlett.

Elling, B., Elling, K., & Rothenberg, M. (2004). *Anatomy and physiology*. Sudbury, MA: Jones and Bartlett.

NetCE. (n.d.). 3426: Systemic Lupus Erythematosus. Retrieved from http://www.netce.com/coursecontent.php?courseid=511

Porth, C. (2006). *Essentials of pathophysiology* (6th ed.). Philadelphia, PA: Lippincott Williams & Wilkins.

Professional guide to pathophysiology (2nd ed.). (2007). Philadelphia, PA: Lippincott Williams & Wilkins.

Resources

www.aarda.org
http://health.howstuffworks.com/immune-system.htm
www.cdc.gov
www.medlineplus.gov
www.nih.gov

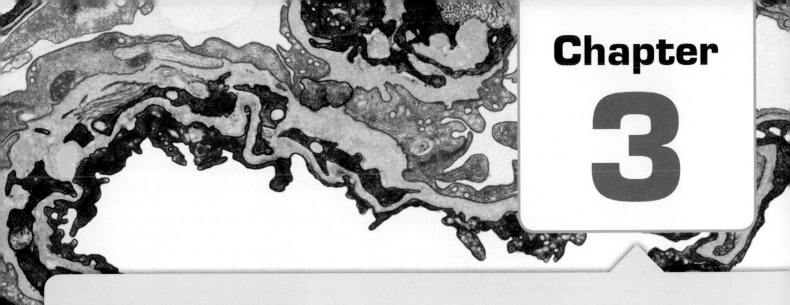

Chapter 3

Hematopoietic Function

KEY TERMS

anemia
disseminated intravascular
   coagulation (DIC)
erythrocyte
hematocrit
hematopoiesis
hemoglobin
hemoglobin S

hemolysis
hemophilia A
idiopathic thrombocytopenic
   purpura (ITP)
infectious mononucleosis
leukemia
leukocyte
leukocytopenia

leukocytosis
multiple myeloma
neutropenia
neutrophil
pancytopenia
plasma
plasmin
pus

thrombocyte
thrombocytopenia
thrombocytosis
thromboplastin
thrombotic thrombocytopenic
   purpura (TTP)
von Willebrand's disease

Blood is the life fluid of the human body, and it is essential for health and homeostasis. The approximately 5 liters of blood continuously circulating in the human body provides nutrients and oxygen to tissues while aiding in the excretion of waste products. Blood is comprised of plasma, blood cells, and platelets. Disease occurs when there are too few, too many, or dysfunctional blood components. These conditions can result from congenital or genetic causes and can be acquired from medical treatment. Healthcare providers, especially nurses, play a pivotal role in identifying those persons at risk and assisting in the management of these diseases.

Normal Hematopoietic Function

Blood is both a viscous fluid and a tissue. Hematopoiesis is the process of blood formation, and it occurs primarily in the bone marrow. Stem cells (primitive cells) differentiate the precursors for the different blood cells. Blood accomplishes its functions through several components—the plasma (liquid protein), leukocytes (white blood cells), erythrocytes (red blood cells), and thrombocytes (platelets) (Table 3-1). Plasma is a transport medium that carries the blood cells as well as antibodies, nutrients, electrolytes, hormones, lipids, and waste products. Leukocytes are key players in the inflammatory response and infectious process

(see Chapter 2). Erythrocytes are disk-shaped cells that carry oxygen to tissues and carbon dioxide for removal. Erythrocytes contain proteins and hemoglobin, which binds to oxygen, giving blood its red color. The brighter the shade of red, the more the blood is saturated with oxygen. Hematocrit refers to how much of the blood volume is being occupied by the erythrocytes. Thrombocytes, along with clotting factors, control coagulation. Carried passively in the blood, thrombocytes are coated with a sticky material that causes them to adhere to irregular surfaces. Clotting is a quick chain reaction stimulated by the release of thromboplastin from damaged cells lining blood vessels (**Figure 3-1**; **Figure 3-2**).

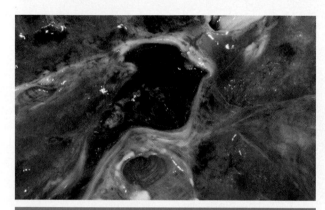

Figure 3-2

Blood clot.

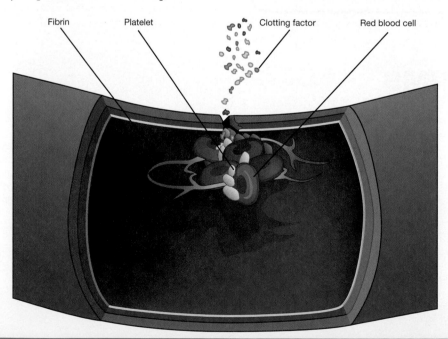

Fibrin Platelet Clotting factor Red blood cell

Figure 3-1

Blood clotting.

Table 3-1 Summary of Blood Cells

Name	Light Micrograph	Description	Concentration (Number of Cells/mm^3)	Life Span	Function
Red blood cells (RBCs)		Biconcave disk; no nucleus	4 to 6 million	120 days	Transport oxygen and carbon dioxide
White blood cells Neutrophil		Approximately twice the size of RBCs; multi-lobed nucleus; clear-staining cytoplasm	3,000 to 7,000	6 hours to a few days	Phagocytize bacteria
Eosinophil		Approximately same size as neutrophil; large pink-staining granules; bilobed nucleus	100 to 400	8 to 12 days	Phagocytizes antigen-antibody complex; attacks parasites
Basophil		Slightly smaller than neutrophil; contains large, purple cytoplasmic granules; bilobed nucleus	20 to 50	Few hours to a few days	Releases histamine during inflammation
Monocyte		Larger than neutrophil; cytoplasm grayish-blue; no cytoplasmic granules; U- or kidney-shaped nucleus	100 to 700	Lasts many months	Phagocytizes bacteria, dead cells, and cellular debris
Lymphocyte		Slightly smaller than neutrophil; large, relatively round nucleus that fills the cell	1,500 to 3,000	Can persist many years	Involved in immune protection, either attacking cells directly or producing antibodies
Platelets		Fragments of megakaryocytes; appear as small dark-staining granules	250,000	5 to 10 days	Play several key roles in blood clotting

Source: Chiras, D. (2008). *Human biology* (6th ed.). Sudbury, MA: Jones & Bartlett Learning.

Along with the initiation of the clotting cascade (**Figure 3-3**), platelets containing contractile proteins pull the edges of the wound together. Blood clots do not stay indefinitely, or they would clog up the entire circulatory system. **Plasmin** is an enzyme that dissolves clots once healing has occurred.

Diseases of the White Blood Cells

Leukocytes are a diverse group of cells that trigger the inflammatory process and combat infections. Normal white blood cell levels range from 5,000 to 10,000 mm³.

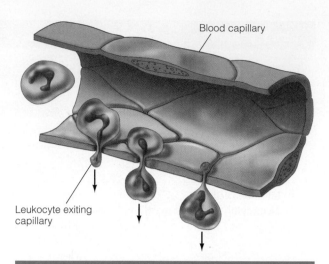

Blood capillary

Leukocyte exiting capillary

Figure 3-4

Leukocyte movement.

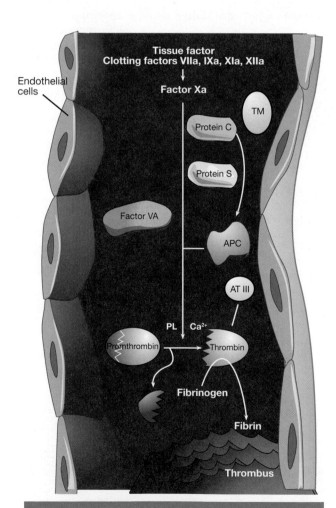

Tissue factor
Clotting factors VIIa, IXa, XIa, XIIa

Factor Xa

Endothelial cells

TM

Protein C

Protein S

Factor VA

APC

AT III

PL Ca²⁺

Promthrombin Thrombin

Fibrinogen

Fibrin

Thrombus

Figure 3-3

Clotting cascades. Notes: Black arrows = activation; red arrows = inactivation; APC = activated protein C; TM = thrombomodulin, a protein bound to endothelial cell membranes to which protein C binds; PL = phospholipid; Ca²⁺ = calcium.

Leukocytosis describes states of increased white blood cell levels, and **leukocytopenia** refers to decreased white blood cell levels. Leukocytosis can indicate an active infectious process, and leukocytopenia can indicate an immune deficiency state (e.g., bone marrow suppression). The blood, by way of the circulatory system, transports leukocytes to the site of the infection. When the leukocytes arrive at the scene, they leak through the capillary wall to the site of trauma or invasion (**Figure 3-4**). Most leukocyte disorders originate from deficiencies of one or more of the varying leukocytes.

Neutropenia

Usually the first to arrive on the scene of an infection, **neutrophils** are attracted by various chemicals released by infected tissue (**Figure 3-5**). Neutrophils escape from the capillary wall and migrate to the site of infection. Once they get to the site, neutrophils phagocytize microorganisms, preventing the infection from spreading. As the neutrophils are fully utilized, the cells die and become part of the yellowish wound drainage, or **pus**.

Neutropenia refers to a decrease in circulating neutrophils to fewer than 1,500 cells/μL (normal range is 2,000–7,500 cells/μL). With fewer of these first responders, the body is poorly equipped to fight infections. The degree to which the body can fight infections, especially bacterial infections, is related to the severity of the neutropenia. In other words, the lower

| 1 | Foreign invaders signal nearby neutrophils to squeeze through endothelial cells that line the blood vessel and enter the infected tissue. | 2 | Through a cell-eating process, known as phagocytosis, the neutrophil ingests the bacteria and releases toxic products that kill the bacteria. |

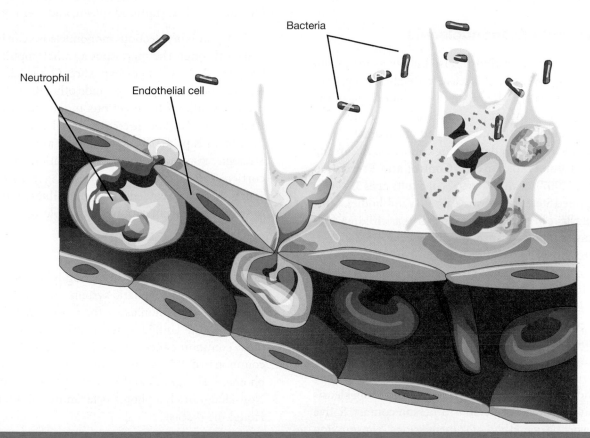

Bacteria

Neutrophil

Endothelial cell

Figure 3-5

The role of neutrophils.

the neutrophil count, the less ability to fight infections. Causes of neutropenia include:

- Increased usage (e.g., infection and inflammation)
- Drug suppression (e.g., immunosuppressants and chemotherapies)
- Radiation therapy
- Congenital conditions (e.g., periodic or cyclic)
- Bone marrow cancers (e.g., leukemias and lymphomas)
- Spleen destruction (e.g., Felty's syndrome)

- Vitamin deficiency (e.g., B_{12} and folate deficiency)

Clinical manifestations of neutropenia initially include signs and symptoms of bacterial and fungal infections (e.g., malaise, chills, and fever). The respiratory tract is the most common site of infections. Mouth ulcerations are also commonly associated with neutropenia, as are ulcerations of the skin, vagina, and gastrointestinal tract.

Diagnostic procedures center primarily on serum neutrophil levels. Additionally, bone marrow biopsy may be conducted to determine cause. Antibiotic therapy is used to treat infections as they develop. Identification and treatment of the cause of the neutropenia is crucial for positive outcomes. Hematopoietic growth factors such as granulocyte colony-stimulating factor may be used to stimulate maturation and differentiation of neutrophils.

Infectious Mononucleosis

Infectious mononucleosis, also known as mono and the kissing disease, is a disease caused by the Epstein-Barr virus (EBV). The EBV is a common virus of the herpes family. Infectious mononucleosis is most frequent in adolescents and young adults in upper socioeconomic classes in developing countries. According to the Centers for Disease Control and Prevention (CDC) (2007), as many as 95% of adults ages 35–40 in the United States test positive for EBV antibodies. Most people have been exposed to the virus as children, and because of the exposure, they have developed immunity to the virus. Most people who are exposed to the EBV do not ever develop infectious mononucleosis. EBV infects the B cells by killing the cell or being incorporated into its genome. The B cells incorporated with EBV produce heterophile antibodies that are used for diagnosis. Once the disease is eliminated, a few B cells remain altered, giving the individual an asymptomatic infection for life and the potential to occasionally spread the EBV to others. Infectious mononucleosis is usually spread by person-to-person contact. Saliva is the primary method of transmission. Transmission can also occur through coughing or sneezing, which causes small droplets of infected saliva and/or mucus to suspend in the air to be inhaled by others. The incubation period for infectious mononucleosis is between 4 and 6 weeks. During an infection, a person is likely to transmit the virus to others for at least a few weeks.

According to the CDC (2007), depending on the method used to detect the virus, anywhere from 20% to 80% of people who have recovered from infectious mononucleosis will continue to secrete the EBV in their saliva for years due to periodic reactivations of the viral infection. Since healthy people without symptoms also secrete the virus during reactivation episodes throughout their lifetime, isolation of people infected with EBV is not necessary. It is currently believed that these healthy people, who secrete EBV particles, are the primary reservoir for transmission of EBV among humans.

Onset of clinical manifestations is usually insidious. The initial manifestations of malaise, anorexia,

and chills can last 1–3 days. Following this period, the manifestations intensify and include severe sore throat, fever, and lymphopathy. The acute phase usually lasts 2–3 weeks. Some patients may not fully recover for 2–3 months, but most people recover without incident. Possible complications of infectious mononucleosis include hepatitis, ruptured spleen, and meningitis.

Diagnosis of infectious mononucleosis can be confirmed through the monospot and heterophils antibody test 2–3 weeks postexposure. Other laboratory tests can be performed to exclude other disorders that present similarly to infectious mononucleosis (e.g., strep throat). Leukocyte counts may also be increased. Treatment is primarily symptomatic and supportive. Strategies may include bed rest, hydration, analgesics, corticosteroids, and antipyretics. Vigorous contact sports should be avoided in the acute illness and recovery phase to prevent rupture of the spleen.

Lymphomas

Lymphomas are cancers involving lymphocyte proliferation in the lymphatic system. According to the CDC (2007), lymphomas are the most common blood cancers in the United States. Lymphoma is the sixth most common cancer in adults and the third most common in children. There are two main types of lymphomas—Hodgkin's and non-Hodgkin's lymphoma. Non-Hodgkin's lymphoma is far more common than Hodgkin's disease.

Hodgkin's Lymphoma

Hodgkin's lymphoma can start in any lymph node of the lymphatic system, but it most often starts in the lymph nodes of the upper body (e.g., the neck, chest, and upper arms). The affected lymph nodes swell and compress surrounding tissue. Systemically, the cancer cells spread from one lymph node to the next through the lymphatic vessels. Rarely, the disease spreads into the blood vessels and other structures until late in the disease. The cancer cells of Hodgkin's lymphoma are unique; they are called Reed-Sternberg cells (or Hodgkin cells) (**Figure 3-6**). These cells are an abnormal type of B lymphocyte that is much larger than normal lymphocytes. The T lymphocytes also appear defected, and the total lymphocyte number decreases.

The two main types are classical Hodgkin's disease (which has several subtypes) and nodular lymphocyte predominance Hodgkin's disease. The types differ in the way the cancer cells appear under a microscope.

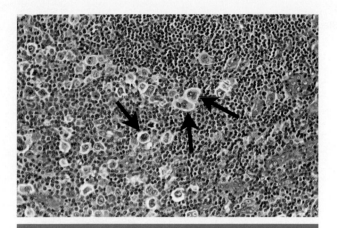

Figure 3-6

Reed-Sternberg cells associated with Hodgkin's disease.

Identification of which type the patient is experiencing is important because each grows and spreads in a different way, and they are often treated differently. Classical Hodgkin's disease will be discussed further because it accounts for 95% of Hodgkin's disease cases.

Though on the decline, the CDC (2007) reports that Hodgkin's disease occurs primarily in adults 20–40 years of age with equal prevalence in both genders. A second peak occurrence is seen in men over 50 years of age. Prognosis is excellent when localized and treated early, with many cases considered cured.

Clinical manifestations of Hodgkin's disease include:

- Swollen, painless lymph nodes
- Weight loss
- Persistent fever
- Night sweats
- Generalized pruritus
- Coughing, trouble breathing, or chest pain
- Malaise
- Recurrent infections
- Splenomegaly

Diagnostic procedures primarily center on a biopsy of the affected lymph node. Biopsy samples reveal the presence of Reed-Sternberg cells. Other diagnostic procedures consist of a physical examination, complete blood count, and chest X-rays. A staging system is used to grade the severity and progression of the disease. The stages of Hodgkin's lymphoma (**Figure 3-7**) include:

- **Stage I:** The lymphoma cells are in one lymph node group (such as in the neck or underarm), or if the lymphoma cells are not in the lymph nodes, they are in only one part of a tissue or an organ (such as the lung).

- **Stage II:** The lymphoma cells are in at least two lymph node groups on the same side of (either above or below) the diaphragm, or the lymphoma cells are in one part of a tissue or an organ and the lymph nodes near that organ (on the same side of the diaphragm). Lymphoma cells may be in other lymph node groups on the same side of the diaphragm.

- **Stage III:** The lymphoma cells are in lymph nodes above and below the diaphragm. Lymphoma cells may be found in one part of a tissue or an organ (such as the liver, lung, or bone) near these lymph node groups. The cells may also be found in the spleen.

- **Stage IV:** Lymphoma cells are found in several parts of one or more organs or tissues, or the lymphoma cells are in an organ (such as the liver, lung, or bone) and in distant lymph nodes.

- **Recurrent:** The disease returns after treatment.

Staging involves computed tomography scan, magnetic resonance imaging, positron emission tomography scan, and bone marrow biopsy. Other staging procedures may include biopsies of other lymph nodes, the liver, or other tissue. After diagnosis, the usual cancer treatment is implemented (combination of chemotherapy, radiation, and surgery).

Non-Hodgkin's Lymphoma

Non-Hodgkin's lymphoma can start at any age and in any lymph node. There are many different types of non-Hodgkin's lymphoma. These types can be divided into aggressive (fast-growing) and indolent (slow-growing) types, and they can be formed from either B cells (80% of cases) or T cells. Non-Hodgkin's lymphoma is similar to Hodgkin's lymphoma in clinical manifestations, staging, and treatment. Differences lie in the spread and diagnosis. Non-Hodgkin's lymphoma involves multiple nodes scattered throughout the body and metastasizes in an unorganized manner. Metastasis is often present at diagnosis. With non-Hodgkin's lymphoma, there are no Reed-Sternberg cells present. Additionally, non-Hodgkin's lymphoma is more difficult to treat, and the prognosis is poor, but improving.

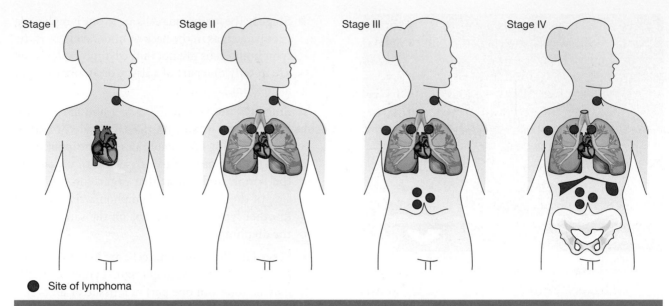

Stage I   Stage II   Stage III   Stage IV

● Site of lymphoma

Figure 3-7

Stages of Hodgkin's lymphoma.

Leukemias

Leukemia is a cancer of the leukocytes. With leukemia, the bone marrow makes abnormal leukocytes, or leukemia cells. Unlike normal blood cells, leukemia cells do not die when they should, sometimes crowding normal leukocytes, erythrocytes, and thrombocytes. This crowding makes it difficult for normal blood cells to function properly. The exact cause of leukemia is unknown. Risk factors include exposure to chemical, viral, and radiation mutagens; use of chemotherapies; certain disease conditions (e.g., Down syndrome); and immunodeficiency disorders.

Leukemias are grouped as either acute or chronic. The four most common types of leukemia include:

1. **Acute lymphoblastic leukemia:** Affects primarily children; responds well to therapy, and carries a good prognosis.

2. **Acute myeloid leukemia:** Affects primarily adults; responds fairly well to treatment, and carries a prognosis somewhat worse than that of acute lymphoblastic leukemia.

3. **Chronic lymphoid leukemia:** Affects primarily adults; responds poorly to therapy, yet most patients live many years after diagnosis.

4. **Chronic myeloid leukemia:** Affects primarily adults; responds poorly to chemotherapy, but the prognosis is improved with allogenic bone marrow transplant.

Clinical manifestations of leukemia include:

- Leukopenia (frequent infections)
- Anemia (pallor, fatigue, dyspnea, and decreased activity tolerance)
- Thrombocytopenia (petechiae, bleeding gums, hematuria, and prolonged bleeding time)
- Lymphadenopathy
- Joint swelling
- Bone pain
- Weight loss
- Anorexia
- Hepatomegaly
- Splenomegaly
- Central nervous system dysfunction

Diagnostic procedures include a history, physical examination, peripheral blood smears, complete blood count, and bone marrow biopsy. Chemotherapy is the mainstay of treatment for leukemia. Several courses may be necessary. Chemotherapy is more effective for the acute types of leukemia than for the chronic types of leukemia. Bone marrow transplants may be attempted if chemotherapy is unsuccessful.

Multiple Myeloma

Multiple myeloma is a cancer of the plasma cells that most often affects older adults. Multiple myeloma is characterized by excessive numbers of abnormal plasma cells in the bone marrow crowding the blood-forming cells and causing Bence Jones proteins to be excreted in the urine. Multiple bone tumors develop and bone destruction occurs, leading to hypercalcemia and pathologic fractures. Hypercalcemia leads to renal impairment and neuromuscular issues. Tumor cells can spread through the lymph nodes and infiltrate organs.

The onset of multiple myeloma is usually insidious, and malignancy is often well advanced upon diagnosis. Clinical manifestations of multiple myeloma include:

- Anemia (pallor, fatigue, dyspnea, and decreased activity tolerance)
- Thrombocytopenia (petechiae, bleeding gums, hematuria, and prolonged bleeding time)
- Leukopenia (frequent infections)
- Decreased bone density
- Bone pain
- Hypercalcemia (neuromuscular dysfunction)
- Renal impairment

The diagnosis of multiple myeloma is often made incidentally during routine blood tests for other conditions. For example, the existence of anemia and a high serum protein may suggest further testing is needed. Diagnostic procedures include serum and urine protein, calcium, renal function tests, complete blood count, biopsy, X-rays, computed tomography, and magnetic resonance imaging. Multiple myeloma is not considered curable, but chemotherapy improves remission rate. Median survival rate is 3 years. Analgesics are used to treat bone pain. Blood dyscrasias, hypercalcemia, and renal impairment are treated as needed.

Diseases of the Red Blood Cells

Erythrocytes are the most prevalent blood cell in the human body—millions can be found in a single drop of blood (normal range is 4.2–5.9 cells/μL). These cells function primarily to transport oxygen to the tissue and the waste products for excretion. Most diseases of the red blood cells are related to the quantity or quality of the erythrocytes.

Anemia

Anemia is a common acquired or inherited disorder of the erythrocytes that impairs the oxygen-carrying capacity of the blood. This condition can result from (1) a decrease in the number of circulating erythrocytes (e.g., blood loss or decreased production), (2) a reduction in hemoglobin content, or (3) the presence of abnormal hemoglobin. Some anemias are treated easily while others can cause lifelong problems. Clinical manifestations of anemia reflect the decreased oxygen-carrying capacity regardless of causes. These manifestations usually include:

- Weakness
- Fatigue
- Pallor
- Syncope
- Dyspnea
- Tachycardia

Anemia is diagnosed when hematocrit is less than 41% in males and 37% in females. Respectively, hemoglobin falls less than 13.5 g/dL in males and 12 g/dL in females. Anemia treatment depends on the specific anemia.

Iron Deficiency Anemia

According to the World Health Organization (2010), iron deficiency anemia is the most frequent anemia in the world. Iron deficiency anemia is most commonly seen in women of childbearing age, children less than 2 years of age, and the elderly. Iron deficiency anemia occurs when the supply of iron necessary to produce hemoglobin is inadequate to meet the demand of hemoglobin production. Iron deficiency anemia is caused by decreased iron consumption, decreased iron absorption, and increased bleeding (e.g., such as occurs during menstruation and as a result of cancers). Iron is ingested through both animal and plant sources. Although the average American absorbs more than 10 mg of iron each day, which is within the recommended daily allowance, only about 10% of ingested iron is actually absorbed. Due to this lack of iron, erythrocytes will become pale (hypochromic) and small (microcytic) (**Figure 3-8**).

In addition to the previously mentioned anemia signs and symptoms, clinical manifestations of iron deficiency anemia include:

- Cyanosis (blue coloration) to sclera of the eyes
- Brittle nails
- Decreased appetite (especially in children)
- Headache

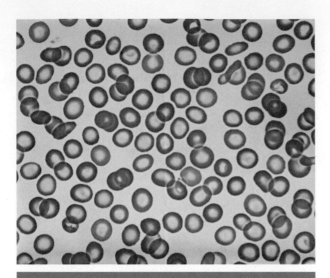

Figure 3-8

Iron deficiency anemia.

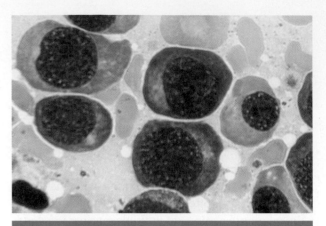

Figure 3-9

Pernicious anemia.

- Irritability
- Stomatitis
- Unusual food cravings (pica)
- Delayed healing

Diagnostic procedures for iron deficiency anemia include a complete blood count, serum ferritin, serum iron, and transferring saturation. Additional tests may be performed to determine cause (e.g., fecal occult blood). Treatment includes the identification and resolution of the underlying cause of the iron deficiency anemia. Other strategies to increase iron levels include increasing iron-rich foods (e.g., liver, red meat, fish, beans, raisins, and green leafy vegetables) or administering iron supplements. Additionally, foods or supplements high in vitamin C should be increased since vitamin C increases the absorption of iron.

Pernicious Anemia

Pernicious anemia is also known as B_{12} deficiency and megaloblastic anemia. This type of anemia is characterized by large (macrocytic), immature erythrocytes (**Figure 3-9**). Pernicious anemia results most often from cyanocobalamin (vitamin B_{12}) deficiency. This deficiency usually occurs gradually and from a lack of intrinsic factor. Intrinsic factor is a protein produced by the stomach that is necessary for B_{12} to be absorbed in the stomach. The lack of intrinsic factor results from autoantibodies. The subsequent immune reaction leads to atrophy of the gastric mucosa and glands.

Vitamin B_{12} is necessary for DNA synthesis and leads to decreased cell division and cell maturation. Too little vitamin B_{12} gradually causes neurologic problems because of a breakdown in myelin. The neurologic effects may be seen before anemia is diagnosed. In addition to the usual signs and symptoms of anemia, clinical manifestations may include:

- Bleeding gums
- Diarrhea
- Impaired sense of smell
- Loss of deep tendon reflexes
- Anorexia
- Personality or memory changes
- Positive Babinski's sign (a pathological reflex where the first toe extends and flexes toward the top of the foot and the other toes fan out when the sole of the foot is firmly stroked)
- Stomatitis
- Paresthesia of hands and feet
- Unsteady gait, especially in the dark

Diagnostic tests for pernicious anemia include serum B_{12} levels, Schilling's test (measures B_{12} absorption), complete blood count, gastric analysis, and bone marrow biopsy. Treatment of pernicious anemia includes vitamin B_{12} injections if no intrinsic factor is being produced, and oral vitamin B_{12} can be administered for those individuals who are producing intrinsic factor.

CLINICAL CASE

Mrs. Williams is a 45-year-old Caucasian woman who sought medical attention for fatigue that developed during the previous month. She reported no chest pain. However, she did feel mildly short of breath with exertion such as after walking up a flight of stairs. She denied any rectal bleeding, but she had heavy menstrual periods for about a year.

Her past medical history included being treated for anemia following her third pregnancy 10 years prior. She was not taking any prescribed medications. Her family history revealed that her parents were born in Italy and died when she was in grade school. She did not know their medical history.

A physical examination revealed that Mrs. Williams's general appearance was pale but with no acute distress. Her vital signs were blood pressure 125/90, heart rate 88 regular, respirations 12/min. There were no significant changes in the blood pressure and heart rate between the supine and upright positions. Other findings included pale conjunctiva and moist mucous membranes without lesions. No adenopathy or hepatosplenomegaly were noted. Breath sounds were clear to auscultation, and the heart had a regular rate and rhythm with a murmur. The abdomen was soft, nontender, and nondistended. A rectal examination revealed no masses and heme-negative brown stool was present. Additionally, Mrs. Williams reported that she was taking aspirin 81 mg daily; she is a vegetarian who eats a lot of cereal, and she did not have an urge to eat ice.

Mrs. Williams's laboratory tests revealed the following results:

CBC	Result	Normal Range
WBC	$8.2 \times 10^3/\mu L$	$4.8–10.8 \times 10^3/\mu L$
Hgb	8.0 g/dL	12–15.6 g/dL
Hct	24%	35–46%
RBC	$4.0 \times 10^6/\mu L$	$3.8–5 \times 10^6/\mu L$
MCV	60 fL/red cell	80–96.1 fL/red cell
MCH	20 pg/red cell	27.5–33.2 pg/red cell
MCHC	33 g/L	33.4–35.5 g/L
RDW	16.5	11.5–14.5
Platelets	500,000/μL	150–400,000/μL
Reticulocyte count	3%	0.5–1.7%
Absolute reticulocyte count	40,000/μL	25,000–75,000/μL
LDH	210 U/L	0–304 U/L

CBC = complete blood count; WBC = white blood cells; Hgb = hemoglobin; Hct = hematocrit; RBC = red blood cells; MCV = mean corpuscular volume; MCH = mean corpuscular hemoglobin; MCHC = mean corpuscular hemoglobin concentration; RDW = red cell distribution width; LDH = lactate dehydrogenase.

Mrs. Williams was diagnosed with iron deficiency anemia and was placed on iron supplements. Her hemoglobin (Hgb) was expected to be normal after about 8 weeks of iron therapy, which should raise the Hgb about 1 g/dL per week. However, her Hgb was 9.5 g/dL after 8 weeks. Following those results, Mrs. Williams was asked whether she was taking the iron supplements as ordered and whether she has been tolerating the medication. Additionally, she was asked whether she was having dark, tarry stools, which indicate gastrointestinal bleeding. Mrs. Williams reported that she had only taken the iron supplement for 2 weeks because it made her nauseated and constipated. Mrs. Williams was instructed to take the iron supplement with a light carbohydrate such as crackers or toast to minimize the nausea and to take measures to prevent constipation (e.g., increasing fiber and water intake). After implementing these measures and taking the iron supplement as ordered for 8 weeks, Mrs. Williams's Hgb returned to normal.

Source: Adapted from Schick (2006).

SICKLE CELL ANEMIA

ickle cell anemia is a genetic type of hemolytic anemia in which the erythrocytes are abnormally crescent- or sickle-shaped (Figure 3-10). Sickle cell anemia is caused by an abnormal type of hemoglobin called hemoglobin S. Hemoglobin S distorts the shape of erythrocytes, especially when there is low oxygen. These fragile, sickle-shaped cells deliver less oxygen to the body's tissues. These cells also can clog easily in small blood vessels and break into pieces that disrupt blood flow.

Sickle cell anemia is an inherited disorder that is neither recessive nor dominant (see Chapter 1). The allele for the sickle cell gene is co-dominant—meaning that if a person inherits the sickle cell gene from one parent and the normal erythrocyte gene from the other parent, both genes will be expressed. Someone who inherits the hemoglobin S gene from one parent and normal hemoglobin (A) from the other parent, meaning a heterozygous pair of alleles, will have sickle cell trait. Persons with sickle cell trait do not have the symptoms of true sickle cell anemia because less than half of their erythrocytes are sickled. Those persons who inherit the hemoglobin S gene from both parents, creating a homozygous allele pair, have sickle cell disease. Sickle cell disease is more severe because almost all the individual's erythrocytes are abnormal. Sickle cell disease is much more common in people of African and Mediterranean descent. Sickle cell disease is also seen in people from South and Central America, the Caribbean, and the Middle East.

Clinical manifestations usually do not appear until approximately 4 months of age. Most patients will experience painful episodes, or crises, that can last for hours to days. Pain is caused by obstruction of small blood vessels as the sickled cells clog up the vessels leading to ischemia and necrosis. Complications of these blood vessel occlusions depend on location (Table 3-2). The number and severity of these crises vary among patients and can be triggered by dehydration, stress, high altitudes, and fever. Because of increased disease understanding and management, patients now live into their 50s.

Clinical manifestations of sickle cell anemia reflect hypoxia and tissue ischemia. These manifestations include:

- Abdominal pain
- Bone pain
- Dyspnea
- Delayed growth and development
- Fatigue
- Fever
- Jaundice (yellowish skin)
- Pallor
- Tachycardia
- Skin ulcers on the lower legs
- Angina
- Excessive thirst
- Frequent urination
- Painful and prolonged erection (priapism)
- Vision impairment

Carriers of the defective gene can be detected by hemoglobin electrophoresis, a simple blood test. Additionally, the sickle cell test can determine whether the hemoglobin is normal or sickled. A complete blood count and bilirubin test is useful in determining diagnosis and progression. There is no cure for sickle cell anemia; however, stem cell research continues to show promise. Medications (e.g., Hydrea [hydroxyurea]) are available to reduce the frequency of crises. Avoidance of sickling triggers is also helpful. Other strategies include:

- Oxygen therapy
- Hydration
- Pain management (e.g., pain medication, relaxation techniques, distraction)
- Infection control measures
- Vaccinations
- Blood transfusions
- Bone marrow transplants
- Genetic counseling for those persons with sickle cell trait

Aplastic Anemia

Aplastic anemia is a type of anemia that is a result of the bone marrow failing to make enough blood cells. This lack of erythrocytes, leukocytes, and platelets is referred to as pancytopenia. A lack of these blood cells leads to a series of complications (e.g., infections, bleeding, hypoxia, fatty replacement of marrow, death).

Aplastic anemia may be temporary or permanent. Causes of aplastic anemia include:

- Idiopathic causes
- Autoimmune causes (e.g., systemic lupus erythematosus)
- Medications and treatments (e.g., chemotherapy and radiation)

Diagnostic tests for aplastic anemia include complete blood count and bone marrow biopsy. Prompt treatment of underlying causes and complications as they arise is crucial for positive outcomes. Treatment of underlying causes may include removal of medications or treatments. Treatment of complications may include:

- Oxygen therapy
- Infection control measures (e.g., hand washing, avoiding groups, avoiding fresh flowers)
- Infection treatment (e.g., antibiotics)
- Bleeding precautions (e.g., electric razors, soft bristle toothbrushes, injury prevention)
- Blood transfusions
- Bone marrow transplants

Hemolytic Anemia

Hemolytic anemia results from excessive destruction, or hemolysis, of erythrocytes. Causes of hemolytic anemia include idiopathic causes, autoimmune causes, genetics, infections (e.g., malaria), blood transfusion reactions, and blood incompatibility in the neonate. There are several types of hemolytic anemia, including sickle cell anemia, thalassemia, and erythroblastosis fetalis. Specifics in regard to pathogenesis, clinical manifestations, diagnosis, and treatment vary based on type.

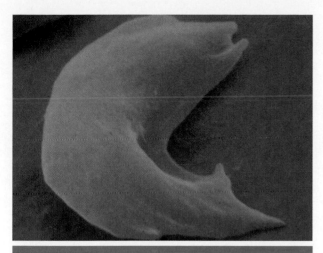

Figure 3-10

Sickle cell anemia.

- Viruses
- Genetic abnormalities (e.g., myelodysplastic syndrome and Fanconi's anemia)

Clinical manifestations include signs and symptoms of general anemia (e.g., weakness, pallor, dyspnea), leukocytopenia (e.g., recurrent infections), and thrombocytopenia (e.g., bleeding). As blood cell levels decline, clinical manifestations worsen.

Table 3-2 Complications of Blood Vessel Occlusions

Area of Occlusion	Result
Bone	Susceptibility to osteomyelitis due to staph infection
Papillae of renal medulla	Gross hematuria Renal tubular concentrating defects
Eye	Retinopathy Blindness
Sinus	Stroke
Spleen	Hyposplenism Susceptibility to infection
Liver	Jaundice Hepatomegaly
Miscellaneous	Enlarged heart Slow-healing leg ulcers

Source: Madara, M., & Pomarico-Denino, V. (2008). *Quick look nursing: Pathophysiology* (2nd ed.). Sudbury, MA: Jones & Bartlett Learning.

THALASSEMIA

Thalassemia is another genetic type of anemia, resulting in abnormal hemoglobin. Thalassemia follows an autosomal dominant inheritance pattern (see Chapter 1). The abnormal hemoglobin is a result of a lack of one of two proteins, which makes up hemoglobin (alpha and beta globin). Thalassemia occurs most frequently in persons of Mediterranean descent. Other ethnic groups affected by thalassemia include those of Asian, Indian, and African descent. Severe cases can lead to death in childhood. Moderate cases and those treated effectively can survive into their 30s.

Clinical manifestations of thalassemia include:

- Abortion
- Delayed growth and development
- Fatigue
- Dyspnea
- Heart failure
- Hepatomegaly
- Splenomegaly
- Bone deformities
- Jaundice

Upon examination, erythrocytes will appear microcytic and hypochromic, and they vary in size. Iron levels may be increased. A complete blood count is also useful in diagnosis (low MCV and MCHC). Treatment may not be necessary in mild cases. If treatment is warranted, it includes blood transfusion, chelation therapy, and splenectomy.

Polycythemia Vera

Polycythemia vera is a disorder in which the bone marrow produces too many blood cells. Polycythemia vera is rare and considered a neoplastic disease. The exact cause of this disease that occurs most frequently in men is unknown. As blood cell numbers increase, so does the blood volume and viscosity. Blood vessels become distended and blood flow is sluggish. Complications include:

- Tissue ischemia and necrosis
- Thrombosis
- Hypertension
- Heart failure
- Hemorrhage

- Splenomegaly
- Hepatomegaly
- Acute myeloblastic leukemia

Clinical manifestations of polycythemia vera include:

- Cyanotic or plethoric (reddish) skin
- High blood pressure
- Tachycardia
- Dyspnea
- Headaches
- Visual abnormalities

Diagnostic procedures for polycythemia vera include complete blood counts, bone marrow biopsy, and uric acid levels. Treatment strategies include chemotherapy, radiation, and phlebotomy (removal of blood). Management for clotting and bleeding disorders will be employed as needed.

Diseases of the Platelets

Platelets are vital components of the coagulation process. Normal platelet levels range from 150,000 to 350,000 mm^3. **Thrombocytosis** refers to increased platelet levels, and **thrombocytopenia** describes decreased platelet levels. Thrombocytosis increases the risk of thrombus formation, while thrombocytopenia increases the risk of bleeding and infection. Capillaries are relatively delicate structures that can leak even from minor injuries. Fortunately, the platelets, along with the coagulation process, quickly halt leaking. Diseases of the platelets include issues in quantity and quality of platelets.

Hemophilia A

Hemophilia A, or classic hemophilia, is an X-linked recessive bleeding disorder (see Chapter 1). Hemophilia A is a deficiency or abnormality of clotting factor VIII (Figure 3-3). Severity of the disorder varies depending on the amount of the factor present in the blood.

Severe forms of hemophilia A become apparent early on. Bleeding is the main symptom of the disease and sometimes, though not always, occurs if an infant is circumcised. Additional bleeding problems are seen when the infant starts crawling and walking. Mild cases may go unnoticed until later in life when they occur in response to surgery or trauma.

Internal bleeding may happen anywhere, and bleeding into joints, or hemarthrosis, is common. Other manifestations include petechia, bruising, gastrointestinal bleeding, and hematuria.

Diagnosis of hemophilia A includes the examination of bleeding studies. Bleeding time and prothrombin time are usually normal, and partial prothromboplastin time, activated partial prothromboplastin time, and coagulation time are prolonged. Serum levels of factor VIII are low. Treatment strategies include replacing clotting factors through transfusions and Advate (antihemophilic factor, a recombinant DNA product). To prevent a bleeding crisis, patients can be taught to give factor VIII concentrates at home at the first signs of bleeding. People with severe forms of the disease may need regular preventative treatment. Mild hemophilia may be treated with desmopressin (DDAVP), which helps the body release factor VIII that is stored within the lining of blood vessels. Additionally, bleeding precautions should be employed (e.g., electric razors, soft bristle toothbrush, and injury prevention).

Von Willebrand's Disease

Von Willebrand's disease is the most common hereditary bleeding disorder. This bleeding disorder results from a deficit of the von Willebrand factor. This factor promotes platelets to come together (aggregate) and stick (adhere) to the vessel wall in times of injury. There are several forms of Von Willebrand's disease:

- **Type 1** is the most common (70–80%) and mildest form. Type 1 follows an autosomal dominant inheritance pattern (see Chapter 1). The level of von Willebrand factor in the blood is reduced. Because this form is often very mild, most cases go undiagnosed. This form does not usually cause spontaneous bleeding, but significant bleeding can occur with trauma or surgery.

- **Type 2** occurs in 15–20% of cases. Type 2 can be either autosomal dominant or recessive, and there are five subtypes. The building blocks (multimers) that make up the von Willebrand factor are smaller than usual or break down easily.

- **Type 3** follows an autosomal recessive inheritance pattern. Severe bleeding problems are seen with this type because of no measurable von Willebrand factor or factor VIII.

- **Aquired type** occurs in those persons with Wilms' tumor, congenital heart disease, systemic lupus erythematosus, and hypothyroidism.

Clinical manifestations of von Willebrand's disease include abnormal bleeding. Diagnosis includes bleeding studies (e.g., bleeding time, prothrombin time, partial prothromboplastin time) and factor VIII levels. Treatment, if needed, includes infusions of cryoprecipitate or administration of desmopressin. Additionally, measures are used to control bleeding and prevent injury (e.g., pressure dressings).

Disseminated Intravascular Coagulation

Disseminated intravascular coagulation (DIC) is a life-threatening disorder that occurs as a complication of other diseases and conditions. Normally, during injury, clotting factors (Figure 3-3) become activated and travel to the injury site to help stop bleeding. However, in persons with DIC, these factors become abnormally active. Often these factors become active as an inappropriate immune reaction. Small blood clots form within the blood vessels. Some of these clots can occlude blood supply to tissue and organs. Over time, the clotting factors become used up. When this happens, the person is then at risk for serious bleeding from even a minor injury.

LEARNING POINTS

In DIC, hypercoagulation uses up all the available clotting factors. Once available clotting factors are utilized, the patient begins excessively bleeding. In other words, the individual clots, clots, clots, and then bleeds, bleeds, bleeds!

It is not clear why certain disorders lead to DIC, but the typical triggers include:

- Blood transfusion reaction
- Cancer (e.g., leukemia, aplastic anemia, and metastatic carcinoma)
- Infection in the blood by bacteria or fungus
- Pregnancy complications (e.g., retained placenta after delivery, abruptio placentae, and eclampsia)
- Recent surgery or anesthesia
- Sepsis (an overwhelming infection)
- Severe liver disease

- Severe tissue injury (e.g., burns and head injury)
- Cardiac arrest
- Poisonous snake bites

Clinical manifestations of DIC include signs and symptoms of tissue and organ ischemia (e.g., angina, confusion, and dyspnea) and abnormal bleeding (e.g., petechiae, epistaxis, and hematuria). Additionally, indicators of complications such as shock and multiple organ failure will appear.

Diagnostic procedures for DIC consist of complete blood counts and bleeding studies (e.g., fibrinogen levels, prothrombin time, partial prothromboplastin time, and fibrinogen degradation products). Management of DIC is complicated but starts with the identification and treatment of the underlying cause. The treatment of the DIC disorder itself is a delicate balance between preventing clots and treating bleeding (**Figure 3-11**).

Idiopathic Thrombocytopenic Purpura

Idiopathic thrombocytopenic purpura (ITP) is a hypocoagulopathy state resulting from the immune system destroying its own platelets. ITP can be acute or chronic. Acute ITP is more common in children. Acute ITP typically has a sudden onset and is self-limiting. Chronic ITP is more common in adults aged 20–50 and women. Circulating immunoglobulin G reacts with the platelets, which are then destroyed in the spleen and liver. Prognosis is usually good for acute and chronic ITP. Causes of ITP include:

- Idiopathic causes
- Autoimmune diseases
- Immunizations with a live vaccine
- Immunodeficiency disorders (e.g., AIDS)
- Viral infections

Clinical manifestations include abnormal bleeding (e.g., petechiae, epistaxis, and hematuria). Diagnostic procedures include complete blood counts, bone marrow biopsy, and humoral studies. Thrombocyte counts will often be less than 20,000/μL. Treatment strategies for acute ITP include:

- Glucocorticoid steroids (prevent further platelet immune destruction)
- Immunoglobulins (prevent further platelet destruction)

- Plasmapheresis
- Platelet pheresis

Treatment strategies for chronic ITP include:

- Glucocorticoid steroids
- Immunoglobulins
- Splenectomy
- Blood transfusions
- Immunosuppressant therapy

Thrombotic Thrombocytopenic Purpura

Thrombotic thrombocytopenic purpura (TTP) is a coagulation disorder resulting from a deficiency of an enzyme necessary for cleaving von Willebrand's factor. This enzyme deficiency leads to increased clotting. This clotting leads to fewer available platelets. Fewer platelets can lead to bleeding under the skin and purple-colored spots called purpura; therefore, TTP is characterized by thromboses, thrombocytopenia, and bleeding. Causes of TTP include:

- Idiopathic causes
- Heredity
- Bone marrow transplants
- Cancer
- Medications (e.g., platelet aggregation inhibitors, immunosupressants, hormone replacement)
- Pregnancy
- HIV

Clinical manifestations of TTP include:

- Purpura
- Changes in consciousness
- Confusion
- Fatigue
- Fever
- Headache
- Tachycardia
- Pallor
- Dyspnea on exertion
- Speech changes
- Weakness
- Jaundice

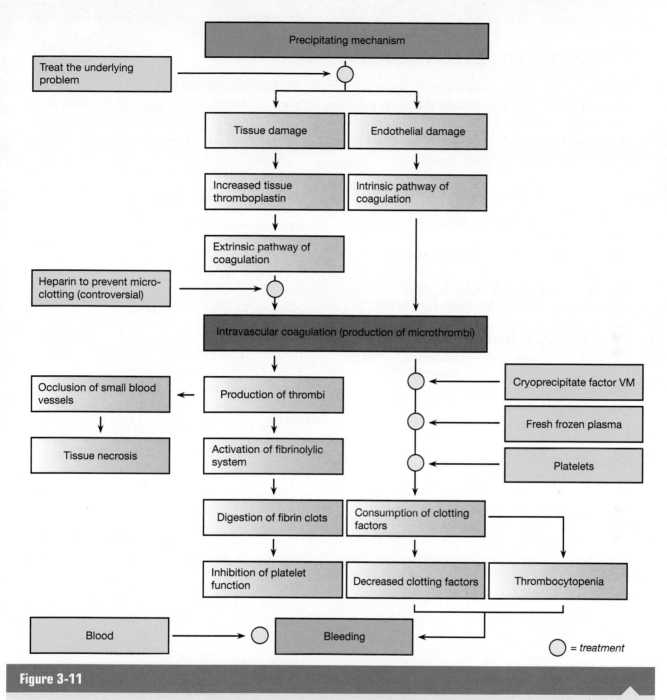

Figure 3-11

Understanding DIC and its treatment.

Diagnostic procedures for TTP include a history, physical examination, complete blood counts, blood smears, and lactate dehydrogenase levels. Plasmaphere-sis is the centerpiece of TTP treatment. Additionally, a splenectomy and glucocorticoid steroids may be necessary.

Chapter Summary

The blood serves many purposes in the body. Without this life fluid functioning properly, the body cannot maintain health and homeostasis; therefore, problems with any of the blood cells can lead to widespread and life-threatening problems. Hematologic problems can result from a variety of origins but usually result in abnormal cell numbers or function. Timely identification and treatment of these disorders is vital for positive healthcare outcomes.

References

Chiras, D. (2008). *Human biology* (6th ed.). Sudbury, MA: Jones and Bartlett.

Copstead, L., & Banasik, J. (2009). *Pathophysiology* (4th ed.). St. Louis, MO: Elsevier.

Elling, B., Elling, K., & Rothenberg, M. (2004). *Anatomy and physiology*. Sudbury, MA: Jones and Bartlett.

Porth, C. (2006). *Essentials of pathophysiology* (6th ed.). Philadelphia, PA: Lippincott Williams & Wilkins.

Professional guide to pathophysiology (2nd ed.). (2007). Philadelphia, PA: Lippincott Williams & Wilkins.

Schick, P. K. (2006). *Anemia*. Retrieved from http://teachingcases.hematology.org/schick06/index.cfm

Resources

www.cancer.org

www.cdc.gov

www.medlineplus.gov

www.nih.gov

www.who.int

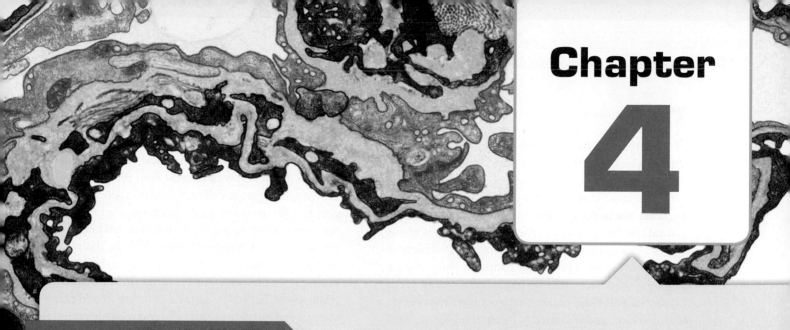

Cardiovascular Function

LEARNING OBJECTIVES

- Discuss normal cardiovascular anatomy and physiology.

- Describe and compare structural alterations of the cardiovascular system.

- Describe and compare electric conduction alterations of the cardiovascular system.

- Explore hypertension, heart failure, and shock.

KEY TERMS

afterload
aldosterone
anaphylactic shock
aneurysm
angina
antidiuretic hormone
aorta
aortic valve
arrythmia
arteriole
artery
atherosclerosis
atrioventricular node
automaticity
baroreceptor
bundle branches
bundle of His
capillary
cardiac output
cardiac tamponade
cardiogenic shock
cardiomyopathy
chemoreceptor
chronotropic

compensatory
  mechanism
conductivity
constrictive
  pericarditis
coronary artery
  disease (CAD)
depolarization
diastole
diastolic dysfunction
dilated
  cardiomyopathy
dissecting aneurysm
distributive shock
dromotropic
dyslipidemia
dysrhythmia
eclampsia
edema
embolus
endocardium
essential
  hypertension
excitability

exsanguination
fatty streaks
fibrous plaque
fusiform aneurysm
heart failure
high-density
  lipoproteins
  (HDLs)
hypertension
hypertrophic
  cardiomyopathy
hypovolemic shock
infarction
infective
  endocarditis
inferior vena cava
inotropic
left atrium
left ventricle
left-sided heart
  failure
lipid
low-density
  lipoproteins (LDLs)

lung
lymph
lymphatic system
lymphedema
malignant
  hypertension
mitral valve
mixed dysfunction
myocardial infarction
  (MI)
myocarditis
myocardium
neurogenic shock
pacemaker
pericardial effusion
pericarditis
pericardium
peripheral vascular
  disease (PVD)
peripheral vascular
  resistance (PVR)
pregnancy-induced
  hypertension (PIH)
preload

primary
  hypertension
progressive
  stage
pulmonary artery
pulmonary
  circulation
pulmonary vein
pulmonic valve
pulse pressure
Purkinje network of
  fibers
Raynaud's disease
regurgitation
renin-angiotensin-
  aldosterone
repolarization
restrictive
  cardiomyopathy
right atrium
right ventricle
right-sided heart
  failure
saccular aneurysm

secondary
  hypertension
septic shock
shock
sinoatrial (SA) node
stable angina
  pectoris
stenosis
stroke volume
superior vena cava
systemic circulation
systole
systolic dysfunction
thromboangiitis
  obliterans
thrombus
tricuspid valve
tunica adventitia
tunica intima
tunica media
unstable angina
varicose vein
vein
venule

The cardiovascular system is comprised of the heart, blood vessels, lymphatic system, and blood (see Chapter 3). This chapter will focus on normal and abnormal states of the heart and blood vessels. All the components of the cardiovascular system work together to maintain life. Additionally, these components play a crucial role in the functioning of other systems. This pivotal role begins early in life when the fetus is about 4 weeks old and lasts until the end of life. Disorders of the cardiovascular system are common and complex as they often affect other systems. Nurses in all areas of practice will likely encounter patients with problems in this system and will need to be equipped to respond to their intricate needs.

Anatomy and Physiology

The cardiovascular system is similar to the plumbing in a house. Both have a pump (the heart), a network of pipes (the blood vessels), and fluid (blood). The cardiovascular system delivers vital oxygen and nutrients to cells, removes waste products, and transports hormones. Circulation is divided into two branches—pulmonary and systemic (**Figure 4-1**). In the **pulmonary circulation**, the waste product of carbon dioxide exchanges with oxygen in the lungs through diffusion (**Figure 4-2**). In the **systemic circulation**, blood carries oxygen and nutrients to all cells and waste products to the kidneys, liver, and skin for excretion. To accomplish

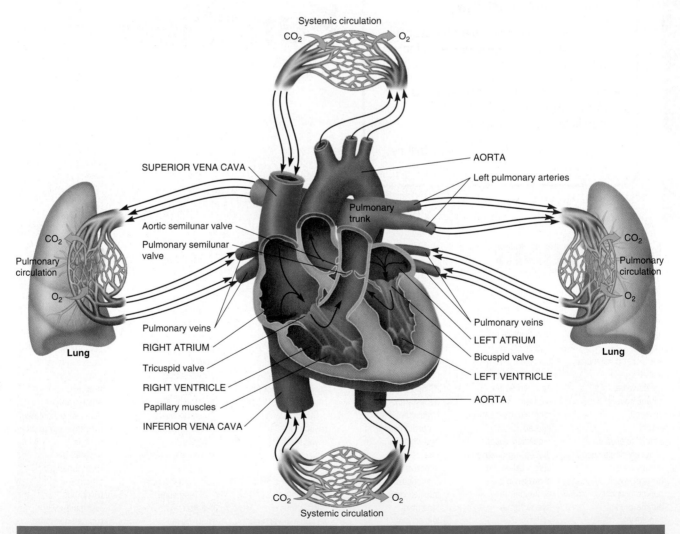

Figure 4-1

The cardiovascular system.

and veins. The lymphatic system assists in maintaining homeostasis by returning excess fluid from the body's tissues back to the circulatory system as well as playing a vital role in the immune system (see Chapter 2). The following sections will review basic anatomy and physiology of the cardiovascular system.

Heart

Roughly the size of a closed fist, the heart is a muscular organ that pumps blood throughout the body (**Figure 4-3**). The heart is the workhorse of the cardiovascular system, pumping blood through the body's 50,000 miles of blood vessels and beating approximately 100,000 times a day. In fact, if you had a dollar for every heartbeat, you would be a millionaire in just 10 days. The heart can quickly adjust its rate to meet the ever-changing needs of the body.

The heart is located in the thoracic cavity between the lungs and behind the sternum. The heart is enclosed by the pericardial sac, or **pericardium**, which provides protection and support. The sac protects the heart

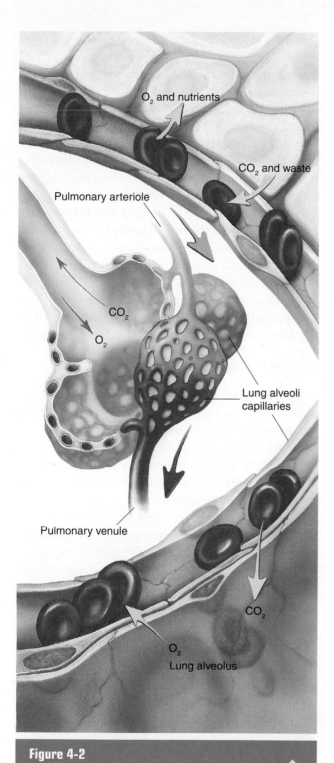

Figure 4-2

Pulmonary gas exchange.

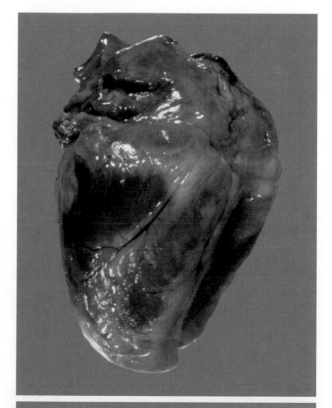

Figure 4-3

A normal heart.

these transportation functions, the cardiovascular system requires a properly functioning heart to propel the blood by rhythmic contractions. The blood circulates through three types of vessels—arteries, capillaries,

against trauma from surrounding structures, invasions of foreign organisms, and friction from the constant movement. The pericardium provides support in terms of anchoring the heart and prevents overdistention. The myocardium, the middle layer of the heart, is the muscle portion of the organ. The walls of the ventricles, especially the left ventricle, are thicker than the atrium because of the distance needed for those chambers to pump. The atria are receiving chambers and pump blood to their respective ventricle while the ventricles are pumping blood outside the heart to the lungs and to systemic circulation. The endocardium is the inner epithelial layer of the heart that makes up the cardiac valves. These valves function to ensure one-way flow of blood through the heart (**Figure 4-4**).

Understanding the blood flow through the heart is essential to understanding structural alterations (**Figure 4-5**). Illustrated in blue, blood low in oxygen and rich in carbon dioxide enters the right side of the heart from systemic circulation through the superior vena cava and the inferior vena cava. These veins empty blood directly into the right atrium. The right

atrium pumps the blood through the tricuspid valve to the right ventricle. The right ventricle pumps blood through the pulmonic valve to the pulmonary arteries. The pulmonary artery carries blood to the lungs for oxygenation. The newly oxygenated blood returns from the lungs to the heart through the pulmonary veins. From the pulmonary vein, blood enters the left atrium. The left atrium pumps blood through the mitral valve to the left ventricle. The left ventricle then pumps blood through the aortic valve to the aorta. The blood is then transported to the body beginning with the coronary arteries (because if the heart's needs are not met first, no other needs will be met) and the carotids (because the brain controls the vital bodily functions). Both atria fill and contract simultaneously, and both ventricles fill and contract simultaneously (**Figure 4-6**) as well. This coordinated contraction occurs due to the internal timing device, or pacemaker, of the conduction system.

Conduction System

Left to their own devices, cardiac muscle cells would contract individually, which would create a disorderly and ineffective contraction. The muscle cells are able to contract in an organized manner due to an internal electrical stimulus initiated by a pacemaker. The brain controls heart rate and contractility through sympathetic and parasympathetic stimulation of the autonomic nervous system. Basically, the heart's pacemaker acts like a generator creating an impulse for every heartbeat. The ability of the cells to respond to electrical impulses is referred to as excitability. Conductivity is the ability of cells to conduct electrical impulses. Cardiac cells possess an ability to generate an impulse to contract even with no external nerve stimulus, a process called automaticity.

All cardiac muscle cells can initiate impulses, but normally the conduction pathway originates in the sinoatrial (SA) node located high in the right atrium (**Figure 4-7**). Impulses originating in the SA node travel through the right and left atrium, resulting in atrial contraction. The SA node automatically generates impulses ranging from 60–100 beats per minute (sinus rhythm). The impulse then travels to the atrioventricular (AV) node, located in the right atrium adjacent to the septum. Though it does not usually initiate impulses unless the SA node begins failing, the intrinsic rate of impulses in the AV node is 40–60 beats per minute. The impulses are delayed, or move slowly through, the AV node to allow for complete ventricular filling. Then the impulses move in rapid succession through the bundle of His, right and left bun-

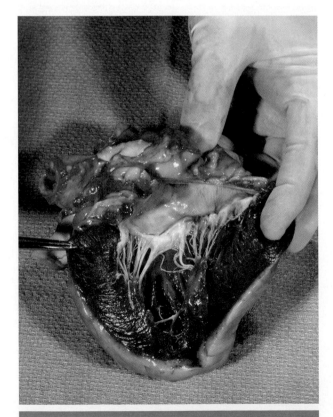

Figure 4-4

Heart valves.

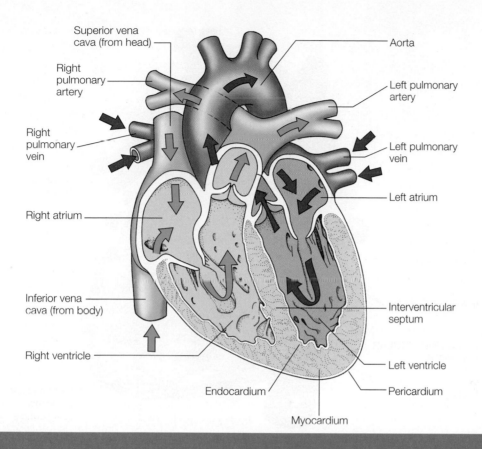

Superior vena cava (from head)

Right pulmonary artery

Right pulmonary vein

Right atrium

Inferior vena cava (from body)

Right ventricle

Aorta

Left pulmonary artery

Left pulmonary vein

Left atrium

Interventricular septum

Left ventricle

Pericardium

Endocardium

Myocardium

Figure 4-5

Blood flow through the heart.

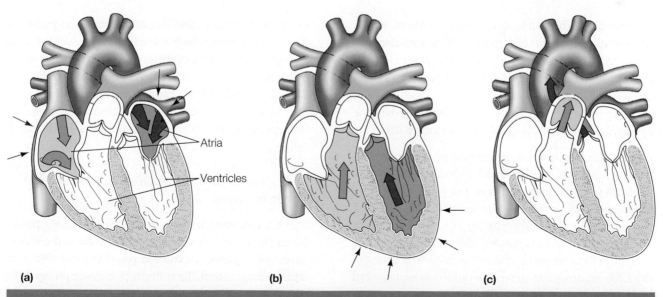

(a)

Atria

Ventricles

(b)

(c)

Figure 4-6

Blood flow through the heart: (a) Blood enters both atria simultaneously from the systemic and pulmonary circuits. When full, the atria pump their blood into the ventricles. (b) When the ventricles are full, they contract simultaneously, (c) delivering the blood to the pulmonary and systemic circuits.

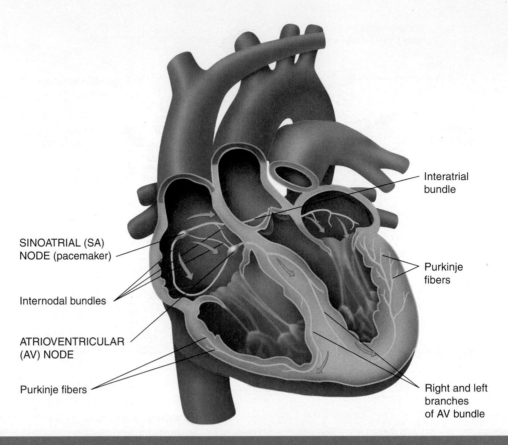

SINOATRIAL (SA)
NODE (pacemaker)

Internodal bundles

ATRIOVENTRICULAR
(AV) NODE

Purkinje fibers

Interatrial
bundle

Purkinje
fibers

Right and left
branches
of AV bundle

Figure 4-7

Electrical conduction through the heart.

dle branches, and Purkinje network of fibers, which stimulates ventricular contraction. If the impulses fail to fire from the SA or the AV node, the ventricles will attempt to pace themselves. The ventricles can generate impulses at 20–40 beats per minute, which may not result in adequate cardiac output. The heart has the optional pacemakers as a fail-safe to sustain life.

The cardiac impulse conduction produces an electric current that can be read by electrodes attached to the skin at various points of the body, producing the electrocardiogram (EKG) (**Figure 4-8**). Organized depolarization (an increase in electrical charge through the exchange of ions across the cell membrane) of the cardiac cells generates cardiac muscle contraction. On the EKG reading, the atrial contraction is represented by the depolarization in the P wave, and the ventricular contraction is represented by the depolarization in the large QRS complex. The more intense the contraction, the higher the wave or complex. Since the force required for the atria to pump blood into the ventricles

is minimal compared to that of the ventricles pumping to the entire body, the P wave is smaller than the QRS complex. The T wave represents repolarization, or the recovery, of the ventricles. In repolarization, the ions line up on both sides of the cell membrane in preparation for depolarization. Repolarization of the atria does not appear on an EKG because it is hidden by the other, more prominent waveforms. Abnormal variations in the EKG, known as arrythmias or dysrhythmias, may indicate acute problems, such as infarction or electrolyte imbalances.

Cardiac muscle cells require sodium (Na^+), potassium (K^+), and calcium (Ca^+) to initiate and conduct electrical signals. To initiate the depolarization that creates contraction, the sodium-potassium pump shifts the ions to generate a charge. Ca^+ balance is required for muscle contractility, especially in a muscle that contracts many times a minute. Additionally, the neurologic system controls cardiac function, and the neurologic system requires Na^+ balance to function

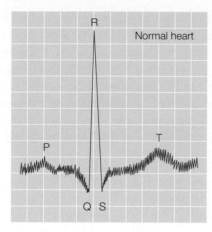

P – atrial depolarization, which triggers atrial contraction.

QRS = depolarization of AV node and conduction of electrical impulse through ventricles. Ventricular contraction begins at R.

T = repolarization of ventricles.

P to R interval = time required for impulses to travel from SA node to ventricles.

Figure 4-8

An electrocardiogram.

properly. The brain (specifically the medulla) monitors and controls cardiac function through the autonomic nervous system, endocrine system, and cardiac tissue. These functions include the rate of contraction (**chronotropic** effect), rate of electrical conduction (**dromotropic** effect), and strength of contraction (**inotropic** effect). Receptors in the brain, heart, blood vessels, and kidneys continuously monitor body functions to maintain homeostasis. **Chemoreceptors** detect chemical changes in the blood, and **baroreceptors**, located in the carotid arteries, detect the pressure in the heart and arteries. If homeostasis is interrupted, receptors begin to fire and neurotransmitters or hormones that activate either the sympathetic nervous system (SNS) or the parasympathetic nervous system are released. Stimulating the SNS will increase heart rate and blood pressure while parasympathetic nervous system stimulation will decrease heart rate and blood pressure.

Blood Pressure

Blood pressure refers to the force that blood exerts on the walls of blood vessels. Blood pressure is noted as a fraction with the **systole** (work) as the top number and

diastole (rest) as the bottom number. According to the American Heart Association, a normal blood pressure reading should be in the range of 120/80 mm Hg to maintain health and limit chronic disease risk. The systolic pressure is the force the blood exerts on the arteries when ejected from the left ventricle. The diastolic pressure is the force in the arteries when the ventricles are relaxed. Blood pressure is commonly measured using a sphygmomanometer and the brachial artery. **Pulse pressure** is the difference between the systolic and diastolic pressures and represents the force that the heart generates each time it contracts.

Blood pressure changes in response to the individual's activity and stress level. Blood pressure also varies at different points of the body. Cardiac output and peripheral vascular resistance significantly affect blood pressure ($BP = CO \times PVR$, where BP is blood pressure, CO is cardiac output, and PVR is peripheral vascular resistance). Other variables that influence blood pressure include blood volume and viscosity, venous return, heart rate, cardiac contractility, and arterial elasticity. Typically, increases in these variables will increase blood pressure with the exception of aterial elasticity. **Cardiac output** refers to the amount of blood the heart pumps in one minute. Cardiac output is determined by stroke volume and heart rate ($CO = SV \times HR$, where CO is cardiac output, SV is stroke volume, and HR is heart rate). **Stroke volume** is the amount of blood ejected from the heart with each contraction. **Peripheral vascular resistance (PVR)** is the force opposing the blood in the peripheral circulation. PVR increases as the diameter of the blood vessels decreases. Stimulation of the SNS can initiate systemic vasoconstriction to raise blood pressure. This vasoconstriction is helpful in times of hypotension, such as with shock. PVR affects **afterload**, the pressure that the left ventricle must exert in order to get the blood out of the heart and into the aorta. The higher the afterload, the harder it is for the heart to eject the blood, thus lowering stroke volume. In addition to afterload, stroke volume is affected by preload. **Preload** refers to the amount of blood returning to the heart for the heart to manage. Additionally, both afterload and preload can affect blood pressure. As afterload and preload increase, blood pressure increases.

Hormones also influence blood pressure. The **antidiuretic hormone** increases water reabsorption in the kidney, which increases blood volume and blood pressure. Additionally, antidiuretic hormone is a vasoconstrictor, which increases PVR. **Aldosterone** increases blood volume by increasing the reabsorption of Na⁺ in the kidneys; Na⁺ attracts water. Increasing renal water reabsorption will increase blood volume. The renin-angiotensin-aldosterone system in the kidneys is another vital control and compensatory mechanism activated when renal blood flow is decreased, often in hypotensive states. When renal blood flow is decreased, renin is released from the kidneys, activating angiotension I to convert to angiotension II (a vasoconstrictor) and stimulating aldosterone secretion. In hypotensive states, this mechanism raises blood pressure and maintains vital organs. In chronic disease states such as hypertension, this mechanism is inappropriately activated because of vasoconstriction to the kidneys, further contributing to the hypertension.

Blood Vessels

Blood vessels are the intricate highway system in which the blood travels. Arteries carry blood away from the heart while veins carry blood back to the heart. Left ventricular contractions project blood through the arteries while valves in the veins assist in moving the blood against gravity back to the heart. Once arteries leave the heart, they begin branching into smaller vessels called arterioles (Figure 4-9). These vessels continue branching into even smaller, thin-walled vessels called capillaries. These thin walls allow oxygen and

nutrients to shift out of the capillaries into the cells. Additionally, carbon dioxide and waste products shift from the cells into the capillaries. This exchange occurs through diffusion (see Chapter 1). Once blood is utilized at the cellular level, the blood moves through the capillaries as they transition into larger vessels known as venules. Venules continue to merge into larger vessels until they become veins, much as small streams unite to form a river.

Generally, arteries carry blood rich in oxygen and nutrients while veins carry blood saturated with carbon dioxide and metabolic waste. One exception to this occurrence is in the pulmonary arteries and veins. The pulmonary arteries carry oxygen-depleted blood away from the right side of the heart to the lungs for gas exchange (Figure 4-2). Following gas exchange in the lungs, the oxygen-saturated blood returns to the left side of the heart through the pulmonary veins.

The walls of the blood vessels consist of three layers (Figure 4-10). The tunica intima is the smooth, thin, inner layer of the blood vessels. The tunica media, the middle layer, is comprised of elastic tissue and smooth muscle that is responsible for the vessel's ability to change diameter. The outer layer, tunica adventitia, consists of elastic and fibrous connective tissue to provide the necessary give to accommodate the rush of blood with each cardiac contraction.

Lymphatic System

The lymphatic system is an extensive network of vessels and glands that returns excess fluid in body tissue to the circulatory system and works with the immune system (see Chapter 2). Cells are surrounded by interstitial fluid that provides a medium through which nutrients, gases, and wastes can diffuse between the capillaries and the cells. Capillaries are continuously replenishing this fluid. Normally, the fluid outflow from the capillaries exceeds the fluid returned. Lymph capillaries absorb the excess fluid (Figure 4-11). This fluid, or lymph, drains from these capillaries into larger vessels and ducts that empty into large veins at the base of the neck. The movement of lymph occurs much in the same way that blood moves through veins, with the assistance of valves and movement.

The lymphatic system also consists of several organs—lymph nodes, the spleen, the thymus, and the tonsils. The lymphatic organs primarily function in the immune response (see Chapter 2). Located in clusters throughout the body, lymph nodes are a network of fibers and irregular channels that slow down

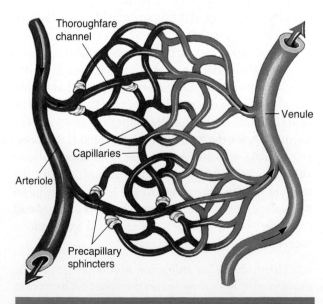

Thoroughfare channel

Venule

Capillaries

Arteriole

Precapillary sphincters

Figure 4-9

The circulatory system.

the lymph flow. As the lymph passes through the nodes, the fibers filter out bacteria, viruses, and cellular debris. Numerous macrophages line the channels to phagocytize microorganisms and other material.

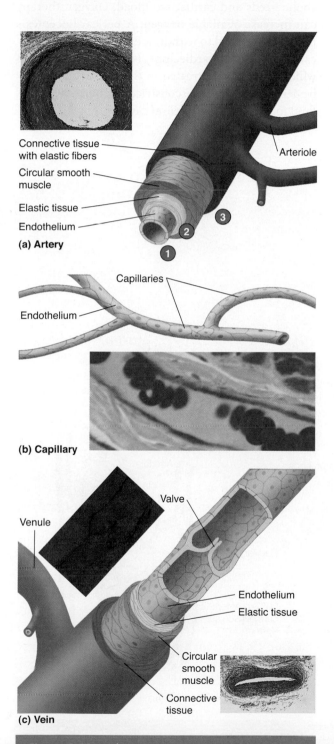

Connective tissue with elastic fibers
Circular smooth muscle
Elastic tissue
Endothelium
Arteriole
(a) Artery

Capillaries
Endothelium
(b) Capillary

Valve
Venule
Endothelium
Elastic tissue
Circular smooth muscle
Connective tissue
(c) Vein

Figure 4-10

The walls of the blood vessels are composed of three layers of tissue: the endothelium, elastic tissue, and the connective tissue. (a) Artery; (b) capillary; (c) vein.

Normally, the rate of lymph produced equals that being removed. In some states, lymph produced exceeds the capacity of the system. For example, burns can cause extensive damage to capillaries, leaking fluid into the tissue. This flooding results in excessive fluid in the tissue, or edema. Additionally, lymphatic vessels may become occluded often because of infection.

Structural Alterations

Pericarditis

Pericarditis refers to an inflammation of the pericardium—the sac that surrounds, protects, and supports the heart. Because it is an inflammatory process (see Chapter 2), fluid shifts from the capillaries to the space between the sac and the heart. The fluid may be serous (resulting from heart failure), purulent (resulting from infections), serosanguineous (resulting from neoplasms or uremia), or hemorrhagic (resulting from aneurysms or trauma). As the pericardial tissue becomes inflamed, the swollen pericardial tissue rubs against the swollen cardiac tissue, creating friction.

Fluid can accumulate in the pericardial cavity, creating a pericardial effusion. This fluid can progress into life-threatening cardiac tamponade (**Figure 4-12**). Cardiac tamponade results when the fluid accumulates in the pericardial cavity to the point that it compresses the heart. This compression prevents the heart from stretching and filling during diastole, resulting in decreased cardiac output. Arterial pressures fall, venous pressures rise, and the pulse pressure narrows as the cardiac tamponade develops. Additionally, the heart sounds are muffled upon auscultation because the fluid drowns out the sound. Heart failure, cardiogenic shock, and death can result from cardiac tamponade.

Chronic inflammation can lead to constrictive pericarditis. In constrictive pericarditis, the pericardium becomes thick and fibrous from the chronic inflammation and adheres to the heart. The pericardium becomes like a restrictive rubber band that has lost its elasticity. The loss of elasticity restricts cardiac filling, decreasing cardiac output and causing systemic congestion.

Clinical manifestations of pericarditis include:

- Pericardial friction rub (grating sound heard when breath is held)

- Sharp, sudden, severe chest pain that increases with deep inspiration and decreases when sitting up and leaning forward

- Dyspnea
- Tachycardia
- Edema
- Flulike symptoms (e.g., fever, chills, myalgia)

Diagnosis of pericarditis is accomplished through a history, physical examination, complete blood count (CBC), EKG, chest X-ray, echocardiogram, computed tomography (CT), and magnetic resonance imaging (MRI). Treatment focuses on treating the underlying cause (by using antibiotics) and reducing inflammation (by using nonsteroidal and steroidal anti-inflammatory drugs). Analgesics may be administered to manage pain. Additionally, bed rest is important to reduce metabolic needs and cardiac workload. Oxygen therapy can increase available oxygen. A pericardiocentesis may be performed to withdraw excess fluid from pericardium, or a pericardiectomy (surgical procedure in which a window is created in the pericardium) may be performed to release constriction and allow excess fluid to drain into the pleural cavity.

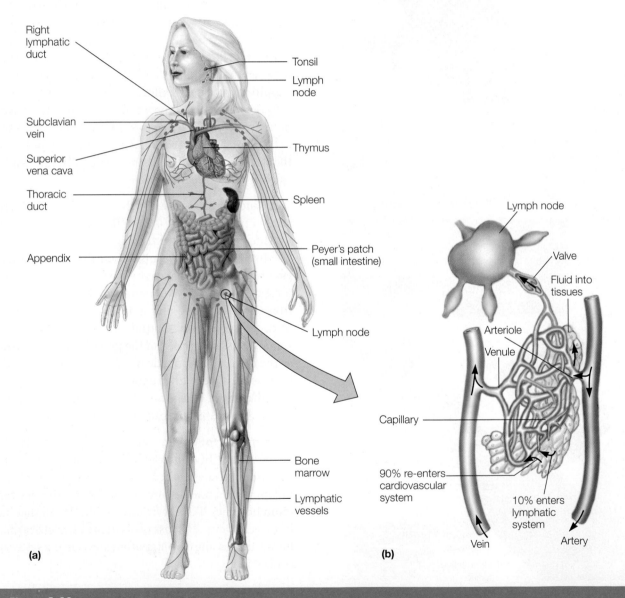

Figure 4-11

The lymphatic system. (a) The lymphatic system consists of vessels that transport lymph, excess tissue fluid, back to the circulatory system. (b) Lymph is picked up by lymphatic capillaries that drain into larger vessels. Like the veins, the lymphatic vessels contain valves that prohibit backflow. Lymph nodes are interspersed along the vessels and serve to filter the lymph.

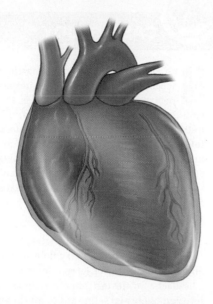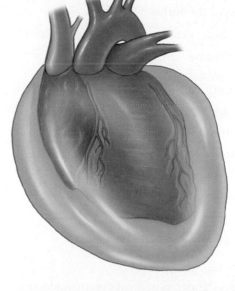

Normal heart   Pericardial tamponade

Figure 4-12

Cardiac tamponade.

Infective Endocarditis

Infective endocarditis (previously called bacterial endocarditis) is an infection of the endocardium (inner layers of the heart) or heart valves. *Streptococcus* viridans, commonly found in the mouth, account for 50% of the infective endocarditis cases (National Institutes of Health, 2008). *Staphylococcus aureus* and *S. enterococcus*, commonly found on the skin and in the gastrointestinal tract, arc also frequent causative agents. The pathogenesis of this condition involves endothelial damage, which attracts platelets and stimulates thrombus formation. Vegetation (including platelets, fibrin, microorganisms, inflammatory cells, and granulomatous tissue) collects on the internal structures because of damage from the infection, much like what occurs when an anchor is placed in a body of water for an extended length of time. With each heart contraction, some of this vegetation is dislodged and ejected from the heart. These small thrombi move throughout the body, collecting in microcirculation and creating microhemorrhages (e.g., petechiae, hematuria). The valves can become scarred and perforated (**Figure 4-13**). If untreated, infective endocarditis is usually fatal, especially when it involves the valvular structures.

Risk factors for development of infective endocarditis include:

- Intravenous drug use
- Valvular disorders
- Prosthetic heart valves

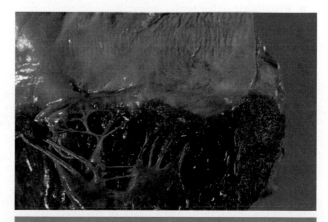

Figure 4-13

Ineffective endocarditis.

- Rheumatic heart disease
- Coarctation of the aorta
- Congenital heart defects (e.g., tetralogy of Fallot)
- Marfan syndrome

Clinical manifestations of infective endocarditis include:

- Flulike symptoms (e.g., fever, chills, myalgia)
- Embolization (e.g., myocardial infarction, pulmonary embolism, stroke, and splenic infarction)
- Heart murmur
- Petechiae
- Splinter hemorrhages under the nails
- Hematuria
- Osler's nodes (tender, raised, subcutaneous lesions on the fingers and toes)

Diagnostic procedures of infective endocarditis include a history, physical examination, blood cultures, CBC, urinalysis, serum rheumatoid factor, erythrocyte sedimentation rate, EKG, and echocardiogram. Treatment focuses on the causative agent (e.g., antibiotics, antifungals). Infective endocarditis often requires long-term therapy (a minimum of 4 weeks). Other treatments are initiated to maintain cardiac function and treat other symptoms. These other strategies include:

- Bed rest
- Oxygen therapy
- Antipyretics
- Surgical repair of cardiac valves
- Prosthetic valve replacement

Myocarditis

Myocarditis is an inflammation of the myocardium, or heart muscle. This uncommon condition is poorly understood because at least several weeks (in some cases a decade) elapse between exposure of the causative agent and the development of symptoms. Penetration of organisms, blood cells, toxins, and immune substances into the myocardium can result in muscle fiber dysfunction and degeneration that can impair contractility and conduction. Most cases of myocarditis are benign, but some cases result in heart failure, cardiomyopathy, dysrhythmias, and thrombi development.

The patient may be asymptomatic, but when present, clinical manifestations of myocarditis include:

CASE STUDY

Mrs. Fulcher is a 58-year-old married homemaker recently discharged from the hospital because of recurrent infective endocarditis. The most recent episodes were a *Staphylococcus aureus* infection of the mitral valve 12 months ago and a *Streptococcus mutans* infection of the aortic valve 1 month ago. During this most recent hospitalization, an echocardiogram showed aortic stenosis, moderate aortic insufficiency, chronic valvular vegetations, and moderate atrial enlargement. In addition, Mrs. Fulcher has a history of chronic joint pain.

After being home for one week, Mrs. Fulcher was readmitted to your telemetry floor with endocarditis. She reports chills, fever, fatigue, joint pain, malaise, and a headache for the last 24 hours. Upon admission, IV infusion of normal saline at 125 mL/hr and vancomycin IV every 8 hours was ordered to be continued over the next 4 weeks. Other routine medications ordered include furosemide (Lasix), amlodipine (Norvasc), and metoprolol (Lopressor). At admission, her blood pressure was 172/48 (supine) and 100/40 (sitting), her pulse was 116, respirations were 20, and her temperature was 101.9°F. Additional assessment findings included a murmur, 2+ pitting tibial edema, but no peripheral cyanosis, lungs sounds clear bilateral, orientation to person, place, and time but drowsiness, hematuria, and multiple petechiae on the skin of her arms, legs, and chest.

1. What is the significance of the orthostatic hypotension, the wide pulse pressure, and tachycardia?
2. What is the significance of the hematuria, joint pain, and petechiae?
3. What complications of embolization should Mrs. Fulcher be assessed for?

- Flulike symptoms (e.g., fever, chills, myalgia)
- Dyspnea
- Dysrhythmias and palpitations
- Tachycardia
- Heart murmurs
- Chest discomfort
- Cardiac enlargement

Diagnosis of myocarditis is accomplished through a history, physical examination, blood cultures, EKG, cardiac enzymes (e.g., troponin and creatinine kinase), CBC, erythrocyte sedimentation rate, chest X-rays, echocardiogram, and myocardium biopsy. Management centers on treating the causative agent (e.g., antibiotics and antifungals). Antipyretics, anticoagulants, antidysrhythmics, and immune suppressive agents (e.g., corticosteriods or nonsteriodal antiinflammatory drugs) may be used to treat symptoms or complications. Increasing bed rest, restricting activity, and limiting fluids can reduce cardiac workload.

Valvular Disorders

Valvular disorders cause disruption of normal blood flow through the heart. These disorders are defined by the valve affected and type of alteration. Two types of alterations can occur—stenosis or regurgitation. Stenosis is a narrowing of a tubular structure, in this case heart valves. When the valves are stenosed, blood moving through the valve is reduced, causing blood to back up in the chamber just before the valve. Pressures in those chambers increase to pump against the resistance of the stenosed valve. Because the heart (specifically the chamber) is working harder, hypertrophy of the chambers develops. Hypertrophy and increased workload escalate the heart's oxygen demands. Decreased cardiac output resulting from the stenosis make it challenging to meet these increased demands. Decreased cardiac output diminishes blood delivery to the coronary arteries that supply the heart. Without adequate blood flow, the heart deteriorates.

Regurgitation, also called insufficiency or incompetence, occurs when the valve leaflets do not completely close. Normally, heart valves allow blood to flow in one direction, but incompetent valves allow blood to flow in both directions. This regurgitation of blood increases the amount of blood that must be pumped and the cardiac workload. This increased workload contributes to hypertrophy developing in the affected chambers. Additionally, the increased blood volume in the heart causes the chambers to dilate to accommodate the volume.

Causes of valvular disorders include:

- Congenital defects
- Infective endocarditis
- Rheumatic fever
- Myocardial infarction
- Cardiomyopathy
- Heart failure

Clinical manifestations of valvular disorders depend upon the valve involved and the nature of the alteration (Table 4-1). Diagnostic procedures for valvular heart disease consist of a history, physical examination, heart catheterization, chest X-rays, echocardiogram, EKG, or MRI. Medications often used to treat valvular disorders include diuretics, antidysrhythmics, vasodilators, angiotension converting enzyme (ACE) inhibitors, beta-adrenergic blockers, and anticoagulants. Additional strategies may include:

- Oxygen therapy
- Low-sodium diet
- Surgical valve repair
- Prosthetic valve replacement

Cardiomyopathy

Cardiomyopathy generally refers to a group of conditions that weaken and enlarge the myocardium. Cardiomyopathies are classified into three groups—dilated, hypertrophic, and restrictive (Figure 4-14).

Dilated cardiomyopathy is the most common type of cardiomyopathy, accounting for approximately 90% of all cases (National Institutes of Health, 2010). Risk for developing dilated cardiomyopathy increases with age, and it is more common in African American men. Most cases are idiopathic, but secondary causes include:

- Chemotherapy
- Alcoholism
- Cocaine abuse
- Pregnancy
- Infections
- Thyrotoxicosis (hypermetabolic syndrome resulting from increased levels of thyroid hormones)
- Diabetes mellitus
- Neuromuscular diseases (e.g., muscular dystrophy)
- Hypertension
- Coronary artery disease
- Hypersensitivity to medications

Dilated cardiomyopathy results from extensively damaged myocardium muscle fibers due to cardiomegaly and ventricular dilation. Consequently, myocardial contractility is decreased resulting in impaired systolic function and decreased cardiac output. Blood can stagnate in the heart, causing thrombi to develop. The SNS and the kidneys attempt to compensate for the

Table 4-1 Clinical Manifestations of Valvular Stenosis and Regurgitation

Manifestation	Aortic Stenosis	Aortic Regurgitation	Mitral Stenosis	Mitral Regurgitation	Tricuspid Regurgitation
Cardiovascular effects	Left ventricular hypertrophy, angina	Left heart hypertrophy, angina	Right ventricular hypertrophy, angina	Left heart hypertrophy, angina	Right heart hypertrophy, angina
General symptoms	Fatigue	Fatigue	Fatigue, edema	Fatigue, dizziness, peripheral edema	Peripheral edema
Respiratory effects	Dyspnea on exertion	Dyspnea on exertion	Dyspnea on exertion, orthopnea, paroxysmal, nocturnal dyspnea, predisposition to respiratory infections, hemoptysis, pulmonary hypertension	Dyspnea; occasional hemoptysis	Dyspnea
Central nervous system effects	Syncope, especially on exertion	Syncope	Neural deficits only associated with emboli	None	None
Gastrointestinal effects	None	None	Ascites; hepatic angina with hepatomegaly	None	Ascites, hepatomegaly (with heart failure)
Heart rate, rhythm	Bradycardia, variety of dysrhythmias	Palpitations, water hammer pulse	Palpitations	Palpitations	Atrial fibrillations
Heart sounds	Systolic murmur	Diastolic and systolic murmurs	Diastolic murmur, accentuated first heart sound	Murmur throughout systole	Murmur throughout systole
Most common cause	Congenital, rheumatic fever	Bacterial endocarditis; aortic root disease	Rheumatic fever	Insufficient valve; coronary artery disease	Congenital

Source: Adapted from Huether, S., & McCance, K. (2000). *Understanding pathophysiology* (2nd ed.). St. Louis, MO: C. V. Mosby Co.

falling cardiac output by increasing the heart rate and the blood volume. Symptoms develop as these compensatory mechanisms begin failing. Deterioration is rapid once symptoms appear. Within a year of the onset of symptoms, 20–50% of patients die, with most deaths occurring within 5 years (National Institutes of Health, 2010).

Clinical manifestations of dilated cardiomyopathy develop insidiously and include:

- Dyspnea
- Fatigue
- Nonproductive cough
- Orthopnea (difficulty breathing while lying down)
- Paroxysmal nocturnal dyspnea (difficulty breathing at night)
- Dysrhythmias

(a) Normal heart

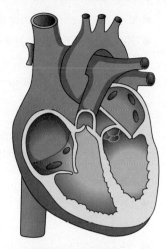

(b) Dilated cardiomyopathy

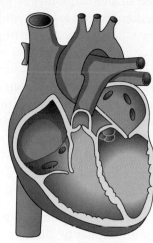

(c) Hypertrophic cardiomyopathy

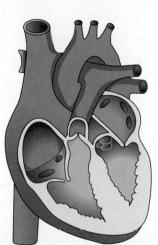

(d) Restrictive cardiomyopathy

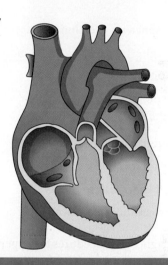

Figure 4-14

Comparing cardiomyopathies.

- Angina (cardiac chest pain that often occurs with exertion)
- Dizziness
- Activity intolerance
- Blood pressure changes
- Tachycardia
- Murmurs
- Abnormal lung sounds (e.g., crackles and wheezes)
- Tachypnea
- Peripheral edema
- Ascites (fluid in the peritoneal cavity)
- Weak pedal pulses
- Cool, pale extremities

- Poor capillary refill
- Hepatomegaly
- Jugular vein distension

Diagnostic procedures for dilated cardiomyopathy include an echocardiogram, EKG, chest X-ray, heart catheterization, and nuclear studies. Treatment is mainly supportive through relieving heart failure symptoms by decreasing afterload and enhancing contractility. Pharmacological treatments usually include ACE inhibitors, diuretics, digoxin (Lanoxin), beta adrenergic blockers, and antidysrhythmics. Other management strategies include an implantable cardiac defibrillator, cardioversion, pacemaker, valvular repair, and heart transplant. Additionally, lifestyle modification includes a low-fat, low-sodium diet, tobacco cessation, physical activity, and abstinence from alcohol.

Unlike dilated cardiomyopathy, which affects systolic function, hypertrophic cardiomyopathy mainly affects diastolic function. Hypertrophic cardiomyopathy is more common in men and those who are more sedentary, and it appears to have an autosomal dominant genetic base. Hypertension, obstructive valvular disease, and thyroid disease increase the risk for developing hypertrophic cardiomyopathy. The hypertrophied ventricle wall becomes stiff and unable to relax during ventricular filling. With a reduction in ventricular filling, cardiac output decreases while artial and pulmonary pressures increase.

Clinical manifestations of hypertrophic cardiomyopathy are similar to dilated cardiomyopathy and include:

- Dyspnea on exertion
- Fatigue
- Syncope
- Orthopnea
- Angina
- Activity intolerance
- Dysrhythmias
- Left ventricular failure
- Myocardial infarction

Diagnostic procedures for hypertrophic cardiomyopathy are similar to those for dilated cardiomyopathy. Treatment goals include reducing ventricular stiffness, improving ventricular filling, and enhancing cardiac output. Beta-adrenergic blockers and calcium channel blockers are often included in the medication regimen. Surgical removal of excess myocardium may be necessary for those who do not respond well to medications. Treatment of any dysrhythmias and hypertension may also be warranted. Additionally, patients should avoid strenuous activity (e.g., running) because most cases of sudden death associated with hypertrophic cardiomyopathy have occurred with this type of activity.

Restrictive cardiomyopathy is the least common of the cardiomyopathies, but it is endemic in parts of South and Central America, India, Asia, and Africa. Restrictive cardiomyopathy is characterized by rigidity of the ventricles, leading to diastolic dysfunction. Causes of restrictive cardiomyopathy include:

- Amyloidosis (buildup of fat and proteins in the heart muscle)
- Hemochromatosis (excess of iron in the heart)
- Radiation exposure to the chest
- Connective tissue diseases
- Buildup of scar tissue after a myocardial infarction
- Sarcoidosis (cellular growths on various organs)
- Cardiac neoplasms

Many cases are asymptomatic, but clinical manifestations of restrictive cardiomyopathy may include:

- Fatigue
- Dyspnea
- Orthopnea
- Abnormal lung sounds
- Angina
- Hepatomegaly
- Jugular vein distension
- Ascites
- Murmurs
- Peripheral cyanosis
- Pallor

Diagnostic procedures include those for the two previously discussed cardiomyopathies. Management focuses on treating the underlying cause, dysrhythmias, and heart failure. A heart transplant may be necessary when the heart can no longer meet the body's demands. The prognosis is generally poor, with death often occurring from heart failure.

Electrical Alterations

As previously mentioned, normal myocardial contraction is accomplished by electrical impulses originating in the SA node, the natural pacemaker of the heart. Normal electric conduction is referred to as sinus rhythm, while deviations from normal are referred to as dysrhythmias or arrhythmias. Dysrhythmias vary in severity and are classified according to their origins (Figure 4-15). Their effects on cardiac output and blood pressure are partially influenced by their site of origin, which also determines the dysrhythmias' clinical significance. Causes of dysrhythmias include:

- Acid–base imbalances
- Hypoxia
- Congenital heart defects
- Connective tissue disorders

- Degeneration of conductive tissues (usually as a result of aging)
- Drug toxicity
- Electrolyte imbalances (especially potassium and calcium)
- Stress
- Myocardial hypertrophy
- Myocardial ischemia or infarction

Clinical manifestations may vary according to the dysrhythmias (Figure 4-15). Some dysrhythmias may be asymptomatic while others can cause sudden death. The danger and symptoms depend on the extent that they reduce cardiac output. Some general manifestations of dysrhythmias include:

- Palpitations
- Fluttering sensation
- Skipped beats
- Fatigue
- Confusion
- Syncope
- Dyspnea
- Abnormal heart rate

Diagnostic procedures for dysrhythmias include a history, physical examination, EKG, and invasive electrophysiologic studies. Additional tests may be performed to identify the underlying cause. Pharmacology is the mainstay of treatment (Figure 4-15). Other interventions may include an internal cardiac defibrillator, pacemaker, cardioversion, defibrillation, and ablation. Avoiding triggers such as caffeine, tobacco, and stress can decrease the occurrence and severity of some dysrhythmias.

Vascular Disorders

Aneurysms

Walls of arteries can weaken because of high pressures, plaque, and infections. These weakened areas balloon outward, a condition known as aneurysm (Figure 4-16). This happens much like a worn spot on a tire or a bulge in an old balloon. Just like the tire and the balloon, an aneurysm can rupture when the pressure builds inside the wall or when the wall becomes too thin. When it ruptures, blood spills out of the circulatory system, also known as exsanguination. Aneurysms may also

develop slow leaks as opposed to rupturing. Risk factors for developing aneurysms include:

- Congenital weakening of the arterial wall
- Atherosclerosis
- Hypertension
- Dyslipidemia
- Diabetes mellitus
- Tobacco
- Advanced age
- Trauma
- Infection (e.g., syphilis)

True aneurysms are those that affect all three layers of the vessel. There are two major types of true aneurysms—saccular and fusiform (**Figure 4-17**). A saccular aneurysm is a bulge on the side of the vessel. With a fusiform aneurysm, the aneurysm occurs the entire circumference of the vessel. A false aneurysm is one that does not affect all three layers of the vessel, and an example of this type is a dissecting aneurysm. With dissecting aneurysms, the weakening occurs in the inner layers (Figure 4-17).

Clinical manifestations of aneurysms may vary by location. Some common locations include the abdominal aorta, thoracic aorta, and the cerebral, femoral, and popliteal arteries. Most aneurysms are asymptomatic until they rupture. If present, symptoms may include a pulsating mass, pain, respiratory difficulty (e.g., dyspnea and cough), and neurologic decline (e.g., confusion or lethargy).

Diagnosis of aneurysms often occurs incidentally during a routine physical examination or X-ray. Other diagnostic procedures include echocardiogram, CT, MRI, and arteriograph. The goal of treatment is to prevent rupture by eliminating or treating causes (e.g., control blood pressure). Surgical intervention is the only effective treatment, and it is performed any time symptoms are present or the diameter is more than 5 cm when asymptomatic. If rupture occurs, immediate surgery is required.

Dyslipidemia

Dyslipidemia, or hyperlipidemia, refers to a raised level of lipids in the blood. These lipids include cholesterol and triglycerides, which are necessary for cellular membrane formation (see Chapter 1). Increased lipid levels have been linked to multiple disease conditions including atherosclerosis, peripheral vascular disease,

Dysrhythmia	Features	Causes
Supraventricular Rhythms		
Sinus bradycardia 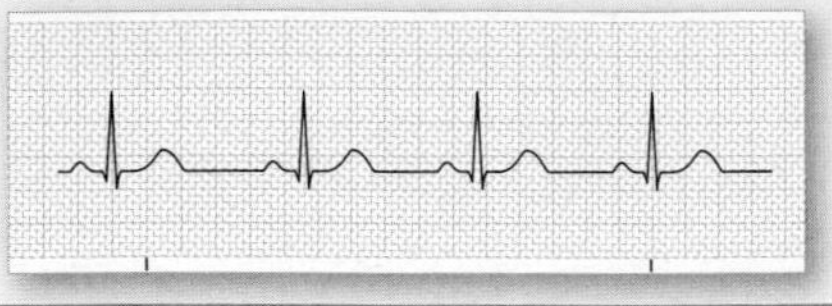	Rate: < 60 bpm Rhythm: Regular P waves: Occur before each QRS complex; look the same in shape and size P-R interval: Normal (0.12 sec to 0.20 sec) QRS complexes: Occur after each P wave; look the same in shape and size; normal (< 0.12 sec)	Normal in a well-conditioned heart (e.g., athletes); increased intracranial pressure; increased vagal tone due to straining during bowel movement, vomiting, intubation, or mechanical ventilation; sick sinus syndrome; inferior-wall MI; may also occur with anticholinesterase, beta-adrenergic blocker, digoxin, or morphine use
Sinus tachycardia 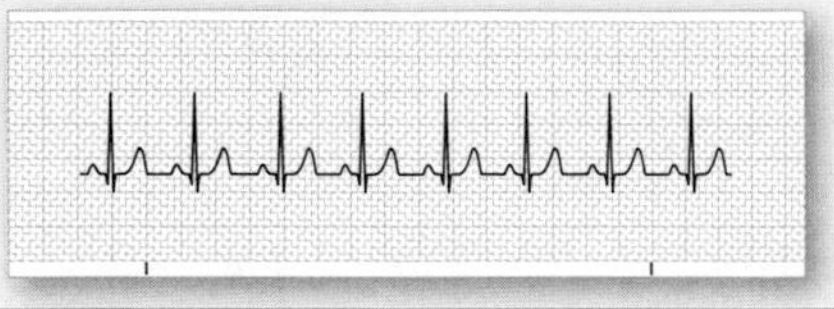	Rate: > 100 bpm Rhythm: Regular P waves: Occur before each QRS complex; look the same in shape and size P-R interval: Normal (0.12 sec to 0.20 sec) QRS complexes: Occur after each P wave; look the same in shape and size; normal (< 0.12 sec)	Normal physiologic response to fever, exercise, anxiety, pain, dehydration; may also accompany shock, left-sided heart failure, anemia, hypovolemia, pulmonary embolism; may also occur with atropine, epinephrine, caffeine, alcohol, and amphetamine or nicotine use
Atrial flutter 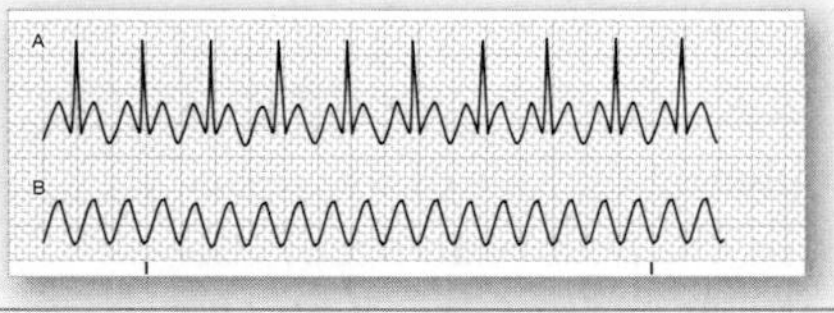	Rate: > 100 bpm Rhythm: Regular (may vary depending on degree of AV block) P waves: Cannot be found; replaced by flutter (F) waves, which may have sawtooth pattern P-R interval: Cannot determine QRS complexes: Look the same in shape and size; normal (< 0.12 sec)	Heart failure, tricuspid or mitral valve disease, pulmonary embolism, cor pulmonale, interior-wall MI, pericarditis; digoxin toxicity
Atrial fibrillation 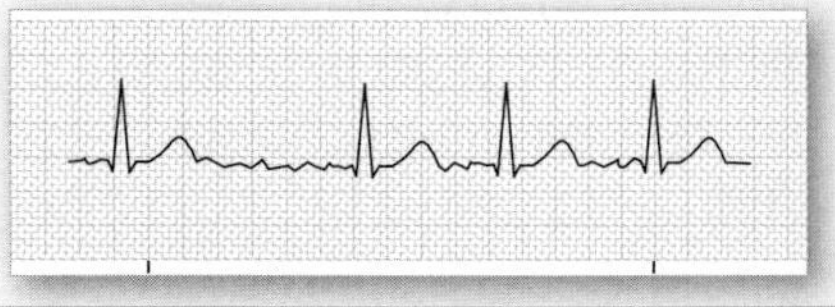	Rate: > 100 bpm (grossly irregular; 350–450 bpm) Rhythm: Irregular P waves: Cannot be found P-R interval: Cannot determine QRS complexes: Look the same in shape and size	Heart failure, COPD, ischemic heart disease, sepsis, pulmonary embolism, rheumatic heart disease, hypertension, mitral stenosis; complication of coronary bypass or valve replacement surgery; nifedipine and digoxin use
Paroxysmal supraventricular tachycardia 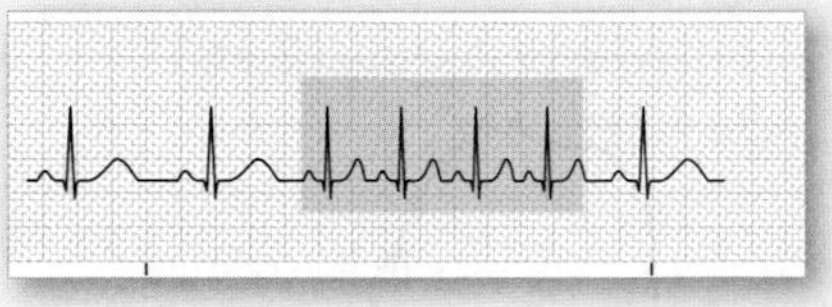	Rate: > 100 bpm Rhythm: Regular P waves: Occur before each QRS complex (may be hidden in preceding T wave); look the same in shape and size (but differs from normal sinus P wave) P-R interval: Normal (0.12 sec to 0.20 sec), but may differ from P-R interval associated with normal sinus beat QRS complexes: Occur after each P wave; look the same in shape and size; normal (< 0.12 sec)	Intrinsic abnormality of AV conduction system; physical/psychological stress, hypoxia, hypokalemia, cardiomyopathy, congenital heart disease, MI, valvular disease, Wolff-Parkinson-White syndrome, cor pulmonale, hyperthyroidism; digoxin toxicity, use of caffeine, marijuana, or CNS stimulants
Junctional rhythm 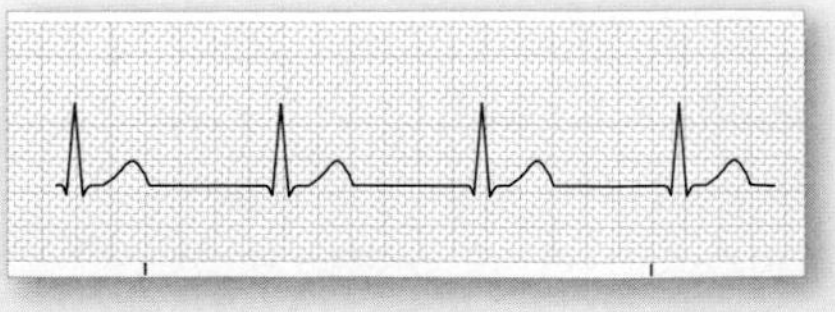	Rate: Atrial rate > 60 bpm, ventricular rate usually > 60 bpm (60–100 bpm is accelerated junctional rhythm) Rhythm: Regular (irregular if escape beats occur) P waves: Cannot be found (nonexistent or hidden; usually inverted if visible) P-R interval: Cannot determine (when present, < 0.12 sec) QRS complexes: Look the same in shape and size; normal (< 0.12 sec) except in abberant conduction	Inferior-wall MI or ischemia, hypoxia, vagal stimulation, sick sinus syndrome; acute rheumatic fever; valve surgery; digoxin toxicity
Ventricular Rhythms		
Premature ventricular contraction (PVC) 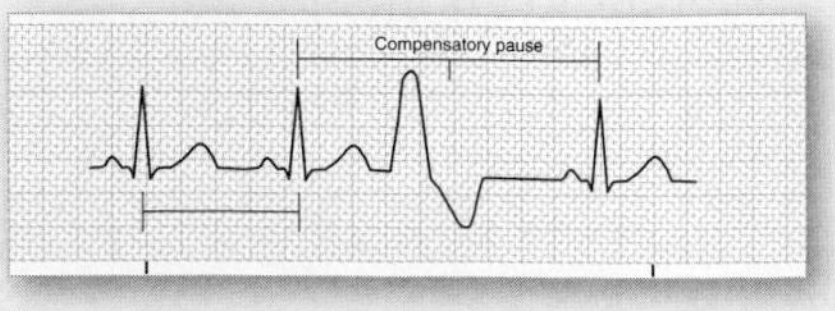	Rate: Irregular Rhythm: Atrial rhythm regular, ventricular rhythm irregular P waves: Cannot be found P-R interval: Cannot determine QRS complexes: Wide and distorted (≥ 0.12 sec); premature QRS complexes occurring alone, in pairs, or in threes, alternating with normal beats; focus from one or more sites; ominous when clustered, multifocal, with R wave on T pattern	Heart failure; previous or acute MI, ischemia, or contusion; myocardial irritation by ventricular catheter or a pacemaker; hypokalemia; hypocalcemia; hypomagnesemia; drug toxicity (digoxin, aminophylline, tricyclic antidepressant, beta-adrenergic blocker, isoproterenol, dopamine); caffeine, tobacco, or alcohol use; psychological stress, anxiety, pain, or exercise

Figure 4-15

Types of cardiac dysrhythmias.

Dysrhythmia	Features	Causes
Ventricular tachycardia 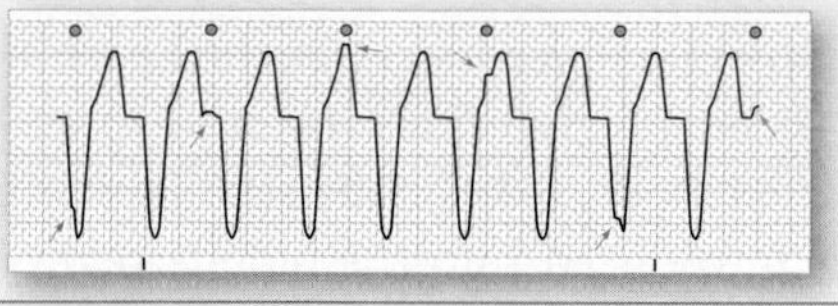	Rate: > 100 bpm Rhythm: Regular P waves: Cannot be found (hidden within QRS complex) P-R interval: Cannot determine QRS complexes: Look the same in shape and size; wide and bizarre (≥ 0.12 sec)	Myocardial ischemia, MI, or aneurysm; coronary artery disease; rheumatic heart disease; mitral valve prolapse; heart failure; cardiomyopathy; ventricular catheters; hypokalemia; hypercalcemia; hypomagnesemia; pulmonary embolism; digoxin, procainamide, epinephrine, or quinidine toxicity; anxiety
Ventricular fibrillation 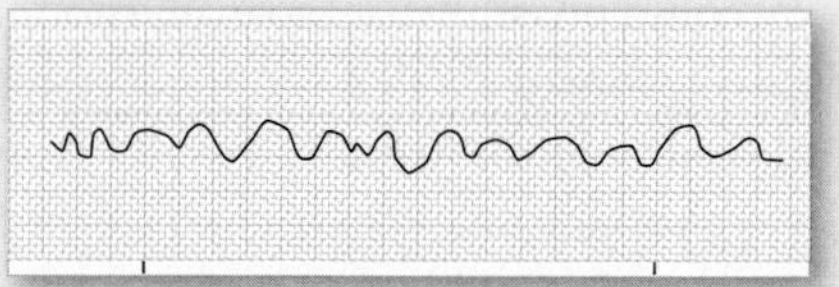	Rate: > 100 bpm Rhythm: Irregular, chaotic, and rapid P waves: Cannot be found P R interval: Cannot determine QRS complexes: Wide and irregular (the ventricle is just "quivering")	Myocardial ischemia, MI, untreated ventricular tachycardia, R-on-T phenomenon, hypokalemia, hyperkalemia, hypercalcemia, hypoxemia, alkalosis, electric shock, hypothermia; digoxin, epinephrine, or quinidine toxicity

Heart Blocks

Dysrhythmia	Features	Causes
First-degree AV block 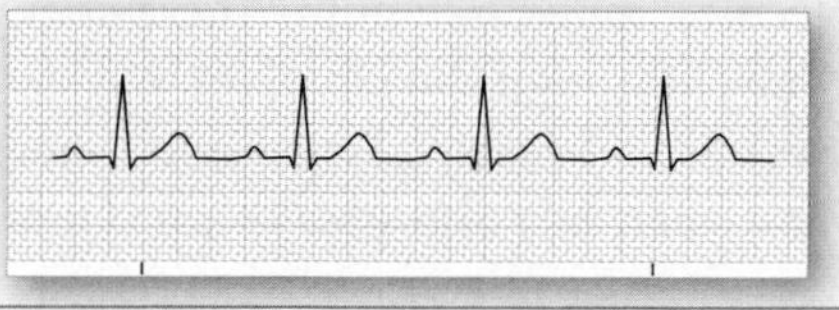	Rate: Varies Rhythm: Regular P waves: Occur before each QRS complex; look the same in shape and size P-R interval: Long (> 0.20 sec) QRS complexes: Occur after each P wave; look the same in shape and size; normal (< 0.12 sec)	May be seen in healthy people; inferior-wall MI or ischemia, hypothyroidism, hypokalemia, hyperkalemia; digoxin toxicity; quinidine, procainamide, beta-adrenergic blocker, calcium channel blocker, or amiodarone use
Second-degree AV block: Mobitz I (Wenckebach) 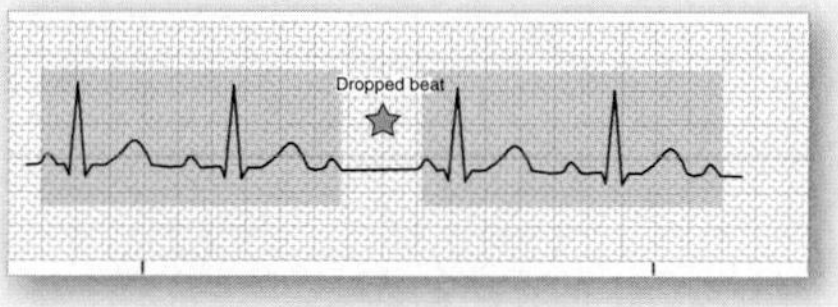	Rate: Slow to normal Rhythm: Atrial rhythm regular, ventricular rhythm irregular P waves: Occur before each QRS complex; look the same in shape and size P-R interval: Normal (0.12–0.20 sec); progressively lengthens until there is a missed beat, then the cycle or grouping repeats itself QRS complexes: Look the same in shape and size; normal (< 0.12 sec)	Inferior-wall MI, cardiac surgery, acute rheumatic fever, vagal stimulation; digoxin toxicity; propranolol, quinidine, or procainamide use
Second-degree AV block: Mobitz II 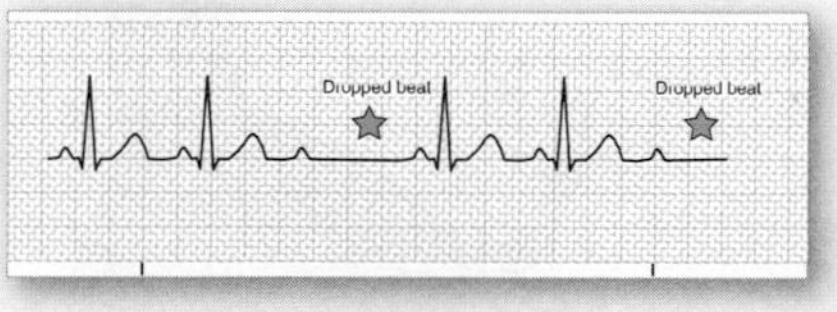	Rate: Slow to normal Rhythm: Atrial rhythm regular, ventricular rhythm regular or irregular, with varying degree of block P waves: Occur before each QRS complex; look the same in shape and size P-R interval: Normal (0.12–0.20 sec); normal P-R interval is key identifier of this rhythm QRS complexes: Look the same in shape and size; normal (< 0.12 sec) if the level of the block is above the bundle of His; wide (≥ 0.12 sec) if the level of the block is below the bundle of His	Severe coronary artery disease, anterior-wall MI, acute myocarditis; digoxin toxicity
Third-degree heart block: Complete heart block 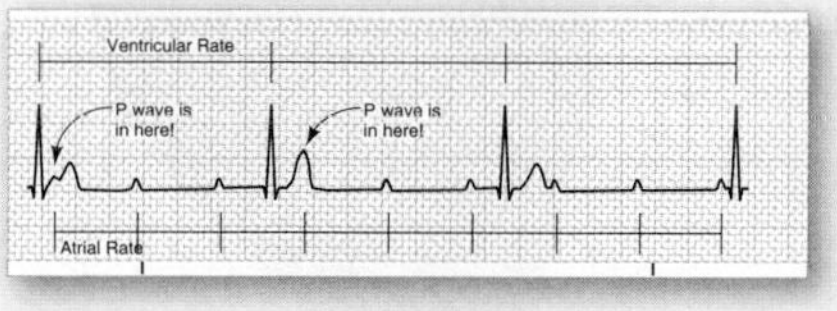	Rate: < 60 bpm Rhythm: Regular (ventricular rhythm rate slower than atrial rate) P waves: Look the same in shape and size (but some are fused into the QRS complex or T wave) P-R interval: Cannot determine QRS complexes: Look the same in shape and size (unless the P wave is fused into the QRS complex); normal (< 0.12 sec) if the level of the block is above the bundle of His; wide (≥ 0.12 sec) if the level of the block is below the bundle of His	Inferior- or anterior-wall MI, congenital abnormality, rheumatic fever, hypoxia; postoperative complication of mitral valve replacement; postprocedure complication of radiofrequency ablation in or near AV nodal tissue; Lev's disease (fibrosis and calcification that spreads from cardiac structures to the conductive tissue); digoxin toxicity
Asystole 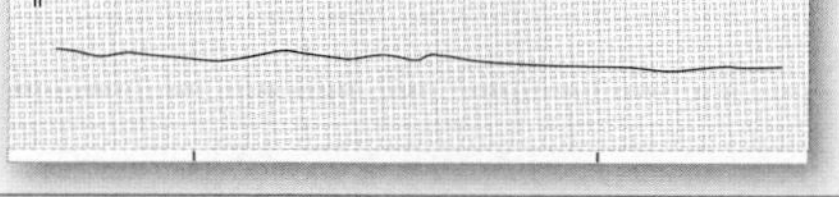	Rate: None Rhythm: None P waves: Not discernable P-R interval: Not discernable QRS complexes: Not discernable	Myocardial ischemia, MI, aortic valve disease, heart failure, hypoxia, hypokalemia, severe acidosis, electric shock, ventricular arrhythmia, AV block, pulmonary embolism, heart rupture, cardiac tamponade, hyperkalemia; electromechanical dissociation; cocaine overdose

Notes: AV = atrioventricular; bpm = beats per minute; CNS = central nervous system; COPD = chronic obstructive pulmonary disease; MI = myocardial infarction.

Figure 4-15 (Continued)

Types of cardiac dysrhythmias.

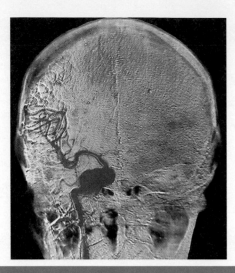

Figure 4-16

Aneurysm: This X-ray shows a ballooning of one of the arteries in the brain. If untreated, an aneurysm can break, causing a stroke.

coronary artery disease, hypertension, and stroke. Lipids are introduced into the bloodstream in two ways—diet and liver production (**Figure 4-18**). Dietary cholesterol is found in animal products (see the Learning Point on p. 89.). Dietary triglycerides are found in saturated fats (e.g., fried foods, cakes). The second way in which lipids are introduced into the bloodstream is through the liver. The human liver makes more cholesterol than the body could possibly use, so even though cholesterol is necessary for survival, it is not necessary to eat it. Familial dyslipidemia usually results from an increase in liver production. When cholesterol is present, it moves through the bloodstream in large molecules much like cooking lard. When triglycerides are present, it moves through the bloodstream in large sticky molecules, much like gum. These sticky, fatty molecules travel through the circulatory system clogging small vessels and coating larger ones, much like what happens when oils and grease are poured down a sink drain.

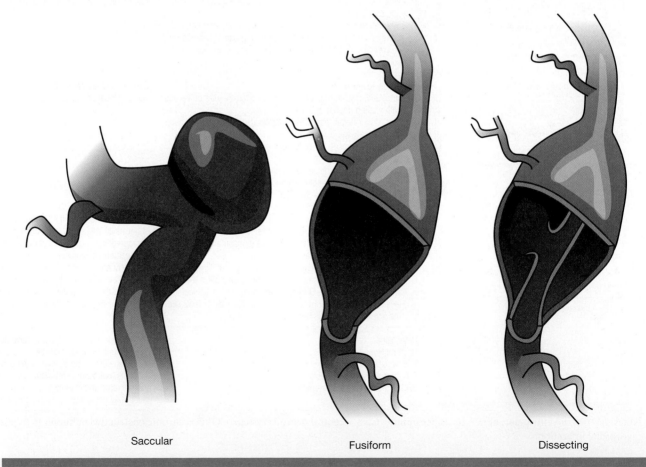

Saccular   Fusiform   Dissecting

Figure 4-17

Types of aneurysms.

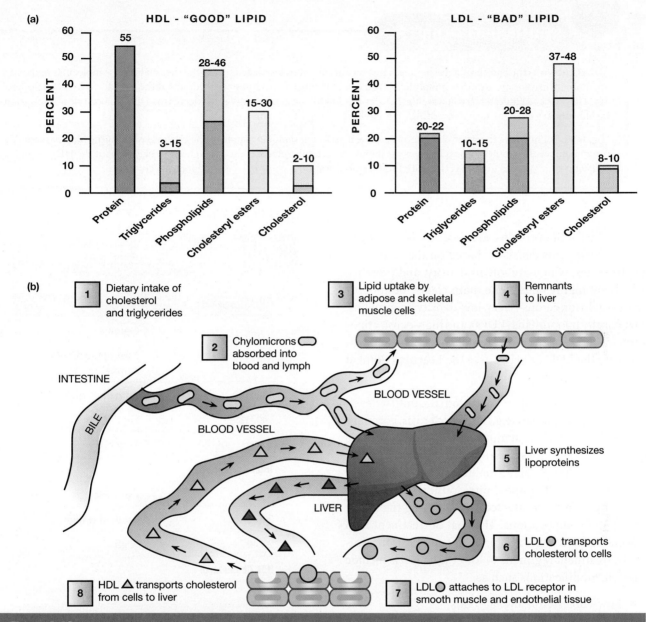

Figure 4-18

Composition and transportation of lipids in the blood. (a) Comparison of HDL and LDL. (b) Transport of lipids.

LEARNING POINTS

Dietary cholesterol comes from animal products. To keep this in mind, remember it *must come from something with a face.* To gauge the amount of cholesterol in the product, think of how many legs the animal has. For example, a cow with four legs has more cholesterol than a chicken with two legs, which has more cholesterol than a fish with no legs. An exception to this rule is deer. A deer has four legs but is a very lean animal; therefore, it has less cholesterol than a cow. When considering pork, it depends on the cut of meat. Bacon has cholesterol content more like beef, and pork chops are more like chicken. Finally, an egg may not have any legs yet, but one yolk has more cholesterol in it than you need all day (the recommended daily allowance is < 200 mg/day). These points create an image that not only helps you remember the cholesterol in foods, but it is great to use with patients because it is easy to remember.

Lipids, or lipoproteins, are classified according to their density. This density is based on the amount of triglycerides, which are low in density, and proteins, which are highly dense. The main classes of lipoproteins are chylomicrons—very-low-density lipoproteins, low-density lipoproteins (LDLs), and high-density lipoproteins (HDLs). The most significant of these lipoproteins are the LDL and HDL (see the Learning Point at the top of this page).

Dyslipidemia is often asymptomatic until it develops into other diseases (e.g., atherosclerosis, coronary artery disease). Then symptoms are related to those diseases. Cholesterol screenings and lipid profiles can identify specific lipid abnormalities (**Table 4-2**). Further testing (e.g., angiography, ultrasounds, and nuclear scanning) can be conducted to determine the development of complications. The goal of treatment is to normalize lipid levels and prevent complications. Initially, treatment regimens to lower lipid levels include lifestyle modifications such as:

- Low-cholesterol, low-fat foods
- Routine exercise
- Weight reduction (if applicable)
- Tobacco cessation (if applicable)

Other treatment approaches are implemented if lifestyle modifications are unsuccessful. These approaches focus on a wide range of lipid-lowering pharmacologic agents (e.g., HMG-CoA reductase inhibitors, bile acid resins, and fibric acid agents). Additionally, other pharmacologic agents (e.g., anticoagulants and antiplatelet agents) may be added to prevent or treat complications.

Atherosclerosis

If lipid levels are not normalized in dyslipidemia, atherosclerosis often develops. Atherosclerosis is a chronic inflammatory disease characterized by thick-

Table 4-2 ATP III Classification of LDL, Total, and HDL Cholesterol (mg/dL)

LDL Cholesterol—Primary Target of Therapy	
< 100	Optimal
100–129	Near optimal/above optimal
130–159	Borderline high
160–189	High
≥ 190	Very high
Total Cholesterol	
< 200	Desirable
200–239	Borderline high
≥ 240	High
HDL Cholesterol	
< 40	Low
≥ 60	High
Triglycerides (mg/dL)	
< 150	Normal
150–199	Borderline high
200–499	High
≥ 500	Very high

ening and hardening of the arterial wall. Lesions (or plaques), comprised of lipids develop on the vessel wall and calcify over time. Development of these lesions causes vessel obstruction, platelet aggregation (collection), and vasoconstriction. Atherosclerosis can lead to peripheral vascular disease, coronary artery disease, thrombi, hypertension, and stroke (**Figure 4-19**).

When arteries are narrowed and hardened, the heart has to work harder to pump the blood through them. In addition to dyslipidemia, other contributing factors to the development of atherosclerosis include diabetes mellitus, hypertension, stress, and tobacco.

Atherosclerosis development is initiated by endothelial injury to the vessel wall (**Figure 4-20**). Dyslipidemia, hypertension, tobacco, diabetes mellitus, elevated homocysteine levels, autoimmune processes, and some bacterial infections can cause this injury. The injured cells become more permeable, suffer from free radical damage, and become inflamed. Leukocytes, macrophages, and cytokines are activated with the initiation of the inflammatory process, which creates more damage. The LDL becomes oxidized and permeates the vessel wall, further contributing to the injury and creating fatty streaks. Fibrous tissue and smooth muscle cells migrate, increasing the size of the lesion and transforming it into fibrous plaque.

Much like dyslipidemia, atherosclerosis is often asymptomatic until complications develop. Then, clinical manifestations will be related to those specific diseases. Diagnostic procedures for atherosclerosis include those that identify contributing factors (e.g., lipid levels). Increased C-reactive protein levels indicate the presence of inflammation and are considered a risk factor. Other diagnostic procedures are used to determine complication development (e.g., angiography, ultrasounds, and nuclear scanning). Treatment is similar to that for dyslipidemia with the addition of angioplasty to open occluded arteries, bypass procedures to detour blood around the occlusions, laser procedures to disintegrate the plaque, and atherectomy to remove the plaque.

Peripheral Vascular Disease

Peripheral vascular disease (PVD) refers to a narrowing in the peripheral vessels (arteries or veins).

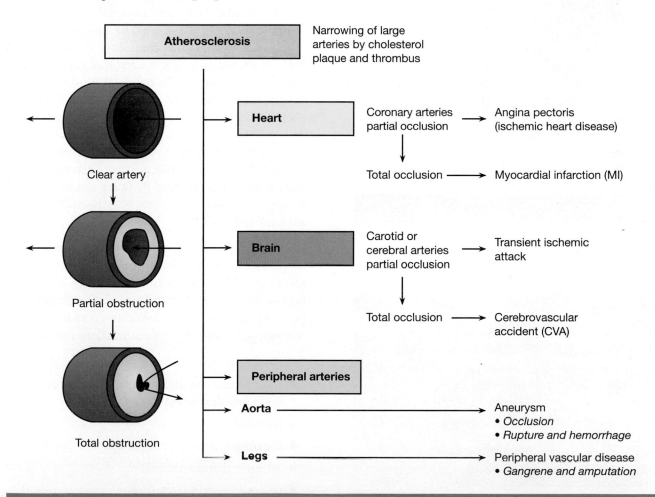

Figure 4-19

Possible complications of atherosclerosis.

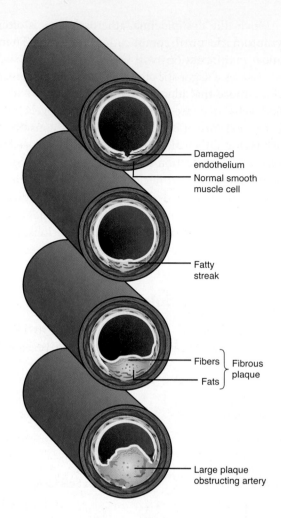

Damaged endothelium
Normal smooth muscle cell

Fatty streak

Fibers } Fibrous
Fats } plaque

Large plaque obstructing artery

☐ Fatty deposits accumulate in the wall of the artery

Figure 4-20

Development of atherosclerosis.

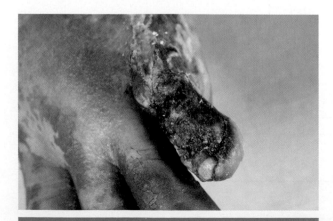

Figure 4-21

Thromboangiitis obliterans.

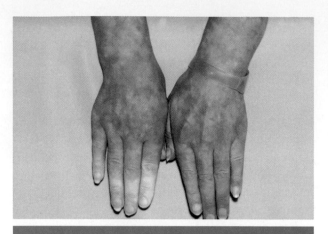

Figure 4-22

Raynaud's phenomenon.

Most often this condition is caused by atherosclerosis, but it can also be caused by a thrombus, inflammation (e.g., thromboangiitis obliterans), or vasospasms (e.g., Raynaud's disease and Raynaud's phenomenon). Thromboangiitis obliterans, or Buerger's disease, is an inflammatory condition of the arteries (**Figure 4-21**). Raynaud's disease is a result of vasospasms of arteries, most often of the hands, that occur because of sympathetic stimulation (**Figure 4-22**). Raynaud's phenomenon describes when these vasospasms occur with an autoimmune disease (e.g., systemic lupus erythemia and scleroderma). As vessel occlusion increases, the ischemia to the affected tissue becomes worse. Risk factors to developing PVD are similar to those for developing atherosclerosis with the addition of an autoimmune disease.

Clinical manifestations of PVD are related to the local tissue ischemia and appear in the extremities. Most symptoms appear in the presence of activity because the oxygen demand exceeds the oxygen supply. The presence of symptoms at rest is an indicator of worsening disease. These manifestations include:

- Pain
- Intermittent claudication (pain that occurs in the lower legs during activity)
- Numbness
- Burning
- Wounds that do not heal
- Changes in skin color (pallor, cyanosis, rubor)
- Hair loss, especially to areas furthest from the heart, like the toes
- Impotency

Diagnostic procedures for PVD include a history, physical examination, ankle/brachial index (compares blood pressure in the arms and the legs), treadmill exercise test, angiography, ultrasounds, and MRI. Treatment strategies for PVD include controlling or reducing contributing factors (e.g., by making dietary changes or by tobacco cessation, physical activity, weight reduction, stress reduction, diabetes management, and hypertension control) in addition to direct intervention of the occlusion (e.g., angioplasty, bypass procedures, laser procedures, and atherectomy). Pharmacologic management includes antiplatelet agents, anticoagulants, thrombolytics, and lipid-lowering medications.

Coronary Artery Disease

When atherosclerosis develops in the arteries supplying the myocardium, coronary artery disease (CAD) develops. In CAD, blood flow temporarily diminishes in the coronary arteries, causing subsequent oxygen reduction to the cardiac muscle. This reduction in oxygen to the cardiac muscle produces chest pain, or angina. Decreased blood flow may or may not cause permanent damage to the myocardium, or infarction. Along with atherosclerosis (the most common cause), vasospasm is another prevalent cause of CAD. Other causes of CAD include cardiomyopathy and thrombi. Additional contributing—some modifiable and some not—factors of CAD are similar to those for atherosclerosis (e.g., diabetes mellitus, hypertension, stress, and tobacco) (Table 4-3). Despite great advancements in treatment, cardiovascular disease (including CAD) is the leading cause of death in the United States for both men and women. CAD is also the leading cause of myocardial infarctions (CDC, 2007).

The left ventricle is the most susceptible to ischemic damage because more arteries supply it to meet its increased needs. With CAD, oxygen supply is insufficient to meet oxygen demand. As ischemia develops, lactic acid and metabolic waste accumulate, causing angina. This accumulation can stimulate other nerves, causing the pain to radiate. Additionally, ischemia causes EKG changes (usually ST segment depression). Reducing oxygen demand reverses ischemia and, in turn, reduces pain. Stable angina pectoris refers to ischemia that is initiated by increased demand (activity) and relieved with the reduction of that demand (rest).

When plaque ulcerates, inflammation occurs, platelets aggregate, and thrombi form. This cascade of events further diminishes the blood supply. As a result, platelets release thromboxane A_2, a potent vasoconstrictor, causing the arteries to spasm. These spasms create an unrelenting cycle of more platelet aggregation and more spasms. Eventually, chest pain becomes unpredictable, occurs at rest, or increases in frequency or intensity. This change in pain is known as unstable angina, and it is considered a preinfarction state.

In addition to causing myocardial infarctions, CAD can cause heart failure, dysrhythmias, and sudden death. Clinical manifestations of CAD include:

- Angina that can radiate to other locations (e.g., jaw, neck, arm, back)
- Indigestion-like sensation
- Nausea and vomiting
- Cool, clammy extremities
- Diaphoresis
- Fatigue

Table 4-3 Risk Factors for Coronary Artery Disease

Nonmodifiable	Modifiable	Negative Risk Factor
Age: men ≤ 45 y; women ≤ 55 y or premature menopause	Tobacco use, obesity, physical inactivity	High HDL cholesterol
Gender	Diabetes mellitus	
Family history: history of premature coronary artery disease in first-degree male relative < 55 y or first-degree female relative < 65 y	Hyperlipidemia	
	Hypertension	

Source: Madara, M., & Pomarico-Denino, V. (2008). *Quick look nursing: Pathophysiology* (2nd ed.). Sudbury, MA: Jones & Bartlett Learning.

Diagnostic procedures for CAD involve identifying contributing factors (e.g., lipid profile, angiography, and nuclear imaging). Additionally, a history, physical examination, exercise stress test, echocardiogram, and EKG will be informative. Treatment focuses on preventing a myocardial infarction by reducing modifiable risk factors through the same strategies to treat dyslipidemia and atherosclerosis (e.g., dietary changes, tobacco cessation, physical activity, weight reduction, stress reduction, diabetes management, hypertension control, angioplasty, bypass procedures, laser procedures, antiplatelet agents, anticoagulants, thrombolytics, and lipid-lowering medications). Additional medications that may be added to the regimen include nitrates, beta-adrenergic blockers, and calcium channel blockers to vasodilate the coronary arteries and increase the oxygen supply. Oxygen therapy may also be used to increase oxygen supply.

Thrombi and Emboli

A **thrombus** is a blood clot that consists of platelets, fibrin, erythrocytes, and leukocytes. These clots can form anywhere in the circulatory system. Three conditions—endothelial injury, sluggish blood flow, and increased coagulopathy—referred to as Virchow's triad, promote thrombus formation (**Figure 4-23**). When a vessel wall is injured, the endothelial damage attracts platelets and inflammatory mediators stimulating clot formation. Stagnant blood flow allows platelets and clotting factors to accumulate and adhere to the vessel wall. Hypercoagulopathy states promote clot formation inappropriately.

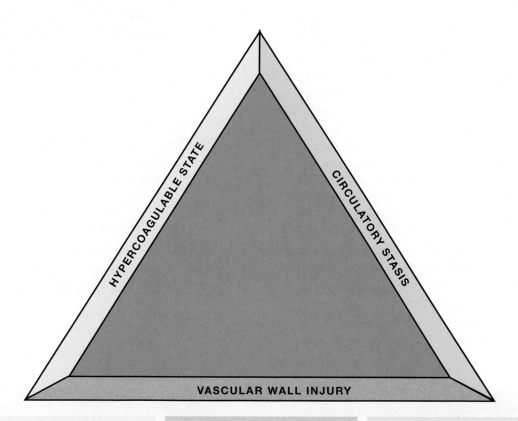

- Malignancy
- Pregnancy and peripartum period
- Estrogen therapy
- Trauma or surgery of lower extremity, hip, abdomen, or pelvis
- Inflammatory bowel disease
- Nephrotic syndrome
- Sepsis
- Thrombophilia

- Trauma or surgery
- Venepuncture
- Chemical irritation
- Heart valve disease or replacement
- Atherosclerosis
- Indwelling catheters

- Atrial fibrillation
- Left ventricular dysfunction
- Immobility or paralysis
- Venous insufficiency or varicose veins
- Venous obstruction from tumor, obesity, or pregnancy

Figure 4-23

Virchow's triad.

The consequences of thrombus formation include the occlusion of a blood vessel or emboli development. An **embolus** occurs when a portion or all of the thrombus breaks loose and travels through the circulatory system until it embeds in a smaller vessel. In addition to thrombi, any other traveling bodies (e.g., air, fat, tissue, bacteria, amniotic fluid, tumor cells, and foreign substances) can become emboli.

Emboli that originate in the venous circulation, such as with deep vein thrombus (**Figure 4-24**), travel to the right side of the heart and then on to the pulmonary circulation, creating a pulmonary embolism (**Figure 4-25**). Most emboli in the arterial system originate in the left side of the heart and travel to other organs such as the brain and heart, causing an infarction.

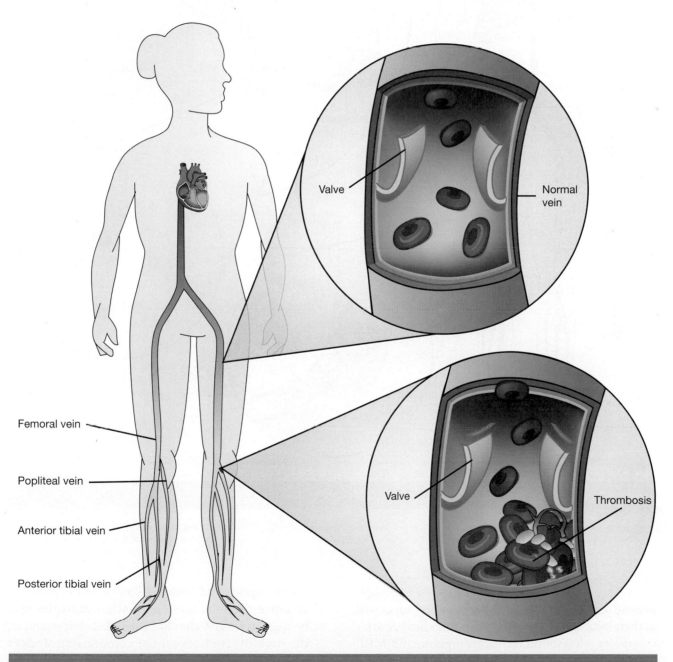

Figure 4-24

Deep vein thrombosis.

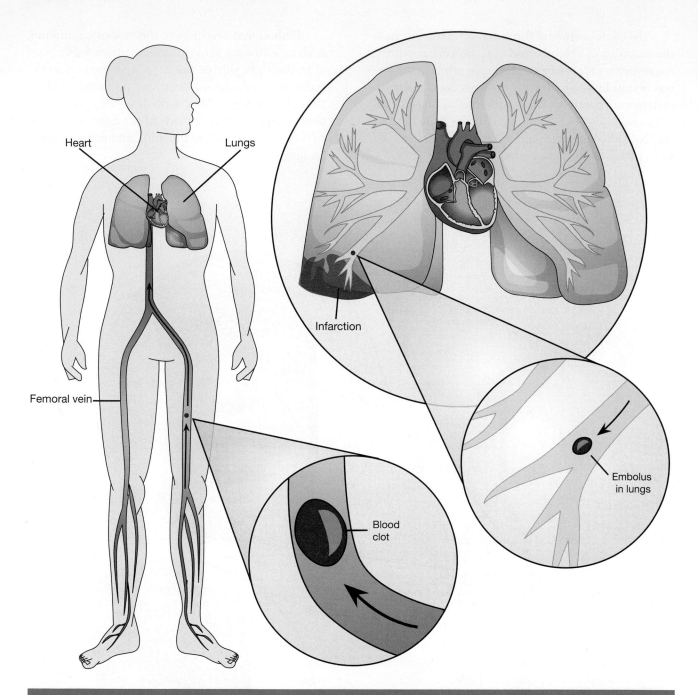

Figure 4-25

Pulmonary embolism.

Clinical manifestations of thrombi and emboli depend on whether they are arterial or venous, as well as their location. Diagnostic procedures include arteriography, ultrasound, echocardiogram, and MRI. Treatment centers on prevention with increasing mobility, hydration, antiembolism hose, sequential compression devices, and medications (e.g., anti-platelet agents and anticoagulants). In the presence of active thrombi, these prevention strategies may be dangerous and should be avoided. For example, the mobility and sequential compression devices may dislodge a stationary clot. Treatment of active thrombi may include thrombolytic agents or an embolectomy.

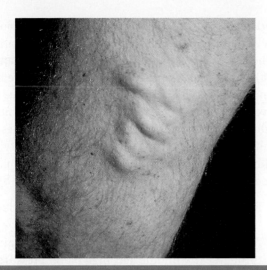

Figure 4-26

Varicose veins.

Varicose Veins

Varicose veins, or varicosities, are dilated, tortuous, engorged veins that develop because of improper venous valve function (**Figure 4-26**). The most common location is the legs, but they can be found in the esophagus (esophageal varices) and the rectum (hemorrhoids). Increased venous pressure and blood pooling cause the veins to enlarge, stretching the valves. The valves become incompetent, blood flow is reversed, and venous pressure and distention are further increased. Capillary pressure increases, causing fluid and pigment to leak out, leading to edema and skin discoloration. As a result, stasis pigmentation (brown skin discoloration), subcutaneous induration (thick, hardened skin), dermatitis (skin inflammation), and thrombophlebitis (vein inflammation resulting from a thrombus) can occur. The pressure caused by the edema can decrease circulation, resulting in metabolic needs not being met. Not meeting cellular oxygen and nutrient needs can lead to necrosis and venous stasis ulcers. Risk factors for developing varicosites include:

- Genetic predisposition
- Pregnancy
- Obesity
- Prolonged sitting or standing
- Alcohol abuse and liver disorders (esophageal varices)
- Constipation (hemorrhoids)

Clinical manifestations are usually minor and include:

- Irregular, purplish, bulging veins
- Pedal edema
- Fatigue
- Aching in the legs
- Shiny, pigmented, hairless skin on the legs and feet
- Skin ulcer formation

Diagnosis of varicosities is usually accomplished through visualization during physical examination. Additional tests may include Doppler ultrasounds and venograms. Treatment ranges from conservative to invasive and includes:

- Rest with the affected leg elevated
- Compression stockings
- Avoiding prolong standing or sitting
- Exercise
- Sclerotherapy (injection of a sclerosing agent that produces fibrosis inside the vessel)
- Surgical removal

Lymphedema

Lymphedema refers to swelling, usually in the arms and legs, because of lymph obstruction (**Figure 4-27**).

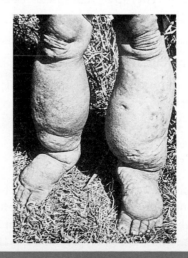

Figure 4-27

Lymphedema.

Lymphedema can occur on its own (called primary) or because of another disease or condition (called secondary). Primary lymphedema is rare and related to a congenital absence or decreased number of lymphatics. Secondary lymphedema is usually related to one of the following:

- Surgery (when lymph nodes and lymph vessels are removed or severed, like with a mastectomy)
- Radiation (causes scarring and inflammation of lymph nodes or lymph vessels, restricting flow of the lymph)
- Cancer (occludes lymphatic vessels)
- Infection (can infiltrate lymph vessels and lymph nodes, restricting the flow of lymph fluid)
- Injury (damages lymph nodes or lymph vessels)

Clinical manifestations of lymphedema include edema and skin changes. The edema may be unilateral or bilateral, and it usually occurs in the extremities. Skin changes include hyperpigmentation, ulcerations, and thickening (referred to as brawny edema). The skin begins to appear like elephant skin, thick and rough. Diagnostic procedures consist of a physical examination, MRI, CT, Doppler ultrasound, and nuclear imaging. Treatment of lymphedema includes:

- Sequential compression devices
- Compression stockings
- Exercise
- Massage therapy (complex decongestive physiotherapy)
- Antibiotics (to treat existing infections)
- Benzopyrone agents (to increase lymphatic flow)
- Diuretics (to remove excess fluid as it returns to the circulatory system)
- Surgery (to remove excess skin)

Hypertension

Hypertension is a prolonged elevation in blood pressure. It is one of the most prevalent chronic health conditions in the United States, affecting about 50 million Americans (CDC, 2008). Hypertension is the leading risk factor for cardiovascular disease (e.g., coronary artery disease, myocardial infarction, and stroke). In hypertension, the heart is working harder than normal to pump the blood to all the parts of the body. This work is due in part to vasoconstriction that increases

afterload. Because of this vasoconstriction, renal blood flow decreases, resulting in an inappropriate activation of the renin-angiotensin-aldosterone system (**Figure 4-28**). A classification scheme for blood pressure has been developed by the Joint National Committee on Prevention, Detection, Evaluation, and Treatment of High Blood Pressure (JNC7) (National Institutes of Health, 2004). JNC7 provides guidelines for classifying children, adolescents, and adults, as well as treatment based on those classifications (**Table 4-4; Table 4-5**).

Risk factors for developing hypertension include:

- Age (vessel compliance decreases with aging; through early middle age, high blood pressure is more common in men, and women are more likely to develop high blood pressure after menopause)
- Race (particularly African Americans)
- Family history
- Being overweight or obese (excessive weight amplifies oxygen and nutrient needs, circulating blood volume increases to meet growing needs, and the increased volume intensifies pressure on artery walls)
- Being physically inactive (increases heart rate, which increases cardiac workload)
- Using tobacco (nicotine immediately raises blood pressure temporarily, and the chemicals in tobacco can damage artery walls)
- High-sodium diet (too much sodium causes fluid retention, which increases blood pressure)
- Low-potassium diet (potassium helps balance the amount of sodium in cells; without enough potassium, too much sodium accumulates in the blood)
- High–vitamin D intake (uncertain; vitamin D may affect the renin-angiotensin-aldosterone system)
- Excessive alcohol consumption (over time, heavy drinking, more than two–three drinks in one sitting, can damage the heart)
- Stress (high levels of stress can lead to a temporary, but dramatic, increase in blood pressure)
- Certain chronic conditions (including dyslipidemia, diabetes mellitus, renal disease, and sleep apnea)

Hypertension is divided into two major forms—primary and secondary. In most hypertension cases in adults, there is no identifiable cause. This type of hypertension, called **primary hypertension** or **essential** hypertension, tends to develop gradually over many years. The other cases of hypertension are caused by an underlying condition. This type of hypertension, called secondary hypertension, tends to appear suddenly and cause higher blood pressure than does primary hypertension. Various conditions and medications can lead to secondary hypertension, including:

- Renal disease (e.g., renal artery stenosis, polycystic kidney disease, and diabetic nephropathy)
- Adrenal gland tumors
- Certain congenital heart defects (e.g., coarctation of the aorta)
- Certain medications (e.g., birth control pills, antihistamines, decongestants, and glucocorticoid steroids)
- Illegal drugs (e.g., cocaine and amphetamines)

An additional form is malignant hypertension. Malignant hypertension is an intensified form that may not respond well to treatment efforts. Occasionally, hypertension is classified as systolic or diastolic, depending which measurement is elevated. Often elderly persons have higher systolic readings and lower diastolic readings because of aging changes.

Hypertension can also occur during pregnancy, which is called pregnancy-induced hypertension (PIH). Other names for PIH include toxemia and preeclampsia. Indicators of PIH include high blood pressure, proteinuria, and edema. PIH can worsen, leading to eclampsia. In eclampsia, seizures often occur because of the PIH. Risk factors for developing PIH include a history of PIH, renal disease, diabetes mellitus, multiple fetuses, and maternal age less than 20 years or greater than 40 years. PIH can lead to multiple problems including miscarriages, poor fetal development, and placental abruption. Management focuses on prevention and nonpharmacologic measures to protect the fetus. Treatment measures include bed rest and magnesium sulfate (to prevent seizures).

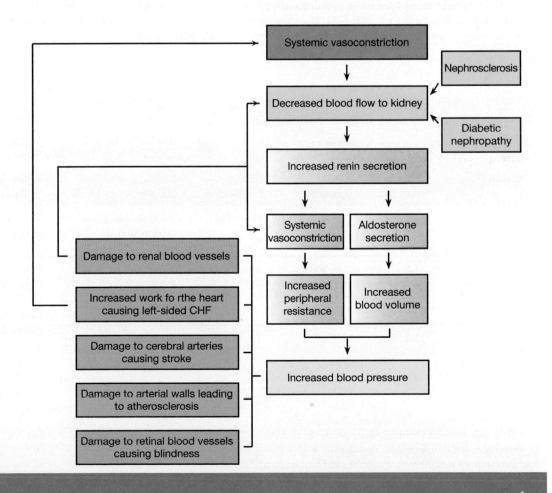

Figure 4-28

Development of hypertension.

Table 4-4 JNC7 Classifications and Treatment for Adults

BP Classification	SBP* (mm Hg)	DBP* (mm Hg)	Lifestyle Modification	Initial Drug Therapy	
				Without Compelling Indications	With Compelling Indications
Normal	< 120	and < 80	Encourage	No antihypertensive drug indicated.	Drug(s) for compelling indications.†
Prehypertension	120–139	or 80–89	Yes		
Stage 1 hypertension	140–159	or 90–99	Yes	Thiazide-type diuretic for most. May consider ACEI, ARB, BB, CCB, or combination.	Drugs for compelling indications.† Other antihypertensive drugs (diuretic, ACEI, ARB, BB, CCB) as needed.
Stage 2 hypertension	≥ 160	≥ 160	Yes	Two-drug combination for most‡ (usually thiazide-type diuretic and ACEI or ARB or BB or CCB).	

*Treatment determined by highest BP category.
†Treat patients with chronic kidney disease or diabetes to BP goal of < 130/80 mm Hg.
‡Initial combined therapy should be used cautiously in those at risk for orthostatic hypotension.
SBP = systolic blood pressure; DBP = diastolic blood pressure; ACEI = angiotensin-converting enzyme inhibitor; ARB = angiotensin receptor blocker; BB = beta blocker; CCB = calcium channel blocker.
Source: National Institutes of Health (www.nih.gov).

Table 4-5 JNC7 Classifications and Treatment for Children and Adolescents

BP Classification	SBP* (mm Hg)	DBP* (mm Hg)	Lifestyle Modification	Initial Drug Therapy	
				Without Compelling Indications	With Compelling Indications
Normal	< 120	and < 80	Encourage	No antihypertensive drug indicated.	Drug(s) for compelling indications.†
Prehypertension	120–139	or 80–89	Yes		
Stage 1 hypertension	140–159	or 90–99	Yes	Thiazide-type diuretic for most. May consider ACEI, ARB, BB, CCB, or combination.	Drugs for compelling indications.† Other antihypertensive drugs (diuretic, ACEI, ARB, BB, CCB) as needed.
Stage 2 hypertension	≥ 160	≥ 100	Yes	Two-drug combination for most‡ (usually thiazide-type diuretic and ACEI or ARB or BB or CCB).	

*Treatment determined by highest BP category.
†Treat patients with chronic kidney disease or diabetes to BP goal of < 130/80 mm Hg. ACE inhibitor or ARB is recommended for chronic kidney disease.
‡Initial combined therapy should be used cautiously in those at risk for orthostatic hypotension.
SBP = systolic blood pressure; DBP = diastolic blood pressure; ACEI = angiotensin-converting enzyme inhibitor; ARB = angiotensin receptor blocker; BB = beta blocker; CCB = calcium channel blocker.
Source: National Institutes of Health (www.nih.gov).

Hypertension is called the silent killer because many people do not have symptoms. Often when symptoms are present, the hypertension is advanced or the blood pressure is remarkably high. When present, clinical manifestations include fatigue, headache, malaise, and dizziness.

Excessive pressure on artery walls caused by hypertension damages blood vessels and organs. The higher the blood pressure and the longer it goes uncontrolled, the greater the damage. Uncontrolled high blood pressure can lead to:

- Atherosclerosis
- Aneurysms
- Heart failure
- Stroke
- Hypertensive crisis (a severe increase in blood pressure that is a medical emergency)
- Renal damage
- Vision loss
- Metabolic syndrome (a cluster of disorders of metabolism—including increased waist circumference, high triglycerides, low HDL, high blood pressure, high blood glucose levels, and insulin resistance)
- Problems with memory or understanding

Prognosis for persons with hypertension depends on treating any underlying causes and maintaining blood pressure control. Early detection and treatment is crucial to preventing or minimizing complications. Diagnosis for hypertension includes a history, physical examination, multiple blood pressure readings at varying times of the day, EKG, and laboratory tests (e.g., urinalysis, CBC, lipid panel, and a creatinine test) to determine the presence of complications. Treatment of hypertension is based on JNC7 standards (Table 4-4; Table 4-5), and adhering to the protocol will increase the likelihood of successful blood pressure control.

Myocardial Infarction

Myocardial infarction (MI) is death of the myocardium from a sudden blockage of coronary artery blood flow (**Figure 4-29; Figure 4-30**). This blockage may be caused by atherosclerosis, thrombus, or vasospasms. Other names for an MI include heart attack and acute coronary syndrome. Risk factors for an MI include those for atherosclerosis (e.g., dyslipidemia, diabetes mellitus, hypertension, stress, and tobacco). Cardiovascular

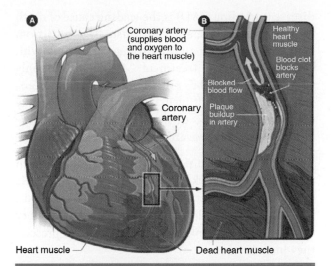

Figure 4-29

Myocardial infarction. (a) An overview of a heart and coronary artery showing damage (dead heart muscle) caused by a heart attack. (b) A cross-section of the coronary artery with plaque buildup and a blood clot.

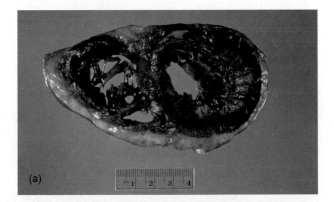

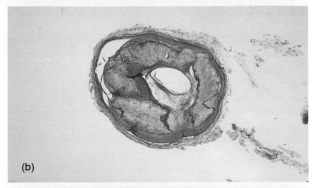

Figure 4-30

Myocardial infarction. (a) Sectioned heart showing myocardial infarction of the posterior left ventricle. (b) Severely occluded coronary artery with calcification from an elderly woman with a fatal myocardial infarction.

disease (including CAD) is the leading cause of death in the United States, and death usually results from cardiac damage after an MI. Prognosis improves with early and aggressive treatment. MIs most commonly occur when a thrombus progresses and occludes coronary blood flow, resulting in myocardial oxygen supply and demand. MIs occur in progressive stages as the blood flow to the myocardium decreases.

Some people do not experience symptoms. An asymptomatic MI is known as a silent MI. Silent MIs generally occur in persons who have diabetes mellitus, neurologic dysfunction (e.g., neuropathy), or history of an MI. When clinical manifestations are present, they include:

- Angina
- Fatigue
- Nausea and vomiting
- Shortness of breath
- Diaphoresis
- Indigestion
- Elevation in cardiac markers (**Table 4-6**)
- EKG changes

Complications are more likely to occur when MIs are not treated early and aggressively. Those complications include heart failure, dysrhythmias, cardiac shock, thrombosis, and death. Diagnostic procedures for MIs consist of a history, physical examination, EKG, cardiac markers, stress testing, nuclear imaging, and

LEARNING POINTS

Initial treatment of an MI can be remembered using the acronym MONA.

Morphine

Oxygen

Nitroglycerin

Aspirin

angiography. Treatment is complex and depends on when the individual sought treatment (**Figure 4-31**). If a patient survives the MI, it is vital that the individual takes steps to prevent another MI through lifestyle modifications and other measures (e.g., dietary changes, tobacco cessation, physical activity, weight reduction, stress reduction, diabetes management, hypertension control, angioplasty, bypass procedures, laser procedures, antiplatelet agents, anticoagulants, thrombolytics, and lipid-lowering medications) to treat atherosclerosis.

Heart Failure

Heart failure, often referred to as congestive heart failure, is a condition in which the heart is unable to pump an adequate amount of blood to meet the body's metabolic needs. This pump inadequacy leads to decreased

Table 4-6 Cardiac Markers		
Marker	**Advantages**	**Disadvantages**
CK-MB	Rapid Cost effective Detected early in infarctions	Loss of specificity with skeletal muscle damage Detection after 6 hours of myocardial necrosis
Myoglobin	Highly sensitive Early detection of MI, within 2 hours Detects reperfusion Most useful in ruling out MI	Low specificity with skeletal muscle injury Rapid return to normal
Troponins	Powerful tool for risk stratification Greater sensitivity and specificity than CK-MB Detects recent MI up to 2 weeks Helpful to determine therapy Detection of reperfusion	Low sensitivity in MI of less than 6 hours Require repeat measures at 8–12 hours if first result is negative Less able to detect late, minor MIs

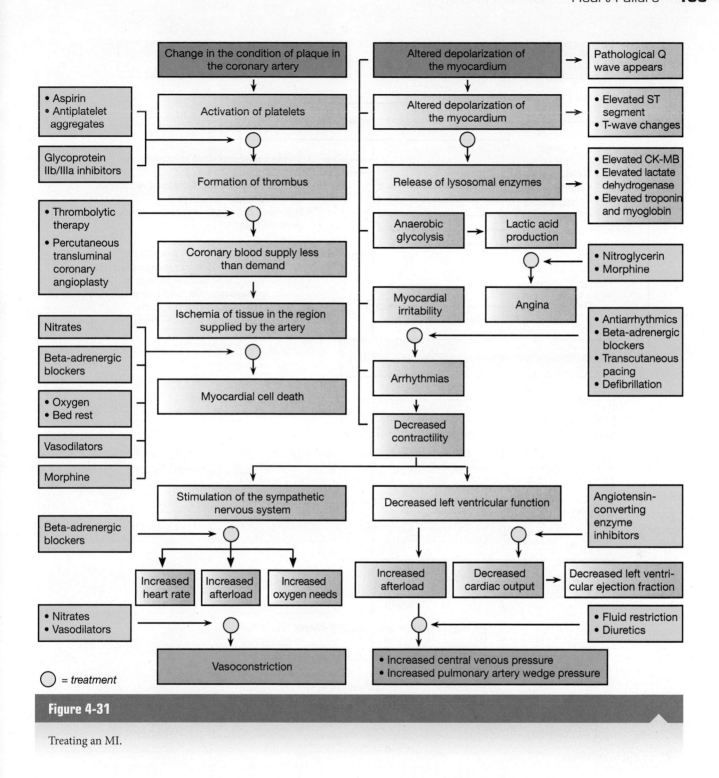

Figure 4-31

Treating an MI.

cardiac output, increased preload, and increased after-load. These three events result in decreased contractility and stroke volume.

Several compensatory mechanisms are activated in times of decreased cardiac output (**Figure 4-32**). Initially, the SNS is stimulated, which increases heart rate, contractility, vasoconstriction, and antidiuretic

hormone secretion. These mechanisms increase cardiac output initially, but they lead to further increased preload and afterload. These compensatory mechanisms maintain metabolic needs until excessive myocardial oxygen demand and preload result in decreased contractility and decompensation. This cycle becomes much like trying to bail water out of a sinking ship. Initially, the efforts to bail the water are able to keep

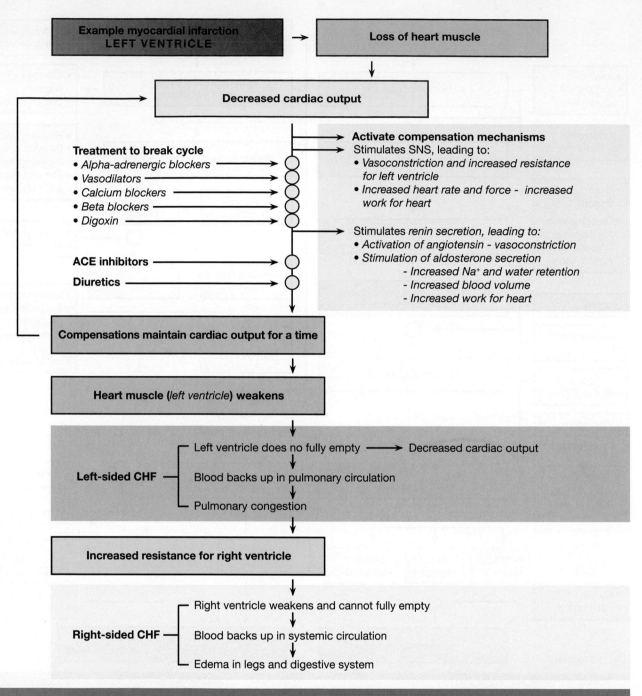

Figure 4-32

Course of heart failure.

the ship afloat, but the incoming water eventually is more than can be removed. Declining cardiac output also leads to decreased renal perfusion, which activates the renin-angiotensin-aldosterone system. This activation further contributes to the vasoconstriction and fluid retention. Ventricular hypertrophy is an additional compensatory mechanism, but this enlarged myocardium eventually outgrows the oxygen supply and decreases contractility. All these compensatory mechanisms are helpful at first, but in the end, they create a vicious cycle.

Heart failure can be categorized in several ways—systolic dysfunction, diastolic dysfunction, and mixed. Systolic dysfunction is characterized by decreased cardiac output due to decreased contractility. The causes of decreased contractility include coronary artery disease (most common), dysrhythmias, dilated cardiomyopathy, chronic alcohol abuse, and myocarditis. **Diastolic dysfunction** is characterized by decreased ventricular filling that results from abnormal myocardial relaxation and increased left ventricular pressure. This type of heart failure is caused by conditions that stiffen the myocardium, such as coronary artery disease, hypertrophic and restrictive cardiomyopathy, and pericardi-

al disease. Most patients have a combination, or **mixed dysfunction**, of systolic and diastolic dysfunction.

Heart failure can be classified as left- or right-sided heart failure (**Figure 4-33**). **Left-sided heart failure** is a result of ineffective left ventricular contractility. As cardiac output falls, blood that is not being pumped out into the body backs up in the left atrium and then the pulmonary circulation. Pulmonary congestion,

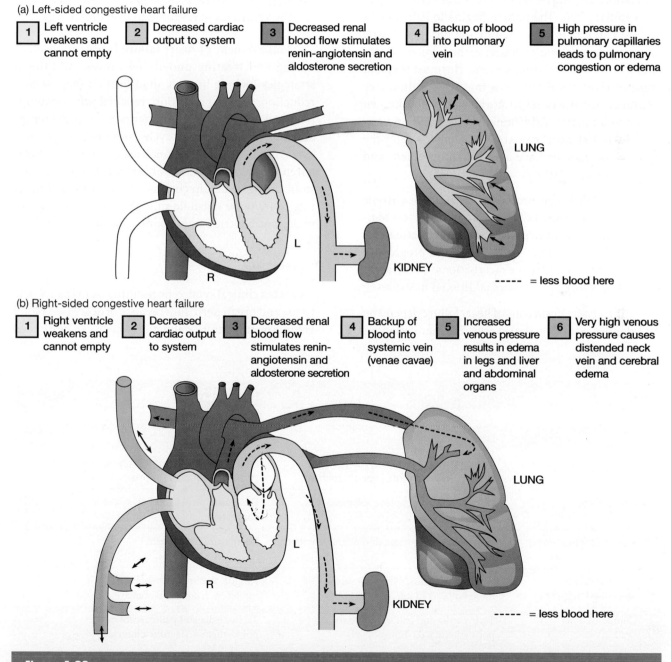

(a) Left-sided congestive heart failure

1 Left ventricle weakens and cannot empty | 2 Decreased cardiac output to system | 3 Decreased renal blood flow stimulates renin-angiotensin and aldosterone secretion | 4 Backup of blood into pulmonary vein | 5 High pressure in pulmonary capillaries leads to pulmonary congestion or edema

----- = less blood here

(b) Right-sided congestive heart failure

1 Right ventricle weakens and cannot empty | 2 Decreased cardiac output to system | 3 Decreased renal blood flow stimulates renin-angiotensin and aldosterone secretion | 4 Backup of blood into systemic vein (venae cavae) | 5 Increased venous pressure results in edema in legs and liver and abdominal organs | 6 Very high venous pressure causes distended neck vein and cerebral edema

----- = less blood here

Figure 4-33

Effects of left and right heart failure.

dyspnea, and activity intolerance develop as blood backs up in the lungs. If blood continues to back up, pulmonary edema and right-sided heart failure will develop. Common causes of left-sided heart failure include left ventricular infarction, hypertension, and aortic and mitral valve stenosis. **Right-sided heart failure** is a result of an ineffective right ventricular contractility. Consequently, blood does not move appropriately out of the right ventricle. Blood backs up into the right atrium and then to the peripheral circulation, causing increased pressures in the peripheral capillary bed. The patient begins to gain weight as fluid is not being excreted by the kidneys. Tissue becomes edematous as pressures in the capillaries push fluid out of the circulatory system. The most frequent cause of right-sided failure is increased pulmonary resistance because of respiratory disease (also known as cor pulmonale). Additionally, pulmonic and tricuspid valve stenosis can strain the right side of the heart. Most patients have a combination of left- and right-sided heart failure.

Heart failure can present as an acute or chronic problem. Acute heart failure may be related to a temporary condition and resolves with the treatment of that condition. Chronic heart failure is a progressive condition that may have exacerbations, or an acute worsening, which will require additional measures.

Clinical manifestations of heart failure depend on the side affected and on the severity. The manifestations of right-sided failure reflect systemic fluid accumulation, while left-sided reflects pulmonary fluid accumulation (**Table 4-7**). Diagnosis of heart failure includes:

- History and physical examination
- Chest X-ray
- Arterial blood gases
- Echocardiogram
- EKG
- Brain natriuretic peptide (a hormone released by the ventricles in response to overstretching)

Management of heart failure begins with identifying and treating underlying causes. Additional strategies include lifestyle modification (e.g., weight reduction, tobacco cessation, reduced salt consumption, and exercise), ACE inhibitors (to stop the renin-angiotensin-aldosterone cycle), diuretics (to remove excess fluid), inotropics (to increase contractility), beta-adrenergic blockers (to slow heart rate to increase diastolic filling), calcium channel blockers (to slow heart rate to increase diastolic filling), biventricular pacemaker, intraaortic balloon pump, and heart transplant.

Shock

Shock is a clinical syndrome resulting from inadequate tissue and organ perfusion because of decreased blood volume or circulatory stagnation. Shock can be divided

Table 4-7 Comparison of Left- and Right-Sided Heart Failure Clinical Manifestations

	Left-Sided CHF	Right-Sided CHF
Causes	Infarction of left ventricle, aortic valve stenosis, hypertension, hyperthyroidism	Infarction of right ventricle, pulmonary valve stenosis, pulmonary disease (cor pulmonale)
Basic effects	Decreased cardiac output, pulmonary congestion	Decreased cardiac output, systemic congestion
Signs and symptoms	Pulmonary congestion, dyspnea, and activity intolerance	Edema and weight gain
Forward effects (decreased output)	Fatigue, weakness, dyspnea, exercise intolerance, cold intolerance	Fatigue, weakness, dyspnea, exercise intolerance, cold intolerance
Compensations	Tachycardia and pallor, secondary polycythemia, daytime oliguria	Tachycardia and pallor, secondary polycythemia, daytime oliguria
Backup effects	Orthopnea, cough, shortness of breath, paroxysmal nocturnal dyspnea, hemoptysis, rales	Dependent edema in feet, hepatomegaly and splenomegaly, ascites, distended neck veins, headache, flushed face

into three categories based on precipitating factors—distributive (neurogenic, septic, and anaphylactic), cardiogenic, and hypovolemic. Shock progresses through three stages that are common to all types of shock—compensatory, progressive, and irreversible. Compensatory mechanisms are bodily activities activated when arterial pressure and tissue perfusion decrease in an effort to maintain cardiac and cerebral function. These compensatory mechanisms include the activation of the SNS and renin-angiotensin-aldosterone system.

The progressive stage begins when the compensatory mechanisms fail to maintain cardiac output. Tissues become hypoxic, cells switch to anaerobic metabolism, lactic acid builds up, and metabolic acidosis develops. This acidotic state further impairs cardiac functioning, causing sluggish blood flow, and increases the risk for disseminated intravascular coagulation (see Chapter 3). Irreversible organ damage occurs as the shock progresses, leading to respiratory and cardiac failure (**Figure 4-34**).

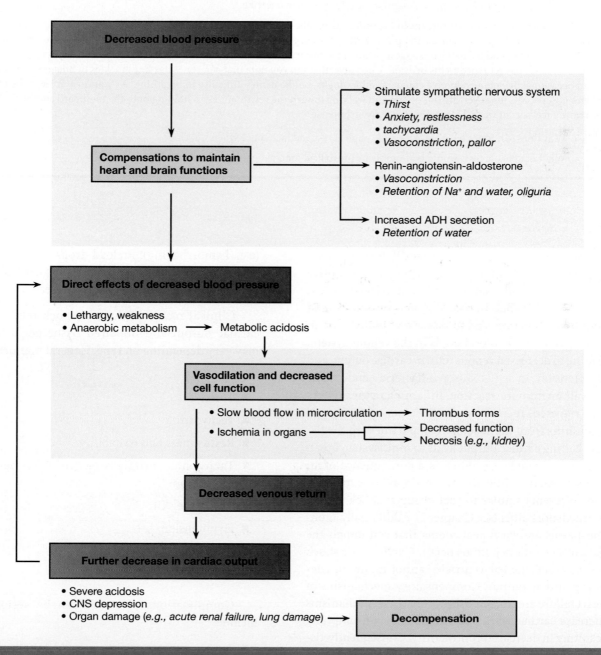

Figure 4-34

Progression of shock.

M r. Jones, a 50-year-old professor, is 5 hours postlaparoscopic cholecystectomy. He is alert and oriented. His physical assessment is within normal limits including active bowel sounds and soft, slightly tender abdomen. He is sipping on clear liquids and conversant. The nurse is performing the final assessment and providing discharge patient education. Mr. Jones states he feels a little tired because of all the excitement about going home and feeling so good after surgery. While checking his vital signs for the discharge form, you notices that his pulse is 110 beats/minute and irregular compared to the 86–90 beats/minute regular pulse, which he had been having since surgery. Mr. Jones states that it is just his excitement; he feels great, and his wife is waiting in the car at the patient discharge area for him.

1. What should you do?

2. Is there any significance in an irregular pulse? If yes, then describe.

The healthcare provider returns to the unit to assess the patient's current condition. The healthcare provider orders a stat EKG and chest X-ray, and cancels the prior written discharge order. The EKG shows atrial fibrillation with a ventricular rate of 118, with QRS and ST patterns suggesting an old anterior wall MI. Mr. Jones continues to rest in semi-Fowler's position in bed. His wife has returned to his bedside. Upon auscultation, you note that Mr. Jones has fine crackles in bilateral lung bases, an occasional dry nonproductive cough, and hiccoughs, but he denies difficulty in breathing. As you turn to leave the room, you observe Mr. Jones getting out of bed and walking toward the restroom. He is holding onto the footboard stating, "I don't know. I feel sort of weak." He appears slightly tachypneic.

3. Why does Mr. Jones have crackles and cough at rest and tachypnea when walking?

4. What diagnostic tests would commonly be prescribed for a patient such as Mr. Jones?

In **distrubutive shock**, vasodilatation causes hypovolemia. There are three types of distributive shock—neurogenic, septic, and anaphylactic. A loss of sympathetic tone in vascular smooth muscle and autonomic function lead to massive vasodilatation in **neurogenic shock**. Blood pools in the venous system, leading to decreased venous return, cardiac output, and hypotension. In **septic shock**, a bacteria's endotoxins activate an immune reaction. Inflammatory mediators are triggered, increasing capillary permeability and fluid shifts from the vascular compartment to the tissue. Falling cardiac output leads to multisystem organ failure. **Anaphylactic shock** is a consequence of an allergic reaction. The allergic reaction leads to a cascade of events similar to that of septic shock, except the mediators differ (see Chapter 2). Additionally, bronchospasms and laryngeal edema that can impair the patient's respiratory status occur. **Cardiogenic shock** results when the left ventricle cannot maintain adequate cardiac output. Compensatory mechanisms of heart failure are triggered; however, these mechanisms increase cardiac workload and oxygen consumption, resulting in decreased contractility. Consequently, tissue and organ perfusion decreases, leading to multisystem organ failure. In **hypovolemic shock**, venous return reduces because of external blood volume losses (e.g., hemorrhaging). Preload drops, decreasing ventricular filling and stroke volume. As cardiac output falls, tissue and organ perfusion decreases.

Clinical manifestations of shock reflect falling cardiac output and impaired tissue perfusion and may vary depending on type. General manifestations include:

- Thirst
- Tachycardia
- Restlessness and irritability
- Tachypnea progressing to Cheyne-Stokes respiration
- Cool, pale skin
- Hypotension
- Cyanosis
- Decreasing urinary output

Complications of shock can be serious and include:

- Acute respiratory distress syndrome (see Chapter 5)
- Renal failure (see Chapter 7)

- Disseminated intravascular coagulation (see Chapter 3)
- Cerebral hypoxia
- Death

Diagnostic procedures for shock consist of a CBC, cultures, coagulation studies, cardiac markers, arterial blood gases, chest X-ray, hemodynamic monitoring, EKG, and echocardiogram. Prompt treatment is crucial for positive patient outcomes. Management of shock includes the identification and treatment of underlying cause, maintaining respiratory status, cardiac monitoring, and rapid fluid replacement.

Chapter Summary

The cardiovascular system is responsible for transporting the body's life fluid to maintain a delicate internal balance. This system has a reciprocal relationship with all the other systems—one in which problems in one create problems in another. Problems in the cardiovascular system are prevalent, and understanding these issues is vital for nurses to provide appropriate care. Prevention of cardiovascular issues often includes lifestyle changes. Early identification and treatment of these conditions are crucial to improve outcomes.

Case Study Answers

Mrs. Fulcher

1. Mrs. Fulcher might have been decompensating and in need of cardiac support.

2. They indicate the presence of microhemorrhages.

3. Signs and symptoms of a stroke (e.g., confusion and paralysis), myocardial infarction (e.g., angina), and pulmonary embolism (e.g., sudden shortness of breath and chest pain).

Mr. Jones

1. Call the healthcare provider to report findings before discharging the patient.

2. Yes, normally the pulse should be regular. An irregular pulse may indicate a dysrhythmia.

3. The dysrhythmia is decreasing cardiac output and causing blood to back up into the lungs.

4. A chest X-ray, echocardiogram, EKG, arterial blood gases, and a brain natriuretic peptide test.

References

Chiras, D. (2008). *Human biology* (6th ed.). Sudbury, MA: Jones and Bartlett.

Elling, B., Elling, K., & Rothenberg, M. (2004). *Anatomy and physiology.* Sudbury, MA: Jones and Bartlett.

Madara, B., & Pomarico-Denino, V. (2008). *Pathophysiology* (2nd ed.). Sudbury, MA: Jones and Bartlett.

Professional guide to pathophysiology (2nd ed.). (2007). Philadelphia, PA: Lippincott Williams & Wilkins.

Resources

www.medlineplus.gov

www.americanheart.org

www.cdc.gov

www.nih.gov

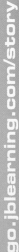

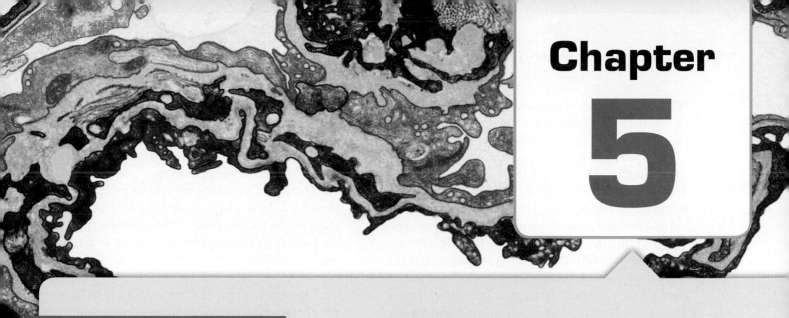

Respiratory Function

LEARNING OBJECTIVES

- Discuss normal respiratory anatomy and physiology.

- Describe and compare infectious disorders of the respiratory system.

- Describe and compare obstructive diseases of the respiratory system.

- Describe and compare restrictive diseases of the respiratory system.

KEY TERMS

active infection
acute bronchitis
acute respiratory distress
  syndrome (ARDS)
acute respiratory failure (ARF)
alveolus
aspiration pneumonia
asthma
atelectasis
bacterial pneumonia
blue bloaters
bronchiole
bronchiolitis
bronchopneumonia
bronchus
chronic bronchitis
chronic obstructive pulmonary
  disease (COPD)
cilium
community-acquired pneumonia
cystic fibrosis

diaphragm
drug-induced asthma
emphysema
epiglottis
epiglottitis
exercise-induced asthma
expiration
expiratory reserve volume
extrinsic asthma
forced expiratory volume in one
  second
forced vital capacity
infectious rhinitis
influenza
inspiration
inspiratory reserve volume
interstitial pneumonia
intrinsic asthma
laryngitis
laryngotracheobronchitis
larynx

legionnaires' disease
lobar pneumonia
lung cancer
minute respiratory volume
mucus
nocturnal asthma
non–small cell carcinoma
nosocomial pneumonia
occupational asthma
perfusion
pharynx
pink puffers
pleural effusion
pleurisy
Pneumocystis carinii pneumonia
pneumonia
pneumothorax
primary TB infection
residual volume
secondary TB infection

severe acute respiratory
  syndrome (SARS)
sinusitis
small cell carcinoma
spontaneous pneumothorax
status asthmaticus
surfactant
tension pneumothorax
tidal volume
trachea
traumatic pneumothorax
tuberculosis (TB)
type A influenza
type B influenza
type C influenza
ventilation
ventilation/perfusion ratio (VQ
  ratio)
viral pneumonia
vital capacity

The respiratory system includes the organs and structures associated with breathing and gas exchange. The structures of the respiratory system are grouped into two branches—the upper respiratory tract (mouth, nasal cavity, pharynx, and larynx) (**Figure 5-1**) and the lower respiratory tract (trachea, bronchi, bronchioles, and alveoli). This chapter will focus on normal and abnormal states of the lungs. The respiratory tract functions automatically to provide cells oxygen and remove carbon dioxide waste. Disorders of the respiratory tract can become serious quickly because of the body's critical need for oxygen. Patients with these disorders will need astute nurses who respond quickly yet thoughtfully.

Anatomy and Physiology

The respiratory system provides vital oxygen and removes toxic carbon dioxide through the act of breathing. The respiratory tract allows one to breathe in and out approximately 23,000 times a day. In fact, if you had a dollar for each breath, you would be a millionaire in a month and a half. The act of breathing allows for gas exchange of oxygen and carbon dioxide. Oxygen is necessary for cells to produce energy through cellular metabolism. Carbon dioxide is the waste product of this process. Through these functions, the respiratory system plays a pivotal role in maintaining homeostasis.

The respiratory system consists of two basic functional divisions—an air-conducting portion and a gas-exchange portion (**Table 5-1**). The air-conducting portion delivers air to the lungs while the gas-exchange portion allows gas exchange to occur between the air and the blood (Figure 5-1). The gas-exchanging portion of the respiratory tract includes the lungs with their millions of **alveoli** and capillaries (**Figure 5-2**).

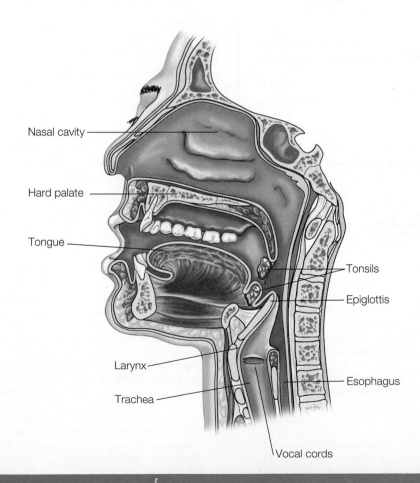

Nasal cavity

Hard palate

Tongue

Tonsils

Epiglottis

Larynx

Esophagus

Trachea

Vocal cords

Figure 5-1

The upper respiratory tract.

Table 5-1 Summary of the Respiratory System

Organ	Function
Air conducting	
Nasal cavity	Filters, warms, and moistens air; also transports air to pharynx
Oral cavity	Transports air to pharynx; warms and moistens air; helps produce sounds
Pharynx	Transports air to larynx
Epiglottis	Covers the opening to the trachea during swallowing
Larynx	Produces sounds; transports air to trachea; helps filter incoming air; warms and moistens incoming air
Trachea and bronchi	Warm and moisten air; transport air to lungs; filter incoming air
Bronchioles	Control air flow in the lungs; transport air to alveoli
Gas exchange	
Alveoli	Provide area for exchange of oxygen and carbon dioxide

Source: Chiras, D. (2008). *Human biology* (6th ed.). Sudbury, MA: Jones & Bartlett Learning.

Air enters the respiratory system through the nose and mouth, traveling to the pharynx. The pharynx joins the larynx, or voice box (**Figure 5-3**). The larynx is made of cartilage and plays a central role in swallowing and talking. When food is swallowed, the larynx rises to be closed by the epiglottis. This process prevents food and liquids from entering the lungs where they would cause severe irritation. Food occasionally enters the lungs, often triggering the cough reflex (a primitive protective reflex). The larynx works much like the strings of a guitar or violin to produce sound—tightening and loosening to change pitch. The larynx opens up into the trachea, or windpipe. From the trachea, the air travels to the mainstem bronchi where it branches into the right and left bronchi, one for each lung (**Figure 5-4**). The left bronchus is narrow and positioned more horizontally than the right. The right bronchus is shorter and wider than the left and extends downward more vertically. Because of the difference in size between the two, objects are more easily inhaled (aspirated) into the right bronchus.

Inside the lungs, the bronchi branch extensively into smaller and smaller tubes, or bronchioles, until reaching the alveoli. This branching from larger to smaller mimics the vessels in the cardiovascular system. The walls of the bronchioles are also like the vessel walls in that they are mostly smooth muscle. The smooth muscle allows for constriction and dilatation of the bronchioles to control airflow. When oxygen needs are higher (e.g., during exercise or stress), the airways open more (dilate) to allow more air to enter the lungs. In times of normal or decreased oxygen needs (e.g., during sleep), the airways may narrow (constrict) slightly. Disease processes may cause constriction to the point of impeding airflow, which becomes dangerous.

The air entering the respiratory tract often contains particles that can be harmful. These particles include infectious organisms (e.g., bacteria, viruses, and fungi) and environmental agents (e.g., dust, pollen, and pollutants). The respiratory system is equipped to filter out some of these particles as well as protect against those that gain entry. The air-conducting portion of the respiratory tract filters many particles by trapping them in the mucous layer (**Figure 5-5**). Mucus is a thick, sticky substance produced by the goblet cells in the epithelial lining of the nose, trachea, and bronchi. This

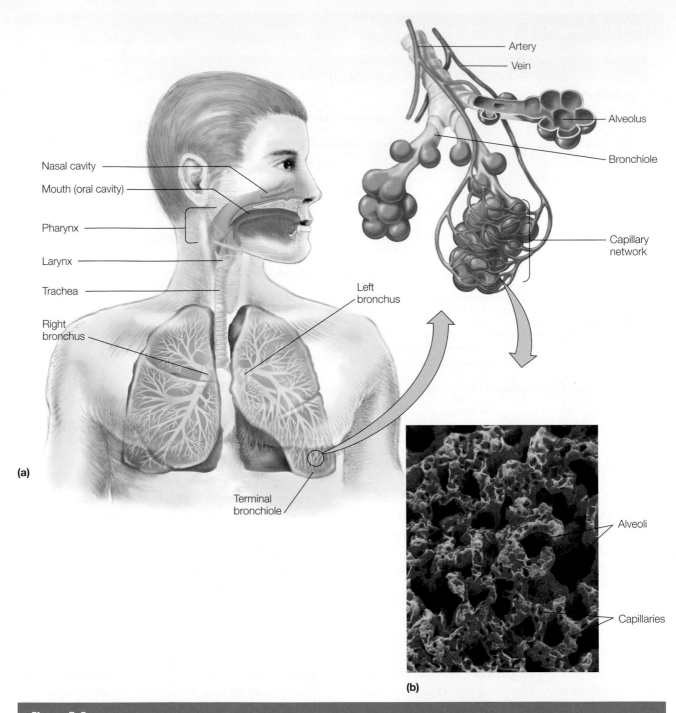

Nasal cavity

Mouth (oral cavity)

Pharynx

Larynx

Trachea

Right bronchus

(a)

Left bronchus

Terminal bronchiole

Artery

Vein

Alveolus

Bronchiole

Capillary network

Alveoli

Capillaries

(b)

Figure 5-2

The respiratory system. (a) This illustration shows the air-conducting portion and the gas-exchange portion of the human respiratory system. The insert shows a higher magnification of the alveoli where oxygen and carbon dioxide exchange occurs. (b) A scanning electron micrograph of the alveoli, showing the rich capillary network surrounding them.

epithelial lining also contains many cilia, hair-like projections, that move in a wavelike motion to propel the mucus and trapped particles upwards to the mouth where they can be expectorated (spit out). Cigarette smoking and air pollution can decrease mucus production and destroy cilia, increasing the risk of respiratory infections. Alcohol consumption can paralyze cilia, also increasing infection risk. Additionally, the immune system is outfitted with IgA cells that prevent the attachment and invasion of bacteria and viruses

on mucous membranes (see Chapter 3). Macrophages are also present around the alveoli in the lungs to keep the lungs clean by phagocytizing particles that gain access (**Figure 5-6**). Once the macrophages fill with particulates, they reside in the surrounding connective tissue. In situations where there are an unusually high number of particulates (e.g., situations that occur with cigarette and marijuana smoking and pollution), the lungs become blackened by the accumulation of the particles.

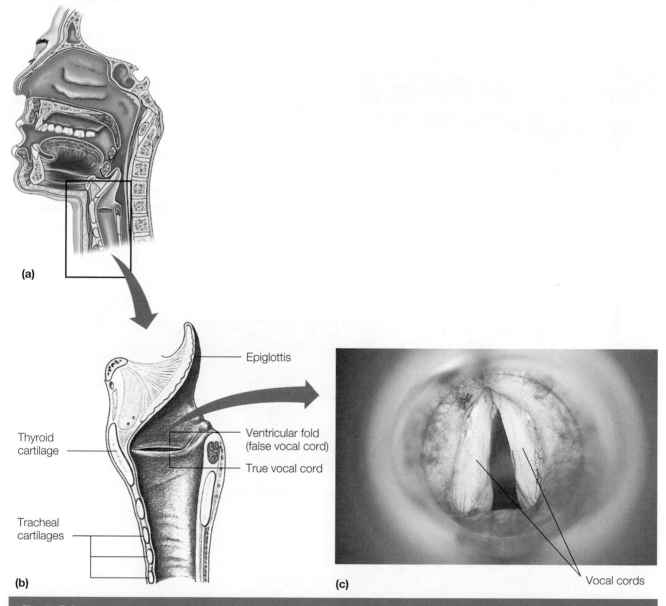

Figure 5-3

The vocal cords. (a) Uppermost portion of the respiratory system, showing the location of the vocal cords. (b) Longitudinal section of the larynx showing the location of the vocal cords. Note the presence of the false vocal cord, so named because it does not function in phonation. (c) View into the larynx of a patient showing the true vocal cords from above.

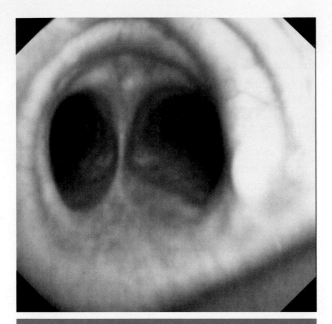

Figure 5-4

The bifurcation of the trachea at the carina into the right and left mainstem bronchi.

The air-conducting portion of the respiratory system also moistens and warms incoming air. An extensive network of capillaries lies beneath the epithelium of the respiratory tract. These capillaries release moisture into the incoming air, humidifying it, to prevent drying of the respiratory tract. The warm blood circulating through the capillaries warms this air prior to entering the lungs, protecting the lungs from cold temperatures. As the air leaves the respiratory tract, much of the water that has been added to the air condenses on the slightly cooler lining of the nasal passages. The condensation is recycled for the next inhalation to conserve water, and contributes to runny noses on cold days.

Alveoli are the site for gas exchange with the bloodstream (**Figure 5-7**). Oxygen is delivered to the alveoli by the air-conducting portion of the respiratory system, and carbon dioxide is brought to the lungs by the circulatory system. Each human lung contains approximately 150 million alveoli that create a surface area that is about the size of a tennis court for gas exchange. The alveoli and capillaries are often a single cell layer thick, which further facilitates gas exchange. The amount of gas exchanged is dependent upon the total surface area and the thickness of the alveoli and capillary walls. The more surface area and the thinner the layers, the more rapidly gas is diffused. Gas exchange in the alveoli requires adequate **ventilation** of air and **perfusion** of blood flow. The **ventilation/ perfusion ratio**, or **VQ ratio**, is a measurement used

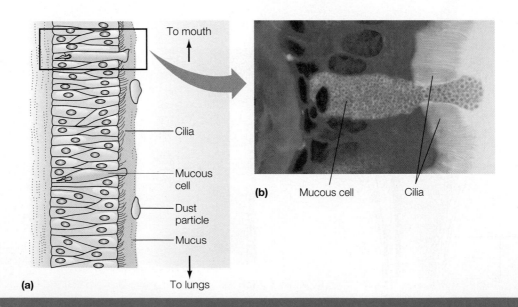

(a)

To mouth

Cilia

Mucous cell

Dust particle

Mucus

To lungs

(b) Mucous cell   Cilia

Figure 5-5

Mucous trap. (a) Drawing of the lining of the trachea. Mucus produced by the mucous cells of the lining of much of the respiratory system traps bacteria, viruses, and other particulates in the air. The cilia transport the mucus toward the mouth. (b) Higher magnification of the lining showing a mucous cell and ciliated epithelial cells.

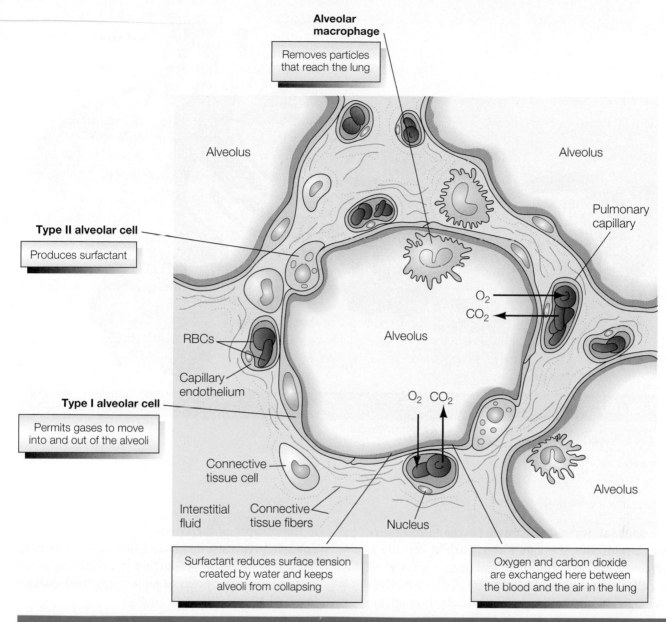

Alveolar macrophage

Removes particles that reach the lung

Alveolus

Alveolus

Pulmonary capillary

Type II alveolar cell

Produces surfactant

O_2

CO_2

Alveolus

RBCs

Capillary endothelium

Type I alveolar cell

Permits gases to move into and out of the alveoli

O_2 CO_2

Connective tissue cell

Alveolus

Interstitial fluid

Connective tissue fibers

Nucleus

Surfactant reduces surface tension created by water and keeps alveoli from collapsing

Oxygen and carbon dioxide are exchanged here between the blood and the air in the lung

Figure 5-6

The alveolar macrophages.

to assess the efficacy and adequacy of these two processes. In the ideal lung, inspired air reaches all the alveoli and all the alveoli have the same blood supply. Actually, neither alveolar ventilation nor capillary blood flow is uniform. The supply of air and blood is never equally matched, even in healthy persons. Because of gravity, the lower parts of the lungs have greater blood flow than the upper parts. Distribution of alveolar ventilation from the top to the bottom of

the lungs is also uneven. Normal ventilation is 4 liters of air per minute, and normal perfusion is 5 liters of blood per minute. This makes the expected VQ ratio 4/5 or 0.8. A VQ ratio higher than 0.8 indicates that ventilation is exceeding perfusion, and a VQ ratio less than 0.8 indicates poor ventilation. Some respiratory disorders are issues with ventilation while others are with perfusion, but regardless, the result is impaired gas exchange.

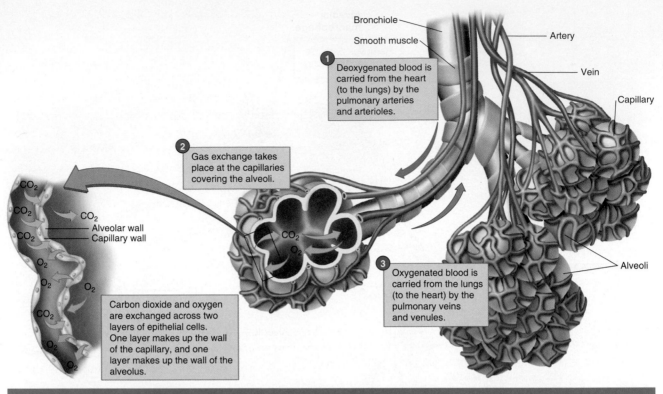

1 Deoxygenated blood is carried from the heart (to the lungs) by the pulmonary arteries and arterioles.

2 Gas exchange takes place at the capillaries covering the alveoli.

3 Oxygenated blood is carried from the lungs (to the heart) by the pulmonary veins and venules.

Carbon dioxide and oxygen are exchanged across two layers of epithelial cells. One layer makes up the wall of the capillary, and one layer makes up the wall of the alveolus.

Bronchiole
Smooth muscle
Artery
Vein
Capillary
Alveoli

CO_2
Alveolar wall
Capillary wall
O_2

Figure 5-7

Gas exchange in the lungs.

Once air is inhaled, gases are exchanged between the alveoli and the capillaries; carbon dioxide is removed through expiration, and oxygen is delivered to cells by the cardiovascular system (**Figure 5-8**). Once hemoglobin carries oxygen to the cells, hemoglobin releases the oxygen. The rate at which hemoglobin binds and releases oxygen is affected by several factors such as temperature, pH, and others (**Figure 5-9**).

The surface of the alveoli contains a substance called **surfactant**. Surfactant is a lipoprotein produced by alveoli cells that has a detergent-like quality. Surfactant is a watery substance that produces surface tension on the alveoli, which enhances pulmonary compliance (elasticity) and prevents the alveoli from collapsing. Because the pressure in the lungs is negative as compared to atmospheric pressure, the walls of the alveoli tend to draw inward, making them collapse. This pressure is much like a vacuum-sealed pack of coffee. This pressure and, therefore, risk of collapse further increase at the end of expiration. Surfactant promotes reinflation of the alveoli during inspiration. Disease states and other conditions can decrease surfactant, leading

to the collapse of the alveoli (called atelectasis). For example, premature infants lack surfactant, and smoking alters surfactant production. Synthetically made surfactant may be given to replace any inadequacies in production.

The process of breathing is largely involuntary and controlled by the medulla oblongata in the brain. This center is located in the brainstem, which controls many vital functions in the body (e.g., heart rate, blood pressure, and temperature). Breathing includes two phases—**inspiration** (inhalation—moving air in) and **expiration** (exhalation—moving air out). Inspiration is an active neural process that begins with nerve impulses traveling from the brain to the **diaphragm**, a dome-shaped muscle that separates the thoracic and abdominal cavities (**Figure 5-10**). These impulses cause the diaphragm to contract, lower, and flatten, which draws air into the lungs. Inspiration also involves the intercostal muscles between the ribs. Nerve impulses cause the intercostal muscles to contract, lifting the ribs up and out. Contraction of the diaphragm and intercostal muscles changes intrapulmonary pressure,

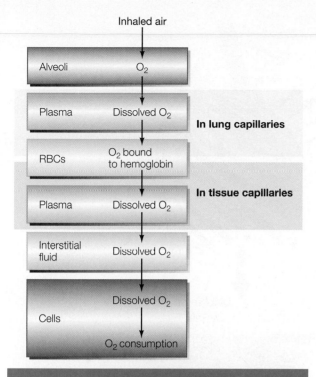

Inhaled air

Alveoli — O_2

Plasma — Dissolved O_2

In lung capillaries

RBCs — O_2 bound to hemoglobin

In tissue capillaries

Plasma — Dissolved O_2

Interstitial fluid — Dissolved O_2

Cells — Dissolved O_2

O_2 consumption

Figure 5-8

Oxygen diffusion: Oxygen travels from the alveoli into the blood plasma, then into the RBCs, where much of it binds to hemoglobin. When the oxygenated blood reaches the tissues, oxygen is released from the RBCs and diffuses into the plasma, then into the interstitial fluid and body cells.

causing air to naturally flow into the lungs. In contrast, expiration is passive—it does not require muscle contraction. As the lungs fill with air, the diaphragm and intercostal muscles relax, returning to their previous position. Returning to their natural position decreases thoracic volume and increases intrapulmonary pressure. Increasing pressure forces air out of the lungs. Elastic fibers in the lungs aid in passive expiration by causing the lungs to recoil. Expiration can also be active by contracting the chest and abdominal muscles. Airflow, both inspiratory and expiratory, can be measured to aid in diagnosis of respiratory disorders (**Figure 5-11**).

The pulmonary function test evaluates lung volumes and capacities. Tidal volume is the amount of air involved in one normal inhalation and exhalation. The average tidal volume is 500 mL, but is less in shallow breathing. The minute respiratory volume is the amount inhaled and exhaled in 1 minute. It is determined by the tidal volume multiplied by the respirations per minute, and the average is 6 liters per minute. The inspiratory reserve volume is the amount of air beyond the tidal volume that can be taken in with the deepest inhalation. Inspiratory reserve volume averages 2–3 liters. The expiratory reserve volume is the amount of air beyond tidal volume that can be forcibly exhaled beyond the normal passive exhalation.

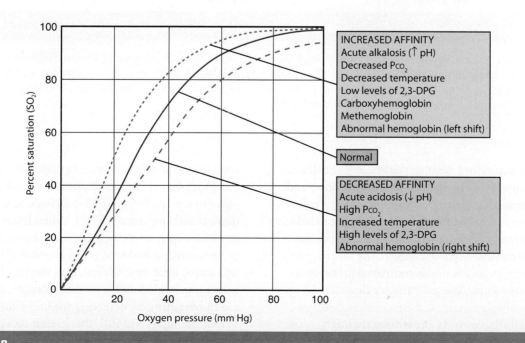

INCREASED AFFINITY
Acute alkalosis ($\uparrow$ pH)
Decreased P_{CO_2}
Decreased temperature
Low levels of 2,3-DPG
Carboxyhemoglobin
Methemoglobin
Abnormal hemoglobin (left shift)

Normal

DECREASED AFFINITY
Acute acidosis ($\downarrow$ pH)
High P_{CO_2}
Increased temperature
High levels of 2,3-DPG
Abnormal hemoglobin (right shift)

Figure 5-9

Oxyhemoglobin dissociation curve.

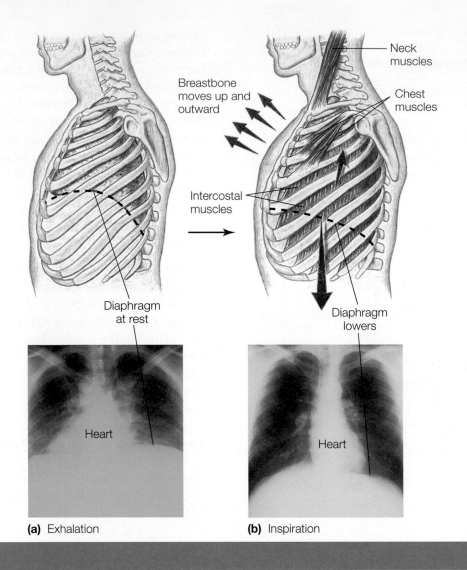

Breastbone moves up and outward

Neck muscles

Chest muscles

Intercostal muscles

Diaphragm at rest

Diaphragm lowers

Heart

Heart

(a) Exhalation

(b) Inspiration

Figure 5-10

Breathing: The rising and falling of the chest wall through the contraction of the intercostal muscles (muscles between the ribs) is shown in the diagram, illustrating the bellows effect. Inspiration is assisted by the diaphragm, which lowers. Like pulling a plunger out on a syringe, the rising of the chest wall and the lowering of the diaphragm draw air into the lungs. Illustrations and X-rays showing the lungs in full exhalation (a) and full inspiration (b).

The average expiratory reserve volume is 1–1.5 liters. The **vital capacity** is the sum of the tidal volume and reserves. There is always air in the lungs, which is called residual volume. Even after the most forceful exhalation, 1–1.5 liters of air remain in the lungs. This ensures efficient and consistent gas exchange. The **forced expiratory volume in one second** is compared to the **forced vital capacity** to diagnose pulmonary disease.

The medulla controls breathing through nerve cells that generate nerve impulses to the respiratory muscles. When the lungs are full, these impulses cease, allowing the muscles to relax. Chemoreceptors inside

the brain and arteries also regulate breathing. These receptors detect carbon dioxide levels and send messages to the medulla. Carbon dioxide levels normally drive breathing (**Figure 5-12**). When levels go up, respiration depth and rate increase to excrete the excess carbon dioxide and vice versa. In some disease states, this drive becomes altered, and oxygen levels drive breathing. Additionally, stretch receptors in the lungs aid in breathing by detecting when the lungs are full. When the lungs are full, the stretch receptors in the lungs send a message to the medulla to cease firing. These stretch receptors prevent overinflation of the lungs (this is called the Hering-Breuer reflex). The body

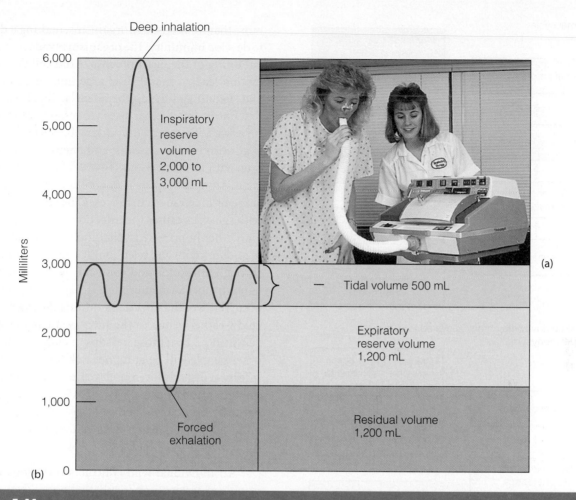

Deep inhalation

Inspiratory
reserve
volume
2,000 to
3,000 mL

Tidal volume 500 mL

Expiratory
reserve volume
1,200 mL

Forced
exhalation

Residual volume
1,200 mL

Milliliters

(a)

(b)

Figure 5-11

Measuring air flow. (a) This machine allows healthcare workers to determine tidal volume, inspiratory reserve volume, and other lung-capacity measurements to determine the health of an individual's lung. (b) This graph shows several common measurements.

LEARNING POINTS

Carbon dioxide is the normal driving force for breathing. This means that breathing is controlled by carbon dioxide levels. How does this translate into action? As carbon dioxide levels rise, the lungs will exhale to expel the excess carbon dioxide. To understand how strong this drive is, consider holding your breath. If you take a deep breath and try to hold it, eventually you have to let the air out. No matter how hard you try, you cannot hold your breath forever. The body can be trained to hold a breath longer and longer (as swimmers and divers do), but no matter the training, you will eventually have to let it out.

also has oxygen receptors, but they are not very sensitive. These receptors do not generate impulses until oxygen levels fall to critical levels.

In addition to regulating oxygen and carbon dioxide levels, the lungs aid in regulating pH by altering breathing rate and depth. Carbon dioxide is a source of acid in the body. Increasing the respiratory rate and depth will excrete more carbon dioxide, making the blood less acidic, and decreasing the respiratory rate and depth will retain more carbon dioxide, making the blood more acidic. This compensatory mechanism allows for a quick fix to pH imbalances to reestablish homeostasis.

(a) Normal cycle

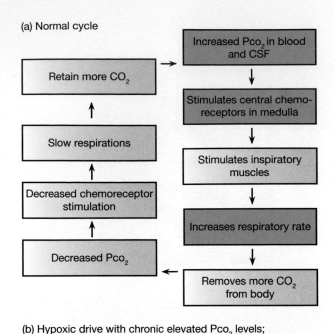

(b) Hypoxic drive with chronic elevated P_{CO_2} levels;
    e.g., emphysema

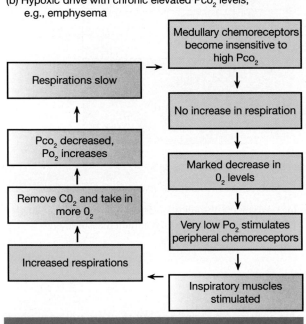

Figure 5-12

Normal respiratory control and hypoxic drive.

Infectious Disorders

Upper Respiratory Tract Infections

Infectious Rhinitis

Infectious rhinitis, or the common cold, is a viral upper respiratory infection. The most frequent culprit is the rhinovirus, but many viruses (e.g., adenovirus, coronavirus, and influenza) can cause it. There are more than 100 causative organisms, making it difficult to develop immunity. The organism invades the epithelial lining of the nasal mucosa. Mild cellular inflammation leads to nasal discharge, mucus production, and shedding of the epithelial cells. This break in the first line of defense increases vulnerability to bacterial invasions. Therefore, secondary bacterial infections (e.g., otitis media, sinusitis, and pneumonia) are common with viral infections (**Figure 5-13**). Despite popular misconceptions, wet and cold conditions do not cause or increase occurrences. Close physical contact with the virus causes the infection through exchanges with other humans (e.g., shaking hands) and surfaces (e.g., doorknobs and telephones). Transmission occurs through inhalation and contact (e.g., hand to hand or hand to mucous membrane). The apparent increase in occurrence of the infectious rhinitis during rainy and cold weather is due to the increased congregation in confined spaces. Those persons in closer contact with other people will be at higher risk for developing the infection (e.g., children in daycare centers, healthcare providers, and teachers). The virus is highly contagious because the virus is shed in large numbers from the nasal mucosa, and the virus can survive for several hours outside the body.

An individual who contracts infectious rhinitis usually experiences an incubation period between the invasion and the onset of symptoms that usually lasts about 2–3 days, but it can last up to 7 days. Clinical manifestations include:

- Sneezing
- Nasal congestion
- Nasal discharge
- Sore throat
- Nonproductive cough
- Malaise
- Myalgia
- Low-grade fever
- Hoarseness
- Headache
- Chills

Diagnosis is primarily made by the presence of symptoms. Treatment is symptomatic. Most over-the-counter cold preparations are ineffective in shortening the course of the infection. Pharmacologic therapies that may be used include antipyretics (for fever), analgesics (for discomfort), antihistamines (for nasal symp-

MYTH BUSTERS

A common misconception is that you get colds from being cold or wet. The fuel for this myth is the increased occurrence of colds during cold and wet weather. The weather conditions themselves do not make you sick. The weather does increase congregation of people indoors to avoid those weather conditions. The congregation of people in close, closed spaces is responsible for the spread of the cold. The virus is virulent and highly contagious through close contact. Misconceptions are hard to change; it usually takes multiple efforts. So do your part to educate the public about the truth of cold transmission and prevention!

Primary viral infection *e.g., influenza or common cold virus*

↓

Virus attaches firmly to respiratory mucosa, invades the tissue, causing necrosis, inflammation, and swelling	→	Congestion Obstructed airways

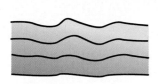 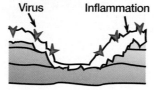 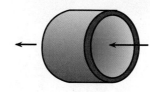 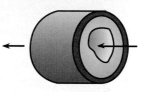

| Healthy mucosa | Necrosis | | Good air flow | Poor air flow |

Virus spreads along continuous mucosa invading ears (*otitis media*), sinuses (*sinusitis*), bronchi and lungs (*pneumonia*)	→	Bacteria, sometimes resistant flora, penetrate the damaged mucous membranes, causing secondary **BACTERIAL INFECTION**

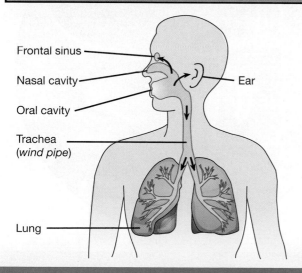

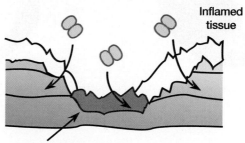

Bacteria invade necrotic area

Figure 5-13

Complications of viral respiratory infections.

toms), decongestants, and antibiotics (only if a bacterial infection is present). Humidifiers can liquefy secretions to aid in expectoration. The benefit of vitamin C in prevention and treatment remains controversial. Proper hand washing remains the long-standing cornerstone of prevention. Other measures will limit the spread of active infections to others, including:

- Covering one's mouth when coughing and sneezing, using tissue or the upper sleeve of one's shirt.

- Disposing of tissue immediately after use.

Sinusitis

Sinusitis is an inflammation of the sinus cavities most often caused by a viral infection. Other causative agents include bacteria and fungi. Sinusitis can be a result of a secondary bacterial infection associated with infectious rhinitis or allergic rhinitis in which the drainage from the sinus cavity has become blocked (**Figure 5-14**). As exudate accumulates, pressure builds in the sinus cavity, which causes facial bone pain. Other clinical manifestations of sinusitis may already be present, such as nasal congestion, fever, and sore throat. Diagnostic procedures for sinusitis include a history, physical

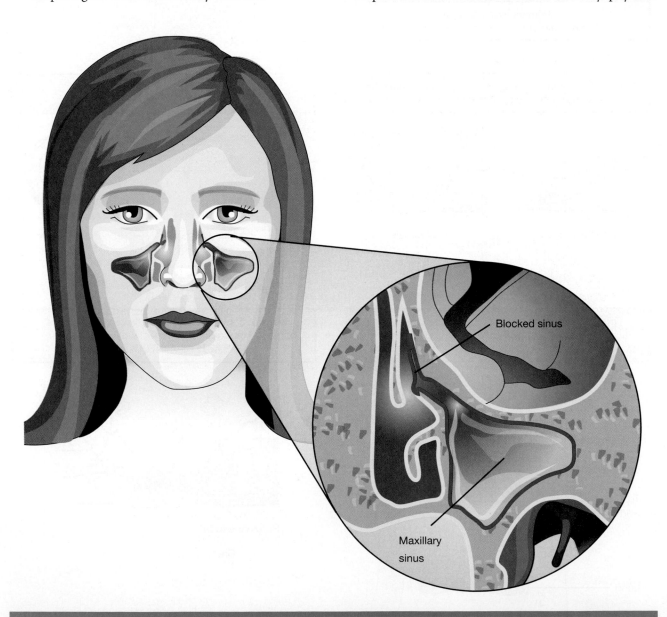

Figure 5-14

Blocked sinus.

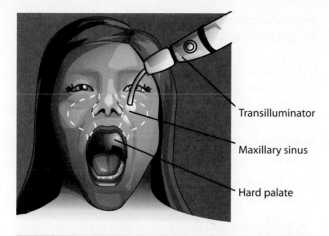

Transilluminator

Maxillary sinus

Hard palate

Figure 5-15

Transillumination of the sinuses.

examination, sinus X-ray, and transillumination (**Figure 5-15**). Treatment usually includes decongestants and analgesics until the sinuses begin draining. Bacterial infections require antibiotic therapy to resolve.

Epiglottitis

Epiglottitis is a life-threatening condition of the epiglottis, the protective cartilage lid covering the trachea opening. Haemophilus influenza type B (Hib) is the most common cause. Hib is a routine infection in children 3–7 years of age, especially those children in daycare centers. Other causes include throat trauma from events such as drinking hot liquids, swallowing a foreign object, a direct blow to the throat, or smoking crack or heroin. The Hib invasion triggers the inflammatory response, causing the epiglottis to quickly swell and block the air entering the trachea, leading to respiratory failure. Hib can also travel to the bloodstream, leading to sepsis, which is also life-threatening because it activates a massive immune response.

The onset of clinical manifestations is typically rapid and includes:

- Fever
- Sore throat
- Difficulty swallowing
- Drooling with mouth open
- Inspiratory stridor (harsh, high-pitched sound made as result of air turbulence)

- Respiratory distress
- Central cyanosis (blue discoloration of the mouth and lips)
- Anxiety (a result of hypoxia)
- Pallor
- Assuming a sitting position (subconscious attempt to facilitate breathing)

If epiglottitis is suspected, maintaining airway and stabilizing respiratory status is a priority before diagnostic procedures are performed. Efforts to preserve respiratory function include oxygen therapy (likely via mask), endotracheal intubation with mechanical ventilation, and a tracheotomy. Once the patient is stabilized, diagnostic procedures include visualization of the epiglottis through a fiber-optic camera, X-rays (throat and chest), cultures (throat and blood), arterial blood gases (ABGs), and a complete blood count (CBC). Intravenous antibiotics will be used to treat infections quickly. Hib vaccinations are available for prevention and should be administered to children, the elderly, and immune-compromised persons. Other prevention strategies include proper hand washing, avoiding crowds, cleaning objects (e.g., toys), and not sharing objects (e.g., pacifiers and bottles).

Laryngitis

Laryngitis is an inflammation of the larynx that is usually a result of an infection, increased upper respiratory exudate, or overuse. With laryngitis, the vocal cords become irritated and edematous because of the inflammatory process. This inflammation distorts sounds, leading to hoarseness and in some cases making the voice undetectable.

Clinical manifestations of laryngitis usually last less than a week and include:

- Hoarseness
- Weak voice or voice loss
- Tickling sensation and raw feeling in the throat
- Sore, dry throat
- Dry cough
- Difficulty breathing (in children)

Diagnostic procedures for laryngitis include a history, physical examination, CBC, and laryngoscopy. A biopsy may be conducted if symptoms persist because throat cancer can mimic acute laryngitis. Treatment depends on the cause, and many times the laryngitis will improve without treatment. Strategies aim to increase comfort or decrease the duration. These strategies include:

- Warm humidity
- Resting the voice
- Increasing fluid intake
- Treating the underlying cause (e.g., infection or gastric reflux)
- Throat lozenges
- Gargling with salt water
- Avoidance of decongestants (they dry out the mucous membranes)

Laryngotracheobronchitis

Laryngotracheobronchitis, or croup, is a common viral infection in children 1–2 years of age. Other children and adults may also contract it. Routine causative agents include parainfluenza viruses and adenoviruses. Croup usually begins as an upper respiratory infection with nasal congestion and cough. The larynx and surrounding area swell, leading to airway narrowing and obstruction. This swelling can lead to respiratory failure.

Clinical manifestations of croup include:

- Nasal congestion
- Seallike barking cough (because of laryngeal swelling)
- Hoarseness
- Inspiratory stridor
- Dyspnea
- Anxiety
- Cyanosis

Diagnostic procedures for croup consist of a history, physical examination, X-rays (throat and chest), throat cultures, ABGs, and CBC. Croup is usually self-limiting but can be life threatening without supportive therapy. Treatment strategies include cool humidity, corticosteroids, and bronchodilators.

Acute Bronchitis

Acute bronchitis is an inflammation of the tracheobronchial tree or large bronchi. This inflammation is most commonly caused by a wide range of viruses (e.g.,

influenza, rhinovirus, coronavirus, and adenovirus). Bacterial invasions, irritant inhalation (e.g., smoke, chlorine, and bromine), and allergic reactions are less frequent causes. Young children, the elderly, and smokers are at the highest risk for developing acute bronchitis. In acute bronchitis, the airways become irritated and narrowed due to the results of the inflammatory process (e.g., capillary dilatation, edema, and exudate).

Clinical manifestations of acute bronchitis are usually mild and include:

- Productive and nonproductive cough
- Dyspnea
- Wheezing
- Low-grade fever
- Pharyngitis
- Malaise
- Chest discomfort

Diagnosis of acute bronchitis is usually based on symptoms. Additionally, a CBC and chest X-ray may be performed for differential diagnosis. A throat X-ray reveals a narrowing of the trachea often referred to as the steeple sign (**Figure 5-16**). Acute bronchitis is generally self-limiting; therefore, treatment is often supportive. Pharmacologic treatment may include antipyretics, analgesics, antihistamines, decongestants, cough suppressants, and bronchodilators. Other strategies include increasing fluid intake, avoiding smoke, and humidifying air.

Influenza

Influenza, or flu, is a viral infection that may affect the upper and lower respiratory tract. There are three types—A, B, and C. The influenza viruses are highly adaptive and constantly mutate, preventing the development of any long-term immune defense. Type A influenza, which includes several subtypes, is the most common type of influenza virus. This type is usually responsible for the most serious epidemics and global pandemics, such as those that occurred in the United States in 1918, 1957, and 1968. A subgroup of type A is H1N1, colloquially referred to as the swine flu, which was responsible for a serious pandemic that started in the United States and Mexico in 2009. Type B influenza outbreaks can also cause regional epidemics, but the disease it produces is generally milder than that caused by type A. Type C influenza causes sporadic

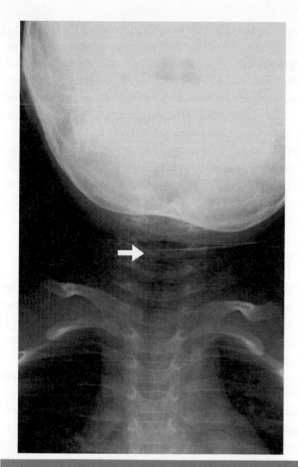

Figure 5-16

Steeple sign.

Severely immunocompromised persons can spread the virus for weeks or months. Flu differs from the common cold in that the flu usually has a sudden onset of symptoms. Clinical manifestations of the flu include:

- Fever
- Headache
- Chills
- Dry cough
- Body aches
- Nasal congestion
- Sore throat
- Sweating
- Malaise

Typically, fever and body aches last 3–5 days while cough and fatigue may last for 2 or more weeks.

Diagnostic procedures for influenza consist of a history, physical examinations, rapid flu screen, and flu culture (a nasal culture that tests for the presence of the virus). Treatment is symptomatic and supportive unless a secondary bacterial infection is present. Antiviral medications can reduce the severity and the duration of the symptoms. These antivirals can also be given postexposure to decrease the likelihood of developing the flu. Other strategies include increasing fluids, rest, antipyretics, and analgesics. Prevention strategies involve those to prevent the common cold (e.g., hand washing and avoiding crowds) and vaccina-

cases and minor, local outbreaks. Type C has never been connected with a large epidemic.

Millions of Americans contract the flu each year. The flu season in the United States, when the incidence is the highest, is typically between November and March. The virus is transmitted through the inhalation or contact with respiratory droplets. Although many people recover from the flu, it does account for about 200,000 hospitalizations and about 36,000 deaths per year (CDC, 2008). Persons at risk for having negative outcomes because of the flu are children, elderly, those who are immune compromised, and those with preexisting chronic diseases. Often deaths associated with the flu are a result of secondary bacterial pneumonia.

The influenza virus has an incubation period of 1–4 days, with peak transmission risk starting at approximately 1 day before onset of symptoms and lasting 4–7 days afterward in adults. Children can be infectious for more than 10 days, and young children can spread the virus 6 days before onset of symptoms.

 MYTH BUSTERS

A common misconception is that you can get the flu from the flu vaccine. What fuels this myth is that some people may experience very mild flulike symptoms (e.g., low-grade fever, aches, malaise) after receiving the vaccination. These symptoms are not because the individual has a mild case of the flu; it is due to the immune system developing antibodies. An additional factor fueling this myth is that people may still have the flu even after receiving the vaccination. This infection is not because of the flu vaccine; rather, it is because they encountered a strain of the flu that was not covered by the vaccination. Remember, the vaccination is based on predictions. Negative outcomes from the flu vaccine are rare and minimal. So get vaccinated and encourage others to do the same!

tions. Currently, vaccinations exist for the seasonal flu and H1N1 flu. Prior to each flu season (usually before the previous season is over), the Centers for Disease Control and Prevention (CDC) develops a seasonal flu vaccine based on predictions of the likely strain to be encountered. In the United States, the seasonal flu vaccine should be administered each year in October. When outbreaks of other types of the flu occur, like with the H1N1 in 2009, the CDC develops vaccinations specific for those strains. Vaccine development can be a lengthy process. In many cases, the vaccines are grown in fertilized chicken eggs for approximately 10 months. Therefore, flu vaccines should not be administered to those persons with egg allergies.

Lower Respiratory Tract Infections

Bronchiolitis

Bronchiolitis is a common viral infection of the bronchioles most frequently caused by the respiratory syncytial virus. The infection most often occurs in children under 1 year of age, and incidence increases in the fall and winter months. When the virus infects the bronchioles, these small airways become inflamed and swollen. As a result of the inflammatory process, mucus collects in these airways. The combination of edema and mucus prevents airflow into the alveoli. Transmission of the respiratory syncytial virus occurs through contact with or inhalation of infected respiratory droplets. Contributing factors to developing bronchiolitis include neonatal prematurity, asthma family history, and cigarette smoke exposure.

Clinical manifestations of bronchiolitis vary in severity and include:

- Nasal drainage
- Nasal congestion
- Cough
- Wheezing
- Rapid, shallow respirations
- Chest retractions
- Dyspnea
- Fever
- Tachycardia
- Malaise

Diagnostic procedures include a history, physical examination, chest X-ray, mucous swab, CBC, and ABGs. Bronchiolitis can progress to atelectasis (col-

lapse of the alveoli) and respiratory failure without aggressive and early treatment; therefore, airway management and respiratory stability are the treatment foci. Hospitalization is often required, and intubation may be necessary if the child decompensates or respiratory failure occurs. Other treatment strategies include oxygen therapy, cool humidity, increased fluids (either by mouth or intravenously), keeping the child calm, bronchodilators, and corticosteroids. Prevention strategies are the same as those previously discussed for other infectious respiratory conditions (e.g., hand washing and avoiding crowds).

Pneumonia

Pneumonia is an inflammatory process caused by numerous infectious agents (e.g., bacteria, viruses, and fungi) and injurious agents or events (e.g., aspiration and smoke). The sixth leading cause of death in the United States, pneumonia can be a primary or secondary infection (CDC, 2008). *Streptococcus pneumoniae* is responsible for 75% of all cases of pneumonia. Viral pneumonia and bacterial pneumonia have some notable differences (Table 5-2). In contrast to bacterial pneumonia, viral pneumonia is usually mild and heals without intervention, but viral pneumonia can lead to a virulent bacterial pneumonia. Irritating agents or events can also lead to pneumonia. Some of these agents or events include aspiration of gastric contents, endotracheal intubation, respiratory suctioning, and inhalation of smoke or chemicals. Aspiration pneumonia frequently occurs when the gag reflex is impaired because of a brain injury or anesthesia. Aspiration can also occur because of impaired lower esophageal sphincter closure secondary to nasogastric tube

Table 5-2 Comparison of Viral and Bacterial Pneumonia

	Viral	Bacterial
Cough	Nonproductive	Productive
Fever	Low grade	Higher
WBC	Normal (low)	Elevated
X-ray	Minimal change	Infiltrates
Severity	Less	More
Antibiotics	No	Yes

placement or disease (e.g., gastroesophageal reflux disease). Additionally, inappropriate tube-feeding placement can lead to tube-feeding formulas entering the lungs rather than the stomach. Gastric contents and tube-feeding formulas irritate the lung tissue, triggering the inflammatory response. The inflammatory response increases mucus production that can lead to atelectasis and pneumonia. Tube-feeding formulas also contain sugar and protein, creating a superior medium for bacteria to grow and flourish. Finally, pneumonia can develop from stasis of pulmonary secretions. Activities such as movement, talking, and coughing normally keep pulmonary secretions moving, and adequate hydrations keep secretions thin. When these secretions become thick and stagnate, ciliary action cannot remove the bacteria-laden mucus, leading to pneumonia.

Pneumonia is classified based on the causative agents or events previously discussed and its location in the lung (**Table 5-3**). **Lobar pneumonia** is confined to a single lobe and is described by that affected lobe (e.g., right upper lobe). **Bronchopneumonia** is the most frequent type and is a patchy pneumonia throughout several lobes. **Interstitial pneumonia**, or atypical, occurs in the areas between the alveoli. Interstitial pneumonia is routinely caused by viruses (e.g., influenza type A and B) or by uncommon bacteria (e.g., *Legionella*). Pneumonia is also classified according to where it is acquired. **Nosocomial pneumonia** refers to

SPECIAL CASES

Legionnaires' disease is a specific type of pneumonia that is caused by *Legionella pneumophila*. The bacteria thrive in warm, moist environments, particularly air conditioning systems and spas. Legionnaires' disease is not contagious. Most people acquire this type of pneumonia from inhaling the bacteria as they are spread by an air conditioning system or spa. Those persons with a weakened immune system are at highest risk for developing legionnaires' disease. Although most people with legionnaires' disease recover without incident, this type of pneumonia can be fatal if untreated. Symptoms are similar to other types of pneumonia and usually appear 10–14 days postexposure. In addition to the usual pneumonia diagnostic procedures, a urine test can be performed to identify the presence of *Legionella* antigens. Treatment of legionnaires' disease follows the usual pneumonia treatment protocol.

pneumonia that develops more than 48 hours after a hospital admission. In contrast, **community-acquired pneumonia** is acquired outside the hospital or healthcare setting.

In addition to previously discussed risk factors, persons at risk for developing pneumonia include children, the elderly, those with immune-compromised states, those with existing chronic disease conditions, smokers, and alcoholics. Otherwise healthy patients

Table 5-3 Types of Pneumonia

	Lobar Pneumonia	Bronchopneumonia	Interstitial Pneumonia
Distribution	All of one or two lobes	Scattered small patches	Scattered small patches
Cause	*Streptococcus pneumoniae*	Multiple bacteria	Influenza virus; *Mycoplasma*
Pathophysiology	Inflammation of the alveolar wall and leakage of cells, fibrin, and fluid into alveoli causing consolidation.	Inflammation and purulent exudates in alveoli often developing from pooled secretions or irritation.	Interstitial inflammation around alveoli. Necrosis of bronchial epithelium.
Onset	Sudden and acute	Insidious	Variable
Signs	• High fever • Chills • Productive cough of rusty sputum • Rales progressing to absent breath sounds in affected lobes	• Mild fever • Productive cough of yellow-green sputum • Dyspnea	• Variable fever • Nonproductive hacking cough • Headache • Myalgia

usually recover completely from pneumonia when treated properly. Those high-risk persons are more likely to develop complications including septicemia, pulmonary edema, lung abscess, and acute respiratory distress syndrome.

Clinical manifestations of pneumonia include:

- Productive or nonproductive cough
- Fatigue
- Pleuritic pain
- Dyspnea
- Fever
- Chills
- Crackles or rales
- Pleural rub
- Tachypnea
- Mental status changes (especially in the elderly)

Early diagnosis and treatment will be paramount to have positive outcomes. Diagnostic procedures may include a history, physical examination, chest X-ray, sputum cultures, CBC, ABGs, and bronchoscopy. Endotracheal intubation may be necessary to provide ventilation support and maintain oxygenation. Additional treatment strategies include antibiotics (if bacterial infection is present), bronchodilators, corticosteroids, antipyretics, analgesics, oxygen therapy, chest physiotherapy, increased fluids (either by mouth or intravenously), and rest. If aspiration is the cause of the pneumonia, additional treatment includes eliminating the causes and not giving the patient anything by mouth until swallowing studies can be performed. Pneumonia prevention strategies include hand wash-

ing, avoiding crowds, vaccinations (e.g., for pneumococcus and influenza), mobilizing secretions (e.g., turning, coughing, deep breathing), and smoking cessation.

Tuberculosis

Once on the decline, tuberculosis (TB) is a potentially serious infectious disease that is increasing globally (Figure 5-17). Significant advances have been made in TB treatment, yet many new cases are detected each year, particularly among AIDS patients in Africa. TB remains a major cause of illness and death worldwide, killing more than 2 million people each year. Person-to-person transmission occurs through the inhalation of tiny infected aerosol droplets. Many people contract TB but do not develop the disease because of an intact, healthy immune system or early treatment. A growing number of multidrug-resistant TB strains are emerging, increasing treatment concerns and prevalence rates. Fifteen percent of persons infected with TB in the United States have a multidrug-resistant strain (CDC, 2008).

TB is caused by *Mycobacterium tuberculosis*, a slow-growing aerobic (requires oxygen) bacillus that is somewhat resistant to the body's immune efforts. The bacillus is capable of surviving in dried sputum for weeks. Ultraviolet light, heat, alcohol, glutaraldehyde, and formaldehyde destroy the bacillus. Although TB most frequently involves the lungs, it can also affect other organs and tissue (e.g., liver, brain, and bone marrow). TB is often considered an opportunistic infection because it is more likely to become active in someone with a weakened immune system. Therefore, at-risk persons include those with immune deficiency (e.g., AIDS and cancer), malnutrition, diabetes mellitus, and alcoholism. Poverty, overcrowding, homelessness, and drug abuse also increase risk for acquiring TB.

There are two stages of TB pathogenesis—primary and secondary infection. Primary TB infection occurs when the bacillus first enters the body. In this phase, macrophages engulf the microbe causing a local inflammatory response. Some bacilli travel to the lymph nodes, activating the type IV hypersensitivity reaction (see Chapter 2). Lymphocytes and macrophages congregate to form a granuloma (an epithelial nodule). The granuloma contains some live bacilli, forming a tubercle. Caseous necrosis, a cottage cheese–like material, develops in the center of the tubercle

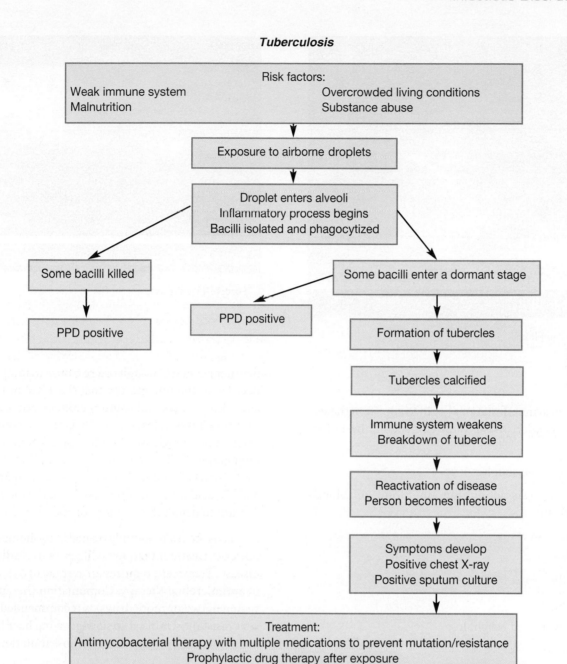

Tuberculosis

Risk factors:

Weak immune system   Overcrowded living conditions
Malnutrition   Substance abuse

↓

Exposure to airborne droplets

↓

Droplet enters alveoli
Inflammatory process begins
Bacilli isolated and phagocytized

Some bacilli killed   Some bacilli enter a dormant stage

↓

PPD positive

PPD positive

Formation of tubercles

↓

Tubercles calcified

↓

Immune system weakens
Breakdown of tubercle

↓

Reactivation of disease
Person becomes infectious

↓

Symptoms develop
Positive chest X-ray
Positive sputum culture

↓

Treatment:
Antimycobacterial therapy with multiple medications to prevent mutation/resistance
Prophylactic drug therapy after exposure
Bacille Calmette-Guérin vaccine after exposure when medications are not available

Figure 5-17

Tuberculosis.

(see Chapter 1). An intact immune system can resist this development, so the lesions remain small, become walled off by fibrous tissue, and calcify. These lesions are referred to as Ghon complexes (**Figure 5-18**). The bacilli can remain dormant and viable in the tubercle for years as long as the immune system is intact. In this phase, the individual has been infected by the bacilli and remains asymptomatic. When the primary infection can no longer be controlled, the infection progresses to the secondary, or active, infection phase. During this phase, TB can spread throughout the lungs and to other organs.

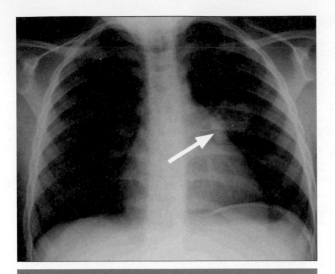

Figure 5-18

Ghon complexes.

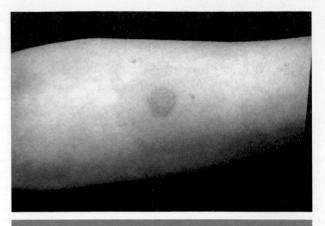

Figure 5-19

Positive TB skin test.

Clinical manifestations begin to appear in the secondary infection phase. These clinical manifestations include:

- Productive cough
- Hemoptysis (coughing up blood or bloody sputum)
- Night sweats
- Fever
- Chills
- Fatigue
- Unexplained weight loss
- Anorexia
- Miscellaneous symptoms depending on other organ involvement

Diagnostic procedures for TB are multifaceted, beginning with a TB skin test (Mantoux test). For the TB skin test, a small amount of a purified protein derivative tuberculin is injected just below the dermis. If the person has been infected by the bacilli, a local reaction (e.g., redness and induration) will occur (**Figure 5-19**). Persons will test positive once the bacilli trigger the inflammatory response (Figure 5-17). A history of the bacillus Calmette-Guérin (BCG) vaccination will produce a false-positive reaction. Additionally, previously treated TB will generate a false-positive reaction. On the other hand, those with immature (e.g., children) or compromised (e.g., AIDS or cancer) immune systems

may not generate enough of a response to test positive. Because of the uncertainty that the TB skin test creates, chest X-rays and sputum cultures are used after a positive TB skin test is noted (whether to confirm an original case or to assess reinfection). A computerized tomography (CT) scan can also be used to visualize TB lesions because it is more sensitive than an X-ray. Nucleic acid amplification may be performed on the sputum to detect the presence of resistant strains.

TB is often successfully treated in the home setting; however, treatment requires diligence to eradicate the disease. Treatment requires an average of 6–9 months of antimicrobial therapy. Combination therapy (consisting of two or more drugs) is recommended to prevent resistant strains. The slow-growing bacilli have a high mutation rate and develop those mutations when

 LEARNING POINTS

TB skin testing is only useful as a screening tool to identify new TB exposure cases. Once a person's immune system has developed antibodies against TB, the person tests positive. This immunity reaction happens after the first exposure and vaccination administration. A person can be treated for TB, and he or she will continue to test positive because the antibodies are still present. Chest X-rays and sputum cultures are better diagnostic procedures once someone has tested positive. So remember . . . once positive, always positive!

exposed to monotherapy. Because TB is a public health risk, antituberculin medications are provided free of charge by the United States Public Health Service. In some states, therapy noncompliance is unlawful, and imprisonment may be used to ensure adherence when other measures fail (e.g., direct observed therapy). Compliance is a common problem in treating TB because of the length of therapy and medication side effects (e.g., nausea, paresthesias, and discolored bodily secretions). Patient education, including an emphasis on taking an entire regimen of drugs as ordered, is crucial to maximize therapy success and prevent resistance. Strategies to prevent the transmission of TB include respiratory precautions (e.g., TB-approved masks, covering one's mouth when coughing, disposing of tissues), adequate ventilation (if the patient is at home), placing the patient in a negative-pressure isolation room (if he or she is hospitalized), and the bacillus Calmette-Guérin vaccination (primarily used in developing countries).

SPECIAL CASES

Severe acute respiratory syndrome (SARS) is a rapidly spreading respiratory illness that presents similarly to atypical pneumonia. First identified in China, prevalence rates remain higher in Asian countries. SARS is caused by a coronavirus, SARS-CoV. Transmission occurs through inhalation of respiratory droplets or close contact, although oral-fecal contact may also be a mechanism of transmission. SARS has high mortality and morbidity rates.

The incubation period for SARS is 2–7 days. The first stage presents as a flulike syndrome (e.g., fever, chills, headache, myalgia, anorexia, and diarrhea) that lasts 3–7 days. Several days later, a dry cough and dyspnea develop as the lungs become damaged and the patient moves into the second stage. Interstitial congestion and hypoxia progress rapidly. Additionally, liver damage can occur. If the patient continues to the third stage, severe and sometimes fatal respiratory distress can develop.

Diagnostic procedures for SARS consist of a history, physical examination, and chest X-ray. Treatment focuses on maintaining oxygenation and respiratory status. Strategies include oxygen therapy, bronchodilators, and antiviral drugs. Endotracheal intubation with mechanical ventilation support may be required as hypoxia worsens.

Obstructive Diseases

Asthma

Asthma is a chronic pulmonary disease that produces intermittent, reversible airway obstruction. Asthma is characterized by acute airway inflammation, bronchoconstriction, bronchospasm, bronchiole edema, and mucus production (**Figure 5-20**). Asthma is the most common chronic illness in children in the United States. Diagnosis, hospitalizations, and death rates associated with asthma have increased from 1996 to 2006 (CDC, 2009). These rate increases may be a result of surging urbanization and pollution.

Asthma is usually classified according to cause (extrinsic, intrinsic, nocturnal, exercise-induced, occupational, or drug-induced) and by severity (mild intermittent, mild persistent, moderate persistent, and severe persistent) (**Table 5-4**). Extrinsic asthma is a result of increased IgE synthesis and airway inflammation, resulting in mast cell destruction and inflammatory mediator release. Extrinsic triggers include allergens such as food, pollen, dust, and medications. The release of the inflammatory mediators cause bronchoconstriction, increased capillary permeability, and mucus production. Extrinsic asthma generally presents in childhood or adolescence. Intrinsic asthma is not an allergic reaction and usually presents after age 35 years. Intrinsic triggers include upper respiratory infections, air pollution, emotional stress, smoke, exercise, and cold exposure. Nocturnal asthma usually occurs between 3:00 and 7:00 a.m. and is thought to be related to circadian rhythms. At night, cortisol and epinephrine levels decrease, while histamine levels increase. Changes in these naturally occurring substances lead to bronchoconstriction.

Exercise-induced asthma is common and usually occurs 10–15 minutes after activity ends. Symptoms can linger for an hour with exercise-induced asthma. The airways can become cool and dry during exercise, and asthmatic symptoms may be a compensatory mechanism to warm and moisten the airways. Following each episode of exercise-induced asthma, a refractory (symptom-free) period begins within 30 minutes and can last 90 minutes. During this time, little or no bronchospasm can be induced even if rechallenged with vigorous exercise. Athletes often take advantage of this fact by warming up vigorously in order to induce a refractory period prior to competition. Occupational asthma is caused by a reaction to substances encountered at work (e.g., plastic or formaldehyde). Symptoms

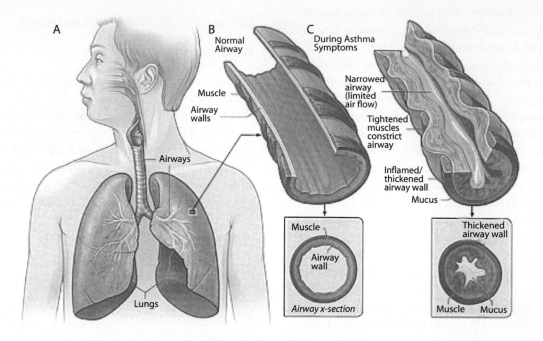

Figure 5-20

Asthma. (a) Location of the lungs and airways in the body. (b) Cross-section of a normal airway. (c) Cross-section of an airway during asthma symptoms.

develop over time, worsening with each exposure and improving when away from work (e.g., on weekends or during vacations). Drug-induced asthma is frequently caused by aspirin and can be fatal. Reactions can be delayed up to 12 hours after drug ingestion. Aspirin and other drugs (e.g., nonsteroidal anti-inflammatory drugs) prevent the conversion of prostaglandins, which stimulate leukotriene release—a powerful bronchoconstrictor.

Regardless of classification, asthma attacks are the body's response to bronchial inflammation. Stage one of an acute asthma attack is primarily related to bronchospasms, and it is usually signaled by cough-

Table 5-4 Classification of Asthma Severity

Step/Classification*	Daytime Symptoms	Nighttime Symptoms	PEF or FEV$_1$†	PEF Variability
Step 1: Mild intermittent	≤ 2/wk	≤ 2/wk	≥ 80%	< 20%
Step 2: Mild persistent	> 2/wk, but < daily	> 2 nights/mo	> 80%	20–30%
Step 3: Moderate persistent	Daily	> 1 night/wk	60–80%	> 30%
Step 4: Severe persistent	Continual	Frequent	≤ 60%	> 30%

*Classification is based on symptoms and lung function before treatment. Patients should be assigned to the most severe step in which any feature occurs.
†Percentage of predicted function.
PEF = peak expiratory flow (rate); FEV$_1$ = forced expiratory volume in 1 second.
Source: National Heart, Lung and Blood Institute (www.nhlbi.nih.gov).

ing. Peaking within 15 to 30 minutes, inflammatory mediators responsible for this stage include leukotrienes, histamine, and some interleukins. Stage two of an asthma attack peaks within 6 hours of symptom onset. This stage is a result of airway edema and mucus production. The alveolar hyperinflation causes air trapping. Bronchospasm, smooth muscle contraction, inflammation, and mucus production combine to narrow the airways.

Clinical manifestations of asthma include:

- Wheezing
- Shortness of breath
- Dyspnea
- Chest tightness
- Cough
- Tachypnea
- Anxiety

Status asthmaticus is a life-threatening, prolonged asthma attack that does not respond to usual treatment. Maintaining a patent airway is critical, and endotracheal intubation with ventilation support may be necessary. In addition, acid–base imbalances—specifically respiratory alkalosis (from expelling too much carbon dioxide because of tachypnea)—can develop. Treatment of these conditions will be crucial to improve outcomes.

Diagnostic procedures can be used to identify those persons with asthma as well as track progression. These diagnostic procedures include a history, physical examination, pulmonary function tests (Figure 5-11), ABGs, CBC, challenge testing, and allergen testing.

Asthma cannot be cured, but symptoms can be controlled. Unless treated promptly, asthma attacks can lead to impaired gas exchange and death. Left untreated, long-term asthma can result in bronchial damage and scarring. The goals of treatment are to minimize the occurrence and severity of asthma attacks. Pharmacologic treatment includes inhaled and systemic corticosteroids, bronchodilators, beta agonists, nebulizer treatments, leukotriene mediators, mast cell stabilizers, and anticholinergics. Additional strategies include:

- Develop an asthma plan (**Figure 5-21**) and teach it to all caregivers
- Avoid triggers
- Keep environment clean
- Limit environmental fabrics

- Filter indoor air
- Maintain a healthy immune system (e.g., exercise, get adequate nutrition)

Chronic Obstructive Pulmonary Disease

Chronic obstructive pulmonary disease (COPD) describes a group of chronic respiratory disorders characterized by irreversible, progressive tissue degeneration and airway obstruction. These debilitating conditions can impair an individual's ability to work and function independently. Severe hypoxia and hypercapnia can lead to respiratory failure. The chronic hypercapnia shifts the normal breathing drive from the need to expel excess carbon dioxide to the need to raise oxygen levels (Figure 5-12). Additionally, COPD can lead to cor pulmonale, right-sided heart failure due to lung disease (see Chapter 4). The most significant contributing factor to developing COPD is cigarette smoking. Other contributing factors include the inhalation of pollution and chemical irritants. Prevalence rates are likely underestimated because COPD is often asymptomatic in early stages or masked by smoking symptoms. Symptoms usually present around 60 years of age. A rare familial type of COPD (emphysema only), alpha-1 antitrypsin deficiency, presents much earlier—in the 30s or 40s. COPD is often one of or a mixture of two diseases—chronic bronchitis and emphysema (**Figure 5-22**). These two diseases are discussed in the upcoming sections.

Chronic Bronchitis

Chronic bronchitis is an obstructive respiratory disorder characterized by inflammation of the bronchi, a productive cough, and excessive mucus production. Chronic bronchitis differs from acute bronchitis in that the chronic type is not necessarily caused by an infection and symptoms persist longer. As previously mentioned, cigarette smoking is the greatest contributing factor for chronic bronchitis. The inflammatory response results in mucous gland hyperplasia, edema, excessive mucus production, bronchoconstriction, and cough in defense against inhaled irritants. Airway resistance affects inspiratory and expiratory airflow. Impaired pulmonary defenses (e.g., cilia damage and decreased phagocytic activity) result in frequent respiratory infections and, in some cases, respiratory failure.

Airway resistance results in hypoventilation, hypoxemia, cyanosis, hypercapnia, polycythemia,

Asthma Action Plan

For: _____ Doctor: _____ Date: _____

Doctor's Phone Number _____ Hospital/Emergency Department Phone Number _____

GREEN ZONE

Doing Well
- No cough, wheeze, chest tightness, or shortness of breath during the day or night
- Can do usual activities

And, if a peak flow meter is used,

Peak flow: more than _____ (80 percent or more of my best peak flow)

My best peak flow is: _____

Before exercise

Take these long-term control medicines each day (include an anti-inflammatory).

Medicine	How much to take	When to take it

☐ _____ ☐ 2 or ☐ 4 puffs _____ 5 to 60 minutes before exercise

YELLOW ZONE

Asthma Is Getting Worse
- Cough, wheeze, chest tightness, or shortness of breath, or
- Waking at night due to asthma, or
- Can do some, but not all, usual activities

-Or-

Peak flow: _____ to _____ (50 to 79 percent of my best peak flow)

First Add: quick-relief medicine—and keep taking your GREEN ZONE medicine.

_____ (short-acting beta₂-agonist) ☐ 2 or ☐ 4 puffs, every 20 minutes for up to 1 hour ☐ Nebulizer, once

Second If your symptoms (and peak flow, if used) return to GREEN ZONE after 1 hour of above treatment:
☐ Continue monitoring to be sure you stay in the green zone.

-Or-

If your symptoms (and peak flow, if used) do not return to GREEN ZONE after 1 hour of above treatment:
☐ Take: _____ (short-acting beta₂-agonist) ☐ 2 or ☐ 4 puffs or ☐ Nebulizer

☐ Add: _____ (oral steroid) _____ mg per day For _____ (3–10) days

☐ Call the doctor ☐ before/ ☐ within _____ hours after taking the oral steroid.

RED ZONE

Medical Alert!
- Very short of breath, or
- Quick-relief medicines have not helped, or
- Cannot do usual activities, or
- Symptoms are same or get worse after 24 hours in Yellow Zone

-Or-

Peak flow: less than _____ (50 percent of my best peak flow)

Take this medicine:

☐ _____ (short-acting beta₂-agonist) ☐ 4 or ☐ 6 puffs or ☐ Nebulizer

☐ _____ (oral steroid) _____ mg

Then call your doctor NOW. Go to the hospital or call an ambulance if:
- You are still in the red zone after 15 minutes AND
- You have not reached your doctor.

DANGER SIGNS ■ **Trouble walking and talking due to shortness of breath** ■ **Take** ☐ 4 or ☐ 6 puffs of your quick-relief medicine AND

■ **Lips or fingernails are blue** ■ **Go to the hospital or call for an ambulance** _____ (phone) **NOW!**

Figure 5-21

Example of asthma action plan.

---

clubbing of fingers, and dyspnea at rest. Additional clinical manifestations include:

- Wheezing
- Edema
- Weight gain
- Malaise
- Chest pain
- Fever

Diagnosis procedures for chronic bronchitis consist of a history (persistent, productive cough for at least 3 months in a year for 2 consecutive years), physical examination, chest X-ray, pulmonary function tests (Figure 5-11), ABGs, and CBC. The goal of treatment is to maintain airway patency. Treatment strategies include oxygen therapy (in limited amounts because too much will knock out the newly oxygen-centered drive for breathing), bronchodilators, corticosteroids, antibiotics (if bacterial infection is present), postural drainage, chest physiotherapy, and increased hydration.

 LEARNING POINTS

Patients with chronic bronchitis are unable to increase ventilatory effort to maintain adequate gas exchange; therefore, they eventually develop cyanosis. This cyanosis coupled with the edema that develops gives these patients the nickname, the blue bloaters.

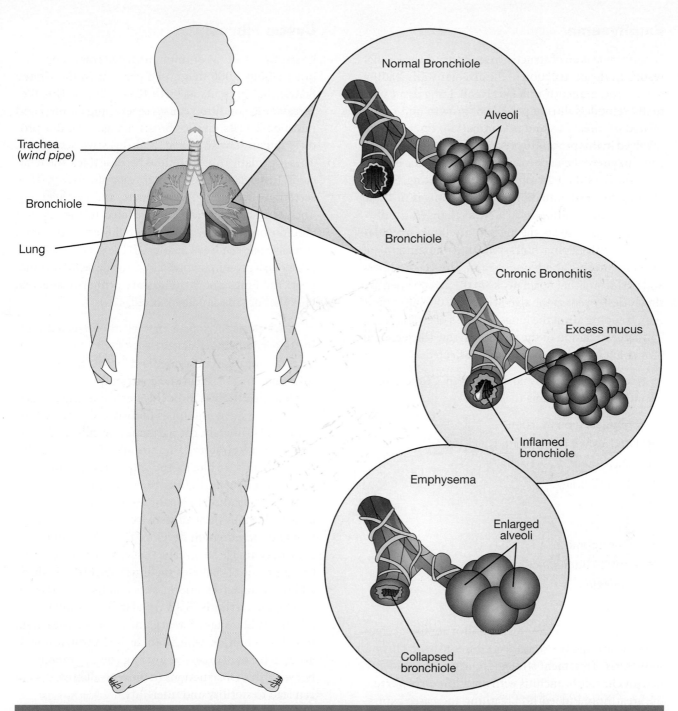

Trachea (*wind pipe*)

Bronchiole

Lung

Normal Bronchiole

Alveoli

Bronchiole

Chronic Bronchitis

Excess mucus

Inflamed bronchiole

Emphysema

Enlarged alveoli

Collapsed bronchiole

Figure 5-22

Chronic obstructive pulmonary disease (COPD) is often one of or a mixture of two diseases—chronic bronchitis and emphysema.

Emphysema

Emphysema is an obstructive respiratory disorder that results in the destruction of the alveolar walls leading to large, permanently inflated alveoli. Lung tissue normally remodels during periods of growth and repair related to infections and inflammation. Enzymes are involved in this process to prevent excessive tissue damage. Enzyme deficiency may result from genetic predisposition (less than 2% of cases) and smoking. Smoking initiates inflammation, causing changes in these enzyme levels leading to structural changes. Emphysema gradually turns the alveoli into large, irregular pockets with gaping holes, limiting the amount of oxygen entering the bloodstream. The elastic fibers and surfactant that normally keep the alveoli open are slowly destroyed, so the alveoli collapse during expiration, trapping air in the lungs. The loss of elastic recoil and hyperinflation of the alveoli narrow the terminal bronchioles, but inspiration is not affected.

Coughing is usually not a symptom. Clinical manifestation of emphysema includes:

- Dyspnea upon exertion
- Diminished breath sounds
- Wheezing
- Chest tightness
- Tachypnea
- Hypoxia
- Hypercapnia
- Activity intolerance
- Anorexia
- Malaise

Diagnosis and progress monitoring are accomplished through the same procedures as with chronic bronchitis. Treatment strategies include those identified for chronic bronchitis with the addition of pursed-lip breathing. Pursed-lip breathing increases expiratory resistance and produces airway back pressure, preventing alveoli collapse.

LEARNING POINTS

Patients with emphysema often hyperventilate, creating a pink appearance to their skin. This pantinglike breathing pattern coupled with the pink skin has earned emphysema patients the nickname, the pink puffers.

Cystic Fibrosis

Cystic fibrosis is a common inherited respiratory disorder (about 1,000 diagnosed per year in the United States) that presents at birth (CDC, 2008). This life-threatening condition causes severe lung damage and nutrition deficits. Cystic fibrosis changes cells that produce mucus, sweat, saliva, and digestive secretions. These normally thin secretions become thick and tenacious. Instead of lubricating the respiratory tract, these secretions occlude airways, ducts, and passageways. The genetic defect has been isolated to the seventh chromosome, and transmission follows an autosomal recessive pattern (see Chapter 1). The genetic deficit is related to a protein involved in chloride cellular transport. The lungs and pancreas are primarily affected, but other organs can be involved.

Atelectasis develops as airways are obstructed, leading to permanent damage (**Figure 5-23**). Mucus stagnates, becoming a prime medium for bacterial growth. Infections are recurrent and contribute to the progressive lung destruction. Bronchiectasis and emphysema-like changes are common as fibrosis and obstructions advance. Ultimately, cor pulmonale (right-sided heart failure) or respiratory failure results. In the digestive tract, the mucus blocks the intestines, producing a meconium ileus in the newborn. Mucus blocks pancreas ducts, leading to a pancreatic enzyme excretion deficit. Without these digestive enzymes, malabsorption and malnutrition develop. The trapped digestive enzymes damage pancreatic tissue, contributing to the development of diabetes mellitus. Blocked bile ducts add to the malabsorption issues and increase risk for developing cirrhosis. Salivary glands are only mildly affected by blockages. Sweat glands produce sweat high in sodium chloride, which can cause electrolyte imbalances in times of excessive loss (e.g., during exercise or hot weather). Obstructions in the reproductive system can lead to sterility and infertility.

Clinical manifestation of cystic fibrosis may appear at birth and progressively worsen throughout the life span. These manifestations include:

- Meconium ileus
- Salty skin
- Steatorrhea (fatty, foul-smelling stools)
- Fat-soluble vitamin deficiency (vitamins A, D, E, and K)
- Chronic cough
- Frequent respiratory infections

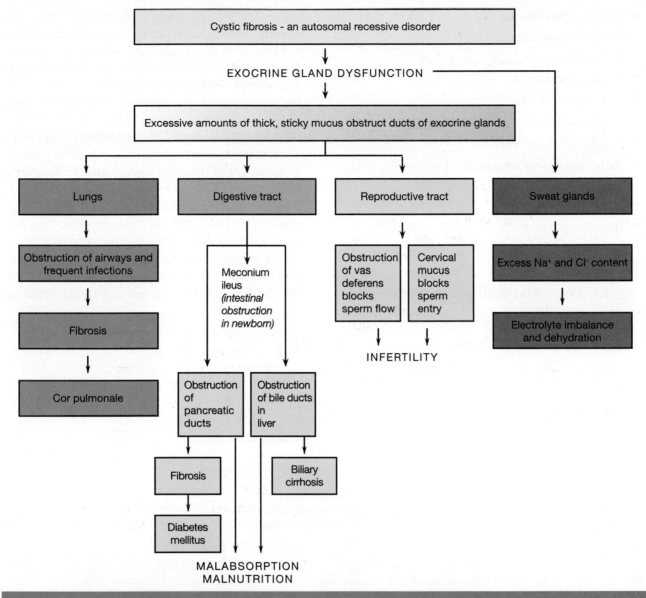

Figure 5-23

Cystic fibrosis.

- Hypoxia
- Fatigue
- Activity intolerance
- Audible rhonchi
- Delayed growth and development

Diagnosis of cystic fibrosis can be accomplished prenatally when family history warrants testing. Sweat analysis can be conducted at about 2–3 weeks of age to detect electrolyte abnormalities. Some states include cystic fibrosis testing as a part of their newborn screening. In addition, stool can be evaluated for the presence of pancreatic content. Other tests that assess lung function include chest X-rays, pulmonary function tests, and ABGs.

Cystic fibrosis treatment requires diligent family involvement and an interdisciplinary approach because of the progressive multisystem nature of the disease. With advances in treatment, the life expectancy of children with cystic fibrosis extends into adulthood. Treatment strategies include:

- Pancreatic enzyme replacement
- Bile salt replacement
- A well-balanced, high-protein, low-fat diet
- Fat-soluble vitamin replacement

- Increased fluid intake
- Intensive chest physiotherapy
- Postural drainage
- Coughing exercises
- Humidified air
- Bronchodilators
- Regular, moderate exercise
- Early, aggressive treatment of infections with antibiotics
- Oxygen therapy
- Heart-lung transplant

Lung Cancer

Lung cancer is the third most common neoplasm that can arise as a primary and secondary tumor (approxi-mately 180,000 new cases per year) (CDC, 2008). Frequently, other cancers, such as breast, liver, and lung, to name a few, metastasize (spread) to the lung tissue. Lung cancer is the deadliest of the cancers among men and women—mortality rates are about 90%. Smoking contributes to the majority (80–90%) of cases. The more than 4,000 chemicals in cigarette smoke include carcinogens and chemicals that paralyze cilia. The risk for developing lung cancer is directly related to the length of time one smokes and the number of cigarettes smoked. Second-hand smoke can also be a significant contributing factor, and in fact, some research has indicated that it may be worse than first-hand smoking. Smoking cessation or removing the smoke exposure will gradually decrease risk. Inhalation of other chemicals (e.g., asbestos, tar, and pollution) and chronic lung disease can also increase risk (**Figure 5-24**).

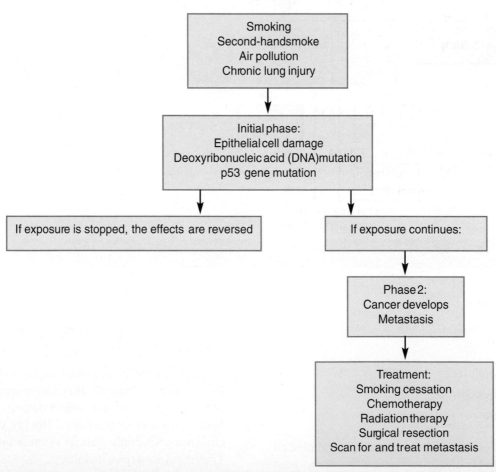

Lung Cancer

Smoking
Second-handsmoke
Air pollution
Chronic lung injury

↓

Initial phase:
Epithelial cell damage
Deoxyribonucleic acid (DNA)mutation
p53 gene mutation

If exposure is stopped, the effects are reversed

If exposure continues:

↓

Phase 2:
Cancer develops
Metastasis

↓

Treatment:
Smoking cessation
Chemotherapy
Radiationtherapy
Surgical resection
Scan for and treat metastasis

Figure 5-24

Lung cancer.

The lungs provide an optimum environment for tumor development and growth. Carcinogens can seek refuge in the many air passages, having an opportunity to cause cellular changes (usually metaplasia). The scores of blood vessels supplying the lungs serve as entrance points for distant cancer cells to gain access, and those vessels furnish the cancer with a rich blood source.

Lung cancers are divided into two types—small cell and non–small cell. Small cell carcinoma, often referred to as oat cell carcinoma, occurs almost exclusively in heavy smokers and is less frequent than non–small cell cancers. Non–small cell carcinoma, often referred to as bronchogenic carcinoma, is the most common type of malignant lung cancer. This very aggressive lung cancer has several subgroups—squamous cell carcinoma, adenocarcinoma, and bronchioalveolar carcinoma. Upon exposure to the carcinogen, irreversible oncogene deoxyribonucleic acid mutations and inactivation of tumor suppressor genes occur. If carcinogen exposure continues, cancer develops (**Figure 5-25**).

Tumors in the lungs lead to several issues, including the following:

- Airway obstruction
- Inflammation of lung tissue eliciting coughing and contributing to infections
- Fluid accumulation in the pleural space (e.g., pleural effusion, hemothorax, and pneumothorax)
- Paraneoplastic syndrome (endocrine dysfunction associated with hormone secretion from the tumor)

Clinical manifestations of lung cancer are insidious because they mimic signs of smoking. These manifestations include:

- Persistent cough or a change in usual cough
- Dyspnea
- Hemoptysis
- Frequent respiratory infections
- Chest pain
- Hoarseness
- Weight loss
- Anemia
- Fatigue
- Other symptoms specific to site of metastasis

Diagnostic procedures of lung cancer include a history, physical examination, chest X-ray, CT, MRI, bronchoscopy, sputum studies, biopsy, positron emission tomography, bone scans, and pulmonary function tests. Treatment is based on staging and follows usual cancer treatment—chemotherapy, surgery, and radia-

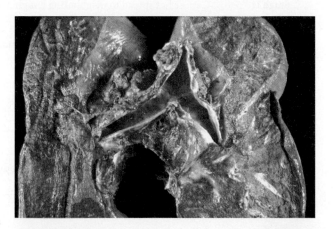

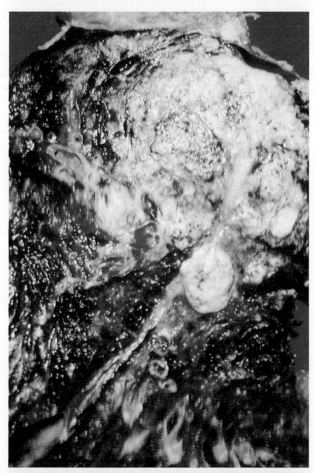

Figure 5-25

The normal (top) and cancerous (bottom) lung.

Table 5-5 Staging and Treatment of Non–Small Cell Lung Cancer

Stage	Description	Usual Treatment Plan
Stage I	Cancer has invaded the underlying lung tissue but has not spread to the lymph nodes.	Surgery
Stage II	Cancer has spread to neighboring lymph nodes or invaded the chest wall.	Surgery, radiation, and chemotherapy
Stage IIIA	Cancer has spread from the lung to lymph nodes in the center of the chest.	Combined chemotherapy and radiation, sometimes surgery based on results of treatment
Stage IIIB	Cancer has spread locally to areas such as the heart, blood vessels, trachea, and esophagus—all within the chest—or to lymph nodes in the area of the collarbone or to the tissue that surrounds the lungs within the rib cage (pleura).	Chemotherapy, sometimes radiation
Stage IV	Cancer has spread to other parts of the body, such as the liver, bones, or brain.	Chemotherapy, targeted drug therapy, clinical trials, supportive care

Table 5-6 Staging and Treatment of Small Cell Lung Cancer

Stage	Description	Usual Treatment Plan
Limited	Cancer is confined to one lung and to its neighboring lymph nodes.	Combined chemotherapy and radiation, sometimes surgery
Extensive	Cancer has spread beyond one lung and nearby lymph nodes, and may have invaded both lungs, more remote lymph nodes, or other organs.	Chemotherapy, clinical trials, supportive care

tion (**Table 5-5; Table 5-6**). The treatment is generally palliative because the tumor does not usually respond favorably to treatment. Early diagnosis and treatment will improve this prognosis. Other strategies include those to maintain optimum respiratory function—oxygen therapy, bronchodilators, and antibiotics (if bacterial infections are present).

Restrictive Diseases
Atelectasis

Atelectasis refers to incomplete alveolar expansion or collapse of the alveoli. Atelectasis occurs when the walls of the alveoli stick together. Atelectasis is caused by the following:

- Surfactant deficiencies (the lipoprotein that coats the inside of the alveoli allowing them to remain open at the end of expiration)

- Bronchus obstruction
- Lung tissue compression (e.g., tumor, pneumothorax, and pleural effusion)
- Increased surface tension (e.g., pulmonary edema)
- Lung fibrosis (e.g., emphysema)

When alveoli become airless, they shrivel much like a raisin. This ventilation issue can in turn impair blood flow through the lung. Ineffective ventilation and perfusion impair gas exchange. Surgery and immobility increase the risk for developing atelectasis for this reason. Atelectasis can occur in small or larger areas. If only a small area is affected, the respiratory rate will increase to control carbon dioxide levels. The larger the area effected, the more severe the symptoms experienced. Necrosis, infection (e.g., pneumonia), and permanent lung damage can occur if the alveoli are not reinflated quickly.

Clinical manifestations of atelectasis are due to impaired ventilation and perfusion. These manifestations include:

- Diminished breath sounds
- Dyspnea
- Tachypnea
- Asymmetrical lung movement
- Anxiety
- Restlessness
- Tracheal deviation
- Tachycardia

Diagnostic procedures for atelectasis include a history, physical examination, chest X-ray, CT, bronchoscopy, ABGs, and CBC. Treatment of atelectasis focuses on treating the underlying causes (e.g., antibiotics, thoracentesis) and reinflating the alveoli. Incentive spirometry (a device to promote ventilation) is effective in reinflating the alveoli. For more severe cases, continuous positive airway pressure or endotracheal intubation may be necessary for ventilation support. Prevention strategies include increasing mobility (e.g., turning and ambulating), coughing, and deep breathing exercises (e.g., incentive spirometry) every 1–2 hours. Effective pain management and postoperative incisional splinting increase the likelihood of performing these interventions adequately.

Pleural Effusion

A **pleural effusion** is the accumulation of excess fluid in the pleural cavity. Normally, a very small amount of fluid drained from the lymphatic system is present in this space to lubricate the constantly moving lungs. Excessive fluid in the pleural cavity can compress the lung and limit expansion during inhalation. Effusions vary in nature and may affect both lungs or one lung. Fluid that can accumulate to create the effusion includes exudates (due to inflammation), transudate (due to increased hydrostatic pressure), blood (due to trauma), and pus (due to infection). The consequence of this effusion depends on type, location, amount, and fluid accumulation rate. Large amounts of fluids can cause the pleural membranes to separate, preventing their cohesion during inhalation (**Figure 5-26; Figure 5-27**). This lack of cohesion impedes full expansion, leading to atelectasis and pneumothorax. Large

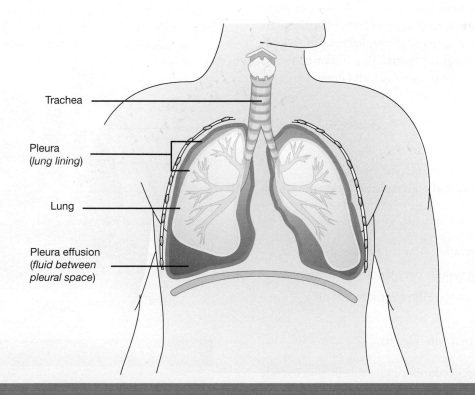

Trachea

Pleura
(*lung lining*)

Lung

Pleura effusion
(*fluid between pleural space*)

Figure 5-26

Pleural effusion is a buildup of fluid in the lining of the lungs.

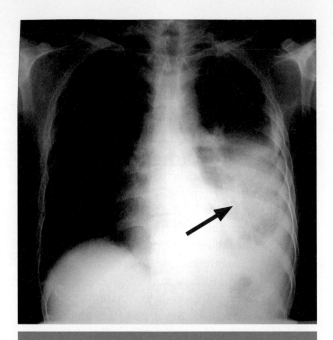

Figure 5-27

X-ray of pleural effusion.

effusions can also impair venous return in the inferior vena cava and cardiac filling by putting pressure on those structures.

Pleurisy, or pleuritis, can precede or follow the effusion, or it may occur independently. Pleurisy refers to inflammation of the pleural membranes, which leads to swollen and irregular tissue. This inflammation is often associated with pneumonia and creates friction in the pleural membranes.

Clinical manifestations of pleural effusion include:

- Dyspnea
- Chest pain (usually sharp and worsening with inhalation)
- Tachypnea
- Tracheal deviation (toward the unaffected side)
- Absent lung sounds over the affected area
- Dullness to percussion over affected area
- Tachycardia
- Pleural friction rub (pleurisy)

Diagnostic procedures for pleural effusion include a history, physical examination, chest X-ray, CT, ABGs, CBC, and thoracentesis (needle aspiration of fluid) with examination of fluid. Treatment focuses on addressing the underlying cause, but regardless of etiology,

removal of the fluid is necessary to promote full expansion of the lungs. Strategies may consist of a thoracentesis, chest drainage tube, and antibiotics.

Pneumothorax

Pneumothorax refers to air in the pleural cavity. The presence of atmospheric air in the pleural cavity and the separation to pleural membranes can lead to atelectasis. The pressure can cause a partial or complete collapse of a lung (Figure 5-28). A small pneumothorax causes mild symptoms and may heal on its own. A larger pneumothorax generally requires aggressive treatment to remove the air and reestablish pulmonary negative pressure. Risk factors for developing a pneumothorax include smoking, tall stature, and history of lung disease or previous pneumothorax.

There are several types of pneumothorax, defined by their cause. A spontaneous pneumothorax develops when air enters the pleural cavity from an opening in the internal airways. Primary spontaneous pneumothorax occurs when a small air blister (bleb) on the top of the lung ruptures. Blebs are caused by a weakness in the lung tissue and can rupture from changes in air pressure, such as occurs in scuba diving, flying, mountain climbing, or listening to extremely loud music. Additionally, a primary spontaneous pneumothorax may happen while smoking marijuana—a deep inhalation, followed by slow breathing out against partial-

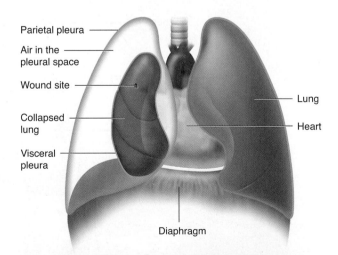

Figure 5-28

A pneumothorax occurs when air leaks into the pleural space between the parietal and visceral pleura. The lung collapses as air fills the pleural space and the two pleural membranes are no longer in contact with each other.

ly closed lips forces the smoke deeper into the lungs. Most commonly, these blebs rupture for no obvious reason, but genetic factors may play a role. A primary spontaneous pneumothorax is usually mild because pressure from the collapsed portion of the lung may in turn collapse the bleb. A secondary spontaneous pneumothorax develops in people with preexisting lung disease (e.g., emphysema, pneumonia, cystic fibrosis, and lung cancer). In these cases, the pneumothorax occurs because the diseased lung tissue is weakened. Secondary spontaneous pneumothorax can be more severe and even life threatening because diseased tissue can create a larger opening, allowing more air into the pleural space. Additionally, pulmonary disease reduces lung reserves, making any further reduction in lung function more serious. A traumatic pneumothorax stems from any blunt (e.g., vehicle air bag deployment) or penetrating injury (e.g., knife or gunshot wounds) to the chest. These injuries can inadvertently occur during certain medical procedures, such as chest tubes insertion, cardiopulmonary resuscitation, and lung or liver biopsies. A tension pneumothorax is the most serious type of pneumothorax; it occurs when the pressure in the pleural space is greater than the atmospheric pressure. This increased pressure is due to trapped air in the pleural space or entering air from a positive-pressure mechanical ventilator. The force of the air can cause the affected lung to collapse completely and shift the heart toward the uncollapsed lung (called a mediastinal shift), compressing the unaffected lung and the heart

(Figure 5-29). Tension pneumothorax progresses rapidly and is fatal if not treated quickly.

Clinical manifestations vary in severity depending on the type of pneumothorax. These manifestations include:

- Sudden chest pain over the affected lung
- Chest tightness
- Dyspnea
- Tachypnea
- Decreased breath sounds over the affected area
- Asymmetrical chest movement
- Trachea and mediastinum deviation toward the unaffected side
- Anxiety
- Tachycardia
- Pallor
- Hypotension

Diagnostic procedures for pneumothorax consist of a history, physical examination, chest X-ray, CT, and ABGs. Treatment usually involves removal of the air and reestablishing negative pressure, allowing for full expansion of the lungs. Such strategies may include a thoracentesis and chest drainage tube with suction (which removes fluid and reestablishes negative pressure).

INSPIRATION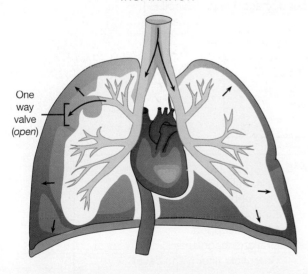

EXPIRATION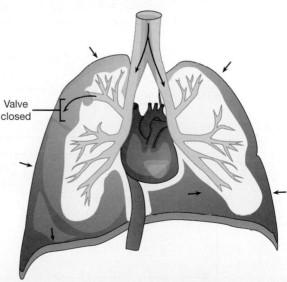

Figure 5-29

Tension pneumothorax: A one-way valve allows air into the pleural space during inspiration, but not out during expiration.

Acute Respiratory Distress Syndrome

Acute respiratory distress syndrome (ARDS) is a sudden failure of the respiratory system often occurring from fluid accumulation in the alveoli. ARDS has many other names, such as shock lung, wet lung, and stiff lung. Multiple conditions can precipitate ARDS, including prolonged shock, burns, aspiration, and smoke inhalation. ARDS involves an acute hypoxemia resulting from a systemic (e.g., trauma, septicemia, pancreatitis, drug overdose) or pulmonary (e.g., illicit drug and toxic gas inhalation, near drowning, fat embolism) event that is not cardiac in origin. ARDS develops rapidly, often within 90 minutes of a systemic inflammatory response or within 48 hours of a lung

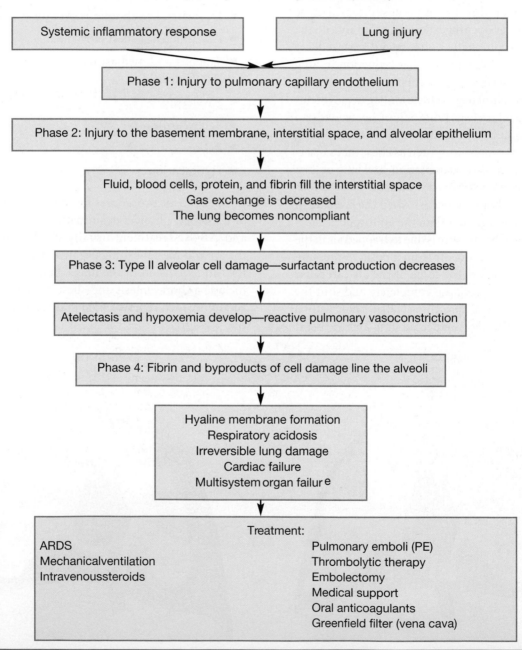

Acute Respiratory Distress Syndrome (ARDS)

Systemic inflammatory response → Lung injury →

Phase 1: Injury to pulmonary capillary endothelium

Phase 2: Injury to the basement membrane, interstitial space, and alveolar epithelium

Fluid, blood cells, protein, and fibrin fill the interstitial space
Gas exchange is decreased
The lung becomes noncompliant

Phase 3: Type II alveolar cell damage—surfactant production decreases

Atelectasis and hypoxemia develop—reactive pulmonary vasoconstriction

Phase 4: Fibrin and byproducts of cell damage line the alveoli

Hyaline membrane formation
Respiratory acidosis
Irreversible lung damage
Cardiac failure
Multisystem organ failure

Treatment:

ARDS
Mechanical ventilation
Intravenous steroids

Pulmonary emboli (PE)
Thrombolytic therapy
Embolectomy
Medical support
Oral anticoagulants
Greenfield filter (vena cava)

Figure 5-30

Acute respiratory distress syndrome (ARDS).

injury. ARDS is fatal in many cases. Those who survive will fully recover, but it may take up to a year to regain complete lung function.

Injury in the alveoli and the capillary membranes lead to the release of chemical inflammatory mediators (**Figure 5-30; Figure 5-31**). These mediators increase capillary permeability, promote fluid and protein accumulation in the alveoli, and damage surfactant-producing cells. These events result in decreased gas exchange, reduced pulmonary blood flow, and limited lung expansion. Diffuse atelectasis and reduced lung capacity ensue. Lung damage progresses as neutrophils migrate to the site, releasing proteases and other mediators. A hyaline membrane, or a thin layer of tissue, forms in the alveoli and causes them to become stiff. Additionally, increased platelet aggregation promotes microemboli development. If the patient survives, scattered necrosis and fibrosis are apparent throughout the lungs.

ARDS is a serious condition that can lead to several complications, including:

- Respiratory failure
- Respiratory and metabolic acidosis
- Pulmonary fibrosis
- Pneumothorax
- Bacterial infections
- Decreased lung function
- Muscle wasting
- Memory, cognitive, and emotional issues

Clinical manifestations of ARDS can develop suddenly and include:

- Dyspnea
- Labored (requiring the use of accessory muscles), shallow respirations
- Rales
- Productive cough with frothy sputum
- Hypoxia
- Cyanosis
- Fever
- Hypotension
- Tachycardia
- Restlessness

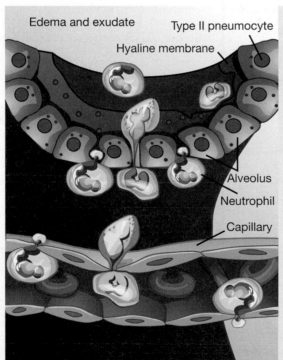

Edema and exudate
Type II pneumocyte
Hyaline membrane
Alveolus
Neutrophil
Capillary

THE ADULT RESPIRATORY DISTRESS SYNDROME:

In ARDS, type I cells die as a result of diffuse alveolar damage.

Intra-alveolar edema follows, after which there is formation of hyaline membrane composed of proteinaceous axudate and cell debris.

In the acute phase, the lungs are markedly congested and heavy.

Type II cells multiply to line the alveolar surface.

Interstitial inflammation is characteristic.

The lesion may heal completely or progress to interstitial fibrosis.

Figure 5-31

Acute respiratory distress syndrome.

- Confusion
- Lethargy
- Anxiety

Diagnostic procedures for ARDS involve a history, physical examination, ABGs, chest X-ray, CT, and CBC. The main goal of treatment is to maintain adequate oxygenation and respiratory status. Such strategies include endotracheal intubation with mechanical ventilator, oxygen therapy, corticosteroids, and antibiotics (if bacterial infections are present), as well as prevention and treatment of emboli (e.g., embolectomy, anticoagulants, and antiplatelet agents).

Acute Respiratory Failure

Acute respiratory failure (ARF) is a serious, life-threatening condition that can be the result of many pulmonary disorders. In ARF, the oxygen levels become dangerously low (less than 50 mm Hg) or carbon dioxide levels become dangerously high (greater than 50 mm Hg). Normally, oxygen levels are 80–100 mm Hg and carbon dioxide levels are 35–45 mm Hg. These low oxygen levels are unable to meet the body's metabolic needs, and the nervous system quickly becomes affected. In ARF, these gas levels progressively change as the patient's condition worsens. Respiratory acidosis develops as the carbon dioxide levels rise (see Chapter 6). The hypoxia and acidosis trigger a reflex pulmonary vasoconstriction, further impairing gas exchange and increasing cardiac workload. The heart decompensates from the lack of oxygen, which could lead to cardiac arrest. Respiratory arrest may occur as the respiratory system ceases all activity from the strain.

Clinical manifestations are usually evident and result from the impaired gas exchange. These manifestations include:

- Shallow respirations
- Headache
- Tachycardia
- Dysrhythmias
- Lethargy
- Confusion

Diagnostic procedures for ARF consist of a history, physical examination, ABGs, chest X-ray, and CBC.

Treatment focuses on resolving the cause and maintaining adequate respiratory status. Strategies include oxygen therapy, endotracheal intubation with ventilation support, bronchodilators, antibiotics (if bacterial infection is present), corticosteroids, and treating emboli (e.g., embolectomy and anticoagulants). Cardiac support is usually inevitable as the heart arrests under the strain (e.g., cardiopulmonary resuscitation, sympathomimetic medications, and inotropic agents).

CASE STUDY

Emma is a 7-year-old girl who has been admitted to the intensive care unit with severe respiratory distress. Her parents report that 3 days ago she developed a fever, aches, and nasal discharge, at which time she was taken to her pediatrician. Her pediatrician diagnosed her with the H1N1 strain of influenza. She was prescribed antiviral drugs, and her parents were given instructions on fever and hydration management. Twenty-four hours ago, her parents said she was improving—her fever was minimal, she was drinking more, and she was beginning to play. Emma's parents brought her into the emergency department because her symptoms suddenly worsened. They reported that over the course of a few hours, her breathing became more and more labored, fever spiked, and coughing started. The emergency department healthcare provider diagnosed her with a secondary bacterial pneumonia that had quickly progressed to acute respiratory distress syndrome.

In the emergency department, Emma was intubated, placed on ventilator support, given bronchodilators, and started on intravenous antibiotics. Upon admission to the intensive care unit, she was stable but fragile. The following are her latest laboratory findings:

- ABG: pH 7.32, PaO_2 72 mm Hg, PaCO 48 mmHg$_2$, HCO_3 23 mm Hg
- CBC: WBC 16,000 mm^3, neutrophils 8,000 mm^3

1. What are the priority nursing interventions for Emma?

2. Describe the progression of this patient's condition from the simple flu to the life-threatening ARDS.

3. What is the significance of her lab findings?

4. What do you think this patient's prognosis is? Give your rationale.

5. What do you expect the treatment plan to include?

Chapter Summary

The respiratory system plays a crucial role in supplying oxygen essential for cellular metabolism as well as excreting the carbon dioxide waste product of that metabolism. Because of this vital function, respiratory disorders can cause extensive and devastating problems throughout the body. Often the healthcare team has a limited amount of time to identify and respond to some of these respiratory disorders to control their negative consequences. Additionally, many of these diseases are preventable; therefore, identifying those at risk and implementing prevention strategies can limit the severity or halt the development of these debilitating conditions. Prevention, early detection, and prompt treatment will improve outcomes of persons suffering from these conditions, and nurses are uniquely positioned to have a positive influence on their health.

Case Study Answers

1. Maintaining oxygen therapy and respiratory treatments through the mechanical ventilator and decreasing anxiety to prevent oxygen consumption (e.g., administering sedatives, limiting stimuli, and having consistent caregivers).

2. The viral infection caused damage to the mucosa of the respiratory tract, allowing the opportunity for bacterial invasion. The massive reaction from both the viral and bacterial infections by the immune system led to fluid accumulation in the alveoli and triggered the ARDS cascade.

3. The significance of the lab findings are as follows:

   - The ABG indicates respiratory acidosis (the pH is low, the $PaCO$ is high), which is likely due to decreased gas exchange because of the ARDS.

   - The respiratory acidosis is uncompensated because the HCO_3 is normal (see Chapter 6).

   - The ABG indicates hypoxemia (PaO_2 is low), which is also due to the impaired gas exchange.

   - The CBC finding indicates a significant infection (WBC and neutrophils are high) (see Chapter 3).

4. Though Emma and her family will have a long recovery ahead of them, she will likely survive this condition because of her age, no preexisting conditions, and early intervention.

5. The treatment plan will likely include the following:

   - Continued oxygen and respiratory support

   - Continued intravenous antibiotics

   - Thrombus prevention strategies (e.g., turning, range of motion, anticoagulants, and antiplatelet agents)

   - Emotional support for both child and parents

   - Possible physical therapy depending on the longevity of the condition

References

Chiras, D. (2008). *Human biology* (6th ed.). Sudbury, MA: Jones and Bartlett.

Elling, B., Elling, K., & Rothenberg, M. (2004). *Anatomy and physiology.* Sudbury, MA: Jones and Bartlett.

Gould, B. (2006). *Pathophysiology for the health professions* (3rd ed.). Philadelphia, PA: Elsevier.

Madara, B., & Pomarico-Denino, V. (2008). *Pathophysiology* (2nd ed.). Sudbury, MA: Jones and Bartlett.

Professional guide to pathophysiology (2nd ed.). (2007). Philadelphia, PA: Lippincott Williams & Wilkins.

Resources

www.the-abg-site.com

www.cancer.gov

www.cancer.org

www.cdc.gov

www.cff.org

www.lungusa.org

www.medlineplus.gov

www.nih.gov

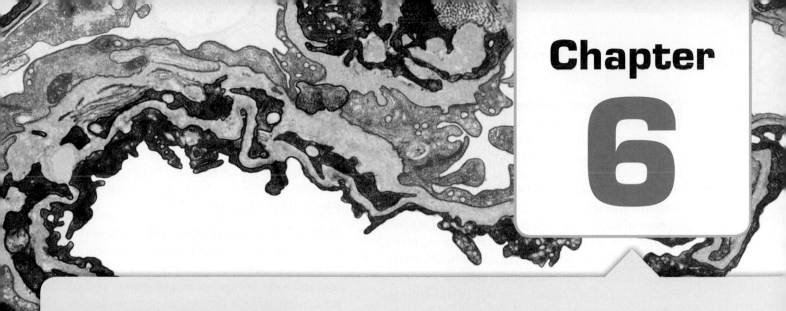

Fluid, Electrolyte, and Acid–Base Homeostasis

LEARNING OBJECTIVES

- Explain fluid distribution and movement.
- Describe and compare fluid imbalance disorders.
- Explain normal electrolyte functions in the body.
- Describe and compare electrolyte disorders.
- Explain normal pH regulation.
- Describe and compare acid–base disorders.
- Analyze arterial blood gases.

KEY TERMS

aldosterone
anasarca
anion
anion gap
antidiuretic hormone (ADH)
arterial blood gas (ABG)
atrial natriuretic peptide
bicarbonate-carbonic acid system
calcium
cation
chloride
Chvostek's sign
dehydration
depolarization
edema
extracellular fluid
fluid deficit

fluid excess
fluid volume deficit
fluid volume excess
fully compensated
hemoglobin system
hypercalcemia
hyperchloremia
hyperkalemia
hypermagnesemia
hypernatremia
hyperphosphatemia
hypertonic solution
hypervolemia
hypocalcemia
hypochloremia
hypokalemia
hypomagnesemia

hyponatremia
hypophosphatemia
hypotonic solution
hypovolemia
interstitial
intracellular fluid
intravascular
isotonic solution
magnesium
metabolic acidosis
metabolic alkalosis
nonvolatile acid
osmolarity
partially compensated
pH
phosphate system
phosphorus

potassium
protein system
repolarization
respiratory acidosis
respiratory alkalosis
sodium
third spacing
thirst mechanism
tonicity
transcellular
Trousseau's sign
uncompensated
volatile acid
volatile gas
water intoxication

The human body requires a delicate balance, or homeostasis, to function optimally (see Introduction to Pathophysiology). The body continuously employs efforts to maintain this balance. Fluids, electrolytes, and pH play a critical role in sustaining homeostasis. Fluids are distributed in various body compartments and move among these compartments to preserve equilibrium. Electrolytes are vital for cellular function, and they work with fluid to maintain stability. Acid–base balance is critical for health and is achieved through a complex buffer system. The fluid, electrolytes, and pH have a dynamic relationship in which imbalances in one area can cause imbalances in the other two. Additionally, the other areas can serve to compensate for those imbalances. When compensatory mechanisms fail to reestablish homeostasis, many bodily functions are impaired, and serious consequences can result. Medical interventions will be necessary to reestablish stability.

Fluid Balance

Distribution

Body fluid is made of water and solutes. Water is the medium within which metabolic reactions and other processes occur. Water carries nutrients into the cells, waste products out of the cells, enzymes in digestive secretions, and blood cells around the body. Fluid also facilitates movement of body parts (e.g., the joints, lungs, and heart). Fluid found inside the cells is referred to as intracellular fluid, and fluid found outside the cells is referred to as extracellular fluid. Extracellular fluid is further divided into interstitial, between the cells, and intravascular, inside the blood vessels, compartments. The cell membrane serves as a barrier for substances and water to move to or from the intracellular compartment. A third compartment of fluid is the transcellular compartment. This compartment includes:

- Fluid in the peritoneal, pleural, and pericardial cavities
- Cerebrospinal fluid
- Fluid in the joint spaces, lymph system, eyes, and gastrointestinal tract

The intracellular fluid accounts for approximately two thirds of the body's water. This intracellular fluid is rich in potassium, magnesium, phosphates, and proteins. The remaining one third of the body fluid makes up the extracellular fluid. About 80% of the extracellular fluid is in the interstitial compartment, and 20%

is in the intravascular compartment. The extracellular fluid is rich in sodium, chloride, and bicarbonate. Blood (serum) electrolyte tests only examine intravascular electrolytes. Transcellular fluid accounts for approximately 1% of the body's fluid.

Fluid Movement

Fluids are constantly circulating throughout the body and moving among compartments to maintain homeostasis. To preserve stability, the body exchanges solutes and water between compartments to compensate for conditions that increase or decrease losses. This movement between compartments is primarily accomplished through osmosis, the movement of fluid (specifically water) across a semipermeable membrane from an area of lower concentration (see Chapter 1). Often water is overlooked as a solvent, but water also has a concentration in any solution. Water moves across the semipermeable membranes to an area of lower water concentration until equilibrium is achieved. Because water moves freely across cell membranes, equilibrium is usually easy to achieve. The movement depends on hydrostatic (push) and osmotic (pull) pressures (**Figure 6-1**). Proteins and electrolytes contribute to the osmotic pressure of a fluid (**Figure 6-2**). At the arteriolar end of the capillary, the blood hydrostatic pressure (blood pressure) exceeds opposing interstitial hydrostatic pressure, moving (pushing) fluid out of the intravascular and into the interstitial compartment. At the venous end of the capillary, the blood hydrostatic pressure is decreased and the osmotic pressure is increased, moving (pulling) fluid from the interstitial to the intravascular compartment. To be an effective osmole, the solute must not be able to pass passively through a semipermeable membrane (e.g., protein).

Tonicity is the osmotic pressure of two solutions separated by a semipermeable membrane. Tonicity is often used to describe the cell's response to an external solution (**Figure 6-3**). Much like osmotic pressure, tonicity is influenced by solutes that cannot cross the membrane. In health care, the external solution that tonicity refers to is intravenous solutions, specifically those containing electrolytes (crystalloids) used to treat a variety of patient conditions (e.g., dehydration, shock). There are three classifications of tonicity for these solutions—isotonic, hypotonic, and hypertonic. Isotonic solutions (e.g., 0.9% saline, lactated Ringer's) have concentrations of solutes equal to those in the intravascular compartment. Because of these solute concentrations, isotonic solutions allow fluid to move equally between compartments and do not cause

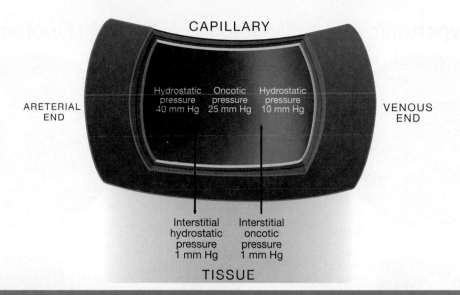

CAPILLARY

ARETERIAL
END

Hydrostatic
pressure
40 mm Hg

Oncotic
pressure
25 mm Hg

Hydrostatic
pressure
10 mm Hg

VENOUS
END

Interstitial
hydrostatic
pressure
1 mm Hg

Interstitial
oncotic
pressure
1 mm Hg

TISSUE

Figure 6-1

Pressures that control fluid balance.

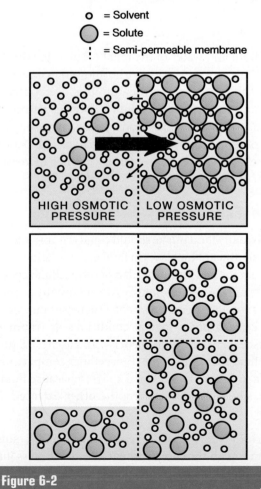

o = Solvent

◯ = Solute

⋮ = Semi-permeable membrane

HIGH OSMOTIC
PRESSURE

LOW OSMOTIC
PRESSURE

Figure 6-2

Osmotic pressure.

notable shifts. **Hypotonic solutions** (e.g., 0.45% saline) have a lower concentration of solutes than those in the intravascular compartment. Hypotonic solutions cause fluid to shift from the intravascular out to the intracellular space. **Hypertonic solutions** (e.g., 5% dextrose in 0.9% saline, 3% saline) have a higher concentration of solutes than those in the intravascular compartment. Hypertonic solutions cause fluid to shift from the intracellular in to the intravascular space.

Additionally, fluid is added to the body through the ingestion of food and fluids and as a cellular byproduct. Approximately 100 mL of water is needed per 100 calories ingested to help with metabolism and waste elimination. Fluid is primarily lost in the urine and feces, but additional insensible (immeasurable) losses occur through the skin (e.g., perspiration) and respiratory tract (e.g., breathing, coughing, talking, and mechanical ventilation). Body fluid intake and output balance is maintained through several mechanisms. The osmoreceptor cells sense intravascular fluid volume. Decreased fluid volume or increased **osmolarity** (solute concentration) triggers the **thirst mechanism** in the hypothalamus to increase oral intake. The thirst sensation occurs with even the smallest water losses and is one of the best regulators of water balance. This thirst sensation can decrease with aging (called hypodipsia). The **antidiuretic hormone (ADH)** regulates fluid volume by controlling water losses in the urine. Released from the pituitary gland in times of decreased

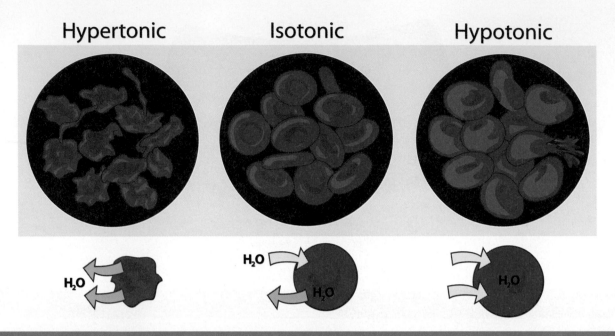

Figure 6-3

Cellular response to tonicity.

fluid volume and increased osmolarity, ADH promotes reabsorption of water into the blood from the renal tubules. **Aldosterone** is a hormone that is released to conserve more water when needed (e.g., when one has low blood pressure) by increasing reabsorption

of sodium and water in the renal tubules. Finally, the **atrial natriuretic peptide** is a hormone that is released when the atria of the myocardium is overstretched, indicating increased fluid volume. The atrial natriuretic peptide stimulates renal vasodilatation, increasing urinary output. Additionally, atrial natriuretic peptide suppresses aldosterone secretion, further increasing urinary output.

Fluid Excess

Ideally, daily fluid intake should equal the amount lost. Most significant increases in fluid accumulation occur in the interstitial, intravascular, or intracellular spaces. Significant daily gains or losses do not usually occur in the transcellular compartments. Increases may occur with certain physiological conditions or traumatic events (e.g., pericarditis, pleurisy, and ascites). Significant fluid increases in the transcellular compartment are often referred to as **third spacing** because fluid is not easily exchanged among the other extracellular fluids.

Fluid excess has several other names, some depending on the compartment affected. Excess fluid in the interstitial space is generally referred to as **edema**. Edema is a problem of fluid distribution, not necessarily of fluid overload. Edema results when hydrostatic and osmotic forces favor fluid moving from the intra-

LEARNING POINTS

Tonicity works by playing on the relationship certain nutrients and electrolytes have with water. Both sodium and glucose attract water—water will go wherever the higher concentrations of sodium and glucose are. In the case of intravenous (IV) fluids, the concentration of sodium and glucose in the intravascular compartment is adjusted to attract or repel water. For example, 0.9% (isotonic) saline has similar sodium concentrations to that in the intravascular space, so no fluid is shifted between compartments. Fluid is just replaced in the intravascular compartment. Hypotonic (0.45%) saline has lower concentrations of sodium than that usually found in the intravascular space, so water moves out of the intravascular to the intracellular compartment. The same occurs when glucose or dextrose is in a solution. Finally, hypertonic (3%) saline has higher concentrations of sodium than is usually found in the intravascular space, so water moves from the intracellular in to the intravascular compartment. So remember that wherever sodium and glucose are, water will follow!

CLINICAL CASE

A demonstration of the severity of water intoxication can be seen in a story familiar to many. A radio station was having a contest. The contestant who could drink the most water without voiding would win the contest. Because water is limited in electrolytes like sodium, excessive water intake in a short period can cause the sodium concentration in the vascular space to drop in relationship to the water. Then, the sodium concentration in the tissue is higher than that in the blood, causing water to move out of the vascular space to the interstitial space. This fluid quickly caused cerebral edema (see Chapter 11), decreased neurological functioning, and death in the individual who consumed the most water in the contest. The sad thing is a nurse called into the radio station to warn them that this contest was dangerous, yet the station went ahead with it. It was a seemingly harmless act that had grave consequences.

vascular to the interstitial space. Edema occurs when hydrostatic forces are greater than osmotic forces. For example, blood stagnates in the periphery with heart failure, increasing hydrostatic pressure and pushing fluid out of the vessel (see Chapter 4). Edema may be localized to one area such as the feet or generalized throughout the body (called anasarca). Excess fluid in the intravascular compartment is frequently referred to as hypervolemia or fluid volume excess. Often hypervolemia results from excessive sodium and/or water intake or insufficient losses. The intake becomes greater than the body's compensatory mechanisms can manage. The excess fluid volume strains the left ventricle, which can cause left-sided heart failure over time (see Chapter 4). Fluid excess can also occur in the intracellular space, also known as water intoxication. Intracellular fluid excess can lead to the rupture, or lysis, of the cells. Cerebral cells are the most sensitive to lysis.

Fluid excess may result from the following conditions:

- Excessive sodium or water intake, including that caused by the following:
  - High-sodium diet (e.g., processed foods, sodas, and certain seasonings)
  - Psychogenic polydipsia (excessive water ingestion)
  - Hypertonic fluid administration
  - Free water
  - Enteral feedings

- Inadequate sodium or water elimination, including that caused by the following:
  - Hyperaldosteronism (which increases sodium retention and, in turn, water retention)
  - Cushing's syndrome (a condition of excessive corticosteroid, which contains high levels of sodium; see Chapter 10)
  - Syndrome of inappropriate antidiuretic hormone (excessive ADH levels, which increases fluid retention)
  - Renal failure (kidneys are unable to eliminate fluid or waste products; see Chapter 7)
  - Liver failure (the liver is unable to synthesize protein, impairing colloidal pressures; see Chapter 9)
  - Heart failure (the heart is unable to pump blood affectively, leading to decreased blood flow to the kidneys and fluid shifts; see Chapter 4)

Clinical manifestations of fluid excess include:

- Peripheral edema (skin usually indents with pressure, referred to as pitting; Figure 6-4)
- Periorbital edema (swelling around the eyes)
- Anasarca (generalized edema; skin may begin to weep fluid)
- Cerebral edema (including headache, confusion, irritability, anxiety, nausea, and vomiting)
- Dyspnea
- Bounding pulse
- Tachycardia
- Jugular vein distension

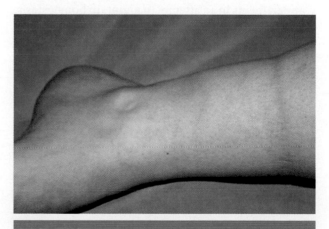

Figure 6-4

Pitting edema.

- Hypertension
- Polyuria (large amounts of pale yellow urine)
- Rapid weight gain (3 pounds in a week or 1–2 pounds in a day; 1 pound approximately equals 500 mL)
- Crackles (adventitious breath sound)
- Bulging fontanelles (in infants)

Diagnostic procedures for fluid excess include a CBC. Urine and blood specific gravity and osmolality will be decreased due to solute dilution. Blood cells, especially the red blood cells and platelets, may be decreased because of the high ratio of fluid. Management focuses on identifying and treating the underlying cause. Strategies may consist of wearing compression stockings, administering diuretics, restricting sodium and fluids, and maintaining high Fowler's position. In severe cases of intracellular and interstitial fluid excess, hypertonic solutions may be given to shift the excess fluid from these spaces to the intravascular space, where it can be excreted. To aid in excretion, a diuretic may be administered.

Fluid Deficit

Fluid deficit occurs when total body fluid levels are insufficient to meet the body's needs. Fluid deficit may be referred to as dehydration. Fluid deficit of the intravascular compartment is often referred to as fluid volume deficit or hypovolemia. Fluid deficit can occur independently or with electrolyte deficits, such as a sodium deficit. As fluid levels decrease, sodium levels, along with other blood solutes (e.g., blood cells, electrolytes), increase because of hemoconcentration. Climbing sodium levels trigger fluid shifts from other compartments in an attempt to maintain homeostasis. When losses are greater than these shifts can accommodate, the cells shrink. Fluid volume levels decrease, causing hypotension.

Causes of fluid deficits include:

- Inadequate fluid intake, such as caused by the following:
  - Poor oral intake (such as that which occurs in the event of stroke or dementia)
  - Inadequate IV fluid replacement
- Excessive fluid or sodium losses, such as those caused by the following:
  - Gastrointestinal losses (such as losses that occur with vomiting, diarrhea, and nasogastric suctioning)

- Excessive diaphoresis (sweating)
- Prolonged hyperventilation
- Hemorrhage
- Nephrosis (also called nephrotic syndrome; a degenerative renal disease that causes excessive protein losses, leading to fluid movement out of the intravascular compartment)
- Diabetes mellitus (which causes renal glucose excretion, and, in turn, results in water losses)
- Diabetes insipidus (an inability to concentrate urine, leading to excessive water losses)
- Burns (heat denatures proteins, which disrupts colloidal pressure)
- Open wounds (increased drainage)
- Ascites
- Effusions
- Excessive use of diuretics
- Osmotic diuresis that can occur with hypertonic tube feedings or administering parenteral feedings too quickly

Clinical manifestations of fluid deficits include:

- Thirst
- Altered level of consciousness
- Hypotension
- Tachycardia
- Weak, thready pulse
- Flat jugular veins
- Dry mucous membranes
- Decreased skin turgor
- Oliguria
- Weight loss
- Sunken fontanelles (in infants)

CLINICAL CASE

An example of osmotic diuresis can be seen in a tragic case in which a newborn was fed concentrated formula by mistake. Often, tube feeding and baby formulas are high in glucose and other electrolytes. Many times these formulas come concentrated for shipping purposes. The newborn's father was unaware that the formula required dilution prior to feeding it to his child. The high concentrations of glucose caused excessive urination. The baby died because of hypertonic dehydration.

Diagnostic procedures for fluid deficit consist of a history, physical examination, measurements of intake and output, daily weights, blood chemistry, urine analysis, and a CBC. Urine and blood specific gravity and osmolality will be increased, indicating a high concentration of solutes. Blood cells, especially red blood cells and platelets, may be increased because of the low ratio of fluid. Management focuses on identifying and treating the underlying cause. Strategies include fluid replacement—oral for mild losses and intravenous fluids for greater losses (either isotonic or hypotonic).

Electrolyte Balance

Electrolytes play a crucial role in homeostasis. Electrolytes are minerals with electrical charges that are found in the blood, urine, and other body fluids. Electrolytes in the body include sodium, chloride, potassium, calcium, magnesium, and phosphorus (**Table 6-1**). Cations are positively charged while anions are negatively charged. Electrolytes are important in muscle and neural activity and in acid–base and fluid balance.

Sodium

Sodium is considered the most significant cation. Sodium is the most prevalent electrolyte of extracellular fluid, and its primary function is to control serum osmolality and water balance. Sodium also has an affinity for chloride and helps maintain acid–base balance when combined with bicarbonate (HCO_3). Sodium is regulated by the kidneys and aldosterone produced by the adrenal cortex. Aldosterone is released, and the kidneys retain sodium in times of high serum osmolality

Table 6-1 Normal Serum Values of the Major Electrolytes*

Electrolyte	Normal Range
Sodium (Na^+)	135–145 mEq/L
Chloride (Cl^-)	98–108 mEq/L
Potassium (K^+)	3.5–5 mEq/L
Calcium (Ca^{++})	4–5 mEq/L
Phosphorus (P)	2.5–4.5 mg/dL
Magnesium (Mg^{++})	1.8–2.4 mEq/L

*Values may vary slightly.

or low blood volume. The opposite is true when serum osmolality decreases and fluid volume increases. The sympathetic nervous system assists the kidneys in sodium regulation by changing the glomerular filtration rate, which is a reflection of renal blood flow. Increasing the glomerular filtration rate increases sodium excretion; decreasing the glomerular filtration rate decreases sodium excretion. The renin-angiotensin-aldosterone mechanism (see Chapter 7) also manipulates sodium in the kidneys, and this mechanism is triggered in times of decreased renal perfusion (e.g., hypovolemia and hypotension). Renin, a protein, converts angiotensinogen to angiotensin I, and angiotensin I is converted to angiotensin II in the lungs. Angiotensin II causes the kidneys to retain sodium and, in turn, water.

The cellular membrane is permeable to sodium, but it is dependent on the sodium-potassium pump (see Chapter 1). Sodium facilitates muscles and nerve impulses through the pump. As sodium moves into the cell, potassium shifts out, resulting in depolarization (increasing membrane potential or excitability) of the cell membrane. When sodium shifts back out of the cell, potassium moves back into the cell, resulting in repolarization (restoring resting potential) of the cell membrane.

Sodium is primarily brought into the body through dietary intake. The recommended dietary allowance (RDA) of sodium is 2–4 grams. Sodium can be found in many sources such as table salt (1 teaspoon has more than 2 grams of sodium), processed or prepackaged foods (e.g., canned foods and deli meats), snack foods (e.g., chips), condiments (e.g., ketchup and hot sauce), and certain cooking seasonings (e.g., garlic salt and seasoning salt).

Normally, sodium losses occur in the kidneys. Excessive losses can occur through the gastrointestinal tract through vomiting, diarrhea, and nasogastric suctioning. Extensive burns can also cause sodium losses through the skin. Finally, sodium losses can occur with excessive sweating (e.g., fever and strenuous exercise).

Hypernatremia

Hypernatremia results from high serum sodium levels (> 145 mEq/L). The excessive sodium levels generally lead to high serum osmolality (> 295 mOsm/kg) because of the imbalance between sodium and water. As sodium levels rise, water shifts from the intracellular and interstitial spaces to the intravascular compartment.

Hypernatremia usually results from ingesting excessive sodium without consuming a proportionate amount of water or through water losses that are greater than the sodium being lost. Causes of hypernatremia include:

- Excessive sodium, such as that caused by the following:
  - Excessive sodium ingestion
  - Hypertonic IV saline (3% saline) administration
  - Cushing's syndrome (a condition of excessive corticosteroid that contains high levels of sodium)
  - Corticosteroid use
- Deficient water, such as that caused by the following:
  - Decreased water ingestion
  - Loss of thirst sensation
  - Inability to drink water (which might occur if one is unconscious or confused)
  - Third spacing
  - Vomiting
  - Diarrhea
  - Excessive sweating
  - Prolonged episode of hyperventilation (increases insensible water losses)
  - Diuretic use
  - Diabetes insipidus (excessive water loss as a result of insufficient ADH levels)

Clinical manifestations of hypernatremia can be subtle to serious, depending on the severity of the hypernatremia itself. These manifestations include:

- Increased temperature
- Warm, flushed skin
- Dry and sticky mucous membranes
- Dysphagia (difficulty swallowing)
- Increased thirst
- Irritability and agitation
- Weakness
- Headache
- Seizures
- Lethargy
- Coma
- Blood pressure changes
- Tachycardia
- Weak, thready pulse

- Edema
- Decreased urine output (can be high with diabetes insipidus)

Diagnostic procedures for hypernatremia include a history, physical examination, blood chemistry, and urine analysis. Other procedures (e.g., computed tomography [CT] and magnetic resonance imaging [MRI]) may be conducted to identify causation. Management of hypernatremia focuses on treating the underlying cause. If the cause is related to water loss, treatment begins with replacing water and any electrolytes. Glucose-electrolyte solutions (e.g., sports drinks) are given orally for less severe cases. More severe cases can be corrected with intravenous hypotonic (e.g., 5% dextrose in water, 0.45% saline) solutions. The healthcare professional must use caution in order to avoid correcting the hypernatremia too rapidly. The brain can become accustomed to the high levels of sodium, and then as the levels drop, water moves into cerebral cells, causing cerebral edema. Generally, one should not correct hypernatremia faster than 1 mEq/L per hour. Diuretics may be necessary if the patient is hypervolemic. Additionally, seizure precautions (e.g., low lighting and decreased stimuli) and neurologic checks should be added to the patient's plan of care.

Hyponatremia

Hyponatremia results from low serum sodium levels (< 135 mEq/L). Serum osmolality levels also fall below 275 mOsm. As sodium levels decrease, water shifts into brain cells, causing cerebral edema. Additionally, nerve conduction becomes impaired as the sodium levels fall.

Hyponatremia results from excessive sodium losses or increased water gains (referred to as dilutional hyponatremia). Causes of hyponatremia include:

- Deficient sodium, including that caused by the following:
  - Diuretic use
  - Gastrointestinal losses (e.g., vomiting and diarrhea)
  - Excessive sweating
  - Insufficient aldosterone levels (Addison's disease)
  - Adrenal insufficiency
  - Dietary sodium restrictions
- Excessive water, including that caused by the following:
  - Hypotonic intravenous saline (0.45% saline)

- Hyperglycemia (excess glucose in the blood attracts water from the intracellular and interstitial spaces)
- Excessive water ingestion
- Renal failure
- Syndrome of inappropriate antidiuretic hormone
- Heart failure (circulation stagnation leads to decreased renal excretion)

Clinical manifestations of hyponatermia may vary in severity depending on the sodium level. These manifestations may include:

- Anorexia
- Gastrointestinal upset (e.g., abdominal cramps, nausea, vomiting, and diarrhea)
- Poor skin turgor
- Dry mucous membranes
- Blood pressure changes (decreased with hypovolemia and increased with hypervolemia)
- Pulse changes (weak with hypovolemia and bounding with hypervolemia)
- Edema
- Headache
- Lethargy
- Confusion
- Diminished deep tendon reflexes
- Muscle weakness
- Seizures
- Coma

Diagnostic procedures for hyponatremia are similar to those for hypernatremia. Management focuses on treating the underlying cause (e.g., administering corticosteroids for Addison's disease). For excessive water, oral intake may be limited. For deficient sodium, oral intake may be increased. Correction of sodium levels should be done slowly so as not to overload the heart from fluid shifting into the intravascular space. Additionally, seizure precautions (e.g., low lighting and decreased stimuli) and neurologic checks should be added to the patient's plan of care.

Chloride

Chloride is a mineral electrolyte and the major extracellular anion. Chloride assists in fluid distribution by attaching to sodium or water. Because of its negative charge, chloride can bind and travel with the positively charged ions (e.g., sodium, potassium, calcium, etc.). Chloride is found in gastric secretions, pancreatic juices, and bile. In the stomach, chloride unites with hydrogen to form hydrochloric acid. Chloride is abundant in cerebrospinal fluid, where it binds with sodium. When bound to sodium, chloride behaves just as sodium in regard to water balance. When bound to hydrogen, chloride plays an important role in acid–base balance. The kidneys are primarily responsible for chloride excretion, but some chloride is also lost through sweating.

Diet is the main source of chloride. The chloride RDA is 3–9 grams. Chloride is easily obtained through a balanced diet. Common sources of chloride include table salt, fruits, vegetables, cheese, milk, eggs, fish, canned foods, and processed meats. Chloride is primarily excreted in the kidneys.

Hyperchloremia

Hyperchloremia is an excess amount of chloride in the blood (> 108 mEq/L). Hyperchloremia is usually a result of an underlying condition and without its own clinical manifestations. Some causes of hyperchloridemia include:

- Increased chloride intake or exchange, including that caused by the following:
  - Hypernatremia
  - Hypertonic intravenous solution
  - Metabolic acidosis
  - Hyperkalemia
- Decreased chloride excretion, including that caused by the following:
  - Hyperparathyroidism (increases calcium levels, which attracts chloride)
  - Hyperaldosteronism (increases sodium levels, which attracts chloride)
  - Renal failure (decreased chloride excretion)

Diagnostic procedures include a history, physical examination, blood chemistry, urine analysis, and arterial blood gases (ABGs). Management of hyperchloremia focuses on treating the underlying cause. Administering diuretics to assist in eliminating sodium will, in turn, assist in the removal of chloride. Administering bicarbonate can correct acidosis if present.

Hypochloremia

Hypochloremia occurs when chloride levels fall below 98 mEq/L. Hypochloremia rarely occurs in the absence of other abnormalities and, therefore, does not have its own set of clinical manifestations. Causative conditions include:

- Decreased chloride intake or exchange such as that accompanied by the following:

  - Hyponatremia
  - 5% dextrose in water intravenous solution
  - Water intoxication
  - Hypokalemia

- Increased chloride excretion, such as that which occurs with the following:

  - Diuretics (sodium loss, which, in turn, increases chloride excretion)
  - Vomiting (excessive loss of hydrochloric acid)
  - Metabolic alkalosis
  - Other gastrointestinal losses (such as those that occur with fistula, ileostomy, nasogastric suction, and diarrhea)

Diagnostic procedures for hypochloremia are similar to those of hyperchloremia. Treatment focuses on correcting the underlying causes. Some of those strategies include increasing oral sodium intake and administering sodium-containing intravenous solutions. Additionally, ammonium chloride can be given with caution to raise chloride levels. Saline solutions can also be used to irrigate gastric tubes.

Potassium

Potassium is the primary intracellular cation. Potassium plays a crucial role in electrical conduction, acid–base balance, and metabolism (carbohydrate, protein, and glucose). Potassium is in huge quantities in the intracellular space and can be utilized if serum levels drop. However, certain circumstances (e.g., lysis) cause excessive shifts of potassium to the intravascular space, which can be dangerous (especially within the heart). Serum potassium has very little room for fluctuations either up or down without causing serious issues. The sodium–potassium pump and the kidneys regulate potassium. Diet (e.g., cantaloupes, raisins, bananas, oranges, green leafy vegetables, and lentils) is the primary source of potassium. The RDA for potassium is 40–60 mEq. In addition to potassium being excreted in the kidneys, it is also lost through the gastrointestinal tract.

Hyperkalemia

Hyperkalemia refers to serum potassium levels greater than 5 mEq/L. Hyperkalemia is unusual in the healthy individual and may be a medical emergency. Gener-

ally, hyperkalemia is caused by conditions that impair excretion, increase intake, or release potassium out of the cells. These conditions include:

- Deficient excretion, such as occurs with the following:

  - Renal failure
  - Addison's disease (decreased levels of aldosterone decreases potassium secretion)
  - Certain medications (e.g., potassium-sparing diuretics, nonsteroidal anti-inflammatory drugs, and angiotensin-converting enzyme inhibitors), which can also alter aldosterone levels
  - Gordon's syndrome (a rare genetic disorder in which the kidneys are unable to respond to aldosterone)

- Excessive intake, such as occurs with the following:

  - Oral potassium supplements
  - Salt substitutes (many contain high amounts of potassium to create a "salty" taste)
  - Rapid intravenous administration of diluted potassium (administering potassium undiluted can be lethal)

- Increased release from cells, including that associated with the following:

  - Acidosis (increased serum hydrogen levels causes potassium to shift out of the cells; lack of insulin in diabetic ketoacidosis impairs the transportation of potassium in the cell)
  - Blood transfusions (can cause blood cell lysis, releasing intracellular potassium)
  - Burns or any other cellular injuries (can cause cell lysis, releasing intracellular potassium)

Hyperkalemia can affect several body systems because of potassium's functions, including the nervous, cardiac, respiratory, and gastrointestinal systems. The severity of these effects depends on the extent of the hyperkalemia. Clinical manifestations of hyperkalemia include:

- Muscle weakness
- Paresthesia (numbness or tingling)
- Flaccid paralysis
- Bradycardia
- Dysrhythmias (some of which can be fatal)
- Electrocardiogram (EKG) changes (long PR interval, wide QRS, peaked T wave, and depressed ST segment [**Figure 6-5**; see Chapter 4])

HYPERKALEMIC EFFECT ON ECG

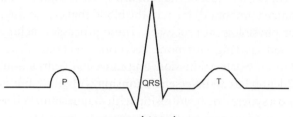

normal tracing
(K⁺ levels between 3.5-5.3 mEq/L)

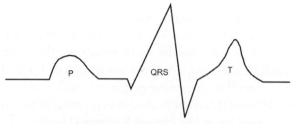

tall peaked T Wave, prolonged PR interval, depressed ST segment, QRS wider with K⁺ > 7 mEq/L

Figure 6-5

Hyperkalemic effects on the electrocardiogram.

- Cardiac arrest
- Respiratory depression (from muscle weakness)
- Abdominal cramping
- Nausea
- Diarrhea

Diagnostic procedures for hyperkalemia include a history, physical examination, blood chemistry, 12-lead EKG, and ABGs. Management focuses on the identification and treatment of the cause (e.g., sodium bicarbonate to treat acidosis). If present, acidosis is treated prior to the hyperkalemia so that potassium can shift back into the cells and a true potassium level can be obtained. Calcium gluconate may be administered to minimize dysrhythmias. Additionally, measures should be taken to decrease intake, increase excretion, and facilitate cellular exchange of potassium. Strategies may include:

- Decrease dietary potassium intake
- Increase excretion, such as by the following methods:
  - Dialysis
  - Kayexalate (sodium polystyrene sulfonate, which increases gastrointestinal potassium excretion)
  - Intravenous fluids
  - Potassium-losing diuretics
- Facilitate cellular exchange by administering insulin (which may be given with intravenous dextrose to prevent blood glucose drops)

Hypokalemia

Hypokalemia occurs when potassium levels drop below 3.5 mEq/L. Hypokalemia typically results from excessive loss, inadequate intake, or increased potassium cellular uptake. These conditions include:

- Excessive loss as a result of one or more of the following:
  - Vomiting
  - Diarrhea
  - Nasogastric suctioning
  - Fistulas
  - Laxatives
  - Potassium-losing diuretics
  - Cushing's syndrome (decreases sodium excretion, which in turn increases potassium excretion)
  - Corticosteroids (decreases sodium excretion, which, in turn, increases potassium excretion)
- Deficient intake, such as occurs with the following:
  - Malnutrition
  - Extreme dieting
  - Alcoholism (can result in inadequate nutrition, nausea, and vomiting)
- Increased shift into the cell as occurs with the following:
  - Alkalosis (decreased serum hydrogen levels causes potassium to shift into the cells)
  - Insulin excess (increases potassium transportation into the cells)

Much like hyperkalemia, hypokalemia can affect several body systems because of potassium's functions including the nervous, cardiac, respiratory, and gastrointestinal systems. The severity of these effects is proportionate to the extent of the hypokalemia. Clinical manifestations of hypokalemia are similar to hyperkalemia and include:

- Muscle weakness
- Paresthesias

HYPOKALEMIC EFFECT ON ECG

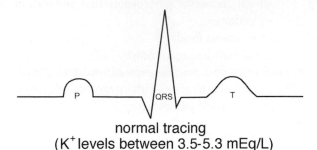

normal tracing
(K$^+$ levels between 3.5-5.3 mEq/L)

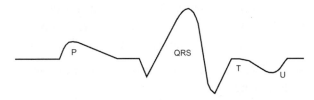

depressed ST segment, T wave
inversion, U waves (K$^+$ level <3.5 mEq/L)

Figure 6-6

Hypokalemic effects on the electrocardiogram.

- Hyporeflexia
- Leg cramps
- Weak, irregular pulse
- Hypotension
- Dysrhythmias (some of which are lethal)
- EKG changes (prolonged PR interval, depressed ST segment, flattened T wave, and a U wave [**Figure 6-6**; see Chapter 4])
- Decreased bowel sounds
- Abdominal distension
- Constipation or ileus
- Cardiac arrest

Diagnostic procedures for hypokalemia include a history, physical examination, blood chemistry, 12-lead EKG, and ABGs. Management focuses on the identification and treatment of the cause (e.g., correct alkalosis). Additionally, strategies are directed at increasing available potassium. Oral potassium is administered for mild cases, while diluted intravenous potassium is administered for more severe deficits.

Calcium

Most of the body's calcium is found in the bones and teeth (99%). Most of the remaining 1% is found in an ionized (unbound) form in the blood that can be used for physiological processes. These processes include blood clotting, hormone secretion, receptor functions, nerve transmission, and muscular contraction. Calcium has an inverse relationship with phosphorus and a synergistic relationship with magnesium. When calcium levels go up, phosphorus goes down and vice versa. Calcium needs magnesium to fully function as well as balance its effects.

Calcium is brought into the body through the absorption of dietary sources in the gastrointestinal tract, specifically the small intestines; therefore, conditions affecting intestinal absorption or surgical procedures that change the gastrointestinal tract (e.g., gastric bypass) can alter calcium absorption. Vitamin D aids in calcium absorption. Vitamin D is primarily obtained from sun exposure and fortified dairy products. Vitamin K also plays an important role in calcium regulation and bone formation (vitamin K binds to calcium in the bone). Vitamin K can primarily be found in green leafy vegetables. Calcium is primarily found in sources such as dairy products, salmon, sardines, green leafy vegetables, pinto beans, almonds, and figs. The RDA of calcium is 800–1,200 mg/day; however, the daily needs vary with certain conditions (e.g., pregnancy, childhood, and osteoporosis).

Calcium is excreted in the urine and stool. Calcium is regulated by the parathyroid hormones and calcitonin (a thyroid hormone). When serum calcium levels are low, the parathyroid hormone mobilizes the bone calcium and pulls it into the bloodstream. To compensate for this shift, parathyroid hormone replaces this calcium by decreasing renal excretion and promoting intestinal absorption. Calcitonin, on the other hand, regulates elevated calcium levels by pushing the excess calcium into the bone, decreasing intestinal absorption and increasing renal excretion.

Hypercalcemia

Hypercalcemia occurs when ionized calcium levels climb above 5 mEq/L. Hypercalcemia results from excessive calcium intake or calcium release from the bone as well as inadequate excretion. These causes include:

- Increased intake or release, including that caused by the following:

- Calcium antacids (e.g., Tums)
- Calcium supplements
- Cancer (especially bone, but also lung, breast, ovarian, prostate, leukemia, and gastrointestinal cancers)
- Immobilization
- Corticosteroids
- Vitamin D deficiency
- Hypophosphatemia
- Deficit excretion, including that caused by the following:
  - Renal failure
  - Thiazide diuretics
  - Hyperparathyroidism

Clinical manifestations of hypercalcemia reflect decreased cell membrane excitability and are often nonspecific. The cardiac, nervous, musculoskeletal, gastrointestinal, and renal systems can be affected by these high calcium levels. Clinical manifestations of hypercalcemia include:

- Dysrhythmias (some of which can be fatal)
- EKG changes (short QT interval)
- Personality changes
- Confusion
- Decreased memory
- Headache
- Lethargy
- Stupor
- Coma
- Muscle weakness
- Decreased deep tendon reflexes
- Anorexia
- Nausea and vomiting
- Constipation
- Abdominal pain
- Pancreatitis
- Renal calculi (stones)
- Polyuria (high calcium levels interfere with ADH, resulting in increased water excretion)
- Dehydration

Diagnostic procedures include a history, physical examination, blood chemistry, and 12-lead EKG. Management of hypercalcemia focuses on identification and treatment of the underlying cause (e.g., dialysis for

renal failure). Additionally, strategies may be implemented to treat clinical manifestations (e.g., antidysrhythmic agents). Oral phosphate, increasing mobility, and administering calcitonin can facilitate the movement of the calcium from the bloodstream and into the bone. Increasing intravenous fluid administration can increase renal excretion of calcium. Diuretics may be necessary to enhance this excretion further.

Hypocalcemia

Hypocalcemia occurs when ionized calcium levels fall below 4 mEq/L. Hypocalcemia occurs from increased losses or decreased intake of calcium. The causes include:

- Excessive losses, including those associated with the following:
  - Hypoparathyroidism
  - Renal failure
  - Hyperphosphatemia
  - Alkalosis (as serum hydrogen levels decrease, calcium levels decrease)
  - Pancreatitis (decreases intestinal absorption of fat; calcium binds to the fat and is excreted)
  - Laxatives (decrease absorption)
  - Diarrhea
  - Other medications (e.g., diuretics, calcitonin, and gentamicin)
- Deficient intake, including that caused by the following:
  - Decreased dietary intake
  - Alcoholism (decreased diet and poor absorption)
  - Absorption disorders (e.g., Crohn's disease)
  - Hypoalbuminemia (much of calcium is bound to protein)

As opposed to hypercalcemia, hypocalcemia increases cell membrane excitability. The low calcium levels affect the cardiac, neurological, musculoskeletal, respiratory, and gastrointestinal systems. Clinical manifestations of hypocalcemia include:

- Dysrhythmias (some of which can be lethal)
- EKG changes (prolonged QT interval)
- Increased bleeding tendencies (e.g., bruising and petechia)
- Anxiety
- Confusion
- Depression
- Irritability

- Fatigue
- Lethargy
- Paresthesia
- Increased deep tendon reflexes
- Tremors
- Muscle spasms
- Seizures
- Laryngeal spasms
- Increased bowel sounds
- Abdominal cramping

In addition to these clinical manifestations, two signs may be present—Trousseau's and Chvostek's signs. To test for the Trousseau's sign, arterial blood flow is occluded using an inflated blood pressure cuff. The cuff is placed on the upper arm and is inflated above the individual's usual systolic pressure measurement. The inflated cuff is left in place for approximately 3 minutes. The test is considered positive for increased neuromuscular irritability if it elicits a carpal spasm (flexed wrist and metacarpophalangeal joints, extended interphalangeal joints, and adducted thumb) (Figure 6-7). To test for the Chvostek's sign, the facial nerve in front of the ear is tapped. A spasm or brief contraction of the corner of the mouth, nose, eye, and muscles in the

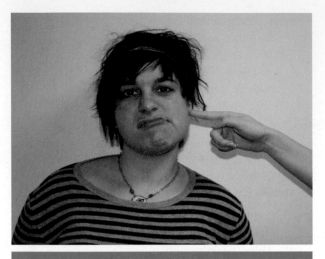

Figure 6-8

Chvostek's sign.

cheek indicates a positive sign and increased neuromuscular irritability (Figure 6-8).

Diagnostic procedures for hypocalcemia are similar to those for hypercalcemia. Management focuses on identification and treatment of the underlying cause. Calcium levels can be increased with oral supplements (mild deficiencies) and intravenous calcium gluconate (moderate to severe deficiencies). Vitamin D supplements can increase intestinal calcium absorption. Additionally, phosphorus intake may be decreased to bring calcium levels up.

Phosphorus

Most of the body's phosphorus, or phosphate, is found in the bones, with smaller quantities found circulating in the bloodstream. As previously mentioned, phosphorus has an inverse relationship with calcium. The functions of phosphorus include bone and tooth mineralization, cellular metabolism, acid–base balance, and cell membrane formation.

Phosphorus primarily enters the body through dietary sources, and elimination mainly occurs in the urine. Foods high in phosphorus include dairy products, protein sources (e.g., chicken, beef, fish, and nuts), grains, and carbonated sodas. The RDA of phosphorus is approximately 1,000 mg/day. Phosphorus absorption is decreased when ingested with foods containing calcium, magnesium, and aluminum—all of which bind with phosphorus.

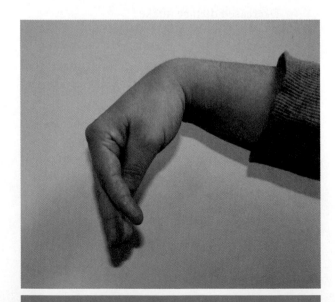

Figure 6-7

Trousseau's sign.

Hyperphosphatemia

Hyperphosphatemia occurs when phosphorus levels climb above 4.5 mg/dL. Hyperphosphatemia usually results from decreased excretion or increased intake of phosphorus. These causes include:

- Deficient excretion, such as that caused by the following:
  - Renal failure
  - Hypoparathyroidism (decreases renal excretion)
  - Adrenal insufficiency
  - Hypothyroidism
  - Laxatives, especially those containing phosphorus (decreases calcium levels, which increases phosphorus levels)
- Excessive intake or cellular exchange, such as that caused by the following:
  - Cellular damage (e.g., burn, trauma, and chemotherapy)
  - Hypocalcemia
  - Acidosis (increased phosphorus shifts from the intracellular to the intravascular compartment)

Clinical manifestations are similar to hypocalcemia and are rarely seen alone. Diagnostic procedures for hyperphosphatemia consist of a history, physical examination, and blood chemistry. Management of hyperphosphatemia includes identification and treatment of the underlying cause (e.g., dialysis for renal failure). Aluminum hydroxide and aluminum carbonate can bind to phosphorus and increase intestinal excretion. Additionally, treatment of hypocalcemia may be necessary.

Hypophosphatemia

Hypophosphatemia occurs when phosphorus levels drop below 2.5 mg/dL. Hypophosphatemia is usually caused by increased excretion or decreased intake of phosphorus. These causes include:

- Excessive excretion or cellular exchange, such as that caused by the following:
  - Renal failure
  - Hyperparathyroidism (increases renal excretion)
  - Alkalosis (increased phosphorus shifts from the intravascular to the intracellular compartment)
- Deficient intake, such as that caused by the following:
  - Malabsorption
  - Vitamin D deficiency
  - Magnesium and aluminum antacids
  - Alcoholism
  - Decreased dietary intake (rare)

Clinical manifestations are similar to hypercalcemia. Diagnostic procedures include a history, physical examination, and blood chemistry. Management of hypophosphatemia focuses on the identification and treatment of the underlying cause (e.g., dialysis for renal failure). Phosphorus levels can be increased with oral supplements (mild deficiencies) and intravenous potassium phosphate (moderate to severe deficiencies).

Magnesium

Magnesium is an intracellular cation that is mostly stored in the bone and muscle. Magnesium helps maintain normal muscle and nerve function, regular cardiac rhythm, a healthy immune system, bones strength, blood glucose levels, and normal blood pressure as well as being involved in energy metabolism and protein synthesis. Magnesium has a direct relationship with calcium and an inverse relationship with phosphorus. Magnesium is excreted through the kidneys and enters the body through dietary intake. Foods high in magnesium include green vegetables, legumes, nuts, seeds, and whole grains. The RDA for magnesium is approximately 400 mg per day.

Hypermagnesemia

Hypermagnesemia occurs when magnesium levels increase above 2.5 mEq/L. Hypermagnesemia is rare and usually results from renal failure as well as excessive laxative or antacid use. Clinical manifestations of hypermagnesemia are similar to hypercalcemia. Diagnostic procedures include a history, physical examination, and blood chemistry. Treatment strategies consist of diuretics and dialysis to promote renal function. Additionally, administering intravenous calcium may be necessary to minimize the effects of magnesium (calcium is a direct antagonist of magnesium).

Hypomagnesemia

Hypomagnesemia results when magnesium levels drop below 1.8 mEq/L. Hypomagnesemia can result from inadequate intake, chronic alcoholism, malnutrition, pregnancy (e.g., preeclampsia), diarrhea, diuretics, and

LEARNING POINTS

Understanding relationships ions have with each other can help you understand what is happening in the body.

- Sodium and potassium have an inverse relationship, so one goes up and the other goes down.
- Calcium and phosphorus have an inverse relationship.
- Calcium and magnesium have a synergistic relationship, so one enhances the other.

stress. Clinical manifestations are similar to those of hypocalcemia. Diagnostic procedures are the same as those with hypermagnesemia. Treatment strategies include magnesium oral supplements for mild deficits and intravenous magnesium for more severe cases.

Acid–Base Balance

Acid–base stability is crucial to sustain life and maintain health. Acid–base balance is achieved through a variety of buffer systems and compensatory mechanisms. Body fluids, the kidneys, and the lungs play a pivotal role in maintaining this balance. Acid–base balance is measured by examining pH, which is the concentration of hydrogen, and there is a narrow safety margin (serum pH is 7.35–7.45). Acid–base imbalances

can vary in severity based on degree of pH change. Death can occur if serum pH levels fall below 6.8 or rise above 7.8. Changes can easily occur because of various conditions including infections, organ failure, or trauma. In many cases, the acid–base fluctuations can cause more negative effects than the causative condition; therefore, the resulting acid–base imbalance is often corrected before treating the underlying condition.

pH Regulation

One way to measure serum hydrogen is by **pH**, which reflects acid–base status. The pH measure is a negative logarithm that reflects hydrogen concentrations; the higher the hydrogen concentration, the lower the pH number (**Figure 6-9**). Hydrogen is necessary for cellular membranes and enzyme activities. Acids are produced as a byproduct of protein, carbohydrate, and fat metabolism. This acidic byproduct occurs in body fluids as a **volatile acid**, such as carbonic acid. Carbonic acid breaks down into hydrogen and bicarbonate. Additionally, acidic **volatile gas** is produced as a byproduct of cellular respiration, such as carbon dioxide. Carbon dioxide (CO_2) is expelled through breathing, and the remaining volatile acid is converted to **nonvolatile acids** (e.g., hydrochloric acid, phosphoric acid, and sulfates) that are then excreted in the urine. Three systems work together to maintain acid–base balance—the buffers, respiratory system, and renal system.

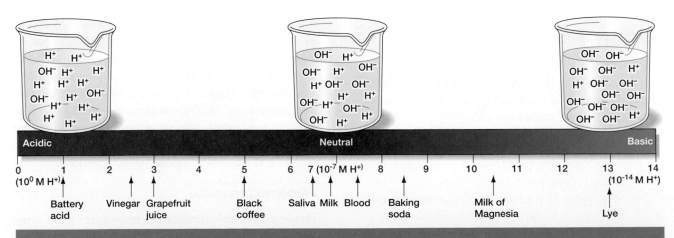

Figure 6-9

The pH scale.

LEARNING POINTS

The blood's pH must remain between 7.35 and 7.45 (**Figure 6-10**). The body's goal is a constant balance between incoming/produced acids and bases (similar to a faucet that is on) and eliminated acids and bases (such as an open drain). Imbalances lead to acidosis (the acid sink overflows) or alkalosis (the base sink overflows). Balance can be restored by increasing elimination (by draining faster) and/or by decreasing flow (slowing down the dripping faucet).

Buffers

Buffers are the chemicals that combine with an acid or base to change pH. Buffering is an immediate reaction to counteract pH variations until compensation is initiated. The body has four major buffer mechanisms—the bicarbonate-carbonic acid system, the phosphate system, the hemoglobin system, and the protein system.

The bicarbonate-carbonic acid system is the most significant in the extracellular fluid. Carbonic acid and bicarbonate (base) are the key players in this system. Carbon dioxide is a byproduct of cellular metabolism. Once produced, carbon dioxide diffuses into the interstitial fluid and blood, where it reacts with water to form carbonic acid. The carbonic acid separates immediately with the presence of the enzyme carbonic anhydrase to form hydrogen ions and bicarbonate. This

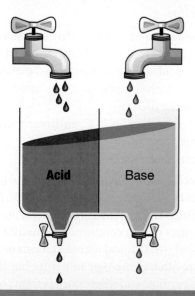

Figure 6-10

Acid–base balance.

enzyme is present in many sites, including the lungs and kidneys. In the lungs, this reaction is reversed so that carbon dioxide can be expired along with water. This process reduces the amount of carbonic acid. In the kidneys, the reaction forms hydrogen ions that are then excreted in the urine, and the bicarbonate is returned to the blood.

The phosphate system acts much like the bicarbonate-carbonic acid system. Phosphates are in high concentrations in the intracellular fluid. Some phosphates act as weak acids, and some act as weak bases. Buffering in this system primarily takes place in the kidneys by accepting or donating hydrogen.

The hemoglobin system is a buffer in the erythrocytes that works by binding to or releasing hydrogen and carbon dioxide. When combined with oxygen, hemoglobin tends to release hydrogen. Exposing hemoglobin to acid and lower oxygen concentrations in the capillaries causes it to release the oxygen. Hemoglobin then becomes a weaker acid, taking up extra hydrogen. This change maintains the pH in the capillaries. An opposite change occurs when hemoglobin is exposed to the higher oxygen concentration in the lung. As hemoglobin binds with oxygen, it becomes more acidic (more prone to release hydrogen). Hydrogen reacts with bicarbonate to form carbonic acid, which is converted to carbon dioxide and released into the alveoli.

The protein system is the most abundant buffering system. Proteins can act as an acid or base by binding to or releasing hydrogen. Proteins exist in intracellular and extracellular fluid but are the most abundant inside the cell. Hydrogen and carbon dioxide diffuse across the cell membrane to bind with protein inside the cell, while albumin and plasma are the primary buffers in the intravascular space.

In addition to these systems, two positively charged ions—potassium and hydrogen—move interchangeably in and out of the cell to balance pH. When there is an extracellular excess of hydrogen, hydrogen moves inside of the cell for buffering, and, in exchange, potassium moves out. As mentioned in a previous section, potassium imbalances can lead to acid–base imbalances, and acid–base imbalances can lead to potassium imbalances.

Respiratory Regulation

The respiratory system manages pH deviations by changing carbon dioxide (acid) excretion. Speeding up respirations will excrete more carbon dioxide, decreasing acidity. Slowing down respirations will excrete less carbon dioxide, increasing acidity. Chemoreceptors that sense pH changes trigger this change in breathing pattern. The only way the lungs can remove acids is through the elimination of carbon dioxide from carbonic acid. The lungs cannot remove other acids. The respiratory system is also a mechanism that can respond quickly to pH imbalances, but its quick action is generally short lived. The respiratory system reaches its maximum response in 12–24 hours and can only maintain the changes in breathing pattern for a limited time before fatiguing.

Renal Regulation

The renal system is the slowest mechanism to react to pH changes, taking hours to days, but it is the longest lasting. The kidneys respond by changing the excretion or retention of hydrogen (acid) or bicarbonate (base). The renal system is effective in balancing pH levels through permanently removing hydrogen from the body. Additionally, the kidneys can reabsorb acids or bases as well as produce bicarbonate to correct pH imbalances.

Compensation

To maintain homeostasis, the body will take actions to compensate for the pH changes. The body never overcompensates; the pH is adjusted so that it is just within the normal range. The cause of the imbalance often

LEARNING POINTS

Compensation can be a challenge to understand. First, make sure you understand what the acids and bases are. Carbon dioxide and hydrogen are acids. Bicarbonate is a base. The body will increase or decrease the excretion of these chemicals to restore pH balance. If the body excretes more acid or produces more bases, then the pH will become more alkaline. If the body retains more acid or produces fewer bases, then the pH will become more acidic. Two body systems can compensate for pH imbalances—the renal and respiratory systems. If the cause of the imbalance originates within one of those systems, then the other system will have to be the primary compensatory mechanism. The system will not be able to resolve its own problem. So, if the problem originates in the lungs, the kidneys will manage it. If the problem originates outside the lungs, the lungs will manage it

determines the compensatory change. For instance, if pH is becoming more acidic because of lung disease that limits gas exchange (e.g., emphysema), then the renal system will have to kick in to compensate for the problem by releasing more bicarbonate and excreting more hydrogen. If a lung disease is increasing carbon dioxide excretion (e.g., hyperventilation), then the kidneys will compensate by decreasing bicarbonate production and hydrogen excretion. On the other hand, if the problem originates outside the lungs, the lungs can compensate for it. For example, if a condition increases the loss of an acid (e.g., vomiting), then the lungs will decrease the rate and depth of respirations to retain more carbon dioxide. If a condition increases the loss of bases (e.g., diarrhea), then the lungs will increase the rate and depth of respirations to excrete more carbon dioxide. If the kidneys and lungs cannot compensate to restore the pH levels to normal range, cellular activities are affected, leading to disease states.

Metabolic Acidosis

Metabolic acidosis results from a deficiency of bicarbonate (base) or an excess of hydrogen (acid) (**Table 6-2**). These conditions drop the pH below 7.35. Causes of metabolic acidosis include:

- Bicarbonate deficit, including that caused by the following:
  - Intestinal losses (e.g., diarrhea and fistulas)
  - Renal losses (e.g., renal failure)
- Acid excess, including that caused by the following:
  - Tissue hypoxia resulting in lactic acid accumulation (e.g., shock and cardiac arrest)
  - Ketoacidosis (e.g., uncontrolled diabetes, excessive alcohol consumption, starvation, and extreme dieting)
  - Drugs and toxins (e.g., antifreeze, aspirin, and hyperalimentation)
  - Renal retention (e.g., renal failure)

Metabolic acidosis exists when the bicarbonate and the pH levels fall below normal (**Table 6-3**). Metabolic acidosis results from an existing problem; therefore, the characteristics of that condition are manifested along with the acidosis. Clinical manifestations of metabolic acidosis are often neurologic in nature but the gastrointestinal, cardiac, and respiratory systems can also be affected. These manifestations include:

- Headache
- Malaise

Table 6-2 Acid–Base Imbalances

	Acidosis	Alkalosis
Respiratory system		
Causes	Slow, shallow respirations Respiratory congestion	Hyperventilation
Effect	Increased $PaCO_2$	Decreased $PaCO_2$
Compensatory mechanism	Kidneys excrete more hydrogen and reabsorb more bicarbonate	Kidneys excrete less hydrogen and reabsorb less bicarbonate
Diagnostic findings	High $PaCO_2$ High bicarbonate Compensated: pH = 7.35–7.4 Decompensated: pH < 7.33	Low PO_2 Low bicarbonate Compensated: pH = 7.4–7.45 Decompensated: pH > 7.47
Metabolic system		
Causes	Diarrhea Renal failure Diabetic ketoacidosis Tissue hypoxia	Vomiting Excessive antacid use
Effect	Decreased bicarbonate	Increased bicarbonate
Compensatory mechanism	Rapid, deep respirations Kidneys excrete more hydrogen and increase bicarbonate absorption (when not involved)	Slow, shallow respirations Kidneys excrete less hydrogen and decrease bicarbonate absorption (when not involved)
Diagnostic findings	Low bicarbonate Low $PaCO_2$ Compensated: pH = 7.35–7.4 Decompensated: pH < 7.33	High bicarbonate High $PaCO_2$ Compensated: pH = 7.4–7.45 Decompensated: pH > 7.47

$PaCO_2$ = partial pressure of carbon dioxide; PO_2 = partial pressure of oxygen.

Table 6-3 Normal Serum Arterial Blood Gas Values*

Blood Gas	Normal Range
pH	7.35–7.45
PaO_2	95–100 mm Hg
$PaCO_2$	35–45 mm Hg
Bicarbonate (HCO_3)	22–26 mEq/L
Base excess	−2.4–+2.5 mEq/L
Arterial O_2 saturation	96–98%

*Values may vary slightly. PaO_2 = partial pressure of oxygen; $PaCO_2$ = partial pressure of carbon dioxide.

- Weakness
- Fatigue
- Lethargy
- Coma
- Warm, flushed skin
- Nausea and vomiting
- Anorexia
- Hypotension
- Dysrhythmias
- Shock
- Kussmaul's respirations (deep, rapid respirations that develop in an attempt to eliminate excess acid by exhaling more carbon dioxide)

- Hyperkalemia (increased serum hydrogen levels cause potassium to shift out of the cells; lack of insulin in diabetic ketoacidosis impairs the transportation of potassium in the cell)

Diagnostic procedures for metabolic acidosis include a history, physical examination, ABGs, blood chemistry, and CBC. Evaluation of the anion gap from the arterial blood gas results can be helpful in determining the cause of metabolic acidosis (**Figure 6-11**). The anion gap is used to identify the anions that are not measured. Conditions that cause metabolic acidosis because of excess acid will increase the anion gap; otherwise, the anion gap is normal. Normally, the sum of cations is approximately equal to the sum of anions in the extracellular fluid. Sodium is the most plentiful cation in the extracellular fluid while bicarbonate and chloride are the most abundant anions. To determine the anion gap, the bicarbonate and chloride results are added together and subtracted from the sodium (sodium – [bicarbonate + chloride]). A normal anion gap is 6–9 mEq/L. Identifying and treating the causative condition (e.g., antidiarrheal agents or dialysis) is vital to successful patient outcomes. Treatment to correct the acidosis merely stabilizes the patient until

the causative condition can be managed. Strategies to correct the acidosis include:

- Administering intravenous bicarbonate
- Correcting of electrolyte disturbances such as hyperkalemia
- Improving oxygenation (e.g., oxygen therapy and mechanical ventilation)
- Administering insulin (probably intravenous) to treat diabetic ketoacidosis

Metabolic Alkalosis

Metabolic alkalosis results from excess bicarbonate or deficient acid or both (Table 6-2). These conditions cause the pH to rise above 7.45. Causes of metabolic alkalosis include:

- Excess bicarbonate, such as that caused by the following:
  - Excessive antacid use
  - Use of bicarbonate-containing fluids (e.g., lactated Ringer's)
  - Hypochloremia (increases bicarbonate reabsorption)

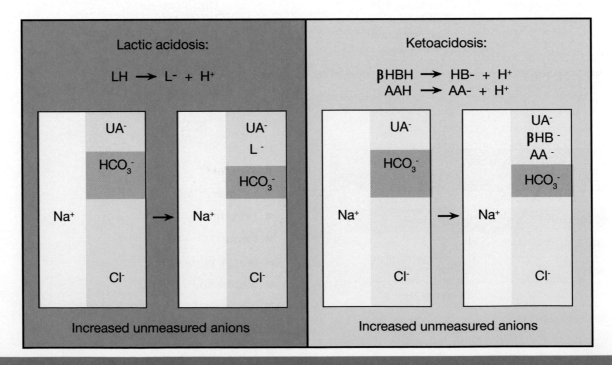

Figure 6-11

Anion gap with metabolic acidosis.

- Deficient acid, such as that caused by the following:
  - Gastrointestinal loss (e.g., vomiting or nasogastric suction)
  - Hypokalemia (low potassium levels cause hydrogen to shift inside the cells)
  - Renal loss (e.g., renal failure or diuretics)
  - Hypovolemia (decreases renal perfusion)
  - Hyperaldosteronism (excessive aldosterone increases renal excretion of hydrogen)

Metabolic alkalosis exists when the bicarbonate and the pH levels rise above normal (Table 6-3). Much like metabolic acidosis, metabolic alkalosis manifestations generally occur in combination with the manifestations of the causative conditions (e.g., hypovolemia). Clinical manifestations of metabolic alkalosis are mostly neurologic in nature but may also involve the respiratory and cardiac systems. These manifestations include:

- Mental confusion
- Hyperactive reflexes
- Paresthesia
- Tetany
- Seizures
- Respiratory depression (respirations will decrease in an attempt to hold in more carbon dioxide)
- Dysrhythmias
- Coma

Diagnostic procedures for metabolic alkalosis include a history, physical examination, ABGs, blood chemistry, and CBC. Identifying and treating the causative condition (e.g., antiemetics or cessation of antacid use) is vital to successful patient outcomes. Treatment to correct the alkalosis merely stabilizes the patient until the causative condition can be managed. Strategies to correct the alkalosis include:

- Adequate hydration, likely including intravenous fluids
- Correcting electrolyte disturbances such as hypokalemia and hypochloremia
- Cautious administration of Diamox (acetazolamide) (which increases bicarbonate excretion but may increase potassium excretion too)
- Administering arginine hydrochloride (which increases chloride levels)
- Administering a weak hydrochloric acid solution

Respiratory Acidosis

Respiratory acidosis results from carbon dioxide retention, increasing carbonic acid and, in turn, decreasing pH level (Table 6-2). This increase in carbon dioxide usually occurs from a state of hypoventilation or decreased gas exchange in the lungs. Many conditions can cause hypoventilation and/or impair gas exchange, including:

- Acute asthma exacerbations
- Chronic obstructive pulmonary disease (emphysema and chronic bronchitis)
- Airway obstructions
- Pulmonary edema
- Pneumonia
- Drug overdose
- Respiratory failure
- Central nervous system depression

Respiratory acidosis exists when the carbon dioxide levels rise and the pH levels fall below normal (Table 6-3). Manifestations generally occur in combination with the manifestations of the causative conditions (e.g. asthma). Carbon dioxide easily diffuses across the blood–brain barrier, causing the neurologic manifestations. Additionally, respiratory acidosis can affect the cardiac system. Clinical manifestations of respiratory acidosis include:

- Headache
- Blurred vision
- Tremors
- Muscle twitching
- Vertigo (dizziness)
- Irritability
- Disorientation
- Lethargy
- Coma
- Tachycardia leading to bradycardia
- Blood pressure fluctuations
- Diaphoresis

Diagnostic procedures for respiratory acidosis include a history, physical examination, ABGs, blood chemistry, CBC, and chest X-ray. Treatment centers on improving respiratory status by relieving hypoxia and hypercapnia. Strategies may include:

- Oxygen therapy
- Mechanical ventilation
- Positioning the patient for optimum ventilation (high Fowler's position)
- Bronchial hygiene measures (e.g., coughing, deep breathing, and chest physiotherapy)
- Bronchodilators
- Treatment of causative conditions (e.g., antibiotics for pneumonia)

Respiratory Alkalosis

Respiratory alkalosis results from excess exhalation of carbon dioxide that leads to carbonic acid deficits and pH increases (Table 6-2). Respiratory alkalosis generally occurs because of conditions that cause hyperventilation. These conditions include:

- Acute anxiety
- Pain
- Fever (which causes excessive oxygen utilization, increasing respirations)
- Hypoxia (e.g., oxygen deprivation and high altitudes)
- Gram-negative septicemia (which triggers the respiratory centers in the brain to increase respirations)
- Aspirin overdose (also triggers the medulla to increase respirations)
- Excessive mechanical ventilation
- Hypermetabolic states such as hyperthyroidism (which causes excessive oxygen utilization, increasing respirations)

Respiratory alkalosis exists when the carbon dioxide levels fall and the pH levels rise above normal (Table 6-3). Clinical manifestations reflect central nervous system irritability. Manifestations of hypercalcemia may be present secondary to calcium binding to protein. Clinical manifestations of respiratory alkalosis include:

- Paresthesia
- Dizziness
- Vertigo (an illusion of motion)
- Syncope

- Muscle irritability, twitching
- Tetany
- Inability to concentrate
- Seizures
- Tachycardia
- Dysrhythmias
- Dry mouth
- Anxiety
- Excessive diaphoresis
- Coma

Diagnostic procedures for respiratory alkalosis include a history, physical examination, ABGs, blood chemistry, CBC, and chest X-ray. Treatment of the underlying cause and increasing carbon dioxide levels is crucial to improving patient outcomes. Often the solution is as simple as breathing into a paper bag. This intervention allows carbon dioxide to be recirculated back to the lungs. Strategies that are more aggressive may be needed if the patient is unable to follow directions or is unconscious. Additional strategies may include controlled mechanical ventilation and anxiety reduction interventions (e.g., sedatives and therapeutic communication).

Mixed Disorders

Mixed disorders occur when respiratory and metabolic disorders result in an acidotic or alkalotic state. This event occurs when both the respiratory and renal systems demonstrate an imbalance of acid or base. The severity of the pH imbalance depends on the degree of acid and base disturbances. Many conditions can create this synergistic effect (**Figure 6-12**). These mixed disorders can make the patient critically ill, and treatment becomes complex to manage.

Arterial Blood Gas Interpretation

Arterial blood gases (ABGs) remain the long-standing, principal diagnostic tool for evaluating acid–base balance (Table 6-2). ABG interpretation has mystified many nursing students and nurses since its invention. Through simple steps, the ABG riddle can be solved, and the patient can receive appropriate care. First, descriptions of the results found on an ABG are in order, some of which have already been discussed.

- The **pH** measures the hydrogen concentration in the plasma.

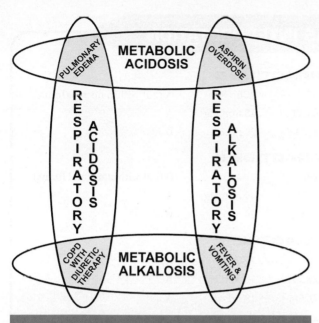

Figure 6-12

Mixed acid–base disorders.

- **PaCO₂** is the partial pressure of carbon dioxide, and it indicates the adequacy of pulmonary ventilation.

- **HCO₃** is bicarbonate, and it indicates the activity in the kidneys to retain or excrete bicarbonate.

- **PaO₂** is the partial pressure of oxygen, and it indicates the concentration of oxygen in the blood.

- **Base excess/deficit** indicates the concentration of buffer, in particular bicarbonate. Positive values indicate an excess of base or a deficit of acid. Negative values indicate a deficit of base or an excess of acid.

When interpreting an ABG result, focus on the pH, PaCO₂, and HCO₃. Interpreting ABGs involves looking for patterns and understanding what those patterns indicate, keeping in mind the patient's total clinical picture. Recall that PaCO₂ is an acid, and HCO₃ is a base. More of the acid will lower the pH, and less of the acid will raise the pH. More of the base will raise the pH, and less of the base will lower the pH.

Now turning to the ABG results, use a systematic approach when examining it. Make note of the patient's pH, PaCO₂, and HCO₃ on a piece of paper. Start with examining the pH. Is it high, low, or normal? This is half of the puzzle. The pH will determine if the condi-

tion is acidosis or alkalosis. If it is high, write a *B* for basic. If the pH is low, write an *A* for acidic beside it. If it is normal, which side of normal is it? For results < 7.4, write an *A*, and for results > 7.4, write a *B*. Next, check the PaCO₂. Is it high, low, or normal? In respiratory disturbances, pH and CO₂ move in opposite directions. If the CO₂ goes up, the pH goes down and vice versa. Because CO₂ is an acidic influence, write an *A* if it is high and a *B* if it is low. If it is within normal range, write an *N* beside it. Then, examine the HCO₃. Is it high, low, or normal? With metabolic disturbances, the pH and HCO₃ move in the same direction. Because HCO₃ is a base influence, write a *B* if it is high and an *A* if it is low. If it is within normal range, write an *N* beside it. Now, you should have three letters written down beside your patient ABG results. At this point, you just match up the *A*s and *B*s you have written down. Finally, determine if the body has been able to compensate. The results with the paired *A* or *B* is the primary change. The third unpaired result indicates the compensation. If the unpaired result is still normal, then it is **uncompensated**. If the unpaired result has changed to the opposite letter of the pairs and the pH is still abnormal, then it is **partially compensated**; if the pH has returned to normal, then it is **fully compensated**. So, to review the steps:

1. Is the pH high, low, or normal?

    a. If it is > 7.4, write a *B* beside it for basic.

    b. If it is < 7.4, write an *A* beside it for acidic.

    c. Make note if it is within normal limits (7.35–7.45).

2. Is the PaCO₂ high, low, or normal?

    a. If it is between 35–45 mm Hg, write an *N* beside it for normal.

    b. If it is > 45 mm Hg, write an *A* beside it for acidic.

    c. If it is < 35 mm Hg, write a *B* beside it for basic.

3. Is the HCO₃ high, low, or normal?

    a. If it is between 22–26, write an *N* beside it for normal.

    b. If it is > 26 mEq/L, write a *B* beside it for basic.

    c. If it is < 22 mEq/L, write an *A* beside it for acidic.

4. Look for patterns:

    a. Two *A*s indicate acidosis. If one of the *A*s is CO₂, then the disorder is respiratory. If one of the *A*s

PRACTICE ARTERIAL BLOOD GAS INTERPRETATION

PRACTICE 1

pH:	7.32	A
PaCO₂:	37 mm Hg	Normal
HCO₃:	14 mEq/L	A

PRACTICE 2

pH:	7.50	B
PaCO₂:	30 mm Hg	B
HCO₃:	24 mEq/L	Normal

PRACTICE 3

pH:	7.33	A
PaCO₂:	55 mm Hg	A
HCO₃:	28 mEq/L	B

PRACTICE 4

pH:	7.47	B
PaCO₂:	48 mm Hg	A
HCO₃:	29 mEq/L	B

PRACTICE 5

pH:	7.38	A (but within normal limits)
PaCO₂:	48 mm Hg	A
HCO₃:	29 mEq/L	B

PRACTICE 6

pH:	7.44	B (but within normal limits)
PaCO₂:	49 mm Hg	A
HCO₃:	29 mEq/L	B

PRACTICE 7

pH:	7.30	A
PaCO₂:	50 mm Hg	A
HCO₃:	19 mEq/L	A

PRACTICE 8

pH:	7.49	B
PaCO₂:	32 mm Hg	B
HCO₃:	30 mEq/L	B

is HCO₃, then the disorder is metabolic. In both cases, the other *A* is the pH.

b. Two *B*s indicate alkalosis. If one of the *B*s is CO₂, then the disorder is respiratory. If one of the *B*s is HCO₃, then the disorder is metabolic. In both cases, the other *B* is the pH.

c. Three *A*s or *B*s indicate a mixed disorder. All *A*s indicate mixed respiratory and metabolic acidosis. All *B*s indicate mixed respiratory and metabolic alkalosis.

5. Determine compensation:

a. If the unpaired result is within normal range, then the disturbance is uncompensated.

b. If the unpaired result is the opposite letter of the pairs but the pH is still abnormal, then the disturbance is partially compensated.

c. If the unpaired result is the opposite letter and the pH has returned to normal range, then the disturbance is fully compensated.

Chapter Summary

Fluid, electrolytes, bases, and acids are constantly moving among body compartments. This movement is influenced by intake, output, cellular metabolism, and pathologic states. The body is equipped with numerous mechanisms to maintain fluid, electrolyte, and pH homeostasis among these compartments. When these mechanisms fail, conditions that threaten the individual's well-being arise. Early identification and action are crucial to improve the prognosis of the person encountering these conditions, and nurses play a pivotal role in managing this patient's plan of care.

Practice Arterial Blood Gas Interpretation Answers

1. Uncompensated metabolic acidosis
2. Uncompensated respiratory alkalosis
3. Partially compensated respiratory acidosis
4. Partially compensated metabolic alkalosis
5. Compensated respiratory acidosis
6. Compensated metabolic alkalosis
7. Mixed respiratory and metabolic acidosis
8. Mixed respiratory and metabolic alkalosis

References

Baumberger-Henry, M. (2008). *Fluid and electrolytes* (2nd ed.). Sudbury, MA: Jones and Bartlett.

Chiras, D. (2008). *Human biology* (6th ed.). Sudbury, MA: Jones and Bartlett.

Elling, B., Elling, K., & Rothenberg, M. (2004). *Anatomy and physiology.* Sudbury, MA: Jones and Bartlett.

Gould, B. (2006). *Pathophysiology for the health professions* (3rd ed.). Philadelphia, PA: Elsevier.

Madara, B., & Pomarico-Denino, V. (2008). *Pathophysiology* (2nd ed.). Sudbury, MA: Jones and Bartlett.

Resources

www.labtestsonline.org/understanding/conditions/acidosis.html

www.the-abg-site.com

www.cdc.gov

www.manuelsweb.com/abg.htm

www.medlineplus.gov

www.nih.gov

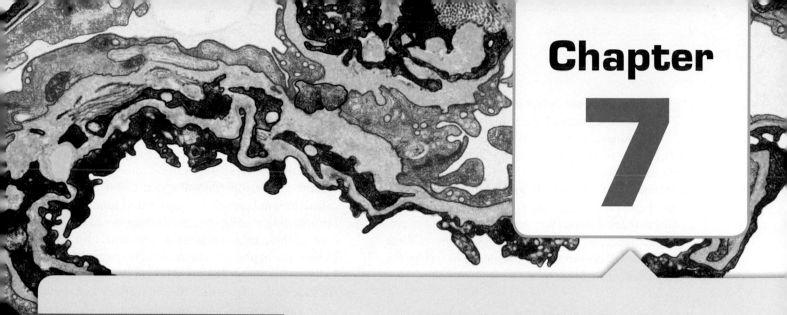

Urinary Function

- Discuss normal urinary anatomy and physiology.

- Explore problems in urination.

- Describe congenital urinary disorders.

- Describe and compare infectious disorders of the urinary system.

- Describe and compare inflammatory disorders of the urinary system.

- Describe and compare obstructive disorders of the urinary system.

- Describe and compare acute and chronic renal failure.

KEY TERMS

acute renal failure (ARF)
afferent arteriole
ammonia
anasarca
azotemia
benign prostatic hyperplasia (BPH)
bladder
bladder cancer
Bowman's capsule
calyx
chronic overdistension
chronic renal failure (CRF)
cystitis
deamination
detrusor hyperreflexia
efferent arteriole

end-stage renal disease
enuresis
erythropoietin
functional incontinence
glomerular filtration rate (GFR)
glomerulonephritis
glomerulus
gross total incontinence
hydronephrosis
intrarenal condition
micturition
mixed incontinence
nephritic syndrome
nephron
nephrotic syndrome
neurogenic bladder
nocturnal enuresis

overactive bladder
overflow incontinence
polycystic kidney disease (PKD)
postrenal condition
prerenal condition
pyelonephritis
reflex incontinence
renal artery
renal capsule
renal cell carcinoma
renal cortex
renal failure
renal hilum
renal impairment
renal insufficiency
renal pelvis
renal sinus

renin-angiotensin-aldosterone
retention
stress incontinence
transient incontinence
urea
uremia
ureter
urethra
urge incontinence
uric acid
urinary incontinence
urinary tract infection (UTI)
urination
urolithiasis
Wilms' tumor

The urinary system plays a pivotal role in homeostasis. Structures of the urinary system include the kidneys, ureters, bladder, and urethra (**Figure 7-1**). This system regulates fluid volume, blood pressure, metabolic waste and drug excretion, vitamin D conversion, pH regulation, and hormone synthesis. This chapter will focus on normal and abnormal states of the urinary system. Disorders of this system can create imbalances in homeostasis quickly. Hence, these disorders will require prompt response to restore the body's delicate balance.

Anatomy and Physiology

The urinary system regulates fluid volume (see Chapter 6), blood pressure (see Chapter 4), metabolic waste and

drug excretion, vitamin D conversion, pH balance (see Chapter 6), and hormone synthesis. The urinary system includes the kidneys, ureters, bladder, and urethra (**Table 7-1**). The kidneys are bean-shaped organs about the size of a person's fists positioned on either side of the vertebrae in retroperitoneal space. Connective tissue called the **renal capsule** surrounds the kidney. The area immediately beneath the capsule is known as the **renal cortex**. This cortex contains the functional units of the kidney, the nephrons. The **renal artery** supplies each kidney with blood. The **renal hilum** is the opening in the kidney through which the renal artery and nerves enter and the renal vein and ureter exit. The hilum opens medially into a cavity called the **renal sinus**. The central portions of the renal sinuses enlarge to form the **renal pelvis**. Urine drains similarly to a funnel

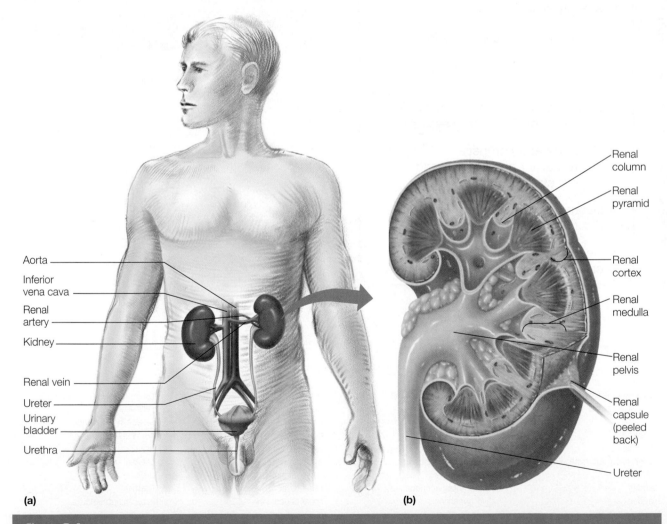

(a)

Aorta

Inferior vena cava

Renal artery

Kidney

Renal vein

Ureter

Urinary bladder

Urethra

(b)

Renal column

Renal pyramid

Renal cortex

Renal medulla

Renal pelvis

Renal capsule (peeled back)

Ureter

Figure 7-1

The urinary system. (a) Anterior view showing the relationship of the kidneys, ureters, urinary bladder, and urethra. (b) A cross-section of the human kidney showing the cortex, medulla, and renal pelvis.

Table 7-1 Components of the Urinary System and Their Functions

Component	Function
Kidneys	Eliminate wastes from the blood; help regulate body water concentration; help regulate blood pressure; help maintain a constant blood pH
Ureters	Transport urine to the urinary bladder
Urinary bladder	Stores urine; contracts to eliminate stored urine
Urethra	Transports urine to the outside of the body

Source: Chiras, D. (2008). *Human biology* (6th ed.). Sudbury, MA: Jones & Bartlett Learning.

into the renal pelvis through tubes called calyces. The calyces drain urine into the ureters, which transport the urine using peristaltic actions to the bladder for storage. The muscular bladder serves as a reservoir for urine until it can be excreted. As the volume of urine in the bladder increases, the urine exerts pressure on the two bladder sphincters (internal and external) and stretch receptors in the bladder. A pressure of 200 to 300 mL on the sphincters and receptors sends nerve impulses to the brain, triggering the urge to urinate (**Figure 7-2**). Urination, or micturition, is a voluntary act; when urination is initiated, the bladder contracts and the external sphincter relaxes, forcing urine out through the urethra. The urethra is approximately 1.5 inches long in women and 6–8 inches long in men. The shorter urethra in women, in combination with sitting for urination, increases women's risk for developing urinary tract infections.

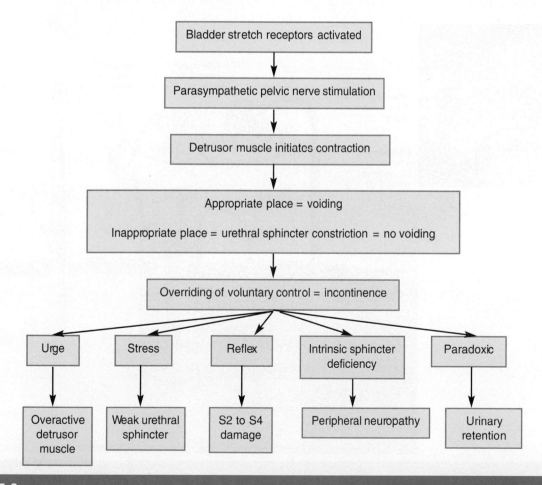

Figure 7-2

Urination.

The kidneys are the primary site for carrying out the urinary system's functions. One kidney contains 1 to 2 million microscopic filtering units, or **nephrons**, to accomplish its functions (**Figure 7-3**). Each nephron is similar to a funnel with a long stem. Each nephron has multiple sections (e.g., loop of Henle, proximal convoluted tubule, and distal convoluted tubule), and each section is responsible for excreting or reabsorbing specific substances (**Table 7-2**). The proximal convoluted tubule enlarges into a double membrane chamber called the **Bowman's capsule**. The Bowman's capsule surrounds a cluster of capillaries referred to as the **glomerulus**. Blood enters the glomerulus through an **afferent arteriole** and exits through an **efferent arteriole** (**Figure 7-4**). This blood supply to the glomerulus determines the amount of urine made and is necessary for healthy renal function. The speed at which blood moves through the glomerulus is termed the **glomerular filtration rate (GFR)**. GFR is the best measure of renal functioning. GFR can be calculated using a formula that incorporates serum creatinine levels, age, gender, and ethnicity. Usually, GFR is approximately 125 mL/minute, and daily urine output is approximately 1,500 mL.

The human body can excrete waste through the kidneys, skin, liver, and intestines, with the kidneys being the primary site for excretion. The kidneys regulate water along with electrolytes by increasing or decreasing their excretion to maintain stability (see Chapter 6). Hormones, such as antidiuretic hormone and aldosterone, alter this excretion (**Figure 7-5**). In part, this water and electrolyte regulation aids in blood pressure management. Other renal mechanisms that contribute to blood pressure control include the **renin-angiotensin-aldosterone** system (see Chapter 4).

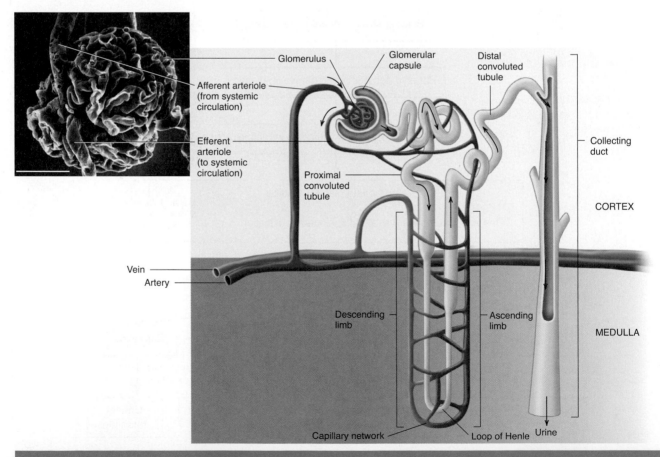

Figure 7-3

Nephrons of the kidney. Part of the nephron is located in the cortex, and part is located in the medulla. The electron micrograph to the left of the illustration is of a glomerulus from a human nephron.

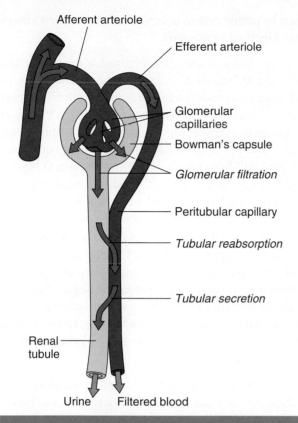

Figure 7-4

The glomerulus of the kidneys. The nephron carries out three processes: glomerular filtration, tubular reabsorption, and tubular secretion. All three processes contribute to the filtering of the blood.

Table 7-2 Components of the Nephron and Their Function

Component	Function
Glomerulus	Mechanically filters the blood
Bowman's capsule	Mechanically filters the blood
Proximal convoluted tubule	Reabsorbs 75% of the water, salts, glucose, and amino acids
Loop of Henle	Participates in countercurrent exchange, which maintains the concentration gradient
Distal convoluted tubule	Site of tubular secretion of II+, potassium, and certain drugs

Source: Chiras, D. (2008). *Human biology* (6th ed.). Sudbury, MA: Jones & Bartlett Learning.

ADH LEVEL	EFFECT ON KIDNEY
Increased ADH levels	Collecting ducts and the distal convoluted tubules become permeable to water; water moves out of ducts and into blood 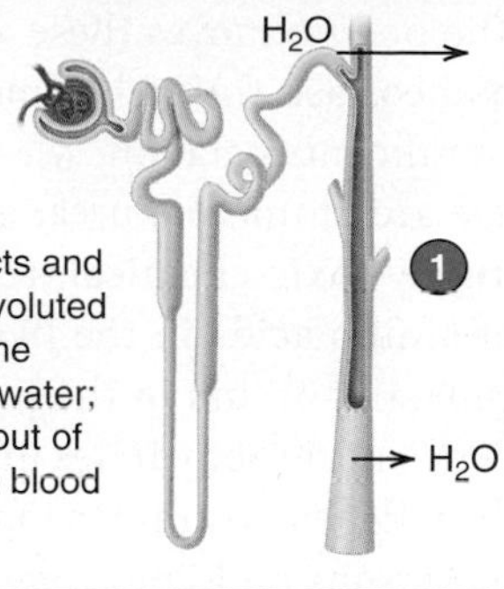
Decreased ADH levels	Collecting ducts become impermeable to water; water is not reabsorbed from the filtrate and is excreted 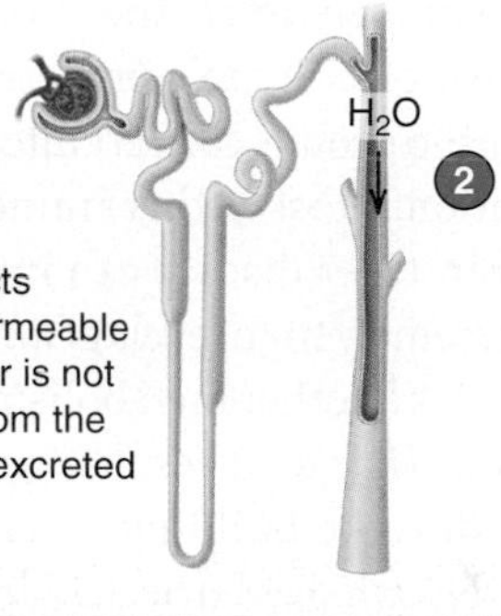

ALDOSTERONE LEVEL	EFFECT ON KIDNEY
Increased aldosterone levels	Tubules increase reabsorption of sodium from the filtrate and decrease reabsorption of potassium; water and sodium thus move from filtrate into the blood, and excess potassium is excreted 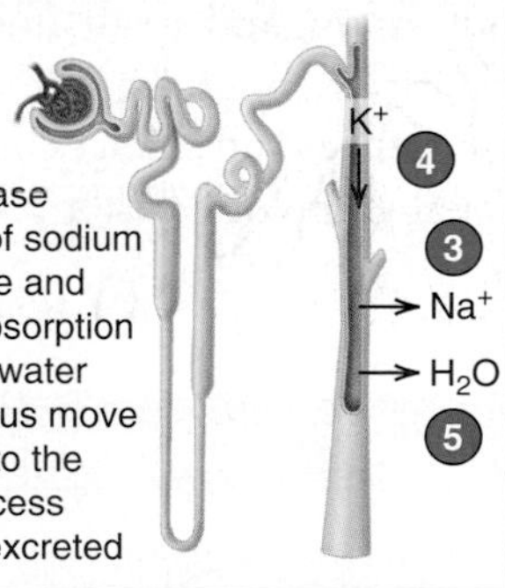
Decreased aldosterone levels	Tubular absorption of sodium and potassium is normal; water is not reabsorbed from the filtrate and is excreted 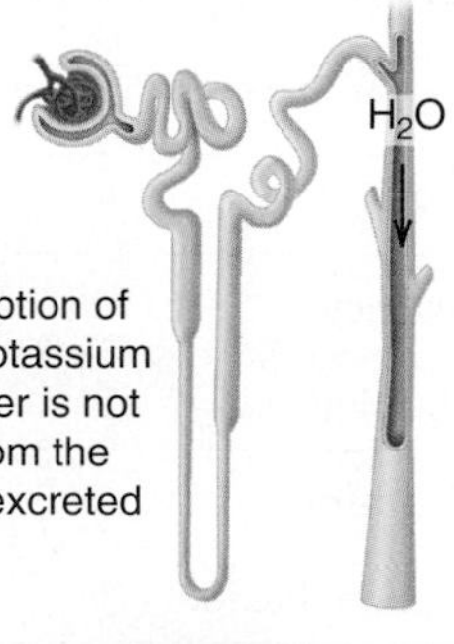

Figure 7-5

Effects of antidiuretic hormone and aldosterone on the kidneys.

Cells continuously produce waste products as they go about conducting their processes (**Table 7-3**). The body removes these waste products to maintain homeostasis through urine formation. The three most significant metabolic wastes that the kidneys manage are ammonia, urea, and uric acid. **Ammonia**, a highly toxic chemical, results from the breakdown of amino acids in the liver. Amino acid breakdown generally occurs in the presence of excess protein or deficient carbohydrates in the diet; however, carbohydrate deficits are rare in industrialized countries except in persons on high-protein diets. When amino acids are broken down, the amino groups are stripped from the molecules in a process called **deamination**. These amino groups convert into ammonia following deamination. Most of this ammonia converts to **urea** in the liver. Liver disease can impair this process leading to extremely high levels of ammonia (see Chapter 9). **Uric acid** is another metabolism byproduct produced by the liver. Uric acid results from the breakdown of nucleotides, the building blocks of deoxyribonucleic acid (DNA). Excess uric acid levels can lead to gout, which results in uric acid crystal deposits in the joints (see Chapter 12). Along with these waste products, other substances normally found in urine include sodium, potassium, and small amounts of protein and bacteria. Urine should be pale yellow and clear. Additional substances and changes in color or clarity can indicate renal pathology (**Table 7-4**). Multiple diagnostic tests can be performed to determine whether the kidneys are functioning properly.

The kidneys are also responsible for converting vitamin D into its active form. The inactive form of vitamin D is produced by the action of ultraviolet rays on cholesterol in the skin or is ingested. Vitamin D requires conversion into its active form to aid in calcium and phosphorus absorption. People with renal disease will have issues converting vitamin D into its active form. Additionally, the kidneys regulate pH by secreting bicarbonate and excreting hydrogen (see Chapter 6). The kidneys synthesize several hormones including atrial natriuretic peptide (see Chapter 6), erythropoietin, and renin (see Chapter 4). The kidneys release **erythropoietin** in a response to hypoxia (e.g., anemia or cardiac or pulmonary disease). Erythropoietin stimulates bone marrow to produce more red blood cells. If iron stores are adequate, an increase in red blood cells increases oxygen-carrying capacity, thus decreasing hypoxia.

With aging, the kidneys begin functioning less efficiently. This decreased functioning can further be exacerbated by the presence of chronic conditions (e.g., diabetes mellitus, hypertension, arterosclerosis). With this decreased renal functioning, the aging individual may experience less filtration capability, leading to waste accumulation and loss of homeostatic regulation (e.g., fluid, electrolyte, and pH balance). Additionally,

Table 7-3 Important Metabolic Wastes and Substances Excreted From the Body

Chemical	Source	Organ of Excretion
Ammonia	Deamination (removal of amine group) of amino acids in liver	Kidneys
Urea	Derived from ammonia	Kidneys, skin
Uric acid	Nucleotide breakdown in liver	Kidneys
Bile pigments	Hemoglobin breakdown in liver	Liver (into small intestine)
Urochrome	Hemoglobin breakdown in liver	Kidneys
Carbon dioxide	Breakdown of glucose in cells	Lungs
Water	Food and water; breakdown of glucose	Kidneys, skin, and lungs
Inorganic ions*	Food and water	Kidneys and sweat glands

*Ions are not a metabolic waste product like the other substances shown in this table. Nonetheless, ions are excreted to maintain constant levels in the body.
Source: Chiras, D. (2008). *Human biology* (6th ed.). Sudbury, MA: Jones & Bartlett Learning.

Table 7-4 Renal Function Tests

Test	Related Physiology
BUN (blood urea nitrogen)	The end product of protein metabolism is urea, which is excreted entirely by the kidneys; therefore, the BUN is an indication of liver and kidney function
Serum creatinine	When creatinine phosphate is used in skeletal muscle contractions, creatinine is formed, which is entirely excreted by the kidneys; therefore, the serum creatinine level is an indication of renal function. The creatinine level is not affected by hepatic function so it is a more precise indication of renal function than is the BUN. A 50% reduction in glomerular filtration rate (GRF) doubles the creatinine level
24-hour urine collection for creatinine clearance	Measures GFR and is dependent upon renal artery perfusion and glomerular filtration (GF)
Urinalysis	Cloudy, foul smelling, white blood cells (WBCs) ˃ urinary tract infection (UTI) Dark yellow ˃ dehydration Acetone odor ˃ diabetic ketoacidosis Presence of protein ˃ injured glomerular membrane Glucose ˃ diabetes mellitus Ketones ˃ fatty acid metabolism Crystals ˃ renal stone formation possible Many hyaline casts ˃ proteinuria Cellular casts ˃ nephrotic syndrome
Intravenous pyelogram (IVP)	IV-administered, radiopaque dye allows the visualization of the kidneys, renal pelvis, ureters, and bladder
PSA (prostatic specific antigen)	PSA is a glycoprotein found in all prostatic epithelial cells. An increase may be indicative of prostatic enlargement, thus this test is used to screen for prostatic cancer and as an indicator of treatment success/failure

Source: Madara, M., & Pomarico-Denino, V. (2008). *Quick look nursing: Pathophysiology* (2nd ed.). Sudbury, MA: Jones & Bartlett Learning.

renal-related complications are common with these aging changes (e.g., anemia, hypertension, and osteoporosis). Aging persons may require alternative medication dosing (usually less of a dose or dosing spaced farther apart) to prevent drug toxicity because of this impaired filtration.

Urination Issues

The act of urination requires (1) a functioning bladder with stretch receptors to sense the filling of urine, (2) an intact parasympathetic pelvic nerve to transmit the signal, and (3) working detrusor muscles to initiate bladder contractions to expel the urine (Figure 7-2). The sympathetic nerve innervations to the detrusor muscle and internal sphincter prevent inappropriate stimulation of urination. Upper motor impulses can delay voiding by tightening the urethral sphincter. Although urination is mostly a voluntary act, void-

ing can only be delayed to a certain point. If the urge to void is ignored too long, bladder contractions take over the neural delaying of urination and involuntary urination occurs.

Incontinence

Urination is a reflex in very young children, but it is controlled consciously in older children and adults. In children up to 3 years of age, urination is completely reflexive—once the bladder expands, it empties. As children grow older, they can control urination. In older children and adults, the external sphincter is under conscious control—it will not relax until deliberately allowed to do so.

Older children and adults sometimes lose control over urination, resulting in a condition referred to as urinary incontinence (Figure 7-2). Urinary incontinence is a common and often embarrassing problem that has many causes. Urinary incontinence can result for a variety of reasons. The types of incontinence and their causes include:

- **Enuresis** is the involuntary urination by a child after 4–5 years of age, when bladder control is expected. Most children have nocturnal enuresis, or bed-wetting, only. Enuresis can have psychological (e.g., anxiety) and structural (e.g., smaller than normal bladder) origins. Multiple strategies and treatments are available (e.g., motivation, support, alarm systems, and medications to concentrate urine at night), but usually the condition resolves in time with or without treatment.

- **Transient incontinence** refers to urinary incontinence resulting from a temporary condition. These conditions include delirium, infection, atrophic vaginitis, medications (e.g., diuretics and sedatives), psychologic factors (e.g., depression and anxiety), high urine output (e.g., overhydration), restricted mobility, fecal impaction, alcohol, and caffeine.

- **Stress incontinence** describes loss of urine from pressure (stress) exerted on the bladder by coughing, sneezing, laughing, exercising, or lifting something heavy. Stress incontinence occurs when the sphincter muscle of the bladder is weakened. In women, physical changes resulting from pregnancy, childbirth, and menopause can weaken the sphincter muscle. Additionally, women may develop a cystocele (bulging of the bladder through the vaginal wall; see Chapter 8) because of these physical changes, which can also increase risk for stress incontinence. In men, prostate removal can lead to this type of incontinence. Additional contributing factors for both genders are obesity and chronic coughing. Obesity increases pressure on the bladder and surrounding muscles, weakening them. Chronic coughing (e.g., that caused by smoking and lung disease) can also increase stress on the urinary sphincter.

- **Urge incontinence** is a sudden, intense urge to urinate, followed by an involuntary loss of urine. The bladder muscle contracts and may only give the individual a few seconds to a minute warning before voiding. With urge incontinence, the need to urinate is felt often, including throughout the night. Urinary tract infections, bladder irritants, bowel conditions, smoking, Parkinson's disease, Alzheimer's disease, stroke, injury, or nervous system damage (e.g., that associated with multiple sclerosis) may cause urge incontinence. Overactive bladder describes urge incontinence with no known cause.

- **Reflex incontinence** refers to urinary incontinence caused by trauma or damage to the nervous system (e.g., that caused by spinal cord injury above the 2nd–4th sacral vertebra, multiple sclerosis, and diabetes mellitus). Detrusor hyperreflexia is increased detrusor muscle contractility that occurs even though there is no sensation to void. With reflex incontinence, urgency is generally absent.

- **Overflow incontinence** is the result of an inability to empty the bladder, or retention. Other indications of overflow incontinence include dribbling urine and a weak urine stream. This type of incontinence may occur due to bladder damage, urethral blockage, nerve damage (e.g., that caused by diabetes mellitus), and prostate conditions. Chronic overdistension, also called nurse's bladder and teacher's bladder, occurs because of a perceived inability to interrupt work to void. This chronic avoidance of emptying the bladder results in detrusor muscle areflexia and overflow incontinence.

- **Mixed incontinence** occurs when symptoms of more than one type of urinary incontinence are experienced.

- **Functional incontinence** occurs in many older adults, especially people in nursing homes. A physical or mental impairment prevents toileting in time. For example, a person with severe arthritis may not be able to undress quickly enough.

- **Gross total incontinence** refers to a continuous leaking of urine, day and night, or the periodic uncontrollable leaking of large volumes of urine. In these cases, the bladder has no storage capacity. This type of incontinence can occur because of anatomic defects, spinal cord or urinary system injuries, or an abnormal opening (fistula) between the bladder and an adjacent structure, such as the vagina.

Generally, risk factors for developing urinary incontinence include:

- *Being female*—Women are more likely than men are to have stress incontinence. Pregnancy, childbirth, menopause, and normal female anatomy account for this difference. However, men with prostate conditions are at increased risk of urge and overflow incontinence.

- *Advancing age*—Bladder and urethra muscles lose some of their strength with age. Changes with age reduce bladder capacity and increase the chances of involuntary urination. However, incontinence is not inevitable with age, and incontinence is not normal at any age, except during infancy.

- *Being overweight*—Being obese or overweight increases the pressure on the bladder and surrounding muscles, weakening them and allowing urine to leak out under stress (e.g., stress caused by coughing or sneezing).

- *Smoking*—Chronic coughing associated with smoking can cause episodes of incontinence or aggravate incontinence that has other causes. Constant coughing puts stress on the urinary sphincter, leading to stress incontinence. Smokers are also at risk of developing overactive bladder.

- *Other diseases*—Renal disease or diabetes mellitus may increase risk for incontinence because of changes in renal function and nerve innervations.

Urinary incontinence can lead to complications that can range from minor to severe. Skin problems (e.g., rashes, skin infections, and ulcers) can result from the constant moisture. Recurrent urinary tract infections can develop from incomplete emptying of the bladder. Additionally, urinary incontinence can negatively affect psychologic health (e.g., it can cause poor self-image, embarrassment, sexual dysfunction, anxiety, and depression), and changes can occur in the individual's usual activities (e.g., work and exercise).

Diagnostic procedures for urinary incontinence include a history, physical examination, bladder diary, urinalysis, urine cultures, cystourethrogram (X-ray of the bladder and urethra), cystoscopy (visualization of the bladder with a small, lighted instrument), pelvic ultrasound, postvoid residual measurement, and urodynamic testing (which measures pressures in the bladder). Treatment for urinary incontinence depends on the type, underlying cause, and severity. Treatment and management strategies range from conservative to aggressive and may include:

- Bladder training
- Scheduled toileting
- Fluid and diet management (e.g., avoiding alcohol, caffeine, or acidic foods; reducing liquid consumption; losing weight; or increasing physical activity)

- Pelvic floor muscle exercises (e.g., Kegel exercises)
- Electric stimulation (electrodes are temporarily inserted into the rectum or vagina to strengthen pelvic floor muscles through gentle electric stimulation)
- Medications (e.g., anticholinergics or estrogen replacement)
- Urethral inserts (small, tamponlike disposable devices or plugs inserted into the urethra)
- Pessary (a stiff ring inserted into the vagina to hold up the bladder)
- Radiofrequency therapy (nonsurgical procedure that uses radiofrequency energy to heat tissue in the lower urinary tract, causing it to become firmer)
- Botulinum toxin type A (Botox) injections into the bladder muscle (research has found this to be a promising therapy for overactive bladder, but the Food and Drug Administration [FDA] has not yet approved this drug for incontinence)
- Bulking material injections (e.g., collagen, carbon-coated zirconium beads, Coaptite) into tissue surrounding the urethra
- Sacral nerve stimulator (an implanted device that emits painless electrical impulses that stimulate the sacral nerve)
- Artificial urinary sphincter (fluid-filled ring implanted around the neck of the bladder that is controlled by a manual subcutaneous valve)
- Sling procedures (surgically constructed pelvic sling or hammock around the bladder neck and urethra created by using strips of tissue, synthetic material, or mesh)
- Bladder neck suspension (surgical procedure to raise and support the bladder in a more normal anatomic position)
- Absorbent pads and protective garments
- Urinary catheter (usually as an intermittent self-catheterization)
- Increased perineal hygiene
- Skin barrier creams
- Safety measures (e.g., move any rugs or furniture out of path to the restroom, adequate lighting, widening the bathroom doorway, and installing an elevated toilet seat)
- Acupuncture

LEARNING POINTS

Here are two easy acronyms to remember the causes of acute urinary incontinence.

DRIP

D = Delirium, dehydration, diapers

R = Retention, restricted mobility

I = Impaction, infection, inflammation

P = Pharmaceuticals, polyuria, Paget's disease (Newman, 2010)

DIAPPERS

D = Delirium

I = Infection

A = Atrophic vaginitis or urethritis

P = Pharmaceuticals (opiates and calcium antagonists cause urinary retention and constipation; anticholinergics cause increased PVR and retention; alpha adrenergic antagonists cause reduced urethral resistance in women)

P = Psychologic problems such as depression, neurosis, or anxiety

E = Excess fluid input or output (diuretics; nocturnal polyuria)

R = Restricted mobility

S = Stool impaction (constipation) (Resnick & Yalla, 1998, p. 1045)

- Hypnotherapy
- Herbal remedies (e.g., *Crataeva nurvala*, horsetail [*Equisetum*], aloe vera extract)
- Coping strategies and support

Neurogenic Bladder

Neurogenic bladder refers to all bladder dysfunction caused by an interruption of normal bladder nerve innervation. Many factors can disrupt bladder nerve innervations, including:

- Brain or spinal cord injury
- Nervous system tumors
- Brain or spinal cord infections
- Dementia
- Parkinson's disease
- Spina bifida

- Diabetes mellitus
- Stroke
- Medications (e.g., antidepressants, antihistamines, analgesics, antihypertensives, and antiemetics)
- Vaginal childbirth
- Multiple sclerosis
- Chronic alcoholism
- Systemic lupus erythematosus
- Heavy metal poisoning
- Herpes zoster

Clinical manifestations of neurogenic bladder include symptoms of an overactive bladder (e.g., frequency and urgency) and an underactive bladder (e.g., hesitancy and retention). Diagnostic procedures for neurogenic bladder consist of a history, physical examination, bladder diary, urinalysis, urine cultures, cystourethrogram, cystoscopy, pelvic ultrasound, postvoid residual measurement, and urodynamic testing. Additionally, other procedures may be conducted to determine the underlying cause (e.g., computed tomography [CT], magnetic resonance imaging [MRI]). Treatment strategies depend on etiology and include those previously discussed for incontinence.

Congenital Disorders

Abnormalities of the urinary and reproductive system are the most common congenital defects (also see Chapter 8). Because of their close relationship with each other, often an abnormality in one system will lead to an abnormality in the other. Numerous congenital disorders of the urinary system are possible, most of which are structural problems. Some defects cause no symptoms (e.g., both ureters draining one kidney, abnormal kidney positioning), while others are life threatening (e.g., renal agenesis [failure of an organ to develop in utero]). Problems with kidney development can be the most severe. The kidneys begin to develop in approximately the 5th week of gestation. Urine formation begins about the 9th–12th week of gestation. Urine is the main component of amniotic fluid, which is vital for normal fetal development.

Polycystic Kidney Disease

Polycystic kidney disease (PKD) is an inherited disorder characterized by numerous, grape-like clusters of fluid-filled cysts in both kidneys (**Figure 7-6**). These cysts enlarge the kidneys while compressing and even-

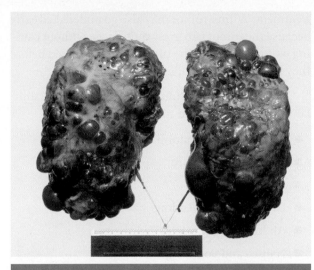

Figure 7-6

Polycystic kidney disease.

tually replacing the functional kidney tissue. The exact trigger for the formation of the cysts is unknown.

Prognosis and progression vary widely depending on the type of PKD. Autosomal dominant (see Chapter 1) PKD has been mapped to the short arm of chromosome 16 and 4. Autosomal dominant PKD occurs in both children and adults, but it is much more common in adults, with symptoms often not showing up until middle age. According to the National Institutes of Health (NIH) (2010), autosomal dominant PKD affects nearly 1 in 1,000 Americans. The actual number of those who have the condition may be more, as some people do not have symptoms. Many cases are discovered inadvertently by performing tests for unrelated reasons. Like most recessive conditions (see Chapter 1), autosomal recessive PKD is far less common. This type appears in infancy or childhood, tends to be extremely serious, and progresses rapidly, resulting in end-stage kidney failure and generally causing death in infancy or childhood. PKD affects men and women equally.

Clinical manifestations depend on age and the type of PKD. These manifestations reflect the structural changes and resulting renal impairment. Manifestations in neonates, adults, and those that occur in both are shown next.

In neonates, manifestations include:

- Potter facies (pronounced epicanthic folds [skin folds at the corner of the eyes on either side of the nose]; pointed nose; small chin; and floppy, low-set ears)

- Large, bilateral, symmetrical masses on the flanks
- Respiratory distress (caused by fluid accumulation from renal impairment)
- Uremia (waste accumulation due to renal impairment)

In adults, manifestations include:

- Hypertension (due to activation of the renin-angiotensin-aldosterone system)
- Lumbar pain
- Increased abdominal girth
- Swollen, tender abdomen
- Grossly enlarged, palpable kidneys

Additional symptoms that may affect both groups include:

- Hematuria (due to impaired glomerular filtration)
- Nocturia (related to an inability to concentrate urine)
- Drowsiness (because of waste accumulation)

Other conditions that may occur with PKD include brain aneurysms, cysts in other organs (especially the liver), and colon diverticula. Because of renal impairment, PKD can lead to critical complications such as pyelonephritis, cyst rupture, retroperitoneal bleeding, and renal failure. Other less serious complications include anemia, hypertension, and renal calculi (kidney stones).

Diagnostic procedures for PKD consist of a history, physical examination, urinalysis, blood chemistry, urography (kidney X-ray), abdominal ultrasound, CT, MRI, and intravenous pyelogram (X-ray of the kidneys, ureters, and bladder with the use of radioactive contrast media). PKD often progresses slowly, leading to end-stage renal disease. Treatment focuses on controlling symptoms and preventing complications. These strategies may involve:

- Pharmacology, including the following:
  - Antibiotics (when infections are present)
  - Analgesics (for pain)
  - Antihypertensive agents
  - Diuretics
- Adequate hydration
- Low-salt diet

- Surgically draining cystic abscesses or retroperitoneal bleeding
- Dialysis
- Kidney transplant

Wilms' Tumor

Wilms' tumor, or nephroblastoma, is a rare kidney cancer that primarily affects children. According to the National Cancer Institute (2010c), 500 new cases of Wilms' tumor are diagnosed each year. Wilms' tumor is the most common malignant tumor in children with the peak incidence around age 3–4 years. Wilms' tumor usually occurs in one kidney, but it can affect both. Wilms' tumor usually grows as a solitary mass that can become quite large (**Figure 7-7**). The exact cause is unknown, but the tumor is thought to arise in utero when the cells that normally form the kidneys fail to develop properly. This type of cancer is associated with several congenital defects including aniridia (absence of the iris of the eye), hemihypertrophy (enlargement of one side of the body), and urinary tract abnormalities (e.g., undescended testes and hypospadias). Even though it is rare, Wilms' tumor tends to run in families, intensifying its genetic connection. Risk also seems to be higher in females and African Americans. On the other hand, Asian Americans have a slightly lower risk than other ethnic groups.

Because of improved diagnostic procedures, Wilms' tumor can be detected early, leading to improved prognosis for children affected with this disease. Long-term survival rate is excellent with early detection and

treatment. Wilms' tumor may also go undetected early because the tumor can grow quite large without causing pain, but most of the tumors are diagnosed before they have metastasized.

Clinical manifestations of Wilms' tumor are similar to other cancers and include:

- Asymptomatic abdominal mass
- High blood pressure
- Hematuria
- Urinary tract infections
- Abdominal pain (late)
- Nausea and vomiting
- Anorexia
- Bowel pattern changes
- Weight loss
- Fatigue

Diagnostic procedures for Wilms' tumor include a history, physical examination, renal ultrasound, and biopsy. Once diagnosed, the following staging system guides treatment:

- *Stage I*—The cancer is only in one kidney and generally can be completely removed with surgery.
- *Stage II*—The cancer has metastasized to the tissues and structures near the kidney, but it can still be completely removed by surgery.
- *Stage III*—The cancer has metastasized beyond the kidney area to nearby lymph nodes or other structures within the abdomen and may not be completely removed by surgery.
- *Stage IV*—The cancer has metastasized to distant structures, such as the lungs, liver, or brain.
- *Stage V*—Cancer cells affect both kidneys.

The standard treatment for Wilms' tumor is surgery (e.g., simple, partial, or radical nephrectomy) and chemotherapy, but radiation may be used if warranted by tumor histology. Coping strategies and support interventions (e.g., allowing playtime and local support groups) will be beneficial for the family and child.

Urinary Tract Infections

Urinary tract infections (UTIs) are extremely common and include any infections that begin in the urinary tract. According to the NIH (2010), UTIs

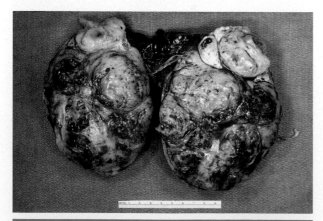

Figure 7-7

Wilm's tumor.

are the second most frequently occurring infection. The lower urinary tract (bladder and urethra) is the most frequent site for the infection. UTIs are caused by a direct invasion of the urinary tract by bacteria. Urine is an excellent medium for microorganism growth because of its protein content. Due to the high concentration of bacteria, most infections invade the urethra from the meatus in the perineal area. The microorganism can then ascend the urethra to the bladder and then move along the ureters to the kidneys. Occasionally, microorganisms can invade the kidney from the blood.

UTIs are most often caused by *Escherichia coli*, which is part of the normal intestinal flora. Virulent forms of *E. coli* can prevent being washed away during urination by attaching to the mucosa along the urinary tract. *E. coli* can gain access to the urinary tract due to the anus's close proximity to the urinary meatus, especially in women. In addition to this close proximity, women are more vulnerable to developing UTIs for the following reasons:

- Women have shorter urethras (the microorganism has a shorter distance to travel).

- Women usually urinate in a sitting position (which prevents full emptying of the bladder).

- Women experience increased perineal tissue irritation from sexual activity, tampons, bubble baths, bathing suits, tight-fitting pants, and deodorants, as well as nylon, lace, and thong underwear.

Other risk factors for developing UTIs include:

- Benign prostatic hypertrophy (causes urinary retention)

- Congenital urinary tract abnormalities

- Immobility (prevents complete bladder emptying)

- Urinary or bowel incontinence

- Renal calculi (obstruct urine output)

- Decreased cognition

- Pregnancy

- Impaired immune response (e.g., diabetes mellitus)

- Urinary catheterization (breaks the first line of defense)

- Improper personal hygiene (which increases the number of microorganisms)

UTIs may be asymptomatic, but when present, general clinical manifestations include:

- Urgency

- Dysuria

- Frequency

- Hematuria

- Bacteriuria

- Cloudy, foul-smelling urine

- Symptoms of infection (e.g., fever, chills, and fatigue)

Diagnostic procedures for UTIs include a history, physical examination, urinalysis, urine culture, cystoscopy, and complete blood count (CBC). Treatment for UTI focuses on eradicating the microorganism with antibiotics. Additional strategies concentrate on prevention and include:

- Increasing hydration, especially water and juices (increases flushing of the urinary tract)

- Avoiding irritants (e.g., bubble bath and deodorants)

- Performing proper perineal hygiene (women should clean front to back, and uncircumcised men should retract the foreskin to clean)

- Wearing cotton underwear

- Not delaying urination

- Adequately emptying the bladder (especially after intercourse)

- Providing appropriate catheter care (when present)

Cystitis

Cystitis refers to inflammation of the bladder. The inflammatory response is triggered, causing the bladder and urethra walls to become red and swollen. Infection most commonly initiates this response, but irritants (e.g., radiation and catheters) occasionally can activate it. In addition to the usual UTI symptoms, clinical manifestations of cystitis include abdominal pain and pelvic pressure. Diagnostic procedures and treatment regimens follow those usually seen for UTIs.

Pyelonephritis

Pyelonephritis refers to an infection that has reached one or both kidneys. The microorganism usually ascends from the lower urinary tract but also can gain access from the bloodstream. *E. coli* is the most common culprit. The kidneys become grossly edematous and structures fill with exudate, compressing the renal artery. Abscesses and necrosis can develop, impairing renal function and causing permanent damage. Pyelonephritis can be acute or chronic.

In addition to the usual UTI symptoms, clinical manifestations are more severe and include flank pain and increased blood pressure. Diagnostic procedures for pyelonephritis consist of a history, physical examination, urinalysis, urine and blood cultures, CBC, cystoscopy, intravenous pyelogram, CT, renal ultrasound, biopsy, and cystourethrogram. With treatment, most cases will improve without any complications. Strategies include the usual UTI treatments, but long-term antibiotics (4–6 weeks) are usually required. Complications, if they occur, can involve renal failure, recurrent UTIs, and sepsis. Surveillance for complication development and treatment for those complications is also necessary.

Inflammatory Disorders

The inflammatory process (see Chapter 2) can cause havoc in the urinary system, especially in the kidneys. The structures can become edematous and damaged due to the inflammatory mediators and their effects. These changes impair the kidneys' ability to function properly, leading to serious consequences.

Glomerulonephritis

Glomerulonephritis is a bilateral inflammatory disorder of the glomeruli that typically follows a streptococcal infection. Affecting men more than women, glomerulonephritis is a leading cause of renal failure in the United States. The inflammatory changes (e.g., congestion and cell proliferation) impair the kidneys' ability to excrete waste and excess fluid. Glomerulonephritis can be acute or chronic. There are many forms of glomerulonephritis, with nephrotic and nephritic syndromes being the most prevalent (**Figure 7-8**).

Nephrotic Syndrome

Nephrotic syndrome results from antibody-antigen complexes lodging in the glomerular membrane, triggering the complement system. Nephrotic syndrome is caused by systemic diseases (e.g., systemic lupus erythematosus, hepatitis B, and diabetes mellitus), as a reaction to gold therapy, and idiopathically. The inflammatory changes result in increased glomerular capillary permeability, leading to marked proteinuria,

lipiduria, hypoalbuminemia, and massive generalized edema (anasarca). The high level of protein in the urine indicates impaired glomerular filtration. The loss of protein in the urine contributes to low serum levels (hypoalbuminemia) and gives the urine a dark and cloudy (smoky or coffee-colored) appearance. Additionally, immunoglobulins are excreted in the urine. This loss of immune cells increases the individual's risk for infection. To compensate for the loss of protein in the urine, the liver increases albumin, triglyc-

CASE STUDY

A 13-year-old boy presented to the clinic complaining of a sore throat that persisted for 2 days. After those 2 days, he developed fever, nausea, and malaise. A throat culture revealed the presence of Group A beta hemolytic streptococci, and the child was started on antibiotic therapy. The child's symptoms gradually improved, but approximately 2 weeks later, he returned to the clinic because the fever, nausea, and malaise returned. He became tachypneic and short of breath. The mother noted that his eyes were puffy, his ankles were swollen, and his urine was dark and cloudy.

On examination, his blood pressure was 148/100 mm Hg, his pulse was 122 beats/minute, and his respirations were 35/minute. Orbital and ankle edema were present. Rales (abnormal breath sounds) were auscultated bilaterally in the chest, but there were no heart murmurs. Slight tenderness to percussion over the flank areas was noted.

A chest X-ray showed evidence of congestion and edema in the lungs. The patient's hematocrit was 37% and WBC 11,200/mm³. Blood urea nitrogen was 48 mg/dL (normal is < 20 mg/dL). Urinalysis results showed his protein was 2+ (24 hours excretion was 0.8 g); specific gravity was 1.012; and there were moderate amounts of RBCs and WBCs in the urine. Serum albumin was 4.1 g/dL (normal is 3.5–4.5).

QUESTIONS

1. What evidence supports that this patient has a kidney disease?
2. What clinical pattern of kidney disease does this patient have? Can you explain the symptoms?
3. What morphologic changes would you expect in the kidney?
4. What is the prognosis? What are the possible short- and long-term complications of this disease? Is it necessary to hospitalize?

Source: University of Colorado (2010).

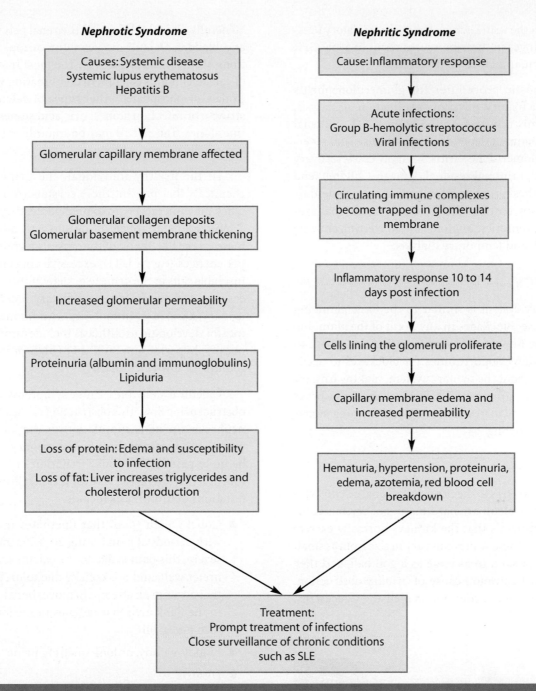

Nephrotic Syndrome

Causes: Systemic disease
Systemic lupus erythematosus
Hepatitis B

↓

Glomerular capillary membrane affected

↓

Glomerular collagen deposits
Glomerular basement membrane thickening

↓

Increased glomerular permeability

↓

Proteinuria (albumin and immunoglobulins)
Lipiduria

↓

Loss of protein: Edema and susceptibility
to infection
Loss of fat: Liver increases triglycerides and
cholesterol production

Nephritic Syndrome

Cause: Inflammatory response

↓

Acute infections:
Group B-hemolytic streptococcus
Viral infections

↓

Circulating immune complexes
become trapped in glomerular
membrane

↓

Inflammatory response 10 to 14
days post infection

↓

Cells lining the glomeruli proliferate

↓

Capillary membrane edema and
increased permeability

↓

Hematuria, hypertension, proteinuria,
edema, azotemia, red blood cell
breakdown

Treatment:
Prompt treatment of infections
Close surveillance of chronic conditions
such as SLE

Figure 7-8

Nephrotic and nephritic syndrome.

eride, and cholesterol production. This response puts the individual at increased risk for atherosclerosis (see Chapter 4).

Nephritic Syndrome

Nephritic syndrome refers to inflammatory injury to the glomeruli that can occur because of antibod-ies interacting with normally occurring antigens in the glomeruli. Diseases that initiate the inflammatory response (e.g., infection) cause nephritic syndrome. Clinical manifestations of nephritic syndrome include gross hematuria, urinary casts and leukocytes, low GFR, azotemia (buildup of waste products), oliguria (decreased urine output), and high blood pressure. The inflammatory injury results in red blood cells being excreted in the urine, which changes circulatory pressures. Changes in these pressures result in a low GFR and, in turn, impair renal function.

Diagnostic procedures for glomerulonephritis consist of a history, physical examination, urinalysis, blood chemistry, serum antibody levels, CT, and renal biopsy. Treatment depends on type, cause, and severity of the glomerulonephritis. In many cases, recovery occurs with minimal residual damage. Children tend to have the best prognosis. Strategies may include antibiotic therapy, corticosteroids, blood pressure management (e.g., diuretics, angiotensin-converting enzyme inhibitors), and temporary dialysis.

Urinary Tract Obstructions

The urinary system is similar to the basic plumbing in any house. Blockages in any point of the plumbing prevent the flow of the liquid, causing the system to back up. Many opportunities for blockages to occur exist throughout the urinary system, making urinary obstructions common. These blockages may be as simple as particulates collecting and forming stones to tumors growing.

Urolithiasis

Urolithiasis refers to the presence of renal calculi (kidney stones). Calculi are hard masses of crystals composed of minerals that the kidneys normally excrete (**Figure 7-9**). These stones can vary in size from as small as a grain of sand to as large as a golf ball, and they are the most common cause of urinary obstruction. Urolithiasis is more common in men and Caucasians.

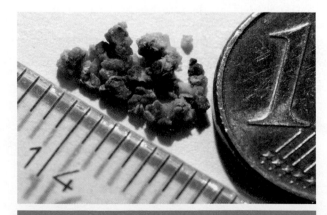

Figure 7-9

Renal calculi.

Generally, the calculi form in the renal pelvis, ureters, and bladder. Calculi may contain various combinations of chemicals (**Table 7-5**). The most frequent type of calculi contains calcium in combination with either oxalate or phosphate. Other types of calculi include struvite or infection stones, uric acid stones, and cystine stones. The calculi may be smooth or jagged and are usually yellow or brown.

In the healthy individual, the urine contains chemicals that prevent these crystals from forming. Once the minerals begin to precipitate, they grow like a snowball being rolled in the snow. Conditions that increase the likelihood of the crystals forming include pH changes (e.g., a UTI), excessive concentration of insoluble salts in the urine (e.g., dehydration, bone disease, gout, renal disease, and dietary increases), and urinary stasis (e.g., immobility). Additional risk factors for developing urolithiasis include family history, obesity, hypertension, and diet (high-protein, high-sodium, or low-calcium diet).

Calculi usually only cause symptoms when they obstruct urine flow. This obstruction can lead to hydronephrosis (urine accumulation in the kidney). The movement of calculi through the urinary system can be quite painful and cause irritation of the urinary mucosa, increasing the risk for a UTI. Clinical manifestations of urolithiasis include:

- Colicky pain (pain that fluctuates in intensity, with periods of pain lasting 20–60 minutes; often severe, this pain is due to the calculi scraping the ureter wall, and it is colicky due to ureter spasms that occur in an attempt to move the calculi along) in the flank area that radiates to the lower abdomen and groin
- Bloody, cloudy, or foul-smelling urine
- Dysuria
- Frequency
- Genital discharge
- Nausea and vomiting
- Fever and chills (if an infection is present)

Diagnostic procedures for urolithiasis consist of a history, physical examination, urine examination (urinalysis, culture, 24-hour urine), kidney-ureter-bladder X-ray, CT, ultrasound, intravenous pyelogram, calculi analysis, and serum studies (calcium, uric acid, etc.). Treatment of urolithiasis is specific to the type of calculi present (Table 7-5); therefore, determining the type of calculi is crucial to resolve

Table 7-5 Types of Renal Stones

Type	Cause	Treatment
Calcium	Causes of renal stones include • Increased absorption of calcium from the small bowel • Hyperparathyroidism • Inability of renal tubules to reabsorb calcium • Dietary excess of calcium • Chronic bowel disease that results in steatorrhea; fat then combines with calcium and renders the calcium unable to bind to oxalate, causing stone formation	Treatment depends on the cause of the stone formation and includes • Cellulose phosphate or thiazide diuretics to decrease dietary absorption of calcium • Surgical resection of the parathyroid gland to reduce hyperparathyroidism • Thiazide diuretic therapy to correct renal tubular defects, resulting in the inability to reabsorb calcium • Purine dietary restrictions to reduce uric acid production • Increased fluid intake and treatment of chronic diarrhea
Struvite (magnesium-ammonium-phosphate)	Caused by urase-producing bacteria Urinary pH around 7.2 Usually large in size Texture is relatively soft Associated with frequent UTI More common in women	Prevention of UTI Percutaneous nephrolithotomy
Uric acid	Urine pH lower than 5.5 encourages insoluble urate salt formation Common causes of uric acid stone formation include rapid and dramatic weight loss, some malignancies	Large calculi can be dissolved by increasing the urine pH above 6.5 with potassium citrate (urate solubility salt is then increased)
Cystine	Abnormal excretion of cystine (amino acid), ornithine lysine, and arginine	Prevention: increase fluid intake and increase urine pH above 7.5

Source: Madara, M., & Pomarico-Denino, V. (2008). *Quick look nursing: Pathophysiology* (2nd ed.). Sudbury, MA: Jones & Bartlett Learning.

the current calculi and prevent future calculus development. To determine the type of calculi, all urine is strained to capture any passed calculi. Small stones can pass through the urinary system. Strategies to assist the passing of these calculi include increasing fluid intake to 2.5–3.5 L throughout the day and physical activity (if possible). The increased presence of fluid in the urinary system will expand the diameter of the ureters and urethra, easing the passing of the calculi. Larger calculi can be broken up to allow for passing of the smaller pieces. Procedures to disintegrate these calculi include extracorporeal shock wave lithotripsy (high-frequency sound waves are directed at the calculi to pulverize them), percutaneous nephrolithotomy (a laser is directed at a calculus with a fiber-optic scope), and ureteroscopy (a forceps is used to grab a calculus and remove it through a fiber-optic scope). Surgical removal of the calculi may be indicated in the following situations:

■ The calculi do not pass after a reasonable period of time and cause constant pain

■ A calculus is too large to pass on its own or is lodged in a difficult location

■ The calculi obstruct urinary flow

■ The calculi cause ongoing UTIs, renal damage, or constant bleeding

■ The calculi have enlarged

Further, treating the underlying cause (e.g., with antibiotics, antigout agents, or urine pH–modifying agents) of the calculi and pain management will be necessary. Recurrence is common with urolithiasis;

MYTH BUSTERS

There are several common myths surrounding renal calculi that warrant addressing.

MYTH 1: **Only men get renal calculi.**

Though calculi formation is more common in men, rates among women are rising.

MYTH 2: **Eating certain foods will cause calculi to form.**

In general, eating certain foods will not cause calculi to form in persons who are not already susceptible to them forming.

MYTH 3: **Most renal calculi form from calcium, so dietary intake of calcium should be reduced.**

For years, the medical community thought a low-calcium diet was the best way to prevent renal calculi, especially in those who already had stones, but recent research has changed that thinking. Studies have shown that low-calcium diets are not effective, and may actually be harmful, since they tend to increase the likelihood of low bone density and osteoporosis. Researchers now believe that more rather than less calcium is better, with normal amounts being best. So, drinking that glass of milk and cutting back on the hamburgers and chips may help reduce your risk of renal calculi!

MYTH 4: **If a person has renal calculi, then he or she is more likely to develop cholelithiasis (gallstones).**

Not even close! Cholelithiasis and urolithiasis are not related at all—they form in different areas of the body. Typically, those at risk for developing cholelithiasis are a different group from those who have renal calculi. Women, Native Americans, and Mexican Americans, people over 60 years of age, and those on frequent diets are more likely to have gallstones.

Source: NIH (2002).

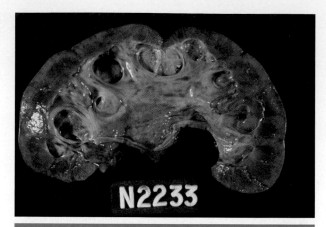

Figure 7-10

Hydronephrosis.

occurs secondary to a disease (**Figure 7-10**). Diseases that obstruct urine flow are commonly associated with this condition, including urolithiasis, tumors, benign prostatic hyperplasia, strictures, and stenosis. Congenital urologic defects can also cause hydronephrosis, including reflux nephropathy, a congenital condition that causes backflow of urine into the kidneys. Unilateral renal involvement indicates an obstruction in one of the ureters, and bilateral renal involvement indicates an obstruction in the urethra.

Because urine is continuously forming, the presence and severity of clinical manifestations are dependent on the degree of urinary obstruction. Partial obstructions with mild hydronephrosis may not yield any initial symptoms. Complete obstruction with severe hydronephrosis applies direct pressure and compression of tissue and blood vessels leading to atrophy, necrosis, and glomerular filtration cessation. When present, clinical manifestations include:

- Colicky, flank pain or pressure
- Bloody, cloudy, or foul-smelling urine
- Dysuria
- Decreased urine output
- Frequency
- Urgency
- Nausea and vomiting
- Abdominal distension
- UTIs

Diagnostic procedures for hydronephrosis include a history, physical examination, urinalysis, renal ultra-

therefore, prevention strategies are essential. Dietary changes are the mainstay of prevention. These changes are specific to the type of calculi (Table 7-5). Additional prevention strategies include adequate fluid intake (2–2.5 L per day) and physical activity.

Hydronephrosis

Hydronephrosis is an abnormal dilation of the renal pelvis and the calyces of one or both kidneys that sound, CT, intravenous pyelogram, and MRI. Prognosis depends on the severity of the hydronephrosis and early treatment. Treatment focuses on resolving the underlying cause and facilitating urine flow will be necessary if UTIs develop. If the hydronephrosis is prolonged, permanent renal damage can occur to one or both kidneys.

Tumors

Benign tumors are rare in the urinary system; most urinary tumors are malignant. These tumors can occur at any point along the urinary system. Regardless of their location, these tumors can obstruct urine flow and impair renal function in addition to the consequences of cancer (e.g., metastasis, pain, and weight loss).

Renal Cell Carcinoma

Renal cell carcinoma is the most frequently occurring kidney cancer in adults (most common in those 50–70 years of age). The National Cancer Institute (2010a) estimates that more than 58,000 new cases of renal cancer will be diagnosed in 2010 with more than 13,000 deaths contributed to this cancer. Renal cell carcinoma is a primary tumor arising from the renal tubule (**Figure 7-11**). Risk factors for developing this type of cancer include being male and smoking. Metastasis to the liver, lungs, bone, or nervous system is common at the time of diagnosis.

Renal cell carcinoma is typically asymptomatic in early stages. When present, clinical manifestations include:

- Painless hematuria (gross or microscopic)
- Abnormal urine color (dark, rusty, or brown)
- Dull, achy flank pain
- Urinary retention
- Palpable mass over affected kidney
- Unexplained weight loss
- Anemia (if the tumor suppresses hormone secretion)
- Polycythemia (if the tumor secretes erythropoietin or an erythropoietin-like substance)
- Hypertension
- Paraneoplastic syndromes such as hypercalcemia (due to ectopic parathyroid hormone production by the tumor or bone metastasis) or Cushing's syndrome (increased adrenocorticotropic hormone)
- Fever

Diagnostic procedures for renal cell carcinoma are used to identify the presence of the tumor and determine metastasis. These procedures include a history, physical examination, urinalysis, CT, MRI, positron emission tomography scan, bone scan, chest X-ray, intravenous pyelogram, cystoscopy, renal arteriogram, biopsy, liver function panel, CBC, and blood chemistry. Partial or complete surgical removal the kidney (nephrectomy) is recommended because the cancer is generally unresponsive to radiation or chemotherapy, although some newer chemotherapy agents are showing promise (e.g., multikinase inhibitors). Hormone and immunotherapy may have modest effects on shrinking the tumor. Prognosis improves if the condition is diagnosed prior to the cancer metastasizing.

Bladder Cancer

Bladder cancer refers to any cancer that forms in the tissue of the bladder. Most bladder cancers are transitional cell carcinomas (cancer that begins in cells that normally make up the inner bladder lining). Other types include squamous cell carcinoma (cancer that begins in thin, flat cells) and adenocarcinoma (cancer that begins in cells that make and release mucus and other fluids). The cells that form squamous cell carcinoma and adenocarcinoma develop in the inner lining of the bladder because of chronic irritation and inflammation. This type of cancer usually develops as multiple invasive tumors that extend through the bladder wall and surrounding structures. Metastasis is common to the pelvic lymph nodes, liver, and bone.

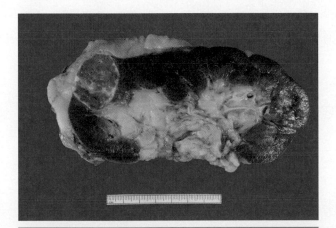

Figure 7-11

Renal cell carcinoma.

The National Cancer Institute (2010b) estimates that nearly 71,000 new cases of bladder cancer will be diagnosed in 2010 with nearly 15,000 deaths attributed to this cancer. Bladder cancer most frequently occurs in older adults although it can occur at any age, and it is more common in men and Caucasians. Other persons at risk include those who work with chemicals (e.g., dye, rubber, and aluminum), smoke, excessively use analgesics, experience recurrent UTIs, have long-term catheter placement, and received chemotherapy or radiation.

Clinical manifestations of bladder cancer include:

- Painless hematuria (gross or microscopic)
- Abnormal urine color (dark, rusty, or brown)
- Frequency
- Dysuria
- UTIs
- Back or abdominal pain

Diagnostic procedures are used to identify the presence of the tumor and determine whether metastasis has occurred. These procedures consist of a history, physical examination, urinalysis, CT, MRI, positron emission tomography scan, bone scan, chest X-ray, intravenous pyelogram, cystoscopy, biopsy, and liver function panel. Even with early diagnosis and treatment, bladder cancer often reoccurs. Treatment strategies include surgical removal of the tumor, radiation, chemotherapy, and immunologic agents.

Benign Prostatic Hyperplasia

Although the prostate is a structure of the male reproductive system, diseases of the prostate can cause significant issues in the urinary system because of its close proximity (**Figure 7-12**). Benign prostatic hyperplasia (BPH) is a common, nonmalignant enlargement of the prostate gland that occurs as men age. The exact cause is unknown, but declining testosterone and increasing estrogen levels are thought to cause prostatic stromal cell proliferation. This increase in proliferation enlarges

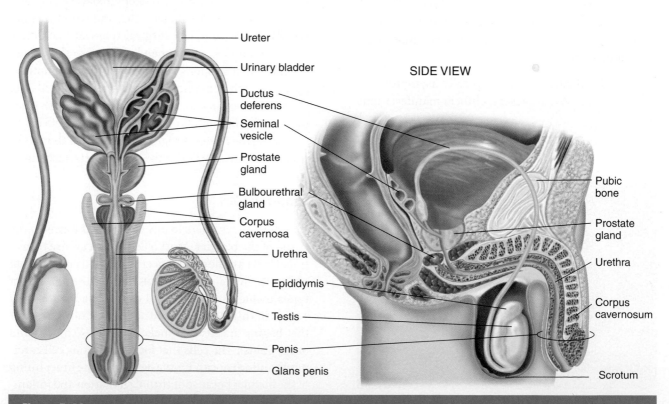

Figure 7-12

Urethra and prostate gland.

the prostate gland. A second theory postulates that stem cells in the prostate do not mature and die as programmed (apoptosis) (see Chapter 1). This imbalance between those cells dying and those reproducing enlarges the prostate over time. As the prostate expands, it presses against the urethra like a clamp on a hose. Clamping the urethra obstructs urine flow, leading to urinary stasis and UTIs. The bladder wall becomes thick and irritated as urine overfills it. The bladder begins to contract with even small amounts of urine, and, over time, the bladder will lose its ability to empty completely.

Clinical manifestations of BPH are primarily urinary in nature. The severity of symptoms depends on the size of the prostate. These manifestations include:

- Frequency
- Urgency
- Retention
- Difficulty initiating urination
- Weak urinary stream
- Dribbling urine

- Nocturia
- Bladder distension
- Overflow incontinence
- Erectile dysfunction

BPH does not increase prostate cancer risk, but the clinical presentation is very similar. Diagnostic procedures can determine whether the enlargement of the prostate is due to BPH or prostate cancer (see Chapter 8). These procedures consist of a history, physical examination (including digital rectal examination), urine flow measures, urinalysis, prostate-specific antigen, rectal ultrasound, biopsy, and cystoscopy. Treatment centers on relieving the urinary obstruction and reestablishing sexual function (if possible). Strategies to improve urine flow include pharmacologic agents (e.g., alpha-blockers and alpha$_5$-reductase inhibitors) to shrink or limit growth of the prostate. Herbal remedies (e.g., saw palmetto) have also been used with limited evidence indicating their effectiveness. Other strategies to improve BPH symptoms include minimally invasive procedures (**Table 7-6**) as well as partial or complete surgical removal of the prostate gland. Additionally,

Table 7-6 Minimally Invasive Benign Prostatic Hyperplasia Treatment

Technique	Description
Laser therapy Advantages • Minimal blood loss • Rare occurrence of transurethral resection syndrome • Outpatient treatment Disadvantages • Lack of tissue for pathological exam • Longer post-op catheterization • Irritation when voiding • Equipment expense	Two main energy sources used • Neodymium:yttrium aluminum garnet (Nd:YAG) • holmium-YAG • TULIP → transurethral laser-induced prostatectomy—ultrasound-guided procedure • Visually directed → coagulation → requires up to 12 weeks for tissue sloughing to complete
TUNA (transurethral needle ablation)	Urethral approach Tissue heated and necrosis results
Transurethral electrovaporization of the prostate	Tissue vaporized in response to heat
Hyperthermia	Microwave hyperthermia technique destroys tissue
HIFU (high-density forced ultrasound)	Short bursts of high-energy ultrasound delivered to the tissue—heats tissue and results in coagulative necrosis
Intraurethral stents	Placed in the prostatic fossa to keep it patent
Transurethral balloon dilation	Most effective if the enlargement is small—rarely used

Source: Madara, M., & Pomarico-Denino, V. (2008). *Quick look nursing: Pathophysiology* (2nd ed.). Sudbury, MA: Jones & Bartlett Learning.

LEARNING POINTS

The urinary system is like a basic household septic system. The kidneys remove waste and unneeded substances from the blood to have them removed. The kidneys collect these products in the form of urine much like a toilet, and flushing the toilet is much like what the kidneys do to send the urine to the bladder. The bladder acts like a septic tank, holding the waste until the tank is full. When full, the bladder and the septic tank must be emptied.

When obstructions occur at any point in the urinary system, urine backs up much like the septic system would do if obstructed. This backflow can cause severe damage in both cases—in the urinary system, the kidneys become damaged by the irritation and pressure of the excess urine, and in the septic system, the house becomes damaged from the corrosive septic contents.

alcohol should be avoided because it can make symptoms worse.

Renal Failure

The pivotal role that kidneys play in maintaining homeostasis (see Chapter 6) becomes clear when the kidneys stop performing that role. Renal failure refers to the kidneys' inability to function adequately. Renal failure is classified as either acute or chronic.

Acute Renal Failure

Acute renal failure (ARF), also termed acute kidney injury, refers to a sudden loss of renal function. This loss is generally reversible and is most common in critically ill, hospitalized patients. ARF has a mortality rate of 10–60% depending on the underlying etiology. Causes of ARF are divided into three categories:

1. Prerenal conditions (which disrupt blood flow on its way to the kidneys), including the following:

   ■ Extremely low blood pressure or blood volume (e.g., hemorrhaging, sepsis, dehydration, shock, and traumatic injury)

   ■ Heart dysfunction (e.g., myocardial infarction and heart failure)

2. Intrarenal conditions (which directly damage the structures of the kidneys), including the following:

   ■ Reduced blood supply within the kidneys (e.g., atherosclerosis)

■ Hemolytic uremic syndrome (associated with certain strains of *E. coli*, in which bacterium toxins damage small blood vessels; it is the leading cause of acute kidney failure in children)

■ Renal inflammation (e.g., glomerulonephritis and acute interstitial nephritis [usually associated with an allergic reaction to certain nephrotoxic medications])

■ Toxic injury (usually from alcohol, cocaine, heavy metals, solvents, fuels, chemotherapy drugs, and contrast dyes)

3. Postrenal conditions (which interfere with the urine excretion), including the following:

   ■ Ureter obstruction (e.g., urolithiasis and tumors)

   ■ Bladder obstruction and dysfunction (e.g., BPH, tumors, and nerve innervation disruption)

In addition to these causes, other factors can increase the risk for developing ARF such as advanced age, autoimmune disorders, and liver disease.

ARF progresses through four phases. The individual is usually asymptomatic in the initial phase. Although renal damage is occurring, those nephrons that are functioning compensate for those that are not. During the second (oliguric) phase, impaired glomerular filtration leads to solute and water reabsorption. This reabsorption decreases daily urine output to approximately 400 mL or less, and waste products accumulate (uremia). The second phase can last a few days to a few weeks. In the third (diuretic) phase, renal function gradually returns as healing and cellular regeneration occur. Diuresis occurs due to tubular damage that impairs the kidneys' ability to concentrate the urine. Daily urine output in this phase can be as much as 5 L. The excessive urine output can lead to dehydration and electrolyte imbalances. The third phase can last days to weeks. In the recovery stage, glomerular function has gradually returned to normal. This final stage can persist for 3–12 months. Depending on the age and overall health of the individual, full renal function may be regained.

As previously mentioned, the initial phase of ARF is asymptomatic. As renal function is lost, symptoms appear. Clinical manifestations vary depending on the ARF phase. In the oliguric phase, manifestations are:

■ Decreasing urine output

■ Electrolyte disturbances

■ Fluid volume excess

- Azotemia
- Metabolic acidosis

In the diuretic phase, manifestations include:

- Increased urine output
- Electrolyte disturbances
- Dehydration
- Hypotension

In the recovery phase, symptoms begin resolving.

Diagnostic procedures for ARF include those to identify the renal injury as well as the underlying cause. These procedures consist of a history, physical examination, blood chemistry, arterial blood gases, urinalysis, CBC, renal ultrasound, and biopsy. Treatment strategies for ARF vary depending on the phase. For instance, the fluid and electrolyte disturbances are different in the second and third phase, requiring alternate strategies. ARF may require temporary dialysis until renal recovery occurs. Other supportive strategies include:

- A diet high in calories and restricted in protein, sodium, potassium, and phosphates
- Hypertension management
- Anemia treatment with synthetic erythropoietin
- Infection prevention strategies (e.g., hand washing, limiting visitors, and aseptic technique)

Chronic Renal Failure

Chronic renal failure (CRF) tends to be a gradual loss of renal function that is irreversible. Nonoperational scar tissue replaces injured nephrons. Several conditions, including those in the following list, can initiate the slow, progressive destruction of the nephrons.

- Diabetes mellitus (type 1 and type 2) is a leading cause of CRF in the United States because of vascular damage (see Chapter 10).
- Hypertension is another leading cause of CRF in the United States; it can damage the glomeruli and ultimately cause the damaged nephrons to lose their ability to filter waste from the blood.
- Urine obstructions (e.g., urolithiasis and BPH) can block urine flow, increasing pressure in the kidneys, reducing their function.

- Renal diseases (e.g., polycystic kidney disease, pyelonephritis, and glomerulonephritis) damage nephrons in a variety of ways.
- Renal artery stenosis (narrowing or blockage of the artery that supplies the kidneys) impairs blood flow and leads to kidney damage.
- Ongoing exposure to toxins (e.g., fuel, solvents, and lead) and nephrotoxic medications (e.g., many antibiotics, chemotherapy, and nonsteroidal anti-inflammatory drugs) can cause direct damage as they circulate through the kidneys.
- Sickle cell disease can damage the kidneys by impairing renal blood flow as the sickled blood cells clump together in the renal arteries.
- Systemic lupus erythematosus causes direct damage to the renal tissue as the autoantibodies destroy the body's own cells.
- Smoking hardens the blood vessel walls throughout the body, especially in the tiny vessels of the kidney, and smoking triggers vasoconstriction; both of these changes cause chronic ischemia and necrosis.
- With aging, the kidneys generally become less efficient and are exposed to more conditions that can cause damage.

CRF generally evolves through three phases as the number of functioning nephrons declines. In the first phase, renal impairment (reduced renal reserve), 60% of nephrons are lost. Clinical manifestations begin to appear slowly as the renal function declines by 50%. Even with the declining GFR, the kidneys can maintain relatively normal function to a point because the surviving nephrons hypertrophy and increase their rate of filtration, reabsorption, and secretion. The kidneys transition into the next phase, renal insufficiency, as 75% of the nephrons are lost and normal GFR reduces by 20%. Waste products begin to accumulate as renal function declines. Additionally, the kidneys lose the ability to concentrate the urine, maintain blood pressure control, and secrete erythropoietin. Multiple systems are affected as these changes develop (Table 7-7). These complications worsen as the renal function further declines. The final phase, end-stage renal disease, is marked by a 90% of nephron destruction and a drop in GFR to 10 mL/min (normal is 125 mL/min). The kidneys lose their ability to maintain any sense of homeostasis. Waste products, fluid, and electrolytes accumulate significantly.

Table 7-7 Complications of Chronic Renal Failure

System	Etiology	Treatment
General appearance	Tired, weak, sallow skin color due to anemia, toxins	Dialysis, Epogen
Integumentary	Itching (uremic frost) occurs in an attempt to remove toxins from the body	Dialysis and palliative care
Sensory	Metallic taste in mouth, fishy breath odor (uremic fetor) due to toxins	Dialysis
Cardiopulmonary	Hypertension • Related to salt and water retention, erythropoietin (20% of patients on this therapy), or increased renin production • Accelerated renal damage if not controlled • Congestive heart failure develops Pericarditis • Result of metabolic toxins • Chest pain, fever, friction rub, decreased cardiac output Congestive heart failure (75% of patients needing dialysis) • Result of increased workload of the heart (left ventricular hypertrophy) secondary to anemia, dialysis (shunting of blood), fluid overload, hypertension, atherosclerosis	 • Limiting salt and fluids • Angiotensin-converting enzyme inhibitors (ACE), angiotensin II receptor blockers, calcium channel blockers, beta blockers • Blood pressure goal is 130/80 mm Hg • Hemodialysis • Salt and fluid restriction • Diuretics (Loop) • Angiotensin-converting enzyme inhibitors, angiotensin II receptor blockers
Hematological	Coagulopathy • Platelet dysfunction due to abnormal aggregation and "stickiness" • Bleeding time increases • Platelet count slightly decreased • May have petechiae or purpura Anemia • Related to decreased erythropoietin production (occurs when glomerular filtration rate falls below 20–25 mL/min) and iron deficiency • Hemodialysis causes some red blood cell destruction	 • Desmopressin (causes release of factor VIII from endothelial cells)—used before surgery • Epogen if hematocrit is below 33% (hemoglobin levels should increase no more than 1 g/dL every 3–4 weeks so hypertension does not develop) • Intravenous iron for patients on dialysis (PO absorption poor)
Gastrointestinal	Anorexia, nausea, vomiting, hiccups—related to metabolic toxins	Dialysis
Endocrine	Decreased libido, impotence, and infertility • Decreased estrogen levels in women—do not ovulate • Decreased testosterone levels in men Glucose intolerance	 • Dialysis and a healthy diet may restore fertility

(Continues)

Table 7-7 Complications of Chronic Renal Failure *(Continued)*

System	Etiology	Treatment
Endocrine *(cont.)*	Peripheral insulin resistance Serum insulin high • Kidneys cannot clear insulin from bloodstream	 • Patients with diabetes may require lower doses of hypoglycemic agents
Mineral metabolism	Renal osteodystrophy (disorder of calcium, phosphorus, and bone) leading to bone pain, fractures, muscle weakness, calcium deposits in blood vessels, soft tissue, heart and lungs • Low glomerular filtration rate = phosphorus excretion slowed so calcium excretion increases → parathyroid hormone secretion rises and causes a high bone turnover • In ESRD, excess hydrogen ions are buffered by leeching large stores of calcium phosphate and calcium carbonate from the bones = bone demineralization	 • Restrict dietary phosphorus • Administer phosphorus-binding drugs such as calcium carbonate • Vitamin D (suppresses parathyroid hormone)
Neurological	Uremic encephalopathy • Appears when glomerular filtration rate falls below 10–15 mL/min or by hyperparathyroidism • Symptoms: poor concentration (first sign) and progresses to confusion, asterixis, weakness, nystagmus, hyperreflexia • Peripheral neuropathy (restless leg syndrome, distal pain, loss of deep tendon reflexes) • Impotence and autonomic dysfunction	 • Dialysis
Metabolic	Hyperkalemia • Glomerular filtration rate falling below 10–20 mL/min • Hemolysis, trauma, acidosis • Diet high in citrus fruits/juices • Medications such as angiotensin-converting enzyme inhibitors, NSAIDs	 • Monitor cardiac status • Administer calcium chlorides, insulin, and glucose (insulin moves K into cells), bicarbonate or an exchange resin • Dietary K restriction
Acid–base disorders	Damaged kidneys • Cannot produce enough ammonia or buffer hydrogen ions • Arterial pH generally between 7.33 and 7.37 • Excess hydrogen ions are buffered by large stores of calcium phosphate and calcium carbonate from the bones	 • Maintain serum bicarbonate above 21 mEq/L by giving alkali supplements such as sodium bicarbonate, calcium bicarbonate, or sodium citrate

NSAIDs = nonsteroidal anti-inflammatory drugs.
Source: Madara, M., & Pomarico-Denino, V. (2008). *Quick look nursing: Pathophysiology* (2nd ed.). Sudbury, MA: Jones & Bartlett Learning.

Clinical manifestations are complex and dependent on the degree of renal function lost. These manifestations also reflect the complications associated with CRF (Table 7-7). As mentioned, CRF is often asymptomatic initially because of the compensation efforts of the remaining nephrons. Clinical manifestations develop insidiously as 50% of the nephrons are destroyed. These manifestations include:

- Hypertension (see Chapter 4)
- Polyuria with pale urine (early)
- Oliguria or anuria (absent urine output) with darkly colored urine (late)
- Anemia
- Bruising and bleeding tendencies
- Electrolyte imbalances, specifically hyperkalemia, hypocalcemia, hypomagnesemia, and hyperphosphatemia
- Muscle twitches and cramps (related to hypocalcemia and hyperphosphatemia; see Chapter 6)
- Pericarditis, pericardial effusion, pleuritis, and pleural effusion (secondary to uremia)
- Congestive heart failure (see Chapter 4)
- Respiratory distress and abnormal breath sounds (due to pulmonary edema associated with congestive heart failure; see Chapter 4)
- Sudden weight change (usually increased because of fluid retention)
- Edema of the feet and ankles (due to fluid retention)
- Azotemia
- Peripheral neuropathy, restless leg syndrome, and seizures

- Nausea and vomiting
- Anorexia
- Malaise
- Fatigue and weakness
- Headaches that seem unrelated to any other cause
- Sleep disturbances
- Decreased mental alertness
- Flank pain
- Jaundice
- Persistent pruritus
- Recurrent infections (due to an impaired immune response because of uremia)

Diagnosis of CRF is often difficult because the initial symptoms are vague and nonspecific. Diagnostic procedures focus on identifying the CRF and any complications that have developed. These procedures include a history, physical examination, urinalysis, blood chemistry (especially the creatinine and blood urea nitrogen), CT, MRI, renal ultrasound, biopsy, CBC, and arterial blood gases. The main goal of CRF treatment of is to stop or slow disease progression, usually by controlling the underlying cause. Additionally, strategies to treat and prevent complications will be necessary (Table 7-7). Dosing of any medications will likely need adjusting; with limited excretion capability, medication toxicity is probable. Without treatment, CRF has a mortality rate of 100%. Conservative management strategies are employed early, progressing to more aggressive measures as renal function declines.

Chapter Summary

The urinary system maintains homeostasis through a complex filter (kidney) that can regulate pH, fluid, electrolytes, and blood glucose. Additionally, the urinary system is the main site for excreting waste products and other harmful substances from the food and water ingested. A functioning urinary system is crucial to maintaining health, and disease in this system can have detrimental effects on other systems and the body as a whole. Prevention and early treatment of these diseases are paramount to avoiding these consequences. Maintaining a healthy lifestyle (e.g., drinking plenty of fluids, avoiding harmful chemicals, preventing sexually transmitted infection, exercising, smoking cessation) can help preserve urinary health.

Case Study Answers

1. Signs and symptoms: edema, hypertension, flank tenderness, dark urine. Laboratory results: elevated blood urea nitrogen. Urinalysis: protein, RBC, and WBC in the urine

2. This is likely acute nephritic syndrome. The elevated blood urea nitrogen indicates decreased GFR. The abnormal urine sediment indicates glomerular inflammation, which is also responsible for the flank tenderness. The edema in this case is not a consequence of proteinuria, since serum albumin is normal. Edema, hypertension, and circulatory congestion are consequences of fluid retention, probably resulting from decreased GFR.

3. Cellular proliferation in the glomeruli, some neutrophils in the glomeruli.

4. In children, the prognosis is excellent, with complete recovery occurring in most cases within a few weeks to a few months. However, in some cases, recovery may take many months to 2 years.

    Short-term complications include:

- *Renal failure*—Decreased GFR may be severe enough to cause azotemia and death.

- *Congestive heart failure*—Can occur when fluid retention and hypertension are severe. May be a cause of death.

- *Nephrotic syndrome*—Rarely, patients have enough proteinuria to cause hypoalbuminemia and have a mixed nephritic–nephrotic clinical picture.

For the first two reasons, patients are often hospitalized.

    Long-term complications include:

- Persistent urinary abnormalities such as hematuria and proteinuria

- Persistent hypertension

- Incomplete return to normal of GFR associated with scarring in the kidney

    Possible resolution of the acute illness followed by slowly progressive chronic glomerulonephritis has been demonstrated in only a handful of cases, most of which were adults who had atypical features.

References

Baumberger-Henry, M. (2008). *Fluid and electrolytes* (2nd ed.). Sudbury, MA: Jones and Bartlett.

Chiras, D. (2008). *Human biology* (6th ed.). Sudbury, MA: Jones and Bartlett.

Elling, B., Elling, K., & Rothenberg, M. (2004). *Anatomy and physiology.* Sudbury, MA: Jones and Bartlett.

Gould, B. (2006). *Pathophysiology for the health professions* (3rd ed.). Philadelphia, PA: Elsevier.

Madara, B., & Pomarico-Denino, V. (2008). *Pathophysiology* (2nd ed.). Sudbury, MA: Jones and Bartlett.

National Cancer Institute. (2010a). Retrieved from http://www.cancer.gov/cancertopics/pdq/treatment/renalcell/HealthProfessional/page2

National Cancer Institute. (2010b). Retrieved from http://www.cancer.gov/cancertopics/types/bladder

National Cancer Institute. (2010c). Retrieved from http://www.cancer.gov/cancertopics/pdq/treatment/wilms/HealthProfessional/page2

National Institutes of Health. (2002). Retrieved from http://www.nih.gov/news/WordonHealth/nov2002/kidneystones.htm

National Institutes of Health. (2010). Retrieved from http://www.genome.gov/20019622

Newman, D. K. (2010). *Causes of acute incontinence.* Retrieved from http://www.seekwellness.com/incontinence/incontinence-causes.htm

Professional guide to pathophysiology (2nd ed.). (2007). Philadelphia, PA: Lippincott Williams & Wilkins.

Resnick, N., & Yalla, S. (1998). Geriatric incontinence and voiding dysfunction. In P. C. Walsh, A. B. Retik, E. D. Vaughan, & A. J. Wein (Eds.), *Campbell's urology* (7th ed., p. 1045) Philadelphia, PA: W.B. Saunders Co.

University of Colorado Health Sciences Center. (2010). *Renal unit: Case 5.* Retrieved from http://www.uchsc.edu/pathology/smallgroups/renal/renc5.htm

Resources

www.labtestsonline.org/understanding/conditions/acidosis.html

www.the-abg-site.com

www.cancer.gov

www.cancer.org

www.cdc.gov

www.kidney.org

www.mayoclinic.com

www.medlineplus.gov

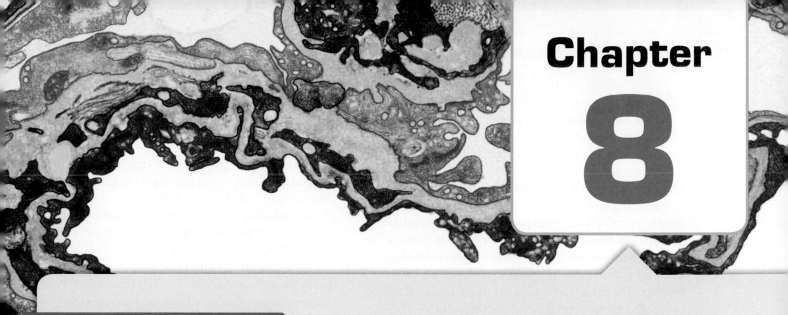

Reproductive Function

LEARNING OBJECTIVES

- Discuss normal reproductive anatomy and physiology.
- Describe congenital reproductive disorders.
- Describe issues with fertility.
- Describe and compare the common menstrual disorders.
- Discuss various disorders of the reproductive structures.
- Describe and compare infectious disorders of the reproductive system.
- Describe and compare cancers of the reproductive system.

KEY TERMS

amenorrhea
ampulla
anteflexed
areola
areolar gland
ascending testicle
Bartholin's glands
breast cancer
candidiasis
cervical cancer
cervix
chancre
chlamydia
chordee
clitoris
condyloma
  acuminatum
Cowper's glands
cryptorchidism
cystocele
dysmenorrhea
ectopic pregnancy
ectopic testes

ejaculation
ejaculatory duct
endometrial cancer
endometriosis
endometrium
epididymis
epididymitis
epispadias
erectile dysfunction
  (ED)
fallopian tubes
fibrocystic breast
  disease
foreskin
genital herpes
gestation
gonorrhea
herpes simplex virus
  (HSV)
human
  papillomaviruses
  (HPV)
hydrocele

hymen
hypospadias
impregnation
infertility
labia majora
labia minora
lactation
latent herpes
  genitalis
latent syphilis
leiomyoma
mammary glands
mastitis
meatus
menopause
menorrhagia
menstrual cycle
menstruation
metrorrhagia
mons pubis
myometrium
nipple
oligomenorrhea

oogenesis
orgasm
ovarian cancer
ovarian cyst
ovaries
ovulation
paraphimosis
parturition
pelvic inflammatory
  disease (PID)
penile cancer
penis
perimetrium
phimosis
placenta
polycystic ovary
  syndrome
polymenorrhea
premenstrual
  dysphoric
  syndrome
premenstrual
  syndrome (PMS)

priapism
primary herpes
  genitalis
primary syphilis
prodrome
prolactin
prostate cancer
prostate gland
prostatitis
recurrent herpes
  genitalis
rectocele
retractile testicle
retroflexed
scrotum
secondary syphilis
semen
seminal vesicles
sexually transmitted
  infection (STI)
shedding herpes
  genitalis
Skene's gland

smegma
spermatic cord
spermatocele
spermatogenesis
syphilis
tertiary syphilis
testes
testicular cancer
testicular torsion
testosterone
trichomoniasis
uterine prolapse
uterus
vagina
varicocele
vas deferens
vestibule
vulva
zygote

The reproductive system is comprised of structures that are responsible for procreation; therefore, a healthy reproduction system is necessary for the survival of the species. This system is responsible for transmitting genetic material to offspring (see Chapter 1). The male reproductive system generates sperm and transports it to the female reproductive system. The female reproductive system produces ovum. When the sperm fertilizes the ovum, the female reproductive system nurtures and safeguards the embryo as it develops into a fetus until birth. The primary difference between the two systems is the varying hormone levels, which cause the reproduction system to develop differently—the male reproductive system is generally external, and the female reproductive system is internal.

Anatomy and Physiology

Normal Male Reproductive System

The male reproductive system includes organs involved in the generation (spermatogenesis) and transportation of sperm. These organs include the penis, scrotum, testes, duct system, and accessory glands (**Figure 8-1; Table 8-1**). In addition to producing sperm, the male reproduction system produces sex hormones (mostly testosterone) that give males their distinct characteristics (e.g., facial hair, increased muscle mass, low voice pitch). Parts of the male reproductive system work with the urinary system to aid in urinary elimination (e.g., the urethra). Because the male reproductive and urinary system is integrated, disorders in one system generally affect the other system (see Chapter 7 for more discussion on the urinary system).

Penis

The penis is part of the male external genitalia; it contains erectile tissue that fills with blood during sexual arousal. The penis deposits sperm in the female reproductive system during sexual intercourse. The penis consists of three cylinders—the corpus spongiosum (which contains the urethra) and two copora cavernosa (**Figure 8-2**). The penis structure includes a root, shaft, and glans (enlarged tip). Penis length can vary considerably, but the average length is 2–5 inches when flaccid and 4–7 inches when erect. Penis appearance can also vary from person to person (**Figure 8-3**). A sheath of loose skin, called the foreskin, covers the glans penis at birth. The foreskin is often surgically removed (circumcision) shortly after birth for hygienic, cultural, or religious reasons. The glans produces an oily secretion that can combine with dead skin to form a cheesy substance called smegma. If the smegma is not regularly removed from under the foreskin, the penis can become irritated and infected. The glans also has an opening, or meatus, that allows for ejaculation (propulsion of sperm-containing fluid) and urination.

Scrotum

The scrotum is a sac of skin just below the penis that contains the testes, epididymides, and lower spermatic cords. The scrotum maintains the proper testicular temperature for spermatogenesis. The scrotum contracts to draw the testes closer to the body to warm them, and the scrotum relaxes to drop the testes further from the body to cool them.

Table 8-1 The Male Reproductive System

Component	Function
Testes	Produce sperm and male sex steroids
Epididymides	Store sperm
Vasa deferentia	Conduct sperm to urethra
Sex accessory glands	Produce seminal fluid that nourishes sperm
Urethra	Conducts sperm to outside
Penis	Organ of copulation
Scrotum	Provides proper temperature for testes

Source: Chiras, D. (2008). *Human biology* (6th ed.). Sudbury, MA: Jones & Bartlett Learning.

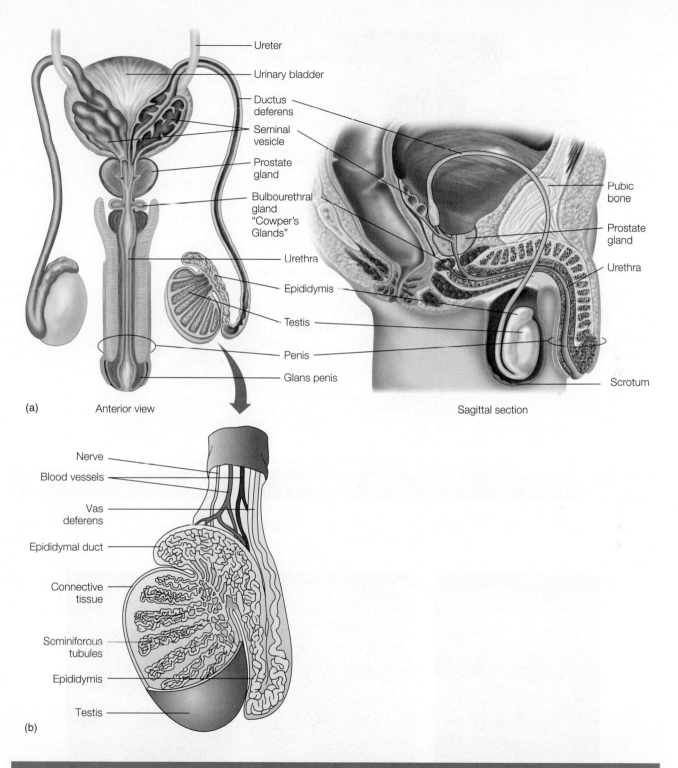

Ureter

Urinary bladder

Ductus deferens

Seminal vesicle

Prostate gland

Bulbourethral gland "Cowper's Glands"

Urethra

Epididymis

Testis

Penis

Glans penis

Pubic bone

Prostate gland

Urethra

Scrotum

(a)   Anterior view

Sagittal section

Nerve

Blood vessels

Vas deferens

Epididymal duct

Connective tissue

Seminiferous tubules

Epididymis

Testis

(b)

Figure 8-1

The male reproductive system. (a) Organs of the male reproductive system. (b) Interior view of the testis.

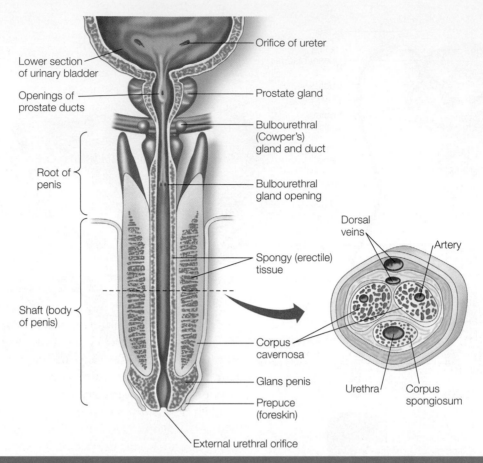

Lower section
of urinary bladder

Openings of
prostate ducts

Root of
penis

Shaft (body
of penis)

Orifice of ureter

Prostate gland

Bulbourethral
(Cowper's)
gland and duct

Bulbourethral
gland opening

Spongy (erectile)
tissue

Dorsal
veins

Artery

Corpus
cavernosa

Glans penis

Prepuce
(foreskin)

Urethra

Corpus
spongiosum

External urethral orifice

Figure 8-2

Anatomy of the penis.

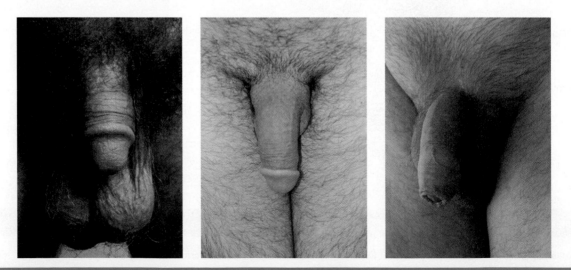

Figure 8-3

Variations of the male genitalia.

Testes

The testes, or gonads, produce sperm and the sex hormones. Spermatogenesis develops in most males by 16 years of age. The testes form in the abdominal cavity in utero and descend into the scrotum in approximately the 7th month of gestation. Seminiferous tubules produce sperm, and the epididymis stores sperm until ejaculation (up to 6 weeks). The sperm mature during storage, making them capable of swimming. The testes can produce approximately 50,000 sperm a minute.

The testes produce hormones (especially testosterone) in its Leydig cells. Exposure to increased testosterone levels gives males their classic secondary sex characteristics (e.g., facial hair, deep voice) and sex drive. Testosterone also regulates metabolism and protein anabolism (encourages skeletal growth and muscle development), inhibits pituitary secretion of the gonadotropins (follicle-stimulating hormone and interstitial cell-stimulating hormone), and promotes potassium excretion and renal sodium reabsorption. Additionally, testosterone contributes to male pattern baldness and acne.

Duct System

The male reproductive system contains a complex tube structure to deliver sperm from the testes to the female reproductive system. This duct system includes the epididymis (which stores the sperm for final maturation), vas deferens, spermatic cord, ejaculatory duct, and the urethra. Once matured, the sperm leaves the epididymis and travels to the vas deferens. The testicular artery and venous plexus, lymph vessels, nerves, connective tissue, and cremaster muscle (which contracts or relaxes the scrotum) surround the vas deferens, which together make the spermatic cord. The vas deferens widens at the prostate, forming a pouch called the ampulla. The ampulla joins the seminal vesicles (a pair of pouches that secrete an alkaline ejaculatory fluid containing sugar, protein, and prostaglandins) to form the ejaculatory duct. The sperm and the ejaculatory fluid join in the vesicles to form semen. The semen flows from the ejaculatory duct to the urethra where it is released from the penis during sexual intercourse.

Accessory Glands

The primary function of the accessory reproductive glands is to facilitate ejaculation. Sexual stimulation initiates the ejaculatory process. Once sexually stimulated, sperm travels from the epididymis to the vas deferens and then to the seminal vesicles. Fluid from the prostate gland (a chestnut-shaped gland at the base of the urethra) mixes with the sperm and secretions of the seminal vesicles. This prostate fluid further decreases acidity, increases sperm motility, and prolongs sperm life. The alkaline medium counteracts the acidity of vaginal secretion that would otherwise kill the sperm. The Cowper's glands (two pea-sized glands adjacent to the urethra) secrete another alkaline fluid into the urethra to neutralize acidity caused by urine transportation. The Cowper's glands' secretions can sometimes be seen at the meatus before ejaculation. This secretion aids in lubrication of the penis during sexual intercourse and may contain some sperm left over from a previous ejaculation; therefore, these secretions can cause pregnancy even if the penis is withdrawn prior to ejaculation.

The actual expulsion of semen from the penis is the result of motor neurons stimulating muscular contractions of the glands and ducts of the reproductive system—particularly the ampulla, seminal vesicles, and bulbocavernosus muscle (muscle surrounding the corpus spongiosum). During ejaculation, a valve at the bladder closes to prevent urine entering the urethra and killing the sperm. An orgasm, the climax of pleasurable sensations, usually accompanies the ejaculation. Ejaculated semen contains sperm (about the volume of a pinhead) and secretions (about a tablespoon) from the seminal vesicles, prostate, and Cowper's glands. One ejaculation contains approximately 300 million sperm.

Normal Female Reproductive System

The female reproductive tract is a complex system that includes organs to manage the generation of eggs (oogenesis), the transportation of the eggs (ovulation) for fertilization (impregnation), the support of fetal development (gestation), the birth of the fetus (parturition), and the feeding of the offspring (through lactation). To accomplish all these functions, the female reproductive system requires a delicate hormone balance and operational organs. These organs include the ovaries, fallopian tubes, uterus, vagina, external genitalia, and mammary glands (**Figure 8-4; Figure 8-5; Figure 8-6; Figure 8-7**). In addition to facilitating the system's function, the hormones (specifically estrogen and progesterone) produced by the female reproductive system give females their distinct characteristics (e.g., enlarged breasts, wide hips, and high-pitched voice). The female reproductive system is located in a hub of activity in the body. The female reproductive system is

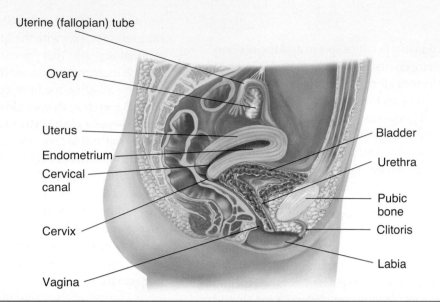

Uterine (fallopian) tube

Ovary

Uterus

Endometrium

Cervical canal

Cervix

Vagina

Bladder

Urethra

Pubic bone

Clitoris

Labia

Figure 8-4

Side view of the female reproductive system.

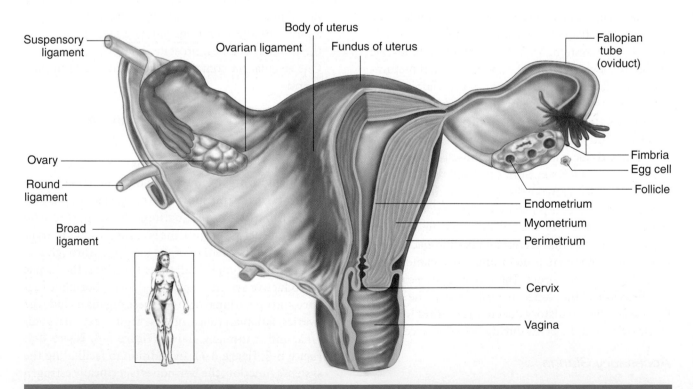

Suspensory ligament

Body of uterus

Ovarian ligament

Fundus of uterus

Fallopian tube (oviduct)

Ovary

Round ligament

Broad ligament

Fimbria

Egg cell

Follicle

Endometrium

Myometrium

Perimetrium

Cervix

Vagina

Figure 8-5

Front view of the female reproductive system.

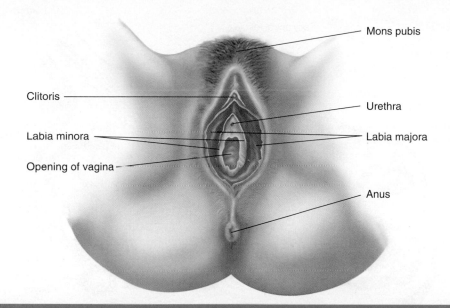

Mons pubis

Clitoris

Urethra

Labia minora

Labia majora

Opening of vagina

Anus

Figure 8-6

The female external genitalia.

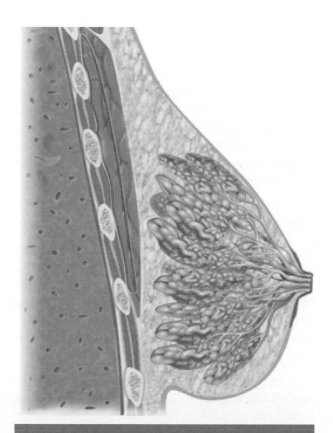

Figure 8-7

The female mammary glands.

interrelated with physiologic functions of nearby structures in the female pelvis. The female pelvis contains organs of the urinary and gastrointestinal system along with organs for reproduction; thus, the female pelvis is the site for urination, defecation, menstruation, ovulation, copulation (sexual intercourse), impregnation, pregnancy, and parturition. Because of the close proximity of these three systems, problems in one can lead to problems in the others.

Ovaries

The **ovaries** are paired, almond-shaped organs located on each side of the uterus (Figure 8-5; **Figure 8-8**). Two ligaments (suspensory and ovarian ligaments) and the mesovarium (fold in the peritoneum) hold the ovaries in place. The ovaries produce hormones (primarily estrogen and progesterone) that regulate reproductive function and secondary sex characteristics (e.g., enlarged breasts, wide hips, high-pitched voice). The ovaries contain the precursors to mature eggs (oocytes). During oogenesis, the oocytes mature into ova (mature eggs). By the 30th week of gestation, the female fetus has about 7 million follicles (biological units, each containing a single oocyte). These 7 million follicles degenerate to about 2 million by birth. By puberty, only about 400,000 follicles remain. During the reproductive years, the follicles mature in response to pituitary hormones (follicle-stimulating hormone

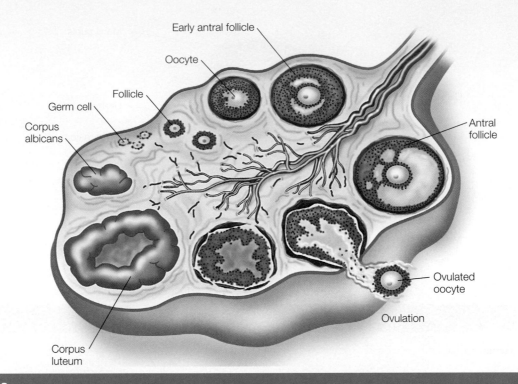

Early antral follicle

Oocyte

Follicle

Germ cell

Corpus albicans

Antral follicle

Ovulated oocyte

Ovulation

Corpus luteum

Figure 8-8

Structure of the ovary.

[FSH] and luteinizing hormone [LH]). During the ovulation phase of the menstrual cycle, the mature follicle ruptures, releasing the mature ovum into the fallopian tubes, through which it travels to the uterus for fertilization by the sperm (**Figure 8-9**). Fewer than 500 of each woman's ova mature and become potentially fertile. Although approximately a dozen follicles begin developing during each cycle, usually only one makes it to ovulation. Multiple births (e.g., twins or triplets) may occur when more than one ovum is produced and released. Once the mature follicle releases the ovum, the empty follicle (called the corpus luteum) secretes progesterone to signal to the endometrium to prepare for fertilization.

Fallopian Tubes

The fallopian tubes are two cylinders that extend from the fundus of the uterus to near the ovaries. The ends of the tubes near the ovaries are fimbriated (fringelike) to capture ovum after ovulation. The tubes use a ciliary and muscular action to move the ovum toward the uterus as well as assist sperm to move from the uterus toward to the ovum that is likely still in one of the tubes. Once fertilized, the same ciliary and muscular

action moves the fertilized egg (zygote) from the tube to the uterus for implantation (**Figure 8-10**). Occasionally, the zygote does not reach the uterus and implants outside the uterus (this is called an ectopic pregnancy). The most common site for ectopic pregnancies is the fallopian tubes. Ectopic pregnancies cannot develop normally and can be life threatening.

Uterus

The uterus is a hollow, pear-shaped organ held in place by the broad, round, and uterosacral ligaments. Usually, the uterus is tilted forward (anteflexed) over the bladder, but approximately 20% are tilted backward (retroflexed). Women with retroflexed uteruses are more likely to experience menstrual discomfort, but these women should have no fertility issues.

During pregnancy, the fetus grows and develops inside the uterus. The thick uterine wall consists of three layers to carry and deliver the fetus. The endometrium is the inner mucosal lining that undergoes hormonal changes to facilitate and maintain pregnancy. During pregnancy, a vascular organ (called the placenta) develops to nourish the fetus through the umbilical cord

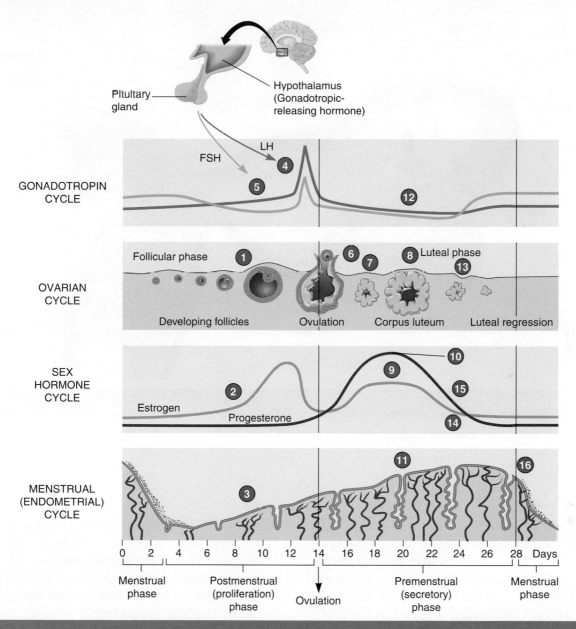

Figure 8-9

The menstrual cycle.

(which contains two arteries and one vein). The placenta attaches to the endometrium on one side and surrounds the fetus on the other (**Figure 8-11**). The uterus expels the placenta within a few minutes after birth. The **myometrium** is the middle layer made up of smooth muscle and a vascular system. During pregnancy, the vascular system radically increases to support the fetus. During childbirth, this layer contracts to push the fetus out through the vaginal canal. After childbirth or abor-

tion (spontaneous or induced pregnancy termination), this layer contracts to constrict blood vessels and control bleeding. The **perimetrium** is the outer, serous layer that covers all of the fundus, part of the corpus, but none of the **cervix** (the narrow opening from the uterus to the vagina). This incomplete coverage of this layer allows for surgical access into the uterus without requiring an incision into the peritoneum (the membrane that lines the abdominal cavity).

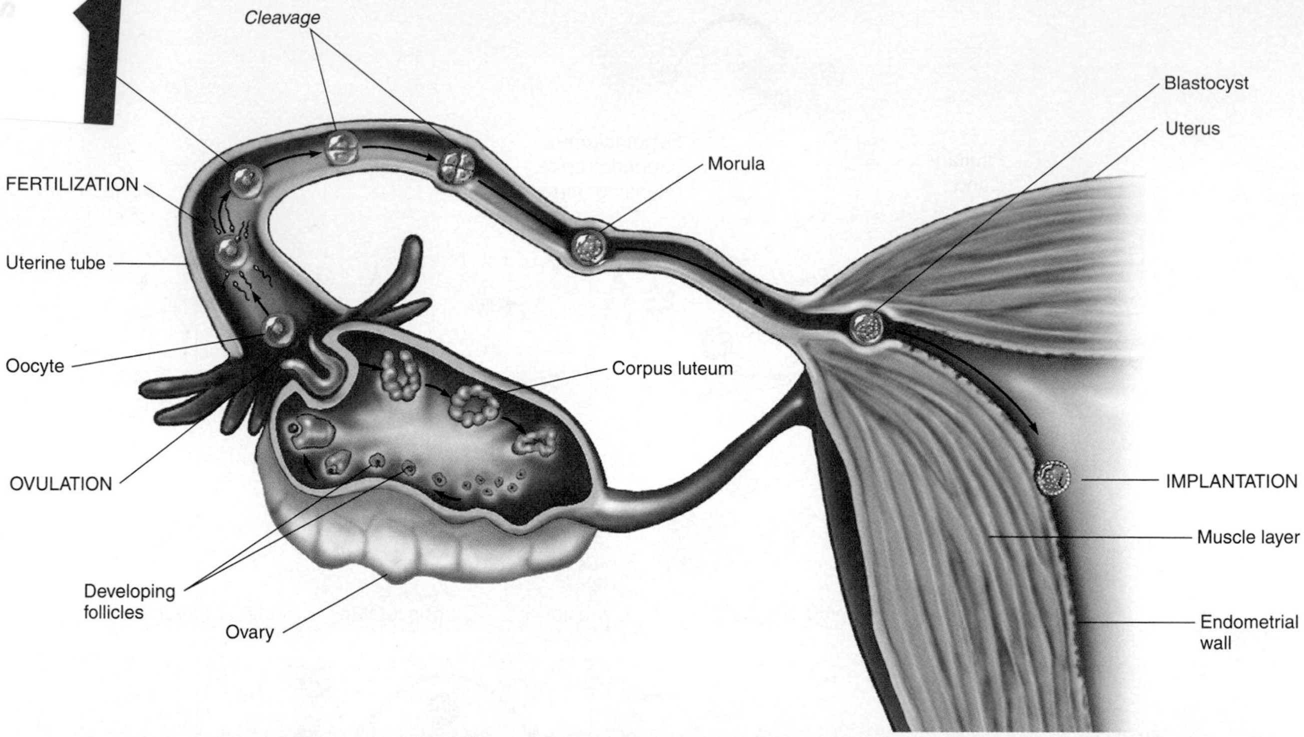

Figure 8-10

Fertilization and implantation of the embryo.

The **menstrual cycle** is a series of monthly changes that begin at puberty and continue through the reproductive years (Figure 8-10). The average age of onset is approximately 13 years of age. Hypothalamus maturation and subsequent hormone increases trigger the menstrual cycle. Initiation of this cycle is marked by the onset of **menstruation** (shedding of the endometrium). The menstrual cycle is usually a 28-day cycle that consists of three phases—the menstrual, proliferative (estrogen dominated), and secretory (progestrogen dominated) phases. At the end of the secretory phase, the uterus is ready to receive and nourish a zygote. If fertilization does not occur, estrogen and progesterone levels increase while FSH and LH levels decrease. Lower FSH and LH levels cause the corpus luteum to atrophy, reducing estrogen and progesterone production. The uterine lining thickens and sloughs off, signaling menstruation. Menstruation expels the unfertilized ovum and maintains a healthy uterine lining that is prepared for fertilization. If fertilization and pregnancy occur, the endometrium thickens and vascularization develops. After implantation of the zygote (5–6 days after fertilization), the placenta

secretes human chorionic gonadotropin to stimulate the corpus luteum to continue estrogen and progesterone production. The continued estrogen and progesterone production will suppress FSH and LH production, preventing further ovulation and menstruation. Human chorionic gonadotropin secretion continues until the placenta fully develops and begins making its own estrogen and progesterone, usually by the end of the first trimester.

The menstrual cycle repeats throughout the reproductive years until estrogen levels begin to decline with age. As the estrogen levels decline, ovulation and menstruation become less frequent and more erratic. This change in the menstrual cycle usually begins between 45 and 55 years of age. **Menopause** refers to the complete cessation of the menstrual cycle. In addition to changes in the menstrual cycle, the declining estrogen levels can cause the following manifestations:

■ Atrophy of the breasts and internal reproductive organs

■ Decreased vaginal secretion (which can make sexual intercourse painful)

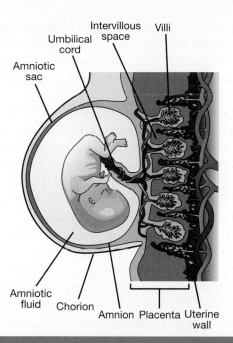

Figure 8-11

The developing placenta and embryo.

- Behavioral changes (e.g., irritability and depression)
- Headaches
- Insomnia
- Hot flashes
- Night sweats
- Decreased bone density

These manifestations can vary in severity, but in most cases, they are mild and improve with time. Hormone replacement therapy can decrease severity of the symptoms, but careful consideration should be given prior to initiating therapy because of the increased risk of breast cancer, thrombus (blood clot), and stroke.

Vagina

The vagina is a hollow, tunnel-like structure that extends from the cervix to the external genitalia. The vagina is located between the bladder and the rectum. The vagina is a muscular canal that is usually 2 to 4 inches in length, and it has the ability to expand in width (like during parturition). The vagina serves as a passageway for sperm to travel to the fallopian tubes, discharging menstrual fluid, and birthing the fetus. The sperm enters the vagina through the insertion of the penis during sexual intercourse. Ejaculation propels the semen into the canal where the sperm begin their journey to the fallopian tubes. The Skene's gland in the mucosal lining of the vagina secretes a protective, lubricating fluid during sexual intercourse. Tactile stimulation of the vagina is generally thought to produce the female orgasm.

The vagina may contain a thin connective tissue that covers the external vaginal opening to some degree, called the hymen (**Figure 8-12**). All hymens have openings large enough to permit menstrual flow passage or tampon insertion, but the openings are generally too small to permit an erect penis to enter without tearing. Tearing of the hymen does not usually cause great discomfort, but it may cause a few drops of

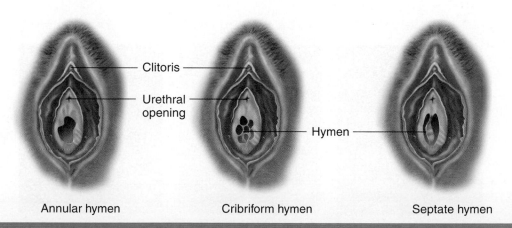

Annular hymen   Cribriform hymen   Septate hymen

Figure 8-12

The various types of hymens.

blood to be noticed. In addition to sexual intercourse, physical activity can partially or completely tear the hymen; therefore, the absence or presence of the hymen is not a reliable indicator of virginity.

External Genitalia

The external female genitalia contain several structures that are collectively referred to as the vulva. These structures include the mons pubis, labia majora, labia minora, clitoris, and vestibule. The size, color, and shape of these structures, as well as hair distribution and skin texture, can vary significantly from person to person (**Figure 8-13**). The mons pubis is the pad of fat over the pubic bone (symphysis pubis) that becomes covered with hair after puberty. The labia majora are the two large, fatty skin folds that protect the perineum and aid in lubrication. The labia majora become prominent and darkened after puberty. The labia minora are two small, firm skin folds just inside the labia majora. The labia minora have a rich blood and nerve supply. The two labia minor connect at their upper portion to form the clitoris. The clitoris is very sensitive to stimulation and becomes filled with blood during sexual arousal. The clitoris contains two corpora cavernosa, similar to the penis. The Bartholin's glands lie just within the labia minor and provide lubrication during sexual intercourse. The vestibule refers to the area that contains the urethral and vaginal opening.

Mammary Glands

The mammary glands are located in the breast. Although both males and females have mammary glands, they are only functioning in females. The mammary glands are not a reproductive organ per se, but they can have a role in sexual arousal and provide nourishment to the newborn. Each breast contains 15 to 20 clusters of milk-secreting mammary glands that open into the nipple. The mammary glands do not make milk unless stimulated to do so. Prolactin, a hormone from the anterior pituitary gland, prompts milk production. During pregnancy, increased estrogen levels trigger prolactin secretion to mature the mammary glands and prepare them for milk production. After childbirth, prolactin initially decreases as the estrogen levels return to nonpregnancy levels, but the newborn's suckling then stimulates prolactin production. Each breast in both sexes contains a nipple surrounded by an areola (area of pigmentation). The areolar gland produces secretions that protect and lubricate the nipple and areola during breastfeeding.

Congenital Disorders

Abnormalities of the urinary and reproductive system are the most common congenital defects. Because of their close relationship with each other, often an abnormality in one system will lead to an abnormality in the other. Additionally, fetal development of both systems is intertwined. The reproductive system continues development until birth, but even though the system is formed at birth, it is incapable of reproduction until it matures during puberty. Numerous congenital disorders of the reproductive system are possible, most of which are structural problems. Some disorders cause mild symptoms (e.g., epispadias and hypospadias), and

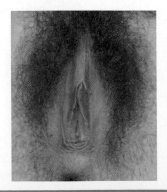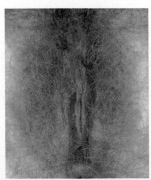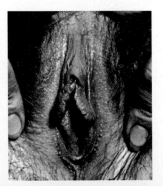

Figure 8-13

Variations of the female genitalia.

others may cause infertility and gender ambiguity (e.g., testicular or ovarian agenesis).

Epispadias

Epispadias refers to the urethral meatus occurring on the dorsal (upper) surface of the penis instead of the end (**Figure 8-14**). The urethral opening may extend the entire length of the penis. According to the National Institutes of Health (NIH) (2007), epispadias is rare (1 in 117,000 newborn boys) and usually develops during the first month of gestation. This malformation can also affect females (1 in 484,000 newborn girls), often placing the meatus in the clitoris. Epispadias is more likely to cause urination problems in men and sexual dissatisfaction in women. Men with epispadias are not necessarily infertile, but they may have trouble propelling the semen adequately during ejaculation. In both male and females, the individual is at risk for urinary

tract infections. Urinary defects, such as exstrophy of the bladder (part or all of the bladder is present outside the body), often occur with this type of congenital condition. Diagnosis of epispadias is typically made through a physical examination. Surgical procedures using the foreskin can repair the defect, but urinary incontinence postoperation is common. Multiple procedures may be required to achieve the desired cosmetic outcome, urine flow control, and sexual function.

Hypospadias

Hypospadias refers to the urethral meatus being on the ventral (under) surface of the penis instead of the end (**Figure 8-15**). According to the NIH (2008), hypospadias is a commonly occurring congenital defect (4 out of 1,000 newborn boys). Like with epispadias, hypospadias can vary in severity, and the opening can extend the length of the penis. Males with this condition may

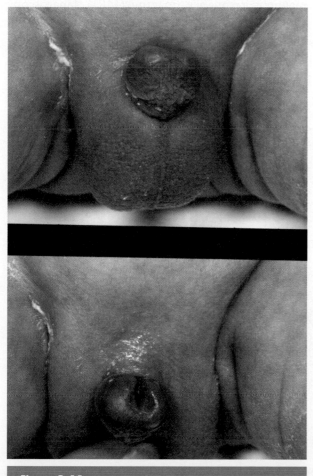

Figure 8-14

Epispadias.

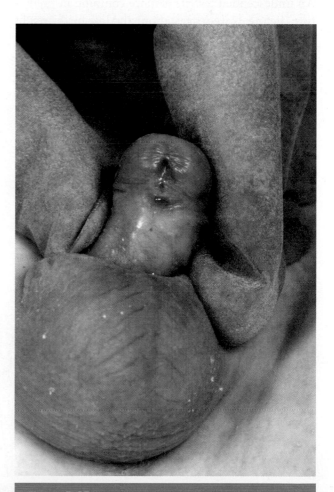

Figure 8-15

Hypospadias.

also have a downward curvature of the penis, called chordee, that becomes apparent with an erection. Hypospadias does not usually affect females, but it can be the cause of gender ambiguity. This ambiguity may lead to inappropriate surgical gender assignment. Genetic studies prior to any gender assignment procedures can minimize this risk. Diagnosis of hypospadias is made through a physical examination. Surgical repair (often in stages) can improve the penis's appearance as well as urinary and sexual function.

Cryptorchidism

Cryptorchidism is a congenital condition in which one or both testes do not descend from the abdomen to the scrotum prior to birth (**Figure 8-16**). Usually the undescended testes remain along the path of descent but can deviate from that path (ectopic testes). About 2–5% of full-term males are born with one or two undescended testicles. Rarely, both testes are undescended. An undescended testicle is more common in premature (before 37 weeks gestation) and low-birth-weight infants. Other risk factors for developing cryptorchidism include:

- Family history of cryptorchidism or other problems of genital development

- Fetal conditions that can restrict growth (e.g., Down syndrome and abdominal wall defects)

- Maternal alcohol use during pregnancy

- Maternal cigarette smoking or secondhand smoke exposure during pregnancy

- Maternal diabetes (type 1 diabetes, type 2 diabetes, or gestational diabetes)

- Parental exposure to some pesticides

Occasionally, a testicle that descended normally by birth may disappear later in childhood, often due to muscular reflexes that develop in puberty. A retractile testicle moves back and forth between the scrotum and the lower abdomen. In this case, the testicle is easily returned to the scrotum through gentle manipulation. An ascending testicle, or acquired undescended testicle, refers to a testicle that has returned to the lower abdomen and cannot easily be guided back into the scrotum.

Diagnostic procedures for cryptorchidism include a history, physical examination, self-testicular examinations (condition places individual at risk for testicular cancer later in life), abdominal ultrasound, magnetic resonance imaging (MRI), laparoscopy (visualization using a small camera through a small abdominal incision), and open abdominal exploratory surgery. Additionally, hormone levels and genetic studies can distinguish potential causes and complications. In most cases, the testes descend by 9 months of age without treatment. Treatment should be considered if both testes are not descended by 1 year of age to prevent permanent damage to the testicles. Testes that do not

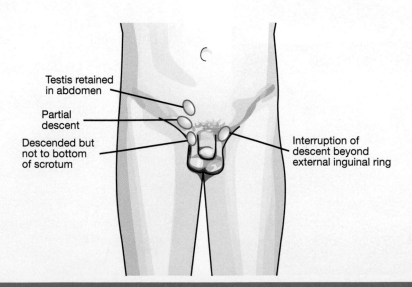

Testis retained in abdomen

Partial descent

Descended but not to bottom of scrotum

Interruption of descent beyond external inguinal ring

Figure 8-16

Potential sites for cryptorchidism.

naturally descend into the scrotum before birth are considered abnormal, and the individual is at increased risk for cancer and infertility even with repair. Treatment strategies include:

- Manual manipulation
- Surgical repair (either laparoscopic or open)
- Orchiectomy (testicle removal)
- Testicle implants
- Hormone replacement (specifically testosterone)

Infertility Issues

Infertility describes a biological inability to contribute to reproduction. The ability to conceive and support a fetus requires functioning male and female reproductive systems. Male problems that can lead to infertility include decreased sperm or sperm abnormalities, hormone deviations, and physical impediments. Female problems include ovulation dysfunction, hormone deviations, physical obstructions (usually in the fallopian tubes), and severe reproductive tract infections. If a couple has been unsuccessful in conceiving after 1 year of actively trying, they should consult a fertility expert.

Erectile Dysfunction

Erectile dysfunction (ED), or impotence, refers to the inability to attain or maintain a penile erection sufficient to complete sexual intercourse. Although ED can occur at any age, this problem is most common in older men. ED can be transient or permanent, depending on the etiology. An erection results from psychologic, neurologic, and vascular processes. ED can result from dysfunctions in any of these areas. Psychologic causes include the following:

- Anxiety
- Depression
- Guilt
- Stress
- Feelings of inadequacy
- Relationship issues

Physiologic causes include the following:

- Circulatory impairment (e.g., arteriosclerosis)
- Diabetes mellitus
- Multiple sclerosis

- Prostate disease (e.g., benign prostatic hypertrophy or prostate cancer)
- Hypertension
- Neurologic dysfunction (e.g., spinal cord injury, Parkinson's disease, or cerebral trauma)
- Certain medications (e.g., antihypertensive agents and antipsychotic agents)
- Low testosterone levels
- Alcohol and tobacco use
- Liver cirrhosis

Diagnostic procedures for ED consist of a history, physical examination, penile ultrasound, dynamic infusion cavernosometry and cavernosography (X-ray of the penis after injecting contrast dye into penile blood vessels), nocturnal tumescence test (tests for nocturnal erections), and specific tests for chronic diseases. A variety of treatment options are available, some of which are costly and are not covered by most insurance plans. In cases with a physiologic origin, identifying and resolving the cause is the priority. Treatment strategies include:

- Psychologic counseling
- Testosterone replacement
- Phosphodiesterase inhibitors (e.g., sildenafil [Viagra], tadalafil [Cialis], and vardenafil [Levitra])
- Other medications (e.g., adrenergic antagonists)
- Herbal remedies (e.g., ginkgo, ginseng, saw palmetto)
- Prostaglandin E injections directly into the corpus cavernosum
- Penis pumps (or vacuum devices)
- Surgical penile implants
- Vascular surgery

Disorders of the Testes and Scrotum

Disorders of the testes and scrotum are usually structural, and some can cause infertility (e.g., cryptorchidism). These disorders can be acquired or congenital, and most can be resolved with minimal residual effects.

Phimosis

Phimosis occurs when the foreskin cannot be retracted from the glans penis. Not being able to retract the foreskin is common during the first 3 years of age, but the foreskin should become retractable as the child grows. Poor hygiene, infections, and inflammation can cause phimosis. Phimosis can lead to urinary obstruction and pain. Paraphimosis refers to a condition in which the foreskin is retracted and cannot be returned over the glans penis. In paraphimosis, the penis becomes constricted and the glans becomes edematous. If paraphimosis is not resolved, the lack of blood flow can lead to gangrene, making it a medical emergency. Treatment strategies for both conditions include circumcision, topical steroid cream, and foreskin stretching.

Priapism

Priapism is a prolonged, painful erection. The unwanted, unrelenting erection is not a result of sexual stimulation. Priapism usually results from too much blood shunting within the corpus cavernosum (referred to as nonischemic or high-flow priaprism) or blood trapping in the penis (referred to as ischemic or low flow priaprism). Priapism is most common in boys between 5 and 10 years of ages and in men 20 to 50 years of ages. Priapism occurs with blood, circulatory, or nervous dysfunctions. These causes include:

- Sickle cell anemia
- Leukemia
- Trauma
- Tumors
- Diabetes mellitus
- Spinal cord injuries
- Neurologic diseases (e.g., multiple sclerosis and stroke)
- Medications (e.g., phosphodiesterase inhibitors, anticoagulants, and antianxiety agents)
- Alcohol and illicit drugs (e.g., cocaine, ecstasy, and marijuana)
- Poisonous venom (e.g., from a scorpion and black widow)

Diagnostic procedures can identify the type of priapism and include a history, physical examination, abdominal and penile ultrasound, penile arterial blood gases (ABGs), complete blood count (CBC), toxicology tests, and computerized tomography (CT). An erection lasting more than 4 hours is considered a urological emergency, warranting immediate medical attention. Without medical attention, priapism can lead to ischemia, necrosis, ED, and infertility. Treatment focuses on managing the underlying cause and varies depend-ing on the type of priapism. Strategies for ischemic (low-flow) priapism include the following:

- Needle aspiration of blood
- Injection of medications directly into the penis (e.g., alpha-adrenergic sympathomimetic agents)
- Surgical placement of a shunt

Strategies for nonischemic (high-flow) priapism include the following:

- Cold application
- Lower abdominal pressure
- Surgical repair of trauma

Additional interventions regardless of type include the following:

- Analgesics
- Sedation
- Hydration
- Urinary catheterization

Hydrocele

A hydrocele refers to fluid accumulation between the layers of the tunica vaginalis (membrane covering the testes) or along the spermatic cord (**Figure 8-17**). This

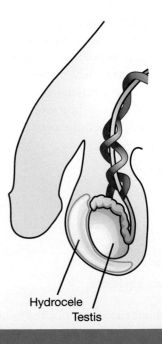

Hydrocele
Testis

Figure 8-17

Hydrocele.

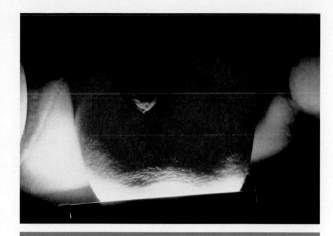

Figure 8-18

Transillumination of hydrocele.

acquire a hydrocele because of inflammation, infection, trauma, and tumors.

Hydrocele is usually painless, but the scrotum feels heavy. The swelling generally worsens over the course of the day. This scrotum enlargement can be differentiated from other testicular disorders (e.g., testicular cancer) through transillumination (transmission of light through tissue). Hydroceles will transilluminate the light, and a solid tumor will not (**Figure 8-18**).

Diagnostic procedures for hydrocele consist of a history, physical examination (including transillumination), and ultrasound. In most cases, the hydrocele resolves without any action other than treating the underlying cause. Strategies to encourage reabsorption of the fluid include scrotal elevation (on a rolled towel), sitz baths (warm water treatments for perineum), and heat/cold application. Large amounts of fluid can compromise testicular blood flow, requiring aspiration or surgical removal (hydrocelectomy) of the fluid.

Spermatocele

A spermatocele is a sperm-containing cyst that develops between the testis and the epididymis (**Figure 8-19**). Usually the cyst is painless and small, but the cyst can

condition can affect one or both testes. Hydrocele can occur as a congenital defect, affecting approximately 10% of newborn males. Congenital hydrocele usually disappears without treatment by 1 year of age. An inguinal hernia, a condition in which a section of intestines passes through the abdominal wall, commonly occurs in infants with hydrocele. Adult men can

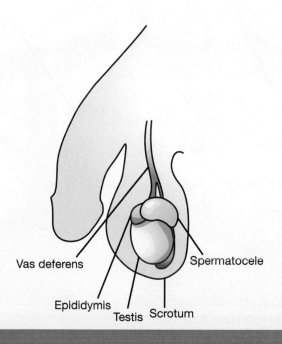

Vas deferens

Spermatocele

Epididymis

Testis   Scrotum

Figure 8-19

Spermatocele.

grow quite large, increasing discomfort. Additionally, the cyst is moveable and may transilluminate. The exact cause of this common condition is unknown, but it is thought to be caused by a blockage of the duct system, infection, inflammation, or trauma. Diagnostic procedures are similar to those of hydrocele. The cyst usually does not cause problems but may require surgical removal (spermatocelectomy) if the cyst is large.

Varicocele

A varicocele is a dilated vein in the spermatic cord (**Figure 8-20**). Much like varicose veins in the leg (see Chapter 4), this condition results from valve issues that allow blood to pool in the veins. These valve issues can be caused by congenital defects (e.g., incompetent or absent valves) or obstructions (e.g., tumors and thrombi). For unknown reasons, varicoceles are more frequent in infertile men (about 40% greater risk). Additionally, varicoceles are the most common cause for low sperm counts and decreased sperm quality because of testicular ischemia. The varicocele may be mild and asymptomatic, while extensive varicoceles can be tender and painful. The dilated veins give the scrotum a "bag of worms" feeling upon palpation, and the blood pooling may give a sense of heaviness in the scrotum. Diagnostic procedures for varicoceles are similar to hydrocele. Treatment is often unnecessary unless the varicocele causes discomfort. Treatment strategies include surgical repair (open or laparoscopic), embolectomy, and sclerotherapy (injection of an irritant into the vein that causes the vessel to harden and fade).

Testicular Torsion

Testicular torsion refers to an abnormal rotation of the testes on the spermatic cord (**Figure 8-21**). Sudden scrotal edema and pain develop as the twisting compresses the blood vessels, leading to ischemia and necrosis. Immediate treatment is required to restore blood flow and minimize testicular damage. Testicular torsion is most common during puberty and is frequently caused by trauma. Testicular torsion can occur spontaneously, especially in persons whose testicles are not secured in the scrotum due to congenital differences. Diagnostic procedures include a history, physical examination, and scrotal ultrasound. Surgery will be required to treat testicular torsion. Manual manipulation may be

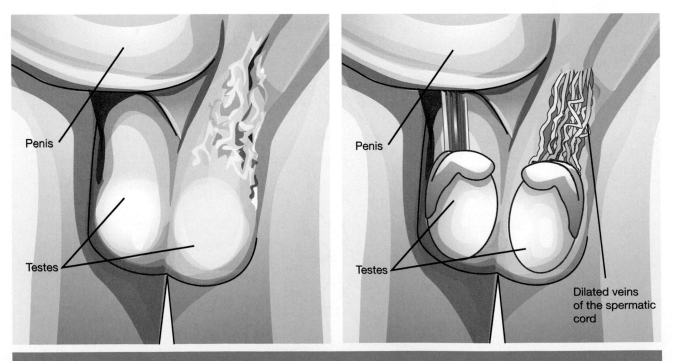

Penis

Testes

Penis

Testes

Dilated veins of the spermatic cord

Figure 8-20

Varicocele.

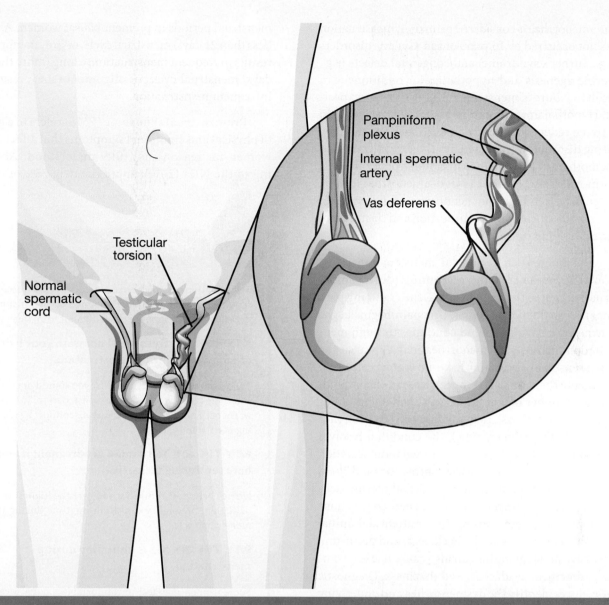

Testicular torsion

Normal spermatic cord

Pampiniform plexus

Internal spermatic artery

Vas deferens

Figure 8-21

Testicular torsion.

used to untwist the testes, but surgery will be required to secure the testicle and prevent reoccurrence.

Menstrual Disorders

The female menstrual cycle can vary from person to person. The duration and the amount of menstrual bleeding fluctuate to some degree, but a standard pattern can be expected. The usual duration of menstrua-

tion is 4–6 days, and the usual amount of bleeding for the entire menstruation is approximately 30 mL. Irregular or abnormal bleeding may be harmless, merely uncomfortable, or an indication of serious problems. These conditions may or may not require treatment.

Amenorrhea refers to the absence of menstruation. With this condition, menstruation may have never occurred (primary) or may have ceased (secondary).

The amenorrhea is considered primary if menstruation has not occurred by 16 years of age. Genetic disorders (e.g., Turner's syndrome) and congenital defects (e.g., uterine agenesis and hypothalamic conditions) can result in failure of menstruation starting when expected. Hypothalamic tumors, stress, sudden weight loss, extreme reduction in body fat (e.g., such as caused by eating disorders or incurred by athletes), anemia, and chemotherapy can halt menstruation from changes in hormone levels. Normal causes of amenorrhea include pregnancy, lactation, and menopause. Management of amenorrhea focuses on identification and treatment of the underlying cause.

Dysmenorrhea is painful menstruation. Most women experience some discomfort during menstruation, but with dysmenorrhea, the cramping pain impairs usual daily activities. The pain begins at the conclusion of ovulation and continues through menstruation. Primary dysmenorrhea may appear at the first menstrual cycle and have no known etiology. Dysmenorrhea may also appear later in life secondary to a number of conditions (e.g., endometriosis or reproductive cancers). In many cases of dysmenorrhea (especially the primary type), the condition resolves following childbirth. Excessive prostaglandin secretion produces strong uterine muscle contractions and blood vessel constriction, intensifying normal uterine ischemia associated with menstruation. These contractions and ischemia generate strong, intermittent abdominal pain that can radiate to the back, legs, and perineum. Excessive prostaglandins can also cause nausea, vomiting, diarrhea, headaches, and dizziness. Diagnostic procedures identify the dysmenorrhea and underlying cause. These procedures consist of a history, physical examination, pelvic ultrasound, laparoscopy, and hysterectomy. Treatment strategies focus on relieving the discomfort and resolving the underlying etiology. These strategies include analgesics (especially nonsteroidal anti-inflammatory drugs because they inhibit prostaglandin secretion), oral contraceptives (which prohibit ovulation), and heat application.

Several abnormal bleeding patterns are possible, and most usually result from a lack of ovulation. However, these conditions can be related to hormone imbalances and pathologic conditions (e.g., reproductive cancers). Any changes in menstrual bleeding pattern warrant investigation. Menorrhagia describes increased menstrual blood flow amount (approximately 80 mL per menstruation) and duration (usually 8–10 days). Metrorrhagia refers to vaginal bleeding between menstrual periods in premenopausal women. A short (less than 21 days) menstrual cycle, or polymenorrhea, results in frequent menstruation; a long (more than 42 days) menstrual cycle, or oligomenorrhea, results in infrequent menstruation.

Premenstrual syndrome (PMS) refers to a group of physical and emotional symptoms that affect many women for reasons not fully understood. According to the NIH (2010), approximately 75% of child-

MYTH BUSTERS

Menstruation has long been a source of myths, misconceptions, and old wives' tales. Because of their history, these misconceptions are often difficult to change.

MYTH 1: **You should not wash your hair or take a bath during menstruation.**

There is absolutely no reason why you should not wash your hair or take a bath during menstruation! In fact, a warm bath may actually decrease discomfort by relaxing uterine muscles.

MYTH 2: **You cannot get pregnant if you have sex during menstruation.**

Do not bet on it! While the odds are the highest near ovulation, pregnancy can occur anytime during the menstrual cycle.

MYTH 3: **Sex is unhealthy during menstruation.**

Some women may feel uncomfortable having sexual intercourse during menstruation, but there is no medical reason not to have sex during menstruation. In fact, sexual intercourse may relieve discomfort.

MYTH 4: **You should not get your feet wet during menstruation.**

There is no medical basis for this one either. This myth was made popular by some historical educational materials.

MYTH 5: **Women menstruating can catch cold easily and should avoid cold water or iced drinks.**

Being cold may make abdominal cramping worse, but there is no increased incidence of colds during menstruation.

There are numerous others. . . . These are just the more popular ones.

bearing women suffer from some degree of PMS. Clinical manifestations of PMS include irritability, depression, fatigue, headache, abdominal bloating, joint pain, breast tenderness, weight gain, and sleep disturbances that usually begin 5 to 11 days before menstruation. Premenstrual dysphoric syndrome (PMDD) is a severe form of PMS that is characterized by severe depression, tension, and irritability. Diagnostic procedures for PMS center on a thorough history (focusing on gynecological complaints) and physical examination. Treatment strategies are individualized and often include hormone therapy, diuretics, antidepressants (especially selective serotonin-reuptake inhibitors), analgesics, and comfort measures (e.g., heat application, warm baths, rest, and light exercise). Additionally, eliminating caffeine, soda, chocolate, fat, processed sugars, and alcohol may improve symptoms.

Disorders of Pelvic Support

Muscles, ligaments, and fascia normally support the bladder, uterus, and rectum in the female pelvis. These supportive structures weaken with age, excessive stretching (e.g., childbirth), and trauma. Decreasing hormone levels at the onset of menopause can further atrophy these structures. With weakened support, the organs can shift out of normal position, and frequently, more than one organ is affected.

Cystocele

A cystocele occurs when the bladder protrudes into the anterior wall of the vagina. For this reason, cystocele may be identified as a prolapsed bladder. The weakened pelvic support that results in a cystocele often results from excessive straining (e.g., childbirth, chronic constipation, heavy lifting). The abnormal positioning prevents the bladder from completely emptying; therefore, recurrent cystitis (bladder infection) is common. Cystoceles vary in severity, and mild cases can be asymptomatic. Clinical manifestations of a cystocele include:

- Visualization of the bladder from the vaginal opening (**Figure 8-22**)
- Feeling of fullness in the pelvis or vagina
- Stress incontinence
- Urinary retention, frequency, and urgency
- Pain or urine leakage during sexual intercourse

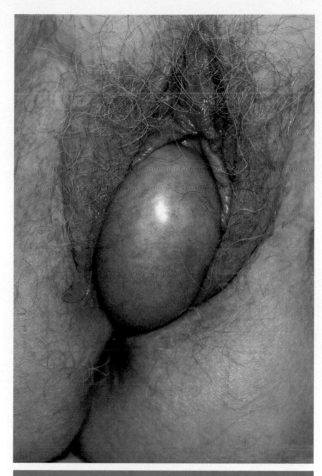

Figure 8-22

Cystocele.

Diagnostic procedures for cystocele consist of a history, physical examination, and voiding cystourethrogram (X-ray of the bladder during urination). Treatment strategies include pessary devices (vaginally inserted rings that support the bladder), surgical repair, estrogen therapy (if postmenopausal), incontinence interventions (e.g., bladder training and protective garments), Kegel exercises (isometric exercises to strengthen the pelvic muscles), and avoidance of straining.

Rectocele

A rectocele occurs when the rectum protrudes through the posterior wall of the vagina. The rectocele may be large enough to bulge through the vaginal opening. Although any condition that strains the fascia can contribute to rectoceles, most occur after menopause because of decreasing estrogen. Rectoceles may be uncomfortable, but they are rarely painful. Mild cases are usually asymptomatic, but when present, clinical manifestations include:

- Visualization of the rectum from the vaginal opening
- Feelings of fullness in the pelvis or vagina
- Difficulty defecating
- Rectal pressure
- Bowel incontinence

Diagnostic procedures for rectoceles are similar to those used for cystoceles. Treatment strategies include surgical repair, estrogen therapy (if postmenopausal), bowel training, and avoidance of straining.

Uterine Prolapse

Uterine prolapse refers to the descent of the uterus or cervix into the vagina. Uterine prolapse results from conditions that stretch or weaken the pelvic support (e.g., childbirth, aging, obesity, chronic cough, and chronic constipation). Uterine prolapse varies in severity and is classified using the following system:

- First degree—the cervix has dropped into the vagina
- Second degree—the cervix is apparent at the vaginal opening
- Third degree—the cervix and uterus bulge through the vaginal opening

Uterine prolapse is usually asymptomatic early, but as the uterus descends, clinical manifestations appear. Those manifestations include:

- Visualization of the cervix or uterus from the vaginal opening
- Feeling of fullness in the pelvis or vagina
- Difficult or painful sexual intercourse
- Vaginal bleeding
- Difficulty with urination and defecation

Diagnostic and treatment strategies for uterine prolapse are similar to those used for cystoceles and rectoceles.

Disorders of the Uterus

The uterus is a crucial organ for reproduction in females. Conditions that affect the uterus include benign or malignant tumors (e.g., leimyomas and cervical can-

cer), congenital disorders (e.g., abnormal uterine positioning), infection (e.g., pelvic inflammatory disease), and hormonal imbalances that may affect menstruation and fertility.

Endometriosis

With endometriosis, the endometrium begins growing in areas outside the uterus. The ectopic endometrial tissue most commonly grows in the fallopian tubes, ovaries, and peritoneum, but the tissue can grow anywhere in the body. The abnormal endometrial tissue continues to act as it normally would during menstruation (e.g., thickening, breaking down, and bleeding) even though it is outside the uterus. Without an outlet, the blood becomes trapped and irritates the surrounding tissue. Pain, cysts, scarring, and adhesions (fibrotic tissue that bind organs together) develop because of the inflammation. The scarring and adhesions often result in infertility.

The exact cause of endometriosis is unclear, but numerous theories exist. One theory holds that menstrual blood containing endometrial cells flows back through the fallopian tubes (retrograde menstruation), takes root, and grows. Another theory proposes that the bloodstream carries endometrial cells to other sites in the body. Other theories speculate that a predisposition toward endometriosis may be carried in the genes of certain families, or an inappropriate immune response may contribute to endometriosis development. Other theories suggest that certain cells (responsible for embryonic reproductive development) present within the abdomen of some women and retain their ability to become endometrial cells with genetic or environmental influences later in life.

Clinical manifestations depend on the severity of the endometriosis and often worsen as the endometriosis progresses (**Figure 8-23**). Endometriosis begins developing at the onset of menstruation and advances over time. Most cases are diagnosed between 25 and 35 years of age. Clinical manifestations of endometriosis include:

- Dysmenorrhea
- Menorrhagia
- Pelvic pain
- Infertility

Diagnostic procedures for endometriosis consist of a history, physical examination, laparoscopy, and pelvic ultrasound. Treatment strategies focus on minimiz-

MILD

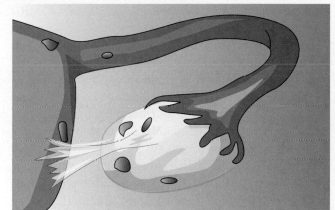

MODERATE

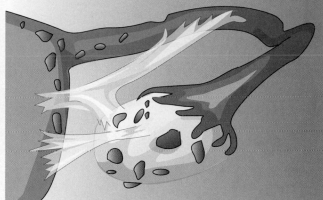

SEVERE

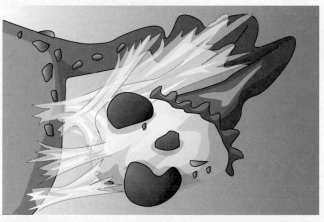

Figure 8-23

Stages of endometriosis.

ing discomfort and maximize childbearing potential (if desired). These strategies include:

- Analgesics
- Hormone therapy (e.g., contraceptive agents, gonadotropin-releasing hormone agonists and antagonists, and androgens)
- Surgical repair (laparoscopy, hysterectomy)

Leiomyomas

A leiomyoma, or uterine fibroid, is a firm, rubbery growth of the myometrium (**Figure 8-24**). Leiomyomas are the most common benign tumors in women, and they are classified according to their location (**Figure 8-25**). According to the NIH (2006), at least 25% of women have symptomatic leiomyomas, but as many

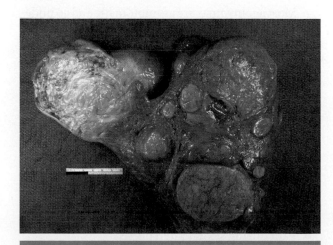

Figure 8-24

Leiomyomas.

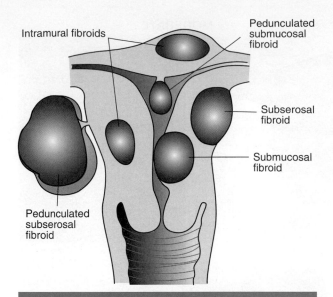

Intramural fibroids

Pedunculated submucosal fibroid

Subserosal fibroid

Submucosal fibroid

Pedunculated subserosal fibroid

Figure 8-25

Leiomyoma classification.

as 77% of women could be affected. Leiomyomas are more frequent in African Americans. The cause of leiomyomas is unknown, but most seem to grow during the menstruation years in the presence of estrogen and shrink after menopause. Tumor growth was thought to increase during pregnancy, but recent research suggests that growth actually levels off during pregnancy. Leiomyomas usually occur as multiple well-defined, unencapsulated masses. Leiomyomas do not usually interfere with fertility, but they do increase the risk of spontaneous abortion and preterm labor slightly. The risk for fertility and pregnancy problems increases as the tumor size increases.

Most leiomyomas are asymptomatic and go undetected. Clinical manifestations depend on the leiomyoma size, which can range from microscopic to weighing several pounds. When present, clinical manifestations include:

- Menorrhagia
- Pain in the pelvis, back, or legs
- Urinary frequency and retention
- Urinary tract infections
- Constipation
- Abdominal distension
- Pain during sexual intercourse
- Anemia

Diagnostic procedures for leiomyomas consist of a history, physical examination, abdominal and trans-

vaginal ultrasound, hysteroscopy (uterine endoscopy), biopsy (to rule out malignancy), laparoscopy, CT, MRI, and CBC. Generally, most leiomyomas are harmless and do not require treatment. Symptom severity and childbearing intentions should be considered when choosing treatment options. Treatment strategies include simple monitoring, hormone therapy (e.g., gonadotropin-releasing hormone agonists, progesterone, and androgen), analgesics (e.g., nonsteroidal anti-inflammatory drugs), surgery (e.g., myomectomy [removal of the fibroid], hysterectomy), myolysis (laparoscopic laser treatment), endometrial ablation (using heat to destroy the uterine lining), and uterine artery embolization (which obstructs uterine blood supply). Additionally, anemia treatment (e.g., iron supplements and blood transfusions) may be necessary.

Disorders of the Ovaries

A variety of benign and malignant conditions can affect the ovaries. Ovarian disorders can be congenital (e.g., hypogonadism, Turner's syndrome) or acquired (e.g., ovarian cancer), but many have a genetic basis. These disorders can affect the women's hormonal balance and fertility status.

Ovarian Cysts

Ovarian cysts are benign, fluid-filled sacs on the ovary. Often the cyst forms in the ovulation process. Instead of the follicle releasing the egg, the fluid stays in the follicle, creating a cyst. In most cases, these cysts are harmless and disappear without treatment. Occasionally, these cysts rupture, causing discomfort. This common condition most frequently occurs during childbearing years. Complications are rare, but ovarian cyst can lead to hemorrhaging, peritonitis, infertility, and amenorrhea.

When present, abdominal pain or discomfort is the most prevalent clinical manifestation. Pain occurs when the cyst bleeds, ruptures, twists, or pushes on nearby structures. Pain may also be associated with bowel movements and sexual intercourse. Other clinical manifestations include abnormal menstrual bleeding and abdominal distension.

Polycystic ovary syndrome is a condition in which the ovary enlarges and contains numerous cysts. The exact cause is unknown, but it has been linked to hormone (e.g., androgen, estrogen, LH increases, and FSH decreases) and endocrine (e.g., hypothalamus and pituitary) abnormalities. Clinical manifestations include infertility (anovulation), amenorrhea, hirsutism (abnormal facial and body hair), acne, and male-pattern baldness. Polycystic ovary syndrome increases the risk for developing obesity, diabetes mellitus, cardiovascular disease, and cancer (especially endometrial and breast cancers).

Diagnostic procedures for ovarian cysts consist of a history, physical examination, abdominal ultrasound, CT, MRI, laparoscopy, biopsy (to rule out ovarian cancer), and hormone levels. When warranted, treatment strategies include:

- Hormone therapy (e.g., oral contraceptives)
- Analgesics
- Management of metabolic (e.g., diabetes mellitus) and other disorders
- Surgery (e.g., laparoscopy)

Disorders of the Breasts

Breast disorders can be benign (e.g., fibrocystic breast disease) or malignant (e.g., breast cancer), but most are not life threatening; however, malignancies should be ruled out. These conditions can affect lactation, breastfeeding, and self-image.

Fibrocystic Breast Disease

Fibrocystic breast disease refers to the presence of numerous benign nodules in the breast. These firm, movable masses become more prominent and painful during menstruation because of hormone fluctuations. This change in breast tissue is so common (affecting over 60% of women) that many healthcare professionals consider it a normal variation. Fibrocystic breast disease is more frequent during childbearing years. Some contributing factors may be family history, high-fat diet, and excessive caffeine intake.

Clinical manifestations vary in severity and include:

- Dense, irregular and bumpy breast tissue (usually more noticeable in the outer upper part of the breast)
- Dull, heavy breast pain and tenderness (usually bilateral; may be constant or intermittent)
- Feeling of breast fullness
- Occasional nonbloody nipple discharge

Diagnostic procedures for fibrocystic breast disease consist of a history, physical examination, mammogram, breast ultrasound, and biopsy (to rule out

breast cancer). Usually no treatment is required. When necessary, treatment strategies are largely symptomatic and include needle aspiration of fluid, surgical removal of cysts, analgesics, a supportive bra, heat/cold application, limitation of dietary fat, and avoidance of caffeine (although research is inconclusive). Vitamin E, vitamin B_6, and evening primrose oil may improve symptoms, but their use is controversial. Additionally, oral contraceptives can minimize symptoms.

Mastitis

Mastitis refers to an inflammation of the breast tissue that can be associated with infection and lactation. Mastitis usually develops within 6 weeks of childbirth. In most cases, a staphylococcal or streptococcal bacterium is introduced to the nipple through the breast-feeding process, but mastitis can occur in the absence of lactation or breastfeeding. Impaired nipple or skin integrity increases the likelihood of mastitis developing. Despite popular belief to the contrary, breastfeeding can occur in the presence of mastitis, but it may be uncomfortable. Additionally, flow of milk may become blocked and abscesses can develop.

Clinical manifestations usually appear suddenly and include:

- Breast tenderness, swelling, redness, and warmth (**Figure 8-26**)
- Malaise
- Pain or a burning sensation continuously or while breastfeeding
- Fever

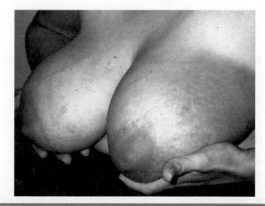

Figure 8-26

Mastitis.

Diagnostic procedures for mastitis include a history and physical examination. Treatment strategies consist of antibiotic therapy, adequate hydration, rest, analgesics, supportive bra, cold application, adequate milk expression, and needle aspiration.

Miscellaneous Infections

Infections can occur at any point along the reproductive tract. Many of these infections originate in the urinary tract. Additionally, reproductive tract infections can migrate to the urinary system. Many of these infections are easily resolved, but if untreated, some can have detrimental effects (e.g., infertility).

Prostatitis

Prostatitis refers to inflammation of the prostate that can be acute or chronic. Prostatitis is caused by conditions (e.g., bacteria, sperm, trauma, stress, and urinary catheter) that trigger the inflammatory process. The prostate has protective mechanisms to prevent ascending infection such as the flushing action of urination and ejaculation. Additionally, the prostate contains secretions that have an antimicrobial action (possibly from its zinc content). With its close proximity, the prostate is often invaded by a pathogen from the urinary system. Immune compromised states also increase the risk of prostatitis developing.

Prostatitis is classified into the following four categories:

1. Category 1: Acute bacterial prostatitis, which has the following characteristics:
   - Usually results from a urinary tract infection
   - Least common
   - Easiest to diagnose and treat
2. Category 2: Chronic bacterial prostatitis, which has the following characteristics:
   - Usually results from recurrent urinary tract infection
   - Relatively uncommon
3. Category 3: Chronic prostatitis/chronic pelvic pain, which has the following characteristics:
   - No clear etiology and may be noninflammatory
   - No bacteria are present, but immune cells can be found
   - Most common and least understood
   - Symptoms last longer than 3 months

4. Category 4: Asymptomatic inflammatory prostatitis, which has the following characteristics:
   - No clear etiology
   - No bacteria are present, but immune cells can be found

Clinical manifestations of prostatitis vary depending on the type. These manifestations include:

- Dysuria
- Difficulty urinating, such as dribbling or hesitancy
- Urinary frequency and urgency
- Nocturia
- Pain in the abdomen, groin, lower back, perineum, or genitals
- Painful ejaculations
- Indications of infection such as fever, chills, and myalgia (with acute bacterial prostatitis)
- Recurrent urinary tract infections (with chronic bacterial prostatitis)

Diagnostic procedures for prostatitis consist of a history, physical examination (including a digital rectal examination), urinalysis, sperm analysis, cultures, cystoscopy, and transrectal ultrasound. Treatment varies depending on the type. These strategies include long-term organism-specific antibiotic therapy, analgesics, antipyretics, adequate hydration, sitz bath, and prostatic massage.

Epididymitis

Epididymitis describes an inflammation of the epididymis, the duct connecting the testes to the vas deferens. Ascending bacterial infections or sexually transmitted infections usually initiate this inflammatory process. Bacteria, most commonly *Escherichia coli*, frequently spread to the epididymis from the urinary system. Gonorrhea and chlamydia are the typical sexually transmitted culprits. Urinary tract infections are the most frequent etiology in older men, and sexually transmitted infections are more frequent in younger men. Rare triggers for the inflammation include tuberculosis and the antidysrhythmic medication amiodarone (Cordarone). Risk factors for developing epididymitis include:

- Being uncircumcised
- Recent surgery or a history of structural problems in the urinary tract

- Urinary catheterization
- Sexual intercourse with more than one partner and not using condoms

The inflammatory and infectious process can lead to abscesses, fistulas (the cutaneous scrotal type), infertility, testicular necrosis, and chronic epididymitis. Clinical manifestations of epididymitis reflect the inflammatory and infectious process. These manifestations include:

- Indicators of infection (e.g., fever, chills, myalgia)
- Scrotal tenderness, erythema, and edema (which can become severe)
- Penile discharge
- Bloody semen
- Painful ejaculation
- Dysuria
- Groin pain

Diagnostic procedures for epididymitis focus on identifying the causative agent and consist of a history, physical examination, CBC, ultrasound, urinalysis, and cultures. Treatment strategies center on eliminating the infection and decreasing discomfort. These interventions include:

- Antibiotic therapy
- Analgesics (especially nonsteroidal anti-inflammatory drugs)
- Bed rest
- Scrotal support (wearing briefs instead of boxer underwear) and elevation (on a rolled towel)
- Cold application
- Screening and treating sexual partners

Candidiasis

Candidiasis is a yeast infection caused by the common fungus *Candida albicans*. The condition usually occurs as an opportunistic infection (see Chapter 2) that can arise anywhere in the body (especially the skin and the gastrointestinal tract), but the focus of this discussion will be the infection's effects on the reproductive system. In the reproductive system, candidiasis most frequently occurs in the vagina and is a common cause of vaginitis (inflammation of the vagina). *Candida* and many other microorganisms are part of the normal flora present in the vagina and usually balance each other. Imbalance often occurs in the presence of vaginal pH changes; normally, the vagina is slightly acidic. Antibiotic therapy can increase vaginal pH (making it more alkaline) leading to yeast overgrowth. Bubble baths and feminine products can also alter the delicate pH balance. Other contributing factors for the imbalance include decreased immune response (e.g., corticosteriod medications) and increased glucose in the vaginal secretions (e.g., pregnancy, oral contraceptives, diabetes mellitus, and obesity). Candidiasis is not sexually transmitted, but men may develop mild symptoms after having sexual intercourse with an infected partner. These symptoms in males will usually resolve without treatment.

Clinical manifestations of candidiasis include:

- A thick, white vaginal discharge that resembles cottage cheese
- Vulvular erythema and edema
- Vaginal and labial itching (can be intense) and burning
- White patches on the vaginal wall
- Dysuria
- Painful sexual intercourse

Candidiasis can mimic other vaginal infections; therefore, diagnostic procedures are used for differential diagnosis. Diagnostic procedures include a history, physical examination (including a pelvic examination), and discharge culture and analysis. Treatment focuses on reestablishing normal flora balance, minimizing tissue irritation, and increasing comfort. Most cases can be treated at home and without medical supervision. Self-management is not recommended in the following situations:

- Symptoms are moderate or severe
- Fever or pelvic pain is present
- Negative history for candidiasis
- Pregnancy
- The presence or possible presence of other vaginal infections

If self-management strategies are not successful, a healthcare provider should be consulted. Treatment strategies can also be used for prevention and include:

- Antifungal agents (available in oral, parenteral, and vaginal cream or suppository forms, some available without a prescription)

- Perineum care, including cleaning from front to back, keeping perineum area clean and dry, avoiding soap and rinsing with water only, and taking warm (not hot) baths

- Avoidance of douching

- Resisting the urge to scratch

- Eating yogurt with live cultures or taking *Lactobacillus acidophilus* tablets (these can also be taken with antibiotics to prevent candidiasis)

- Practicing safe sex (tissue irritation increases risk for contracting a sexually transmitted infection)

- Avoiding use of feminine hygiene sprays, fragrances, or powders in the genital area

- Avoiding wearing extremely tight-fitting clothing (which may cause irritation)

- Wearing cotton underwear or cotton-crotch panty hose and avoiding underwear made of silk or nylon (these materials are not very absorbent and restrict airflow, increasing sweating in the genital area and irritation)

- Using feminine pads instead of tampons during menstruation

- Controlling blood glucose (if diabetic)

Pelvic Inflammatory Disease

Pelvic inflammatory disease (PID) is a general term that refers to an infection of the female reproductive system. Bacteria usually ascend through the reproductive tract from the vagina. PID can be either acute or chronic, and most commonly results from a sexually transmitted infection (usually gonorrhea and chlamydia). According to the NIH (2009), 1 in 8 sexually active adolescent females will develop PID before 20 years of age. Bacteria may also breach the reproductive tract during childbirth, endometrial procedures (e.g., surgery or intrauterine implants), and abortions (spontaneous or induced). Acute bacterial invasions are more likely to occur immediately following menstruation, when the endometrium is more vulnerable. Less frequently, bacteria can invade from the circulatory system or surrounding structures. The infection triggers the inflammatory response resulting in mucosal irritation, edema, and purulent exudate. The edema and exudate can obstruct the reproductive structures, and the exudate can migrate to the peritoneal cavity, increasing the risk of peritonitis (see Chapter 9). Abscesses and septicemia (bacterial blood infection) can develop and become life threatening. Adhesions and strictures frequently result, leading to chronic pel-

vic pain, ectopic pregnancies, infertility, and problems with surrounding structures.

Clinical manifestations of PID vary slightly depending on whether the infection is acute or chronic. These manifestations include:

- Indications of infection such as fever, chills, myalgia, and leukocytosis (with acute forms)

- Pain or tenderness in the pelvis, lower abdomen, or lower back (sudden and severe with acute form)

- Abnormal vaginal and cervical discharge (usually purulent)

- Bleeding after sexual intercourse

- Painful sexual intercourse

- Urinary frequency

- Dysuria

- Dysmenorrhea

- Amenorrhea

- Metrorrhagia

- Anorexia

- Nausea and vomiting

Diagnostic procedures for PID consist of a history, physical examination, discharge culture, Papanicolaou (Pap) smear, CBC, pelvic ultrasound, CT, and laparoscopy. Treatment is aggressive to prevent complications. Treatment strategies include:

- Antibiotic therapy

- Screening and treating sexual partners (to prevent spreading and reinfection)

- Practicing safe sex (to prevent spreading and reinfection)

- Avoiding douching (which spreads infection to the upper reproductive tract)

- Treating abscesses (needle aspiration or surgical removal)

- Follow-up reexamination (to ensure that infection is completely resolved)

- Infertility evaluation

Sexually Transmitted Infections

Sexually transmitted infections (STIs), sometimes referred to as sexually transmitted diseases (STDs), encompass a broad range of infections that can be contracted through sexual contact (includes oral–genital contact, anal contact, and vaginal intercourse). More than 30 different sexually transmissible bacteria, viruses, and parasites have been identified; some of these pathogens can also be transmitted from mother to child during pregnancy and childbirth as well as through blood contact (e.g., human immunodeficiency virus [HIV] [see Chapter 2] and syphilis). Some of these are easily eradicated with appropriate treatment (e.g., chlamydia and gonorrhea) while others remain for a lifetime (e.g., genital herpes and condylomata acuminata). The Centers for Disease Control and Prevention (CDC) (2008) estimates approximately 19 million new STIs are diagnosed each year in the United States—almost half of them among people 15–24 years of age. Many STIs are required by law to be reported to the CDC (e.g., chlamydia, gonorrhea, and syphilis), but some are not required to be reported (e.g., genital herpes and condylomata acuminata); therefore, these numbers may be much higher. STI prevalence rates vary depending on geographical region within and outside the United States. With the exception of gonorrhea, STI rates have been increasing in the United States despite education efforts. Some of this increase may be attributed to changes in societal attitudes toward sex and pregnancy (e.g., less fear and media inundation) as well as changes in screening practices.

Bacterial STIs

Bacterial STIs are common but are usually treated with minimal residual effects. Screening generally focuses on identifying the causative organism through cultures of exudate, rapid assay tests, and fluorescent antibody tests. Treatment of bacterial STIs usually requires a simple course of antibiotics. If taken properly, the antibiotics will resolve the infection. Reinfection is common, but it can be minimized by refraining from sexual activity until bacteria are eradicated by practicing safe sex (e.g., using condoms), and by sexual partners receiving treatment.

Chlamydia

Chlamydia is caused by *Chlamydia trachomatis*, an intracellular parasite that requires a host cell to reproduce. Chlamydia is one of the most prevalent STIs; more than 1.2 million cases were reported to the CDC in 2008. Chlamydia prevalence rates have been on a steady incline in the United States for the past 20 years (**Figure 8-27**). According to the CDC (2008), chlamydia rates are high across all groups and regions in the United States, but the burden of chlamydia is the highest in women, African Americans, and those living in Mississippi.

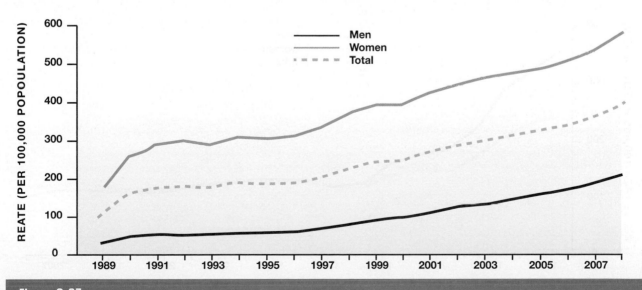

Figure 8-27

United States chlamydia prevalence rates.

Chlamydia can be transmitted through sexual contact and from mother to child during childbirth. Many times, chlamydia is transmitted to the child in the form of neonatal conjunctivitis (an eye infection that can lead to blindness) and pneumonia. Complications of chlamydia include PID, epididymitis, prostatitis, infertility, and ectopic pregnancy. Additionally, the bacterium invades the epithelial lining of the reproductive tract, causing inflammation that can increase the risk for contracting other STIs.

Often called the silent STI, chlamydia is usually asymptomatic in males and females. When present, clinical manifestations include:

- Dysuria
- Penile, vaginal, or rectal discharge (usually purulent)
- Testicular tenderness or pain
- Rectal pain
- Painful sexual intercourse

Because of its prevalence and potential neonatal complications, it is recommended that all pregnant women be screened and treated for chlamydia. Diagnostic procedures include a history, physical examination, and cultures. Treatment usually consists of antibiotics such as azithromycin (Zithromax), doxycycline, or erythromycin. Sexual partners should also

be screened and treated. Additionally, avoiding vaginal childbirth by electing to have a cesarean section delivery may decrease transmission rates.

Gonorrhea

Gonorrhea (referred to colloquially as the clap) is caused by *Neisseria gonorrhoeae*, an aerobic bacterium with many drug-resistant strains. Although rates have been declining for the past 20 years (**Figure 8-28**), those numbers have reached a plateau; gonorrhea remains the second most reported disease to the CDC (second only to chlamydia). According to the CDC (2008), gonorrhea rates are highest in men, African Americans, and those living in Mississippi. The bacterium attaches to the epithelial mucosa of the vagina, mouth, or anus, causing irritation and inflammation. Gonorrhea is transmissible through sexual contact and from mother to infant during childbirth. Mother-to-child transmission usually results in neonatal conjunctivitis. Outside the body, the bacterium dies within a few seconds.

Complications of gonorrhea include PID, epididymitis, prostatitis, infertility, and ectopic pregnancy. Additionally, gonorrhea can spread to other locations in the body. These complications entail arthritis (usually of the hands, wrists, ankles, knees, and elbows), dermatitis (usually of the hands and lower extremities), and endocarditis. Gonorrhea is often

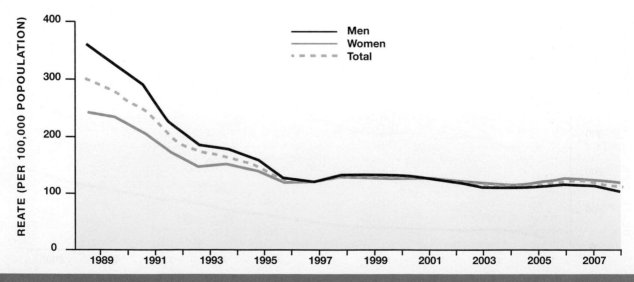

Figure 8-28

United States gonorrhea prevalence rates.

asymptomatic, and when present, clinical manifestations usually do not appear until 2–10 days after the infection. Men are more likely than women to experience symptoms. When present, clinical manifestations include:

- Dysuria

- Urinary frequency or urgency

- Penile, vaginal, or rectal discharge (white, yellow, or green) (colloquially referred to as the drip) (**Figure 8-29**)

- Redness or edema at urinary meatus (in men)

- Testicular tenderness or pain

- Rectal pain

- Painful sexual intercourse

- Sore throat

- White blisters that darken and disappear (Figure 8-29)

Diagnostic procedures include a history, physical examination, and cultures. Treatment usually consists of antibiotics such as azithromycin (Zithromax), doxycycline, or erythromycin.

Syphilis

Syphilis is an ulcerative infection caused by *Treponema pallidum*, a spiral-shaped (spirochete) bacterium that requires a warm, moist environment to survive (**Figure 8-30**). Syphilis is transmitted from skin or mucous membrane contact with infected, ulcerative lesions (chancres). Additionally, the bacterium can

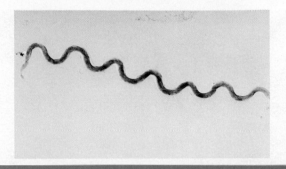

Figure 8-30

Treponema pallidum, the spirochete that causes syphilis.

cross from the mother through the placenta barrier to the fetus after the 4th month of gestation (congenital syphilis). These lesions also provide an opportunity for other STIs to invade.

Syphilis occurs in several stages, each with its own clinical manifestations. Those stages include:

- Primary syphilis is the first stage. Painless chancres (usually one) form at the site of infection about 2–3 weeks after initial infection (**Figure 8-31**). The chancres often go unnoticed and disappear about 4–6 weeks later, even without treatment. The bacteria become dormant, and no other symptoms are present. The individual may not test positive during this stage, so the test should be repeated at a later date. Even if tested negative, the infected individual is contagious during this stage.

- Secondary syphilis occurs about 2–8 weeks after the first chancres form. About 33% of those who do not receive treatment for primary syphilis will develop this second stage. A generalized, non-pruritic, brown-red rash characterizes this stage (**Figure 8-32**). Other symptoms include malaise, fever, and patchy hair loss. These symptoms will often go away without treatment, and again, the bacteria become dormant. The individual will test positive (if untreated) and is contagious during this stage, especially with direct contact with the rash.

- Latent or tertiary syphilis is the final stage of syphilis. The early latency stage begins when the secondary symptoms disappear and lasts 1–4 years. The late latency stage can last for years as the infection spreads to the brain, nervous system, heart, skin, and bones. The infection can cause blindness, paralysis, dementia, cardiovascular disease,

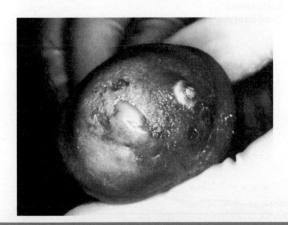

Figure 8-29

Characteristic lesions and discharge associated with gonorrhea.

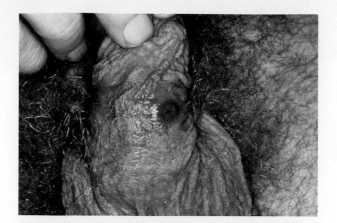

Figure 8-31

Chancre characteristic of primary syphilis.

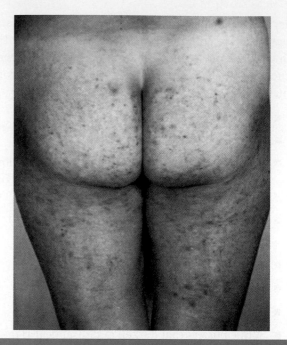

Figure 8-32

Skin rash characteristic of secondary syphilis.

pathological fractures, and death. The individual will test positive (if untreated) and is only contagious during the early part of this stage.

Syphilis prevalence rates in the United States have remained constant for the last 40 years for all three stages (**Figure 8-33**). According to the CDC (2008), syphilis rates are highest in men, African Americans, and those living in Louisiana.

Diagnostic procedures include a history, physical examination, and serum antibodies. In utero, the fetus is protected from syphilis by a membrane known as Langhans layer for the first 4 months of the pregnancy. Screening and treating the mother prior to the 4th month of gestation can significantly decrease the likeli-

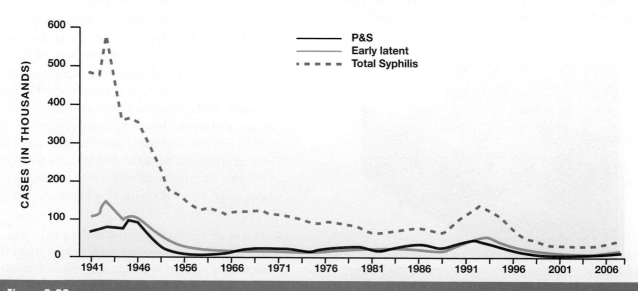

Figure 8-33

United States syphilis prevalence rates.

hood of the fetus contracting the infection. However, positive (if treated) and high-risk women should be retested in the last trimester of the pregnancy. Untreated early maternal syphilis infections can also lead to fetal demise in approximately 40% of cases. Congenital syphilis can lead to multiple defects affecting the bones, teeth, liver, lungs, and nervous system. For nonpregnant women and men, treatment should begin early at the first sign of a suspicious lesion. Treatment usually consists of antibiotics such as penicillin or a penicillin derivative. Antibiotics are useless in the latent phase.

Viral STIs

STIs caused by viruses are common. These infections can range from minor (e.g., condylomata acuminata) to life threatening (e.g., HIV). Viral STIs can also lead to several reproductive cancers (e.g., human papillomavirus). These viral infections are the most difficult STIs to treat because viruses are highly adaptive and elusive. Treatment options for these infections depend on the causative virus.

Genital Herpes

Genital herpes is an infection that causes blisters (vesicles) on the genitals and in the reproductive tract. Genital herpes is caused by the herpes simplex virus (HSV), which belongs to a family of more than 70 herpes viruses. Some more common viruses in this family

include the cytomegalovirus (which can cause mental retardation and fetal demise with maternal infections), varicella-zoster virus (causes chickenpox and shingles), and the Epstein-Barr virus (which can cause lymphoma). HSV occurs in two forms—HSV type 1 and HSV type 2. Generally, HSV type 1 occurs above the waist, and HSV type 2 occurs below the waist. HSV type 1 most frequently manifests as a cold sore (a small blister on the mouth or nose). Most cases of genital herpes are caused by HSV type 2 (70%). HSV type 2 can also spread above the waist, and HSV type 1 can spread below the waist through oral–genital sexual contact. HSV type 2 is also transmissible through direct skin-to-skin contact. Risk of transmission is the greatest when lesions are present, but HSV can be spread when lesions are not apparent. HSV type 2 is also transmissible from mother to child.

Contracting genital herpes during pregnancy creates the greatest risk to the fetus (e.g., spontaneous abortion). HSV can also be transmitted to the infant during childbirth if an active genital herpes infection is present at the time of delivery. Transmission during childbirth can result in encephalitis and brain damage. If lesions are present at the time of birth, a cesarean section should be preformed. Rarely, HSV can be transmitted to the fetus through the placenta, causing an infection prior to birth. Pregnant women should be monitored for genital herpes throughout their pregnancy.

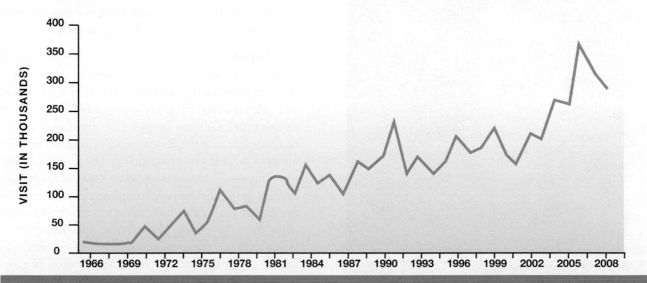

Figure 8-34

Genital herpes–related clinic visits in the United States.

Genital herpes is not a reportable disease to the CDC; however, healthcare clinic activities indicate that genital herpes has been rising for the last 40 years (**Figure 8-34**). According to the CDC (2008), genital herpes rates are highest in women and African Americans.

Both types of HSV are characterized by recurrent episodes of the lesions. Most people with HSV type 2 will experience reoccurrence of the lesions; however, recurrence is much less frequent with HSV type 1. Reoccurrence occurs by the virus causing an initial infection at the entry site, and then the virus travels along the dermatome to the nerve root where it remains protected and dormant until the next outbreak, which will occur at the same site. In either case, the lesions appear and progress similarly. These episodes begin with a tingling or burning sensation at the site just before the lesion appears (**prodrome**). The lesions first appear as a vesicle surrounded by erythema. These vesicles rupture, leaving a painful ulcerative lesion with watery exudate (**Figure 8-35**). Ultimately, a crust forms over the ulcer, and it heals spontaneously in 3–4 weeks. Because genital herpes creates a break in the first line of defense, the individual is at risk for contracting other STIs.

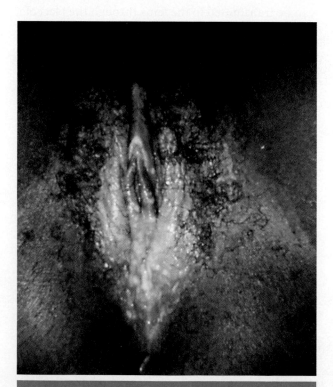

Figure 8-35

Genital herpes blisters on the external genitalia and inner thigh.

Genital herpes progresses through the following four stages:

1. **Primary herpes genitalis** is the first stage. This stage begins at the actual time of infection and antibody development. The time from exposure to this primary infection can range from 2–20 days. This first occurrence of the infection can be very painful or completely asymptomatic (75% of cases). When present, clinical manifestations associated with this stage include a painful lesion, malaise, low-grade fever, and groin lymph node enlargement.

2. **Latent herpes genitalis** begins once the antibodies are formed. Antibodies do not protect against reinfection, but they do tend to make the recurrent episodes less severe. During this phase, the virus travels up the nerve root and becomes dormant (**Figure 8-36**). The individual is asymptomatic while the virus is dormant.

3. **Shedding herpes genitalis** is the third stage. During this stage, the virus is reactivated but produces no symptoms. The virus is being excreted from the body and can be transmitted to another person through sexual contact. This stage occurs infrequently—in fewer than 1% of cases.

4. **Recurrent herpes genitalis** is characterized by the reactivation of the virus and clinical manifestations. During this stage, the virus travels back down the nerve root to the skin and causes a blister at the same site as with the first stage. The number of reoccurrences varies from none to many in a lifetime. Factors that can trigger a reoccurrence include stress, menstruation, and illness.

Diagnostic procedures for genital herpes include a history, physical examination, tissue and secretion cultures, Pap smears, and polymerase chain reaction test (which detects the presence of HSV and determines type). Genital herpes is a significant public concern because the lesions and symptoms are not always apparent, transmission can occur with or without symptoms, and no cure exists. Genital herpes can cause a great deal of psychological stress because of the fear of outbreaks and disclosing the information to partners. Treatment options (e.g., antiviral medications) that can suppress the number of outbreaks as well as minimize the severity and duration of reoccurrences are available. Avoiding reoccurrence triggers, especially stress, can also prevent outbreaks. Implementing stress reduction strategies (e.g., yoga, meditation, journaling, and distraction) is advised.

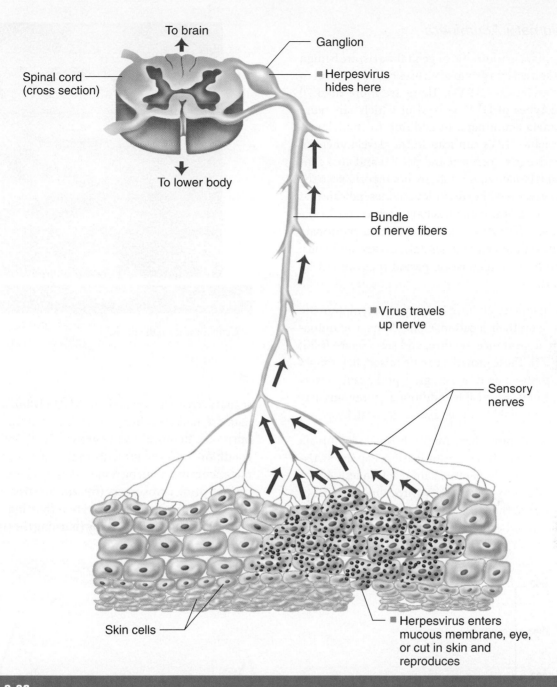

To brain

Spinal cord
(cross section)

Ganglion

■ Herpesvirus
hides here

To lower body

Bundle
of nerve fibers

■ Virus travels
up nerve

Sensory
nerves

Skin cells

■ Herpesvirus enters
mucous membrane, eye,
or cut in skin and
reproduces

Figure 8-36

Herpes simplex virus movement in the nervous system.

Secondary bacterial infections can develop from the lesions, so proper hygiene (e.g., washing the area with soap and water several times a day, keeping the area dry, and wearing loose-fitting clothing and cotton underwear) is advised during outbreaks. Additionally, genital herpes increases the risk for reproductive cancers (especially cervical), so Pap smears should be performed every 6–12 months. Since transmission is highest when lesions are present, sexual activity should be avoided during outbreaks. Due to the life-long implications of genital herpes, prevention is the best treatment strategy. Prevention strategies center on safe sex practices (e.g., using condoms, limiting sexual partners).

Condylomata Acuminata

Condylomata acuminata, or genital warts, are benign growths caused by a group of viruses called the **human papillomaviruses (HPVs)**. There are more than 70 different types of HPV, several of which can cause condylomata acuminata. In addition to condylomata acuminata, HPVs can lead to the development of reproductive (e.g., cervical and penile) and anal cancers. Condylomata acuminata are not reportable to the CDC; however, healthcare clinic activities indicate that condylomata acuminata rates have been rising for the last 40 years (**Figure 8-37**). Condylomata acuminata can occur on the external genitals, cervix, and anus. HPV can have an incubation period that can last up to 6 months.

Condylomata acuminata may be asymptomatic depending on their location. Condylomata acuminata vary in appearance, texture, and size (**Figure 8-38; Figure 8-39**). These growths can be raised, flat, rough, smooth, flesh-colored, white, grey, pink, cauliflower-like, large, or barely visible. Additional symptoms may include abnormal bleeding, discharge, or itching.

Diagnostic procedures for condylomata acuminata include a history, physical examination, Pap smear, tissue biopsy, and polymerase chain reaction test. A vaccine is available to prevent HPV infections. Because of the cancer risk, the HPV vaccine is recommended for all females (it is best if one receives the vaccine before

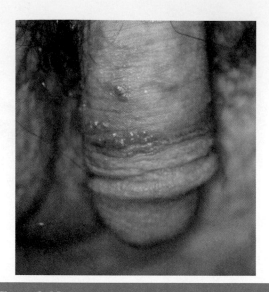

Figure 8-38

Genital warts on the penis.

sexual activity is initiated). Most condylomata acuminata are harmless but can be removed for aesthetic purposes. Removal of the growths will not cure the condition, and the growths may reappear. Condylomata acuminata can be removed using chemicals (e.g., podophyllin), cryosurgery (freezing the tissue with liquid nitrogen), electrocauterization (heating the tissue with electricity), laser therapy (burning the tissue with

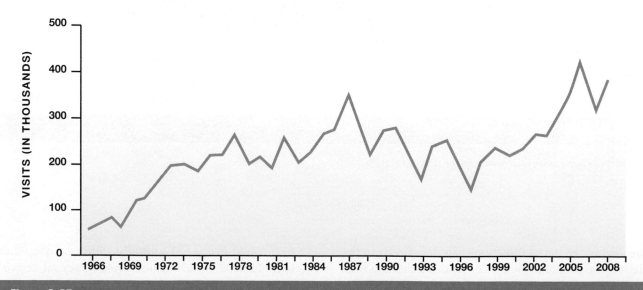

Figure 8-37

Genital warts–related clinic visits in the United States.

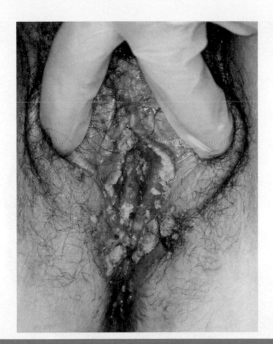

Figure 8-39

Genital warts on the vagina.

a light), or surgical excision. As with other STIs, sexual partners should also be screened and treated. Condylomata acuminata can be fatal if transmitted to infants at birth, so cesarean section deliveries are advised.

Protozoan STIs

Like candidiasis infections, protozoan infections often arise when the body's natural defenses are altered, but unlike candidiasis, some of these protozoa infections can be transmitted through sexual contact. These conditions are usually easily treated and resolve with minimal issues.

Trichomoniasis

Trichomoniasis (colloquially referred to as the trick) is caused by *Trichomonas vaginalis*, a one-celled anaerobic organism. This extracellular parasite can burrow under the mucosal lining. In men, the organism primarily resides in the urethra and causes no symptoms. In women, the organism resides in the vagina and becomes symptomatic when vaginal microbial imbalance occurs. The organism cannot survive in the mouth or the rectum. In addition to sexual contact, trichomoniasis can be contracted through prolonged moisture exposure (e.g., bathing suits and protective garments). Trichomoniasis is not reportable to the CDC, but healthcare clinic activities indicate that trichomoniasis rates in women have been controlled for the last 40 years (**Figure 8-40**). In men, trichomoniasis does not usually generate symptoms and resolves in a few weeks without treatment. In women, the primary clinical manifestation is copious amounts of odorous, frothy, white or yellow-green vaginal discharge. This

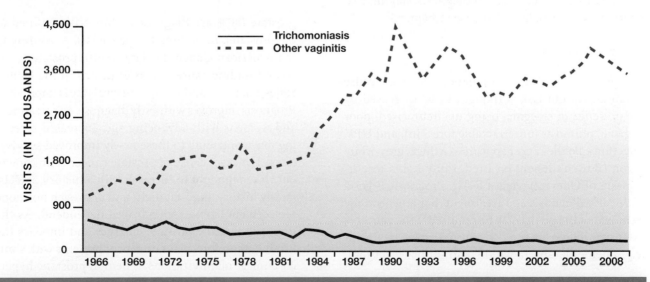

Figure 8-40

Trichomoniasis–related clinic visits in the United States.

MYTH BUSTERS

A common misconception is that condoms protect against all STIs. While condoms are highly effective against most STIs, some STIs have been known to spread despite condom use. STIs that can spread through skin-to-skin contact even with a condom in place include HPV, HSV, and syphilis. Additional strategies such as taking the HPV vaccine, receiving genital herpes suppression therapy, and treating syphilis early can decrease the likelihood of contracting and spreading these infections.

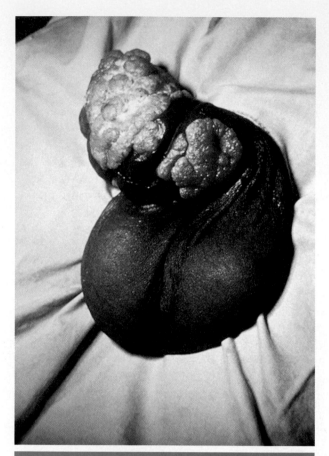

Figure 8-41

Penile cancer.

discharge can irritate the vagina and vulva. Additional symptoms may include itching, painful intercourse, and dysuria. Diagnostic procedures for trichomoniasis include a history, physical examination, and Pap smear. Trichomoniasis is easily treated with metronidazole (Flagyl), an antibiotic that treats bacteria and parasite infections. Sexual partners should also be treated to prevent reinfection. Untreated or prolonged infections can increase the risk of cervical cancer.

Cancers

Malignancies of the reproductive system originate in the reproductive tract or spread from other sites. Some of these cancers have high treatment rates (e.g., testicular cancer), while others have high mortality rates (e.g., ovarian cancer). Typical cancer diagnosis, staging, and treatments are usually utilized (see Chapter 1).

Penile Cancer

Penile cancer is a rare malignancy. The exact cause is unknown, but risk is thought to be increased by the presence of smegma, being uncircumcised, poor hygiene, phimosis (unretractable foreskin), and HPV infections. Penile cancer appears as a thick, grey-white lesion (Bowen's lesion) or a red, shiny lesion (erythroplasia of Queyrat) (**Figure 8-41**). Prognosis is good with early diagnosis and treatment, but a penectomy (removal of the penis) may be required if the cancer is extensive or does not respond to usual cancer treatment (e.g., chemotherapy, radiation, and surgical excision).

Prostate Cancer

Prostate cancer is the most common cancer among men, particularly African Americans (CDC, 2006). The slow-growing tumor is often confined to the prostate (80% are diagnosed while still confined to the prostate), improving the prognosis. According to the American Cancer Society (2010), prostate is the second leading cause of cancer deaths in the United States, but the 5- and 10-year survival rate is improving. Prognosis improves with early diagnosis and treatment and worsens with advancing age. Increased screening may contribute to these newly improved survival rates. The exact cause of prostate cancer is unknown, but risk is thought to increase with a history of STIs, family history, high-fat diets, and androgen hormone replacement (some are androgen dependent). As the tumor grows, the prostate enlarges and impedes the urethra; therefore, prostate cancer presents with similar clinical manifestations as benign prostatic hyperplasia (e.g., urinary difficulties and erectile dysfunctions) (see Chapter 7). Additional manifestations may include bloody semen and hematuria. In addition to the usual cancer diagnostic procedures (e.g., biopsy), the prostate-specific antigen (which is high in any prostate enlargement) test, free prostate-specific antigen test (which can differentiate between benign prostatic hypertrophy and prostate cancer), and the prostatic acid phosphatase (which is high in prostate cancer) test may be performed. Prostate cancer treatment follows the usual cancer treatments and can vary depending on the cancer stage. An aggressive management approach including a combination of a radical prostatectomy (complete prostate removal), radiation, and orchiectomy (removal of the testes) or antitestosterone drug therapy is often taken to improve patient outcomes. Urinary and erectile dysfunctions are possible complications of treatment.

Testicular Cancer

Testicular cancer is an uncommon cancer. Young (15–35 years old) and Caucasian men are at slightly higher risk than other groups. Testicular cancer can occur as a slow-growing (seminoma) or fast-growing (nonseminoma) tumor. Risk for developing testicular cancer is thought to be increased by family history, infection, trauma, and cryptorchidism. Testicular cancer usually affects one testicle, but can affect both. Metastasis usually occurs to the nearby lymph nodes, lungs, liver, bone, and brain. Testicular cancer is often asymptomatic. When present, clinical manifestations usually include a hard, painless, palpable mass that does not transilluminate; testicular discomfort or pain; enlargement of the testicle; and gynecomastia (female-like breast). Testicular cancer is highly curable even when metastasized to other sites. Early diagnosis and treatment enhance prognosis. Monthly self-testicular examinations are the cornerstone to early detection. Other diagnostic procedures include tumor markers such as alpha-fetoprotein, beta human chorionic gonadotropin, and lactate dehydrogenase. In most cases, an orchiectomy is advised, but chemotherapy and radiation may also be used. Testicular cancer can reoccur in the remaining testicle, so self-testicular examinations and follow-up are crucial.

Breast Cancer

Breast cancer is the most common malignancy in women and the second leading cause of cancer death in women (American Cancer Society, 2010). Breast cancer rates are highest in Caucasian women, but African American women are most likely to die from it. Breast cancer can occur in men, but it is rare. Other contributing factors include advancing age, early onset of menstruation, family history (although not always present), genetic predisposition (defects on the BRCA1 and BRCA2 genes), obesity, chest wall radiation, and excessive alcohol consumption (more than 1 to 2 drinks a day). Exogenous estrogen exposure (e.g., oral contraceptives, hormone replacement therapy) may increase risk, but current formulations have minimized this risk. Most breast cancers originate in the duct system, but it may arise in the lobules (structures that produce milk). The tumor can infiltrate the surrounding tissue and adhere to the skin, causing dimpling. Early, the tumor is freely moving, but the tumor becomes fixed as the cancer progresses. Most tumors are estrogen dependent, and metastasis usually occurs to nearby axillary lymph nodes. Metastasis can occur early, and in most cases, several nodes are affected at the time of diagnosis. Widespread metastasis quickly follows to the lungs, brain, bone, and liver.

In early stages, breast cancer is often asymptomatic. Symptoms arise as the tumor grows. In men, symptoms usually include a breast mass and breast tenderness or pain. Clinical manifestations of breast cancer in women include:

- Mass in the breast or axillary that is hard, has uneven edges, and is usually painless

- Change in the size, shape, or feel of the breast or nipple (e.g., redness, dimpling, or puckering that looks like the peel of an orange)

- Nipple drainage that may be bloody, clear to yellow, green, or purulent

Indications that the cancer has metastasized include bone pain, skin ulcers, edema in the arm next to the affected breast, and weight loss.

Early diagnosis and treatment are crucial to positive outcomes. Monthly self-breast examinations are the cornerstone to early detection. Women discover most tumors during this examination. Another diagnostic procedure specific to breast cancer is the mammogram. Currently, the American Cancer Society (2009) recommends annual mammograms for all women over 40 years of age; even though U.S. Preventive Services Task Force controversially stated that screening between ages 40 to 49 "may not be worthwhile" (http://pressroom.cancer.org/index.php?s=43&item=201, paragraph 2). Women in high-risk groups should start annual mammograms sooner. Recent advances in breast cancer treatments (especially in chemotherapies) have increased survival rates significantly. Treatment strategies vary depending on the stage, but usually breast cancer requires an aggressive, multimethod treatment (e.g., chemotherapy, radiation,

MYTH BUSTERS

There are several misconceptions around breast cancer that warrant discussion.

MYTH 1: Breast implants, using antiperspirant, and wearing underwire bras increase breast cancer risk.

There is *no* evidence that links these factors to breast cancer. Breast implants can make it more difficult to detect tumors with a self-breast examination depending on the surgical technique used to insert the implants. Placing the implants behind the muscle wall can improve the ability to detect any tumors. But breast implants, antiperspirant, and underwire bras do *not* increase breast cancer risk.

MYTH 2: Only older women need to worry about breast cancer.

Breast cancer risk does increase in age, but women of *all* ages can develop breast cancer.

MYTH 3: Breast cancer always runs in families.

Family history does increase the likelihood of developing breast cancer, but *most* women who develop breast cancer *do not* have a family history of breast cancer.

MYTH 4: There is no need to worry about breast cancer if no BRCA1 and BRCA2 mutation is present.

BRCA1 and BRCA2 mutations do increase breast cancer risk, but 90–95% of women who are diagnosed with breast cancer *do not* have either a family history or this genetic mutation.

Source: American Cancer Society, 2009.

surgery, and hormone therapy) to improve outcomes. The life-threatening nature of breast cancer, along with the changes in body image that result from treatment, can increase the need for coping and support interventions (e.g., support groups and counseling).

Cervical Cancer

Cervical cancer rates have been declining in recent years with advancements in screening. The Pap smear, the long-standing cervical screening method, can now detect precancerous changes (dysplasia). Procedures can be performed to remove these precancerous cells, limiting the likelihood of these changes progressing to permanent malignant changes (**Figure 8-42**).

The precancerous cells are 100% treatable; however, malignant changes can return if carcinogen exposure continues. Almost all cervical cancers are caused by HPV; therefore, most risk factors are those that increase the risk of contracting HPV (e.g., having multiple sex partners and not practicing safe sex). According to the National Cancer Institute (2009), African American women have the highest cervical cancer prevalence and mortality rates.

Early cervical cancer is usually asymptomatic. When present, clinical manifestations include:

- Continuous vaginal discharge, which may be pale, watery, pink, brown, bloody, or foul smelling
- Abnormal vaginal bleeding between menstruation, after intercourse, or after menopause
- Menorrhagia

Indications of advanced cervical cancer include:

- Anorexia
- Weight loss
- Fatigue
- Pelvic, back, or leg pain
- Unilateral lower extremity edema
- Heavy vaginal bleeding
- Leaking of urine or feces from the vagina
- Bone fractures

The Pap smear remains the cornerstone for early cervical cancer detection. The HPV vaccine may prevent the cancer. Precancerous and early malignant changes can be treated using a loop electrosurgical excision procedure, cryotherapy, and laser therapy. Advanced cancer will require chemotherapy, radiation, and surgery (usually a hysterectomy). The survival rate is usually 100% when treated early, but the rate decreases as the cancer advances.

Endometrial Cancer

Endometrial cancer, or cancer of the uterus, is a common malignancy in women. According to the American Cancer Society (2010), endometrial cancer is the fourth most frequent cancer in women, and the eighth leading cause of cancer death in women, with a 5-year survival rate of approximately 95% in most cases. Caucasian women have the highest prevalence rates, but African American women have the highest mortality rates. The exact cause is unknown, but excessive estrogen exposure may be a major factor. Additional

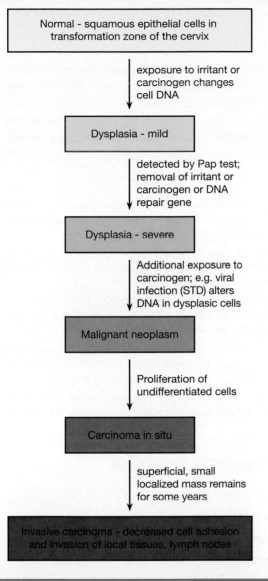

Figure 8-42

Development of cervical cancer.

the endometrium), especially after menopause. Additional clinical manifestations include nonbloody vaginal discharge, pelvic pain, weight loss, palpable abdominal mass, and pain during sexual intercourse. The Pap smear does not detect cancers above the cervix. A simple screening test is not available for endometrial cancer. Biopsy is the diagnostic procedure of choice. If diagnosed early, endometrial cancer can be successfully treated with chemotherapy, radiation, surgery (hysterectomy), and hormone therapy.

Ovarian Cancer

Ovarian cancer is a relatively common cancer in women. According to the American Cancer Society (2010), ovarian cancer is the ninth most frequent cancer in women and the fifth leading cause of cancer death in women. Prevalence and mortality rates are the highest in Caucasian women. Ovarian cancer causes concern because there is no reliable screening test, it is difficult to treat, and it often has metastasized at the time of diagnosis. However, advances in treatment are improving the survival rates (5-year survival rates are approximately 46%). Risk factors for developing ovarian cancer include genetic predisposition (defects on the BRCA1 and BRCA2 genes), advancing age, infertility, excessive estrogen exposure, obesity, and androgen hormone therapy. Early clinical manifestations are vague and include abdominal distention, pelvic pain, and eating disturbances. Additional symptoms consist of bowel pattern changes, gastrointestinal discomfort (e.g., gas, indigestion, and nausea), pain during sexual intercourse, malaise, urinary frequency, and menstruation changes. CA 125, a protein that is produced in response to several conditions including ovarian cancer, is often examined as a part of the diagnostic and treatment process. Because it is not specific to ovarian cancer, a biopsy is still required for definitive diagnosis. During treatment, a declining CA 125 level is considered a favorable response to interventions. Surgery and chemotherapy are the preferred treatment strategies. Surgery may include a bilateral salpingo-oophorectomy (removal of both ovaries and fallopian tubes) and a hysterectomy.

risk factors for developing endometrial cancer include obesity, diabetes mellitus, and hypertension. The most significant finding indicating endometrial cancer is abnormal painless vaginal bleeding (the cancer erodes

Chapter Summary

The reproductive system in males and females is responsible for procreation and hormone balance. Disorders of the reproductive system range from harmless to life threatening. These disorders are most often infections or tumors (benign and malignant). Reproductive function is closely connected with the endocrine, cardio-vascular, and nervous systems and, therefore, can affect those systems. Maintaining reproductive health can decrease the likelihood of issues within this system. Strategies to promote reproductive health include practicing safe sex; abstaining from alcohol, smoking, and illicit drug use; maintaining a healthy weight; and limiting exposure to radiation and chemicals.

References

American Cancer Society. (2009). What are the risk factors for breast cancer? Retrieved from http://www.cancer.org/Cancer/BreastCancer/DetailedGuide/breast-cancer-risk-factors?rnav=cri

American Cancer Society. (2010).Cancer facts and figures 2010. Retrieved from http://www.cancer.org/acs/groups/content/@nho/documents/document/acspc-024113.pdf

Centers for Disease Control and Prevention. (2006). Prostate cancer fast facts. Retrieved from http://www.cdc.gov/cancer/prostate/basic_info/fast_facts.htm

Centers for Disease Control and Prevention. (2008). Sexually transmitted disease surveillance. Retrieved from http://www.cdc.gov/std/stats08/default.htm

Chiras, D. (2008). *Human biology* (6th ed.). Sudbury, MA: Jones and Bartlett.

Elling, B., Elling, K., & Rothenberg, M. (2004). *Anatomy and physiology.* Sudbury, MA: Jones and Bartlett.

Gould, B. (2006). *Pathophysiology for the health professions* (3rd ed.). Philadelphia, PA: Elsevier.

Greenger, J., Bruess, C., & Conklin, S. (2007). *Exploring the dimensions of human sexuality* (3rd ed.). Sudbury, MA: Jones and Bartlett.

National Institutes of Health. (2006). Uterine fibroids. Retrieved from http://www.nichd.nih.gov/publications/pubs/fibroids.cfm

National Institutes of Health. (2007). Epispadis. Retrieved from http://www.nlm.nih.gov/medlineplus/ency/article/001285.htm

National Institutes of Health. (2008). Hypospadis. Retrieved from http://www.nlm.nih.gov/medlineplus/ency/article/001286.htm

National Institutes of Health. (2009). Pelvic inflammatory disease. Retrieved from http://www.nlm.nih.gov/medlineplus/ency/article/000888.htm

National Institutes of Health. (2010). Premenstrual syndrome. Retrieved from http://www.nlm.nih.gov/medlineplus/ency/article/001505.htm

Professional guide to pathophysiology (2nd ed.). (2007). Philadelphia, PA: Lippincott Williams & Wilkins.

Resources

www.cancer.gov

www.cancer.org

www.cdc.gov

www.mayoclinic.com

www.medlineplus.gov

www.nih.gov

www.who.int

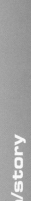

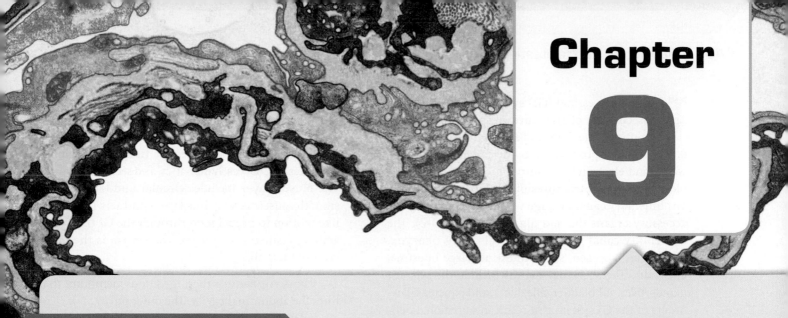

Chapter 9

Gastrointestinal Function

KEY TERMS

achlorhydria
acute gastritis
appendicitis
appendix
ascites
aspiration
atrophic gastritis
bile
cecum
celiac disease
cholecystitis
cholelithiasis
chronic gastritis
chyme
cirrhosis
cleft lip
cleft palate
colon
colorectal cancer
constipation
Crohn's disease
Curling's ulcer
Cushing's ulcer

defecation
diarrhea
diverticular disease
diverticulitis
diverticulosis
diverticulum
duodenal ulcer
dysphagia
emesis
esophageal cancer
esophagus
feces
frank blood
gallbladder
gastric cancer
gastric ulcer
gastritis
gastroenteritis
gastroesophageal reflux disease
 (GERD)
hematemesis
hepatic artery
hepatitis

hepatobiliary system
hiatal hernia
inflammatory bowel disease
intestinal obstruction
irritable bowel syndrome
jaundice
large intestine
liver
liver cancer
lower esophageal sphincter (LES)
mastication
melena
mesentery
mucosa
mucus
muscle layer
nausea
occult blood
oral cancer
pancreas
pancreatic cancer
pancreatitis
paralytic ileus

parietal peritoneum layer
peptic ulcer disease (PUD)
peristalsis
peritoneal cavity
peritoneum
peritonitis
portal hypertension
portal vein
pyloric sphincter
pyloric stenosis
rectum
retching
rugae
serosa
small intestine
stomach
stress ulcer
submucosa layer
ulcerative colitis
visceral peritoneum layer
vomiting
vomitus

The gastrointestinal (GI) system, or digestive system, consists of structures responsible for consumption, digestion, and elimination of food (**Figure 9-1**). These processes provide essential nutrients, water, and electrolytes required for the body's physiologic activities. Structures of the GI system include an alimentary canal through which food is passed and accessory organs that aid digestion (**Figure 9-2**). The alimentary canal includes the oral cavity, pharynx, esophagus, stomach, small intestine, large intestine, and anus. The accessory organs include the salivary glands, liver, gallbladder, bile ducts, and pancreas. Disorders of the GI system can result in nutritional deficits and metabolic imbalances. These conditions vary from mild (e.g., constipation) to life threatening (e.g., pancreatitis) and often present as vague, nonspecific manifestations that reflect a disruption in the system's normal functioning.

Anatomy and Physiology

The GI tract is divided into upper and lower divisions, which will be further discussed in upcoming sections. Additionally, the liver, gallbladder, and pancreas are collectively referred to as the hepatobiliary system because of their close proximity to each other and their complementary functions. The walls of the GI tract have four layers (**Figure 9-3**). The mucosa is the innermost layer that produces mucus. Mucus facilitates movement of GI contents and protects the GI tissue from the extreme pH (pH is 1 to 2 in the stomach) conditions of the GI tract necessary for diges-

tion. The epithelial mucosa cells have a high turnover rate because of erosion associated with food passage and the highly acidic environment. The submucosa layer is comprised of connective tissue that includes blood vessels, nerves, lymphatics, and secretory glands. The muscle layer includes circular and longitudinal smooth muscle layers. This layer contracts in a wavelike motion to propel food through the GI tract (this action is called peristalsis). The serosa is the outer layer of the wall.

The peritoneum is the large serous membrane that lines the abdominal cavity. The outer parietal peritoneum layer covers the abdominal wall as well as the top of the bladder and uterus. The inner visceral peritoneum layer encases the abdominal organs. This double-walled membrane is similar to the pericardial sac (see Chapter 4) and pleural (see Chapter 5) membrane. The peritoneal cavity is the space between these two layers. This space contains serous fluid to decrease friction and facilitate movement. The mesentery is a double-layer peritoneum containing blood vessels and nerves that supplies the intestinal wall. The mesentery supports the intestines while allowing flexibility to accommodate peristalsis and varying content volumes.

Upper Gastrointestinal Tract

The upper GI tract includes the oral cavity, pharynx, esophagus, and stomach (Figure 9-2). Food usually enters the GI tract through the mouth (consumption) where chemical and mechanical digestion begins. Issues with the mouth or swallowing can create a need

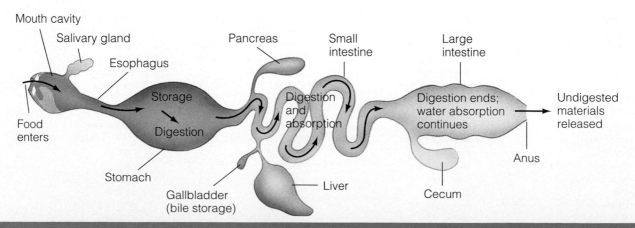

Figure 9-1

Functions of the gastrointestinal system.

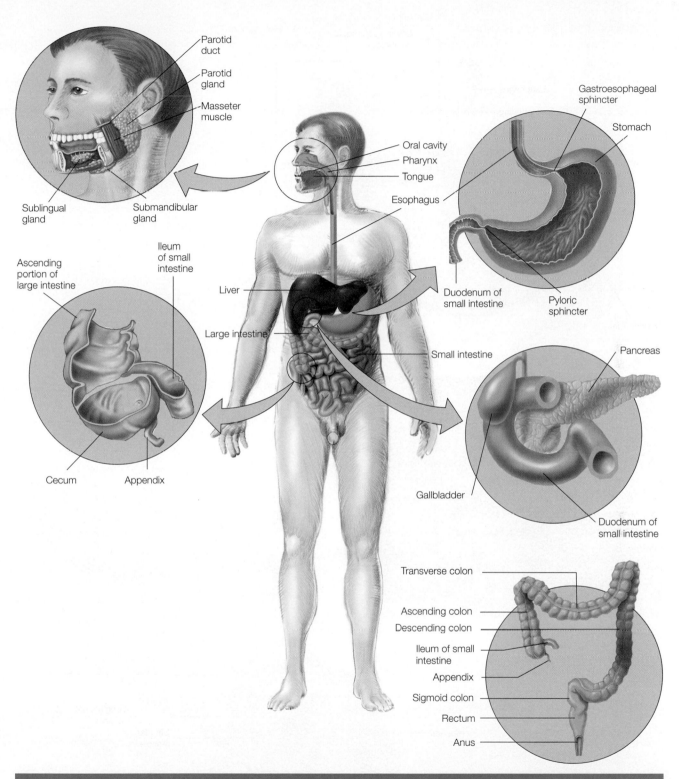

Parotid duct
Parotid gland
Masseter muscle
Sublingual gland
Submandibular gland

Oral cavity
Pharynx
Tongue
Esophagus

Gastroesophageal sphincter
Stomach
Duodenum of small intestine
Pyloric sphincter

Ascending portion of large intestine
Ileum of small intestine
Liver
Large intestine
Small intestine
Cecum
Appendix

Pancreas
Gallbladder
Duodenum of small intestine

Transverse colon
Ascending colon
Descending colon
Ileum of small intestine
Appendix
Sigmoid colon
Rectum
Anus

Figure 9-2

The structures of the gastrointestinal system.

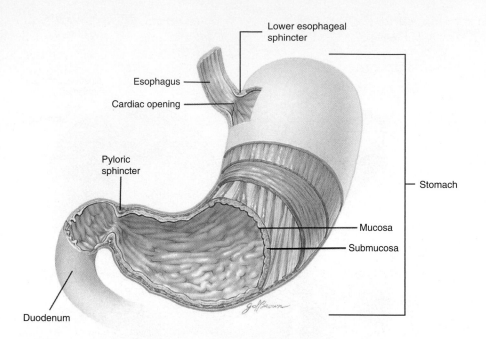

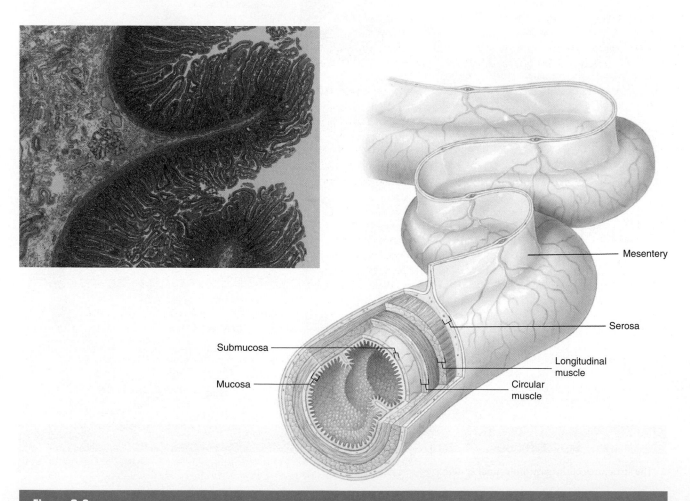

Figure 9-3

The layers of the gastrointestinal tract.

to bypass the mouth and esophagus and introduce the food or a food supplement directly into the stomach or small intestine. Chewing, or *mastication*, pulverizes the food into small pieces, and saliva from the salivary glands moistens and further breaks down the food (**Table 9-1**). Saliva contains enzymes and antibodies that can kill or neutralize bacteria. The smell, taste, feel, and thought of food trigger saliva secretion. Healthy teeth and gums play a key role in maintaining adequate nutrition.

Table 9-1 Digestive Juices and Actions

Diagnostic Studies

- Barium enema—Barium study of colon mucosa to identify structural abnormalities. It is able to show neoplasms, inflammatory bowel disease, fistulas, and diverticulitis.
- Barium swallow—Fluoroscopic examination of pharynx and esophagus, looking at filling patterns, mucosa, size, contour, and peristaltic motion.
- Brush cytology—Uses an endoscope, gastroscope, cystoscope, or bronchoscope to access the site, then a brush is used to gather cell samples for examination.
- Cholescintigraphy (HIDA scan)—A radioactive dye is injected into an intravenous line to evaluate gallbladder and common bile duct function.
- Colonoscopy—Fiber-optic study providing visual access to the mucosa of the colon and terminal ileum to look for growths, inflammation, or bleeding and to biopsy and remove diseased areas.
- Enteroclysis—Barium study of the small bowel to determine the site of an obstruction, metastatic disease, extent of Crohn's disease, or small bowel obstruction. It is used in patients with persistent gastrointestinal (GI) bleeding but with normal upper GI and colonic studies.
- Esophageal acidity test ("Tuttle test")—A probe attached to a catheter is used to measure the pH of gastric and esophageal contents as an indicator of the integrity of the esophageal sphincter. It is often used in conjunction with esophageal manometry.
- Esophageal manometry—Uses a multilumen catheter to measure pressure along the esophagus while the patient is swallowing. It identifies abnormal peristalsis and spasms of the esophagus.
- Esophageal reflux study—A sensitive radionucleotide study to evaluate heartburn and regurgitation.
- Flat-plate X-ray—Screening film used to locate abnormalities of the GI or renal system. It can determine the size, shape, and location of vessels, structures, and gas patterns.
- GI bleeding scan—Labeled red blood cells are scanned during a period of active bleeding to find the bleeding site. Because the images are taken over a longer period of time, it is possible to locate sites that bleed either intermittently or persistently.
- Gastric acid analysis—After a substance is given to stimulate the parietal glands to secrete gastric acid, a Levin tube is inserted and specimens obtained to measure the rate and volume of gastric acid secretion. It is used to diagnose peptic ulcer disease, gastric carcinomas, gastritis, and pernicious anemia.
- Gastric emptying studies—Radionuclide study to evaluate gastric outlet obstruction due to inflammatory or neoplastic disease, dumping syndrome, or gastroparesis.
- Gastroscopy—A fiber-optic endoscope is inserted through the esophagus and the stomach up to the jejunum to visualize mucosal irregularities, varices, ulcers, perforations, or tears. It can be used to obtain brushings of gastric mucosa to identify the presence of *H. pylori*.
- Mesenteric angiography—Used with conscious sedation to localize and possibly perform therapeutic embolization of a bleeding site that does not respond to conservative therapy and cannot be visualized by endoscopy.
- Peroral pneumogram—After ingested barium has reached the cecum, air is passed into the rectum to allow for evaluation of the terminal ileum. This can be performed concurrently with an upper GI series.
- Sigmoidoscopy—A fiber-optic endoscope is inserted through the rectum to visualize the mucosa of the sigmoid colon. It can detect obstruction, carcinoma, inflammatory disease, and other irregularities.
- Upper GI series—Fluoroscopic study used to evaluate the upper GI tract. Films are taken at timed intervals to observe barium as it passes through structures. Different contrast media are used depending on the diagnoses being considered. It can identify, for example, hiatal hernias, esophageal varices, carcinomas, GI perforations, and GI reflux.

Laboratory Tests

- Ca 50 (carbohydrate antigen)—Tumor marker used to plot progression of many types of tumors, but it is especially useful for those of the GI tract.

(Continues)

Table 9-1 Digestive Juices and Actions *(Continued)*

- Carcinoembryonic antigen (CEA)—An antigen released during rapid proliferation of epithelial cells, particularly of the GI tract. Although not diagnostic, frequent measurement can help to guide management and evaluate success of treatment measures. Levels rise 3 months before clinical symptoms of recurrent colorectal cancer are present.
- Colorectal cancer allelotyping for chromosomes 17p and 18q—Blood and tissue samples are used to determine the presence of cellular *p53* and *DCC* genes located on chromosomes 17p and 18q, respectively. These genes are known to suppress the development of tumors in various locations. In the process of a normal cell becoming a colorectal cancer cell, predictable changes take place, including the suppression of these genes.
- Fecal fat—Stool samples are taken after ingestion of a diet with a predetermined amount of fat to measure the amount passed. It is used to diagnose conditions associated with poor fat absorption (i.e., pancreatic disorders, Crohn's disease, and hepatobiliary diseases).
- Fecal antigen assay—One test of choice to verify eradication of the *H. pylori* bacteria after treatment for the disease.
- *Helicobacter pylori*—Initially diagnosed by blood test or upper endoscopy. Breath test and stool samples obtained to determine cure.
- Ki-67 proliferation marker—Marker used to help determine prognosis and outcomes in patients with specific types of cancers, including colorectal cancer. Proliferation refers to the numbers of cells involved in a cycle and the time it takes to complete a cycle. Aggressive rapidly growing tumors have a poorer prognosis. This can also aid in managing inflammatory bowel conditions.
- Urea breath test/C-Urea—Breath samples are taken 10 to 30 minutes after ingestion of radiolabeled urea to stimulate *H. pylori* bacteria to release labeled carbon dioxide if it is present. It is noninvasive and one of the studies of choice to verify eradication of the disease after treatment.
- Vitamin B_{12} absorption test (Schilling test)—A 24-hour urine is collected after oral ingestion of Co-B_{12} and unlabeled intramuscular B_{12}; 5 days later the test is repeated with active intrinsic factor added to the oral dose. Intrinsic factor is secreted by the parietal cells in the stomach antrum, and normal ileal absorption is needed for adequate amounts of vitamin B_{12} to be absorbed into the body. Ileal disease or resection, Crohn's disease, pancreatitis, postgastrectomy, and cystic fibrosis are some conditions that affect this process.

Digestive Juices and Actions

Source	Type	Action
Salivary glands	Bicarbonate	Moistens food
	Salivary lipase	Digests fat
Stomach	Hydrochloric acid	Digests protein
	Pepsin	Kills bacteria
	Gastric lipase	Digests protein
	Intrinsic factor	Digests fat
	Mucus	Aids in absorption of vitamin B_{12} in the small intestine
		Protects stomach lining
Liver	Bile acids	Dissolve fats
	Cholesterol	Excreted in bile
	Phospholipids	Aid in absorption of fats
	Immunoglobulins	Act as antibodies
Pancreas	Bicarbonate	Protects digestive enzymes
	Water	Neutralizes acid
	Amylase	Carries enzymes
	Lipases	Digest starch and glycogen
	Proteases	Digest fats
		Digest protein

Source: Madara, M., & Pomarico-Denino, V. (2008). *Quick look nursing: Pathophysiology* (2nd ed.). Sudbury, MA: Jones & Bartlett Learning.

The tongue pushes the semisolid food mass to the back of the throat, where it is swallowed (**Figure 9-4**). Food passing the trigeminal and glossopharyngeal nerves initiates the swallowing reflex. These nerves relay the information to the swallowing center in the medulla. The swallowing center coordinates the movement of the food from the mouth through the esophagus to the stomach with cranial nerves V, IX, X, and XII. This orchestrated movement prevents food from entering the nearby trachea and lungs (which is called aspiration). The esophagus has muscular rings to move the food toward the stomach (**Figure 9-5**). As the food nears the stomach, the lower esophageal sphincter (LES) relaxes to allow the food to enter the stomach. The LES also prevents the stomach contents from refluxing into the esophagus.

The stomach is an expandable food and liquid reservoir. When empty, the stomach wall shrinks, forming wrinkles called rugae (**Figure 9-6**). As the stomach fills, the rugae unfold and the wall stretches to accommodate up to 2 to 4 liters. Inside the stomach, hydrochloric acid and enzymes (Table 9-1) further chemically digest the food, and peristaltic churning further mechanically digests the food. This new food mixture is referred to as chyme. The highly acidic nature of the chyme aids in digestion and destroys bacteria. The epithelial cells of the stomach's inner lining are densely packed together to prevent tissue damage from the acidic stomach contents. For additional protection, numerous glands are located in the stomach to coat the inner lining with a thick layer of mucus. Nutrients are not absorbed in the stomach; the food is just prepared for absorption. However, alcohol is absorbed in the stomach. Chyme leaves the stomach through the pyloric sphincter in small (1–3 mL), intermittent amounts. As the chyme passes through the pyloric sphincter into the duodenum, liver and pancreatic secretions (Table 9-1) are added to continue the digestion process. Much like the LES, the pyloric sphincter prevents reflux of bile from the small intestines into the stomach.

Liver

The liver is an organ that is a hub of activity. The large organ performs as many as 500 different functions. Some of the liver's primary roles are vital for homeostasis and include the following:

- Metabolize carbohydrates, protein, and fats
- Synthesize glucose, protein (albumin), cholesterol, triglycerides, and clotting factors

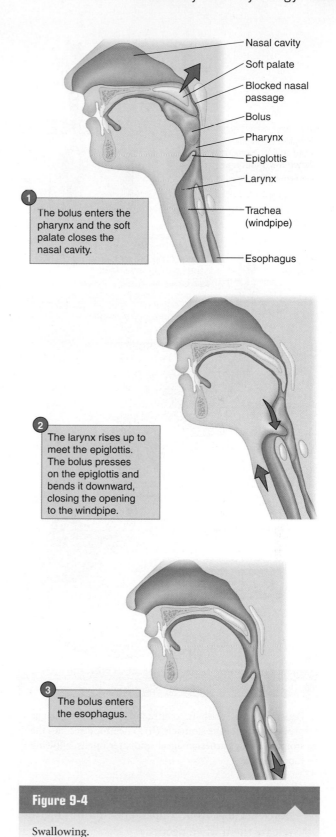

1 The bolus enters the pharynx and the soft palate closes the nasal cavity.

Nasal cavity
Soft palate
Blocked nasal passage
Bolus
Pharynx
Epiglottis
Larynx
Trachea (windpipe)
Esophagus

2 The larynx rises up to meet the epiglottis. The bolus presses on the epiglottis and bends it downward, closing the opening to the windpipe.

3 The bolus enters the esophagus.

Figure 9-4

Swallowing.

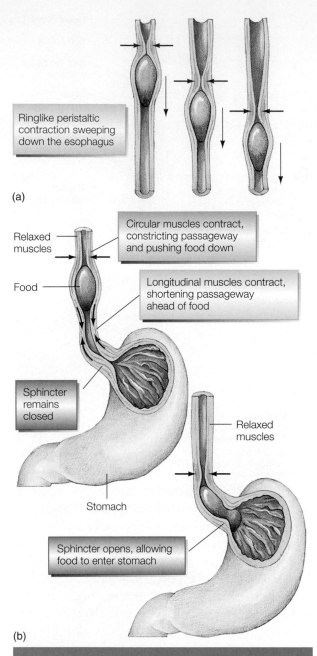

(a)

Ringlike peristaltic contraction sweeping down the esophagus

Relaxed muscles

Circular muscles contract, constricting passageway and pushing food down

Food

Longitudinal muscles contract, shortening passageway ahead of food

Sphincter remains closed

Stomach

Relaxed muscles

Sphincter opens, allowing food to enter stomach

(b)

Figure 9-5

Peristalsis. (a) Peristaltic contractions in the esophagus propel food into the stomach. (b) When food reaches the stomach, the gastroesophageal sphincter opens, allowing food to enter.

- Store glucose (glycogen), fats (lipids), and micro-nutrients (e.g., iron, copper, and vitamin B_{12}) and release them when needed
- Detoxify blood of potentially harmful chemicals (e.g., alcohol, nicotine, and medications)
- Maintain intravascular fluid volume through the production of circulating proteins (see Chapter 6)

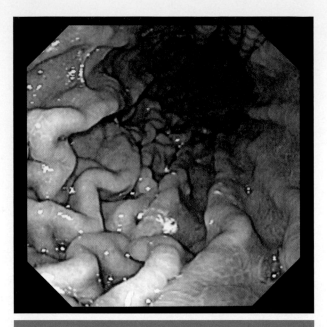

Figure 9-6

Rugae of the stomach.

- Metabolize medications to prepare them for excretion
- Produce bile (necessary for emulsification of fat and fat-soluble vitamins)
- Inactivate and prepare hormones for excretion
- Remove damaged or old erythrocytes from blood to recycle iron and protein
- Serve as a blood reservoir (stores approximately 450 mL that can be used at when needed)
- Convert fatty acids to ketones

A tough membrane (Glisson's capsule) protects this crucial organ. The liver has a dual blood supply. The **hepatic artery** carries oxygenated blood from the general circulation to the liver at a rate of approximately 300 mL per minute to nourish the liver. The **portal vein** carries partially deoxygenated blood from the stomach, pancreas, and spleen, as well as from the small and large intestines to the liver at a rate of approximately 1,000 mL per minute so that the liver can process nutrients and digestion byproducts.

The liver is one of the body's few organs that can regenerate. As much as 75% of the liver tissue can be lost or removed, and the remaining liver tissue can slowly regenerate into a whole liver again. This regeneration occurs primarily due to certain liver cells (hepatocytes) that act as stem cells. A single hepatocyte can divide into two daughter cells. During this time of regeneration, steps should be taken to protect the liver from damage (e.g., avoiding hepatotoxic medications and substances).

In addition to providing regeneration capabilities, the hepatocytes produce bile and perform most of the liver's other activities. The hepatocytes constantly produce bile at a rate of approximately 600–1200 mL per day. Bile is a green or yellowish liquid that contains water, bile salts (formed from cholesterol), conjugated bilirubin, cholesterol, and electrolytes (including bicarbonate). Bile salts are necessary to emulsify fats and fat-soluble vitamins (A, D, E, and K) so that they can be absorbed in the small intestine. The distal ileum reabsorbs most of the bile and returns it to the liver through the portal vein for recycling. The bicarbonate ions in the bile neutralize the acidic gastric contents so that the intestinal and pancreatic enzymes can function. The bile flows from the liver through a duct system to either the gallbladder for storage or on to the duodenum. The gallbladder is a small (usually no larger than a golf ball), saclike organ located on the under surface of the liver that is a reservoir for bile. In addition to storing the bile, the gallbladder concentrates the bile by removing water. The presence of chyme in the small intestine triggers the gallbladder to contract, releasing bile into another duct system where it travels to the small intestine. If the gallbladder requires surgical removal, the bile constantly flows directly from the liver to the small intestine.

Pancreas

The pancreas is an organ that is nestled underneath the stomach and liver. The pancreas has exocrine and endocrine functions. The exocrine functions include producing enzymes, electrolytes (e.g., bicarbonate ions), and water necessary for digestion (Table 9-1). A duct system carries these substances to the duodenum to join the chyme. The endocrine function (see Chapter 10) includes producing hormones (insulin and glycogen) to help regulate blood glucose and, thus, maintaining homeostasis.

Lower Gastrointestinal Tract

The lower GI tract is comprised of the small intestine (duodenum, jejunum, and ileum), large intestine (cecum, colon, and rectum), and anus (Figure 9-2). The small intestine is the longest section of the GI tract (approximately 20 feet long in adults). This length allows for adequate nutrient absorption as the small intestine continues the digestion process. In the small intestine, the enzymes that have been secreted into the GI tract break the large food molecules into smaller molecules that are then absorbed. These smaller molecules are transported to the circulatory and lymphatic system. Muscular rings slowly move the food mixture through the small intestine using a peristaltic wave motion. The wall of the small intestine contains numerous circular folds (plicae circulars) covered with villi and microvilli (Figure 9-7). These projections increase the surface area for absorption of nutrients. Each villus contains capillaries, nerves, and lymphatic vessels for absorption. The small intestine also contains cells that secrete fluid to neutralize pH and enzymes to facilitate digestion. Much like the stomach, the small intestine produces a large amount of protective mucus.

The chyme makes its long journey through the small intestine until it reaches the large intestine (which takes approximately 3–5 hours). The large intestine is about 5 feet long and does not contain villi. The small intestine ends in a pouch called the cecum. The appendix is also attached to the cecum. The appendix is a small, wormlike structure with seemingly no function but plenty of potential to cause harm. The colon makes up most of the large intestine. Unlike the coiled small intestine, the colon has three relatively straight sections—ascending, transverse, and descending. The mixture entering the colon includes water, unabsorbed food molecules, indigestible food remnants (e.g., cellulose), and electrolytes (sodium and potassium). The colon absorbs 90% of the water and electrolytes, and *Escherichia coli* feed off the undigested or unabsorbed food remnants. *E. coli* is a large population of bacteria normally found in the GI tract. These bacteria synthesize several key vitamins (e.g., B_{12}, B_1, B_2, and K) that are later absorbed by the large intestine. As the chyme moves through the colon, it is referred to as feces. Feces contain the remaining undigested or unabsorbed remnants along with bacteria (one third of the feces). Feces also introduce mucus (approximately 300 mL daily) to aid in bowel movements, even in times of decreased dietary intake. Because the feces are more dense than the contents in the small intestines, the colon's muscular rings are thicker to propel the feces until they reach the rectum (this usually takes approximately 18 hours). The rectum serves as a reservoir to store the feces.

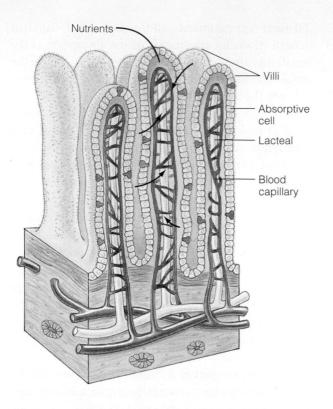

(a)

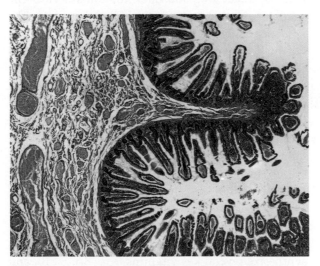

(b)

Figure 9-7

Villi of the small intestines.

Much like the bladder (see Chapter 8), the rectum expands, stimulating the stretch receptors in the wall. These receptors send an impulse through the spinal cord to elicit the defecation reflex. During defecation, the internal and external anal sphincters relax and the rectum contracts to expel the feces. Defecation is consciously controlled (except in infants) and may require assistance from abdominal muscles. Defecation control requires both appropriate muscular and nervous function. The urge to defecate can be delayed up to a point, but the longer the feces remain in the large intestine, the more water will be absorbed, making feces difficult to expel. In addition to the nerves that control defecation, the sympathetic and parasympathetic nervous system innervate the GI tract. Activation of the sympathetic nervous system slows digestive activity, and activation of the parasympathetic nervous system speeds digestive activity.

Gastrointestinal Changes Associated With Aging

The GI system undergoes a few, usually minor, changes with aging. The stomach lining may shrink and become inflamed, leading to atrophic gastritis. Stomach acid production can decrease (achlorhydria), occasionally because of atrophic gastritis. Achlorhydria can cause B_{12} deficiency and slow digestion. The liver changes associated with age include reduced blood flow, delayed drug clearance, and a diminished capacity to regenerate damaged liver cells. Additionally, changes in the metabolism and absorption of lactose, calcium, and iron can occur. The small intestine absorbs less calcium with advancing age. Therefore, increased calcium intake is needed to prevent bone mineral loss and osteoporosis. Some enzymes, such as lactase (which aids in the digestion of lactose, a sugar found in dairy products), decline with age. Peristalsis also decreases with age, increasing the risk of constipation.

LEARNING POINTS

The GI tract is another system in the body that is much like basic household plumbing. Normally, food enters the tubular system and moves in one direction until the waste products are expelled. Peristaltic movement keeps the system flowing in the right direction, but conditions can occur to slow, cease, or reverse this movement. Problems can occur when food moves too fast or too slowly through the system. Much like household plumbing, if an occlusion occurs, the whole system backs up and overall health can be significantly impacted. If the system is backing up, intake should cease until functioning returns. Remember, *what goes in must come out!*

Disorders of the Upper Gastrointestinal Tract

Disorders of the upper GI tract range from mild to life threatening. These disorders can be congenital (e.g., cleft lip/palate or pyloric stenosis) or acquired (e.g., peptic ulcers). Depending on their severity, most of these disorders can be resolved or managed with minimal residual effects.

Congenital Defects

Congenital defects of the digestive system often affect the upper GI tract. These congenital disorders are common and not usually life threatening, but they may cause nutritional and self-image issues.

Cleft Lip and Palate

Cleft lip and cleft palate are common (about 1 in 700) congenital defects of the mouth and face that are apparent at birth (Centers for Disease Control and Prevention, 2009). These conditions usually develop in the 2nd or 3rd month of gestation and are multifactorial in origin. The defects have been associated with genetic mutations, drugs, toxins, viruses, vitamin deficiencies, and cigarette smoking. Clefts are most frequent in children of American Indian, Hispanic, and Asian descent. African American children are the least likely to have a cleft. Males are twice as likely as females to have a cleft lip. Females, however, are about twice as likely as males to have a cleft palate. A cleft lip and palate can affect the appearance of one's face and may lead to problems with feeding, speech, ear infections (otitis media), and hearing problems. The conditions may vary in severity from a small notch in the lip to a complete groove that runs into the roof of the mouth and nose (Figure 9-8). These defects may occur separately or together.

Cleft lip may appear unilaterally or bilaterally (on either side of the midline of the upper lip). This defect results from failure of the maxillary processes and nasal elevations or upper lip to fuse during development. Cleft palate results from failure of the hard and soft palate to fuse in development, creating an opening between the oral and nasal cavity. In addition to lip and palate deformities, teeth and nose malformations may be present. Feeding problems result from these deficits due to an insufficient ability to suck. An infant with a cleft lip and/or palate is also at high risk for aspiration when the nasal cavity is open. The inability to make sounds using the lips and tongue impairs speech development.

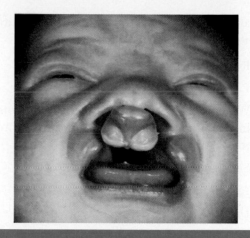

Figure 9-8

Cleft lip and palate.

Diagnostic procedures for cleft lip/palate consist of a history, physical examination, and prenatal ultrasound. Treatment strategies for cleft lip/palate include temporary measures (e.g., special nipples or dental appliances) until surgical procedures are recommended. Surgical repair of the defect is necessary to close the gap. Cleft lip repair is recommended before age 3 months, and cleft palate repair is recommended by 1 year of age. Follow-up procedures are often necessary from 2 years through the adolescent years. Cosmetic plastic surgery can improve the appearance of the defect. Surgical repair in utero is currently being explored. The major advantage of surgical repair before birth is little or no scarring. Speech therapy, including language and eating interventions, and orthodontist consultation can promote normal growth and development. Additionally, a multidisciplinary team (including an audiologist and a pediatrician) is frequently required to manage severe cases.

Pyloric Stenosis

Pyloric stenosis is a narrowing and obstruction of the pyloric sphincter. The pyloric sphincter muscle fibers become thick and stiff, making it difficult for the stomach to empty food into the small intestines. This condition can be present at birth or develop later in life. The exact cause of pyloric stenosis is unknown, but genetics is thought to play a role. Pyloric stenosis is most common in Caucasians and males.

Clinical manifestations of pyloric stenosis usually appear within several weeks after birth. In the congenital form, the hypertrophied pyloric muscle can be palpated as a hard mass in the abdomen. Additional manifestations include:

- Regurgitation
- Projectile vomiting
- Wavelike stomach contractions (results from the increased peristaltic effort to pass food through the narrowing)
- Small, infrequent stools
- Failure to gain weight
- Dehydration
- Irritability (caused by persistent hunger)

Diagnostic procedures for pyloric stenosis include a history, physical examination, abdominal ultrasound, barium X-ray, and blood chemistry (to identify fluid and electrolyte imbalances). Surgical repair called pyloromyotomy is recommended to open the sphincter, but balloon dilatation may be used in high-surgical-risk infants. Signs and symptoms usually resolve within 24 hours of surgical repair.

Dysphagia

Dysphagia, or difficulty swallowing, usually develops secondary to a condition that causes mechanical obstruction of the esophagus or impaired esophageal motility (**Figure 9-9**). Conditions that can lead to dysphagia include:

- Mechanical obstructions, including those caused by the following:
  - Congenital atresia (congenital separation of the upper and lower esophagus)
  - Esophageal stenosis or stricture (may be developmental or acquired)
  - Esophageal diverticula (outpouching of the esophageal wall)
  - Tumors (esophageal or of nearby structures)
- Neurologic disorders, including those caused by the following:
  - Stroke
  - Cerebral damage (e.g., traumatic brain image)
  - Achalasia (failure of the LES to relax because of loss of innervations)
  - Parkinson's disease
  - Alzheimer's disease
- Muscular disorders, including those caused by muscular dystrophy

Clinical manifestations include a sensation of food being stuck in the throat, choking, coughing, "pocketing" food in the cheeks, difficulty forming a food bolus, delayed swallowing, and painful swallowing (odynophagia). Diagnostic procedures focus on identifying the underlying cause and consist of a history, physical examination, barium swallow, chest and neck X-ray, esophageal pH measurement, esophageal manometry (pressure measurement), and esophagogastroduodenoscopy (EGD; visualization of the esophagus, stomach, and duodedum using a small, lighted camera). Treatment strategies are specific for the causative condition but usually include speech therapy.

Vomiting

Vomiting, or emesis, is the involuntary or voluntary forceful ejection of chyme from the stomach up through the esophagus and out the mouth. Vomiting is a common event that often results from a wide range of conditions. Vomiting may be protective (e.g., drug overdose or infections) or result from reverse peristalsis (e.g., intestinal obstructions). Increased intracranial pressure (see Chapter 11) can cause sudden projectile vomiting. Additionally, vomiting may be associated with other symptoms such as severe pain (e.g., migraines or renal calculi). The medulla coordinates vomiting, and drugs, toxins, and chemicals can stimulate this vomiting center. Regardless of the cause, vomiting requires several structures collaborating (**Figure 9-10**). Involuntary vomiting occurs through the following sequence:

1. A deep breath is taken.
2. The glottis closes and the soft palate rises.
3. Respirations cease to minimize the risk of aspiration.
4. The gastroesophageal sphincter relaxes.
5. Abdominal muscles contract, squeezing the stomach against the diaphragm and forcing the chyme upward into the esophagus.
6. Reverse peristaltic waves eject chyme out of the mouth.

Vomiting may be preceded by nausea (a subjective urge to vomit) or retching (a strong unproductive effort to vomit). Recurrent vomiting can be exhausting because of the strong muscular contractions. Additionally, recurrent vomiting can lead to fluid, electrolyte, and pH imbalances (see Chapter 6). Aspiration of the chyme into the lungs can cause serious damage and inflammation. Aspiration can occur if the individual is supine or unconscious when vomiting occurs. Aspiration can also result when the vomiting or cough reflex

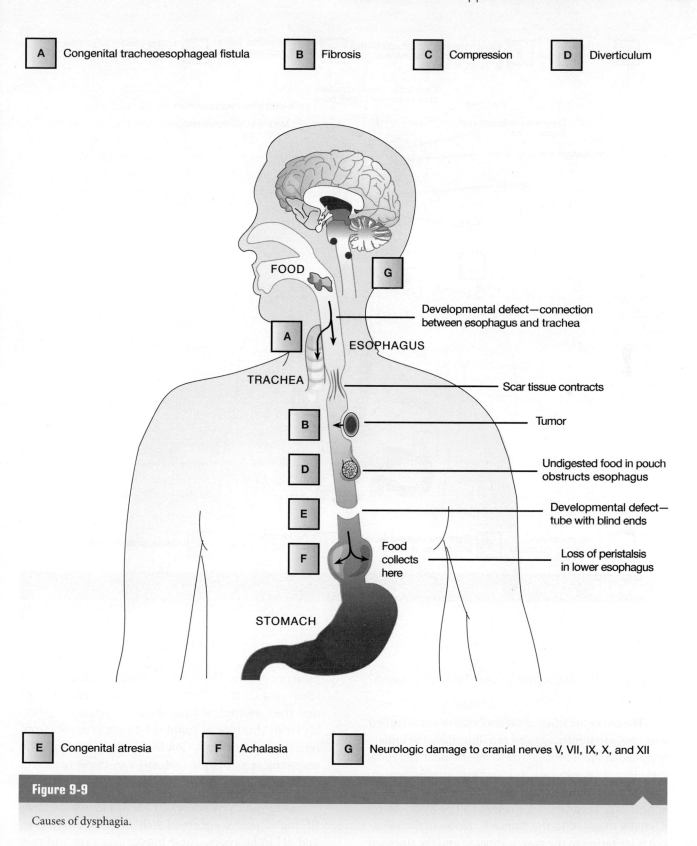

A	Congenital tracheoesophageal fistula
B	Fibrosis
C	Compression
D	Diverticulum

FOOD

G

Developmental defect—connection between esophagus and trachea

A

ESOPHAGUS

TRACHEA

Scar tissue contracts

B

Tumor

D

Undigested food in pouch obstructs esophagus

E

Developmental defect— tube with blind ends

F

Food collects here

Loss of peristalsis in lower esophagus

STOMACH

E	Congenital atresia
F	Achalasia
G	Neurologic damage to cranial nerves V, VII, IX, X, and XII

Figure 9-9

Causes of dysphagia.

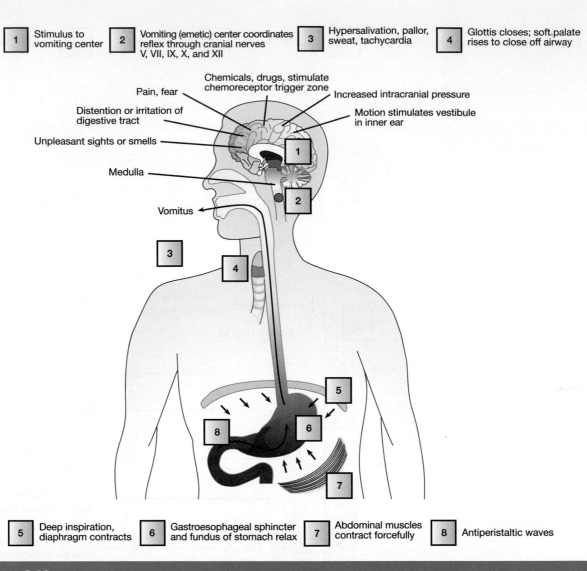

| 1 | Stimulus to vomiting center | 2 | Vomiting (emetic) center coordinates reflex through cranial nerves V, VII, IX, X, and XII | 3 | Hypersalivation, pallor, sweat, tachycardia | 4 | Glottis closes; soft palate rises to close off airway |

| 5 | Deep inspiration, diaphragm contracts | 6 | Gastroesophageal sphincter and fundus of stomach relax | 7 | Abdominal muscles contract forcefully | 8 | Antiperistaltic waves |

Figure 9-10

Vomiting reflex.

is suppressed from drugs (e.g., anesthesia or narcotics) or disease (e.g., stroke).

The characteristics of the contents vomited (called **vomitus**) are significant and can illuminate the underlying cause. **Hematemesis** describes blood in the vomitus. Blood in vomitus has a characteristic brown, granular appearance similar to coffee grounds. This appearance results from protein in the blood being partially digested in the stomach. Blood in the stomach is irritating to the gastric mucosa and the stomach attempts to expel it. Hematemesis can occur from a number of conditions that are capable of causing upper GI bleeding (e.g., gastric ulcers and esophageal varices). Yellow- or green-colored vomitus usually indicates the

presence of bile. This type of vomitus can occur as a result of a GI tract obstruction. A deep brown color may indicate content from the lower intestine, possibly fecal. This type of vomitus frequently results from intestinal obstruction. Conditions that impair gastric emptying (e.g., pyloric stenosis) can cause recurrent vomiting of undigested food.

Diagnostic procedures for vomiting focus on identifying causative agents as well as fluid, electrolyte, and pH imbalances. These procedures vary and may include a history, physical examination, and blood chemistry among others. Treatment strategies center on the cessation of vomiting, maintaining hydration, restoring acid–base balance, and correcting electrolyte alterations. These strategies may vary depending on the severity and include:

- Antiemetic medications (e.g., dimenhydrinate [Dramamine], ondansetron [Zofran], and promethazine [Phenergan])
- Oral or intravenous fluid replacement
- Correcting electrolyte imbalance (see Chapter 6)
- Restoring acid–base balance (see Chapter 6)

Hiatal Hernia

A hiatal hernia occurs when a section of the stomach protrudes upward through an opening (hiatus) in the diaphragm toward the lung. The hiatus develops from weakening of the diaphragm muscle, frequently resulting from increased intrathoracic pressure (e.g., coughing, vomiting, or straining to defecate) or increased intra-abdominal pressure (e.g., pregnancy and obesity). Additional causes of the hiatus include trauma and congenital defects. Risk factors associated with hiatal hernias include advancing age and smoking. Small hiatal hernias may go undetected and rarely cause problems. Large hiatal hernias can cause chyme to reflux into the esophagus, irritating the mucosa. When the stomach protrudes through the diaphragm, it creates a pouch. Chyme collects in this pouch, causing mucosa inflammation.

Clinical manifestations of hiatal hernias reflect inflammation of the esophagus and stomach. These manifestations include indigestion, heartburn (pyrosis), frequent belching, nausea, chest pain, strictures, and dysphagia. Manifestations worsen with recumbent positioning, eating (especially after large meals), bending over, and coughing. Additionally, a soft upper abdominal mass (protruding stomach pouch) may be visualized.

Diagnostic procedures for hiatal hernia consist of a history, physical examination, barium swallow, upper GI tract X-rays, and EGD. Treatment strategies focus on relieving inflammation by decreasing regurgitation of chyme and healing the mucosa. These strategies include eating small frequent meals (six small meals a day), avoiding alcohol, assuming a high Fowler's position after meals, ceasing smoking, reducing stress (stress increases gastrointestinal ischemia), as well as taking antacids, acid-reducing agents (e.g., histamine$_2$ blockers, proton pump inhibitors), and mucosal barrier agents. Surgical repair may be necessary for hiatal hernias not relieved by these strategies.

Gastroesophageal Reflux Disease

Gastroesophageal reflux disease (GERD) is a condition where chyme periodically backs up from the stomach into the esophagus. Occasionally, bile can back up into the esophagus. The presence of these gastric secretions irritates the esophageal mucosa. This gastric backflow occurs because the LES opens from decreases in LES pressure or increases in stomach pressure. Causes of these pressure changes include:

- Certain food (e.g., chocolate, caffeine, carbonated beverages, citrus fruit, tomatoes, spicy or fatty foods, and peppermint)
- Alcohol consumption
- Smoking
- Hiatal hernia
- Obesity
- Pregnancy
- Certain medications (e.g., corticosteroids, beta blockers, calcium channel blockers, and anticholinergics)
- Nasogastric intubation
- Delayed gastric emptying

GERD varies in severity depending on the degree of LES weakness. Clinical manifestations include heartburn, epigastric pain (usually after a meal or when recombinant), dysphagia, dry cough, laryngitis, pharyngitis, regurgitation of food, and sensation of a lump in the throat. The pain associated with GERD is often confused with angina (see Chapter 4) and may warrant ruling out cardiac disease. GERD can result in esophagitis, strictures, ulcerations, esophageal cancer, and chronic pulmonary disease.

Diagnostic procedures for GERD consist of a history, physical examination, barium swallow, EGD, esophageal pH monitoring, and esophagus manometry. Treatment strategies focus on balancing pressures and reducing acid. These strategies include:

- Avoiding triggers (e.g., trigger foods, alcohol, and smoking)
- Avoiding clothing that is restrictive around the waist
- Eating small, frequent meals
- Assuming high Fowler's position for 2–3 hours after meals
- Losing weight

- Reducing stress
- Elevating the head of the bed approximately 6 inches
- Antacids
- Acid-reducing agents
- Mucosal barrier agents
- Herbal therapies (e.g., licorice, slippery elm, and chamomile)
- Surgery (e.g., Nissen fundoplication)

Gastritis

Gastritis refers to an inflammation of the stomach's mucosal lining. Gastritis can be acute or chronic; each type has its own presentation. Acute gastritis can be a mild, transient irritation, or it can be a severe ulceration with hemorrhage. Acute gastritis usually develops suddenly and is likely to be accompanied by nausea and epigastric pain. Chronic gastritis, on the other hand, develops gradually and is likely to be accompanied by a dull epigastric pain and a sensation of fullness after minimal intake. In some cases, chronic gastritis can be asymptomatic. Gastroenteritis refers to inflammation of the stomach and intestines usually because of an infection or allergic reaction.

Helicobacter pylori infections are the most common causes of chronic gastritis. The common bacterium spreads from person to person, but the majority of those infected do not experience gastritis. In other cases, *H. pylori* erode the stomach's protective mucosal barrier, causing inflammation. Why some people experience complications from *H. pylori* infections and others do not is not clear; however, genetic vulnerability and lifestyle behaviors (e.g., smoking and stress) may increase the susceptibility to the bacterium. Several other organisms can be transmitted through food and water contamination (e.g., *E. coli*, *Salmonella*, rotavirus, amoebas). Long-term use of nonsteroidal anti-inflammatory drugs (e.g., ibuprofen [Advil, Motrin], and naproxen [Aleve]) can cause acute and chronic gastritis by reducing cyclooxygenase, a key substance that helps preserve the mucosal lining. Excessive alcohol use can also irritate and erode the mucosal lining. Severe stress due to major surgery, traumatic injury, burns, or severe infections can cause acute gastritis because of tissue ischemia and decreased gastric motility. Autoimmune conditions (see Chapter 2) (e.g., Hashimoto's disease, Addison's disease, type 1 diabetes, and pernicious anemia) can create autoantibodies that attack the cells of the stomach lining. Other chronic diseases (e.g., HIV/AIDS, Crohn's disease, parasitic infections, scleroderma, and liver or renal failure) may be associated with chronic gastritis.

Clinical manifestations of gastritis reflect inflammation of the mucosal lining. Manifestations include indigestion, heartburn, epigastric pain, abdominal cramping, nausea, vomiting, anorexia, fever, and malaise. The presence of hematemesis and dark, tarry stools can indicate ulceration and bleeding. Chronic gastritis increases the risk for peptic ulcers, gastric cancer, and hemorrhage.

Diagnostic procedures for gastritis consist of a history, physical examination, upper GI tract X-ray, EGD, serum *H. pylori* antibodies levels, *H. pylori* breath test, and stool analysis (*H. pylori* and occult blood). Acute gastritis is often self-limiting and resolves within 3 days. Treatment strategies vary depending on the underlying etiology. For instance, bacterial infections require antibiotic therapy. Chronic disease management is important to limit any complications associated with chronic gastritis. In addition to etiology-specific interventions, pharmacologic management may include antacids, acid-reducing agents, and mucosal barrier agents. Other strategies include those for GERD.

Peptic Ulcers

Peptic ulcer disease (PUD) refers to lesions affecting the lining of the stomach or duodenum (accounts for approximately 80% of cases) (**Figure 9-11**). According to the CDC (2008), roughly 8% of adults in the United States have been diagnosed with PUD, and

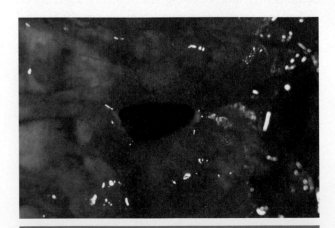

Figure 9-11

Peptic ulcer.

incidence is slightly greater in men. Risk factors for developing PUD include advancing age, nonsteroidal anti-inflammatory drug use, *H. pylori* infections, and certain gastric tumors (e.g., those associated with Zollinger-Ellison syndrome). Other contributing factors include those for GERD (e.g., smoking and alcohol use). Ulcers vary in severity from superficial erosions to complete penetration through the GI tract wall. Regardless of etiology, PUD develops because of an imbalance between destructive forces (e.g., excess acid production) and protective mechanisms (e.g., decreased mucus production).

Duodenal ulcers are most commonly associated with excessive acid or *H. pylori* infections. Patients with duodenal ulcers typically present with epigastric pain that is relieved in the presence of food. Gastric ulcers (stomach ulcers), on the other hand, are less frequent but more deadly. Gastric ulcers typically are associated with malignancy and nonsteroidal anti-inflammatory drug use. In contrast to duodenal ulcers, pain associated with gastric ulcers typically worsens with eating. Stress ulcers describe PUD that develops because of a major physiological stressor on the body (e.g., large burns, trauma, sepsis, surgery, or head injury). Stress ulcers associated with burns are generally called Curling's ulcers, and stress ulcers associated with head injuries are generally called Cushing's ulcers. Stress ulcers develop due to local tissue ischemia, tissue acidosis, bile salts entering the stomach, and decreased GI motility. Stress ulcers most frequently develop in the stomach, and multiple ulcers can form within hours of the precipitating event. Often hemorrhage is the first indicator of a stress ulcer because of the ulcer's rapid development and being masked by the primary problem.

Complications of PUD involve GI hemorrhage, obstruction, perforation, and peritonitis. Clinical manifestations of PUD resemble other conditions of GI inflammation (e.g., gastritis, GERD). These manifestations include:

- Epigastric or abdominal pain
- Abdominal cramping
- Heartburn
- Indigestion
- Nausea and vomiting

Diagnostic procedures for PUD consist of a history, physical examination, upper GI tract X-ray, EGD, serum *H. pylori* antibodies levels, *H. pylori* breath test, and stool analysis (*H. pylori* and occult blood). Treatment strategies include those discussed for gastritis. Additionally, surgical repair may be necessary for perforated or bleeding ulcers. Prevention is crucial with stress ulcers to improve patient outcomes. Prophylactic medications (e.g., acid-reducing agents) are administered to persons at risk for developing stress ulcers.

Cholelithiasis

Cholelithiasis, or gallstones, is a common condition that affects both genders and all ethnic groups relatively equally. Cholelithiasis risk increases with advancing age. The stones, called calculi, vary in size and shape (**Figure 9-12**). Three types of calculi can develop in the gallbladder or nearby ducts (**Table 9-2; Figure 9-13**), and the presence of calculi can cause inflammation or infection in the biliary system (cholecystitis).

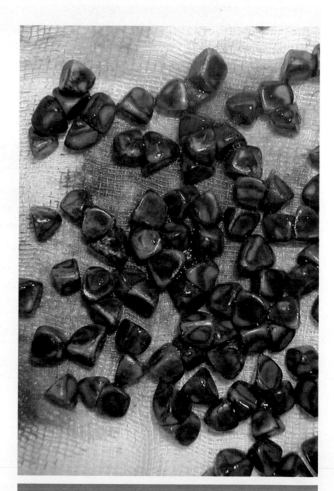

Figure 9-12

Cholelithiasis.

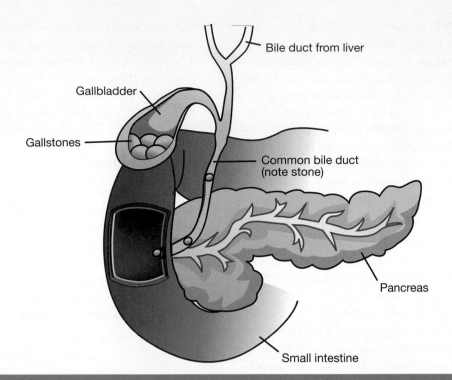

- Bile duct from liver
- Gallbladder
- Gallstones
- Common bile duct (note stone)
- Pancreas
- Small intestine

Figure 9-13

Location of cholelithiasis.

Table 9-2 Types of Cholelithiasis

Type	Characteristics
Cholesterol	Can be small or large, single or multiple
	Can cause obstruction, pain (biliary colic), and jaundice
	Strong association with female hormones
	Increased incidence with obesity, extreme dieting, and hypercholesterolemia
Bilirubin (pigmented)	Usually multiple, small, black stones
	More common in Asians and those persons with chronic diseases
Mixed	Most common
	Usually found in large numbers
	Bilirubin center surrounded by cholesterol and calcium

Small calculi are often asymptomatic and excreted with the bile. Larger calculi are likely to obstruct bile flow and cause clinical manifestations. Prolonged obstruction of bile flow can lead to gallbladder rupture, fistula formation, gangrene, hepatitis, pancreatitis, and carcinoma. Manifestations of cholelithiasis include:

- Biliary colic (abdominal cramping and pain that worsens after a fatty meal)
- Abdominal distension
- Nausea and vomiting
- Jaundice (yellowing of the skin)
- Fever
- Leukocytosis

Diagnostic procedures for cholelithiasis consist of a history, physical examination, abdominal X-ray, gallbladder ultrasound, and laparoscopy. Treatment strategies focus on removing the calculi, restoring bile flow, and preventing reoccurrence. These strategies include:

- Low-fat diet
- Medications to dissolve the calculi (e.g., bile acids)
- Antibiotic therapy (if infection is present)
- Nasogastric tube with intermittent suction (to facilitate abdominal decompression in the presence of an obstruction)
- Lithotripsy (e.g., extracorporeal shock wave)
- Surgically created opening for drainage (choledochostomy)
- Laparoscopic removal of calculi or gallbladder

Disorders of the Liver

Disorders of the liver are usually serious and often life threatening. The liver's involvement in so many activities results in a complex situation to manage. These disorders are often acquired through ingestion of hepatotoxic substances (e.g., medications or alcohol) or infections.

Hepatitis

Hepatitis is an inflammation of the liver that can be caused by infections (usually viral), alcohol, medications (e.g., acetaminophen [Tylenol], antiseizure agents, and antibiotics), or autoimmune disease (e.g., systemic lupus erythematosus, rheumatoid arthritis, and scleroderma). Hepatitis can be acute, chronic, or fulminant (such as in liver failure). Additionally, hepatitis can be active or nonactive. People with nonviral hepatitis usually recover, but some people develop liver failure, liver cancer, or cirrhosis. Nonviral hepatitis is not contagious; whereas viral hepatitis is contagious. People with viral hepatitis also usually recover in time with no residual damage. However, advancing age and comorbidity increase the likelihood of liver failure, liver cancer, or cirrhosis. Viral and nonviral hepatitis can result in hepatic cell destruction, necrosis, autolysis, hyperplasia, and scarring. According to the CDC (2007), rates of all types of viral hepatitis declined from 1996 to 2006. There are five types of viral hepatitis, each with its own characteristics (Table 9-3).

Table 9-3 Types of Viral Hepatitis

Characteristic	Type A	Type B	Type C	Type D	Type E
Mode of transmission	Waterborne	Perinatal	Venereal	Venereal	Waterborne
	Fecal-oral	Blood/skin	Blood/skin	Blood	Fecal-oral
	Venereal	Venereal			
Incubation period (range in days)	15 to 42	42 to 160	14 to 160	28 to 49	14 to 56
average	30	90	50	35	40
Onset	Abrupt	Insidious	Insidious	Insidious	Abrupt
Symptoms					
Fever	Common	Uncommon	Uncommon	Common	Common
Nausea/ vomiting	Common	Common	Common	Common	Common

(Continues)

Table 9-3 Types of Viral Hepatitis *(Continued)*

Characteristic	Type A	Type B	Type C	Type D	Type E
Jaundice	More common in adults than children	Occasionally	Uncommon	Common	Common
Outcome					
Severity	Mild	Moderate	Mild	Moderate to Severe	Severe
Fulminating hepatitis	> .5%	< 1%	Rare	3% to 4% with coinfection with hepatitis B	.3% to 3% 20% in pregnant women
Mortality rate	Low (< 1%)	Low (1% to 3%)	Low (2%)	High (5%)	Moderate; high with pregnancy
Chronic hepatitis	No	Yes (5% to 10%)	Yes (80%)	< 5% with coinfection 80% with superinfection	No
Carrier state	No	Yes (1 million in United States)	Yes	Yes	No
Relapse	Yes	Yes	Persistent	Unknown	Unknown
Carcinoma	No	Yes (25% to 40%)	Yes (25% to 30%)	No increase above that for hepatitis B	Unknown but not likely
Develop cirrhosis	No	40%	30%	Yes, with superinfection	No
Source of virus	Feces	Blood/blood-derived body fluids	Blood/blood-derived body fluids	Blood/blood-derived body fluids	Feces
Route of transmission	Fecal-oral	Percutaneous permucosal	Percutaneous permucosal	Percutaneous permucosal	Fecal-oral
Chronic infection	No	Yes	Yes	Yes	No
Prevention	Pre-/post-exposure immunization	Pre-/post-exposure immunization	Blood donor screening; risk behavior modification	Pre-/post-exposure immunization; risk behavior modification	Ensure safe drinking water

Source: Madara, M., & Pomarico-Denino, V. (2008). *Quick look nursing: Pathophysiology* (2nd ed.). Sudbury, MA: Jones & Bartlett Learning.

Acute hepatitis has four distinct phases—an asymptomatic incubation phase and three symptomatic phases (**Table 9-4**). Chronic hepatitis is characterized by continued hepatic disease lasting longer than 6 months. Chronic hepatitis symptom severity and disease progression varies depending on degree of liver damage. An individual can live with chronic hepatitis for years but can quickly deteriorate with declining liver integrity. Fulminant hepatitis is an uncommon, rapidly progressing form that can quickly lead to liver failure, hepatic encephalopathy, or death within 3 weeks.

Table 9-4 Clinical Manifestations of Acute Hepatitis

Prodromal phase: viral symptoms such as nausea, vomiting, malaise, anorexia, low-grade fever, headache; 2 weeks after exposure to virus, which ends with the onset of jaundice

Icteric phase: jaundice, dark tea-colored urine or clay-colored stools, hepatomegaly and right upper quadrant pain; begins 1–2 weeks after prodromal phase and lasts up to 6 weeks

Recovery phase: resolution of jaundice approximately 6–8 weeks after exposure; liver may remain enlarged for up to 3 months

Source: Madara, M., & Pomarico-Denino, V. (2008). *Quick look nursing: Pathophysiology* (2nd ed.). Sudbury, MA: Jones & Bartlett Learning.

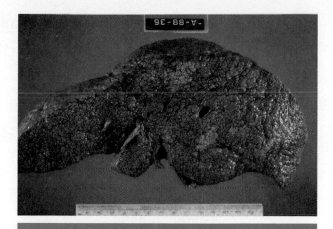

Figure 9-14

Cirrhosis.

Diagnostic procedures for hepatitis include a history, physical examination, serum hepatitis profile, liver enzyme panel, clotting studies, liver biopsy, and abdominal ultrasound. Treatment strategies concentrate on prevention, and vaccinations are the cornerstone of hepatitis prevention. Vaccinations are available for hepatitis A and B. Hepatitis A vaccination is recommended for all children starting at age 1 year, travelers to certain countries, men who have sex with men, intravenous drug users, persons with long-term liver disease, persons requiring repeated blood transfusions (e.g., hemophilia), and others at risk for exposure (e.g., living with someone who is hepatitis A positive). Hepatitis B vaccination is recommended for all infants beginning at birth, older children and adolescents who were not vaccinated previously, and adults at risk (e.g., healthcare workers, men having sex with men, and intravenous drug users). Prevention also includes limiting exposure to the virus (e.g., by limiting exposure to blood, body fluids, and feces). Once viral hepatitis is contracted, there is no method of destroying the virus. Most cases of hepatitis A and E will resolve with no treatment. The other types of viral hepatitis can be treated with interferon injections to improve the immune response (see Chapter 2) and antiviral medications to decrease viral replication. Additional strategies include rest, adequate nutrition (a diet high in carbohydrates, protein, and vitamins), increased hydration, paracentesis (needle aspiration of fluid accumulation in the abdomen), and liver transplant.

Cirrhosis

Cirrhosis refers to chronic, progressive, irreversible, diffuse damage to the liver resulting in decreased liver function (**Figure 9-14**). Cirrhosis can be caused by hepatitis and all those factors that can lead to hepatitis (e.g., alcohol, hepatotoxic medications, and autoimmune conditions). Chronic alcohol abuse is the most frequent cause of cirrhosis in the United States. Hepatitis is the most common etiology in developing countries. Eventually, the damage leads to fibrosis, nodule formation, impaired blood flow, and bile obstruction that can result in liver failure. Cirrhosis may take up to 40 years to develop, and it can develop even with the removal of the underlying cause.

Clinical manifestations of cirrhosis are similar regardless of the underlying cause. These manifestations reflect failure of the liver to accomplish its many functions (**Figure 9-15**). Pressures rise as the hepatic artery and the portal vein become constricted by scar tissue (**portal hypertension**). Veins engorge and varicosities (see Chapter 4) commonly develop in the esophagus (**Figure 9-16**) and abdomen. Nearby organs utilizing the same circulation (e.g., the spleen, pancreas, and stomach) enlarge as pressures rise. Bleeding, either slow or severe, can occur along these overstretched vessels—particularly in the esophagus. Esophageal bleeding has a high mortality and reoccurrence rate. Fluid accumulates in the peritoneal cavity (referred to as **ascites**) as the portal hypertension pushes fluid back into the abdominal cavity and the damaged liver can no longer produce sufficient amounts of albumin (a protein responsible for maintaining fluid balance

Effects of Hepatic Failure and Portal Hypertension

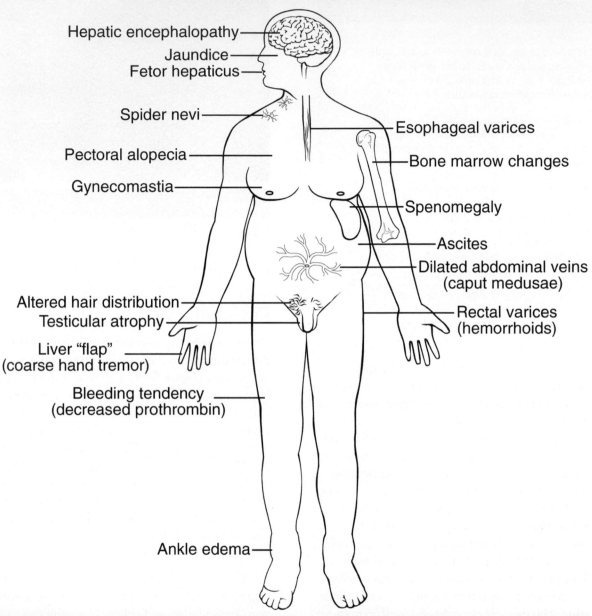

Hepatic encephalopathy
Jaundice
Fetor hepaticus

Spider nevi

Pectoral alopecia

Gynecomastia

Esophageal varices

Bone marrow changes

Spenomegaly

Ascites

Dilated abdominal veins
(caput medusae)

Altered hair distribution
Testicular atrophy

Liver "flap"
(coarse hand tremor)

Rectal varices
(hemorrhoids)

Bleeding tendency
(decreased prothrombin)

Ankle edema

Figure 9-15

Effects of cirrhosis.

in the vessels; see Chapter 6). Changes in protein metabolism result in decreased protein clotting factors, muscle wasting, and hyperlipidemia. Changes in glucose metabolism can lead to hyperglycemia or hypoglycemia. Bile accumulation in the liver causes inflammation and necrosis. Without an ability to flow through the duct system to the intestine, bile enters the bloodstream and causes jaundice. Fats cannot be digested and fat-soluble vitamins cannot be absorbed without the presence of bile. Additionally, the stools become clay colored without the presence of bile. The kidneys attempt to compensate for the excessive bile in the blood by increasing excretion, causing the urine to become dark. The excessive bile also excretes in the sweat, causing bile salts to accumulate on the skin. These bile salts cause intense itching. Estrogen builds up in both sexes, as the liver can no longer inactivate the hormone. Excessive estrogen produces female characteristics in men and irregular menstruation in women. Numerous toxins and waste products accumulate as the liver fails to detoxify the blood. One in particular, ammonia, produces neurologic impairment that presents as confusion, disorientation, and hand tremors. Ulcers and GI bleeding occur as the excessive bile and inflammation impair the mucosa. GI bleeding, along with a high-protein diet, renal failure, and infection can cause protein levels to increase. Excessive protein levels lead to the rapid onset of encephalopathy. Spontaneous bacterial peritonitis may also occur because of compromised host defenses and bacterial overgrowth common in persons with cirrhosis.

Diagnostic procedures for cirrhosis include a history, physical examination, liver biopsy, abdominal X-ray, liver enzyme panel, EGD, clotting studies, and stools examination (for occult blood). Treatment strategies for cirrhosis are complex and vary depending on the underlying cause. Hepatitis-related cirrhosis will be treated with antiviral agents and interferon. Alcohol, drugs, and hepatotoxic medications should be completely avoided. Nutritional imbalances (usually treated with total parenteral nutrition [TPN]) and metabolic dysfunction are corrected to manage complications and promote optimal health. Bile acid-binding agents can aid bile excretion. Portal hypertension is treated with a surgically implanted shunt. Fluid restriction, a low-sodium diet, diuretics, paracentesis, and shunts may be used to treat ascites. Esophageal varices are treated with endoscopic bands, shunts,

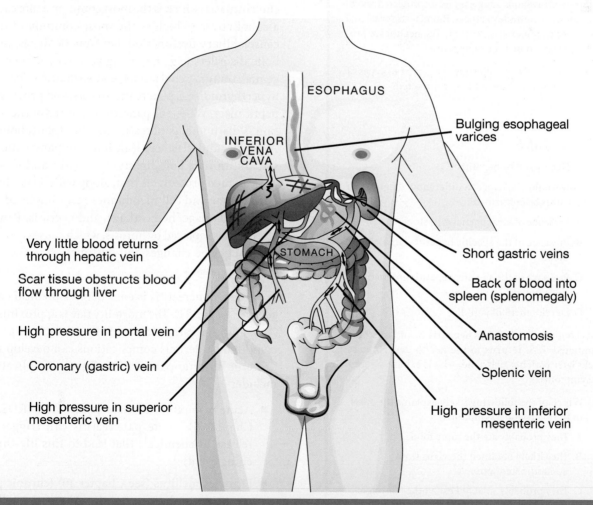

ESOPHAGUS

Bulging esophageal varices

INFERIOR VENA CAVA

Very little blood returns through hepatic vein

Scar tissue obstructs blood flow through liver

High pressure in portal vein

Coronary (gastric) vein

High pressure in superior mesenteric vein

STOMACH

Short gastric veins

Back of blood into spleen (splenomegaly)

Anastomosis

Splenic vein

High pressure in inferior mesenteric vein

Figure 9-16

Development of esophageal varices.

or sclerose procedures. Antacids and acid-reducing agents can minimize GI inflammation. Strategies to treat encephalopathy are directed at eliminating the source of protein breakdown. Lactulose, a type of laxative, can promote ammonia excretion in the stools. Antibiotics can be given to suppress intestinal flora and decrease endogenous ammonia production. A liver transplant usually offers the best outcome, but not all patients are candidates. Alcoholics must refrain from all alcohol consumption for a minimum of 6 months

CASE STUDY

K.S. is a 35-year-old man who has been homeless for the past 5 years. He presents to the health department complaining of flulike symptoms and abdominal pain. He has multiple tattoos and piercings. He admits to intravenous drug use and unprotected sexual behavior with multiple partners. Blood tests reveal that K.S.'s liver enzymes are elevated. The healthcare provider suspects some type of hepatitis.

1. Considering K.S.'s lifestyle, what type or types of hepatitis has he most likely contracted?

    A. Hepatitis A

    B. Hepatitis B

    C. Hepatitis C

    D. Hepatitis B or hepatitis C

2. How would you expect a differential diagnosis of hepatitis be confirmed?

    A. Presence of viral particles in stool

    B. Presence of the specific hepatitis virus in the blood

    C. Presence of the specific hepatitis antibodies in the blood

    D. Development of jaundice

Tests confirm that K.S. has hepatitis B, and treatment is initiated. K.S. returns to the health department 2 weeks later with his girlfriend, who is exhibiting similar symptoms.

3. Which of the following likely explains the onset of the girlfriend's symptoms?

    A. They probably ate the same food.

    B. They likely obtained the virus from contaminated water.

    C. They probably infected each other through sexual contact or drug activity.

    D. They likely became infected because of poor living conditions.

to be considered for transplant. Some hepatitis infections (hepatitis B more so than C) can return after transplant, so those patients may not be considered. Additionally, patients with any evidence of cancer are not considered transplant candidates.

Disorders of the Pancreas

Disorders of the pancreas are frequently grave. The pancreas has a significant role in maintaining homeostasis by regulating electrolytes, water, and glucose. Conditions affecting the pancreas can have a global impact on the individual's health. Most often, the gallbladder is affected by pancreatic disorders because of their intricate relationship.

Pancreatitis

Pancreatitis is an inflammation of the pancreas that can be acute or chronic. Causes of pancreatitis include cholelithiasis (which is the most common acute cause), alcohol abuse (which is the most common chronic cause), biliary dysfunction, hepatotoxic drugs, metabolic disorders (e.g., hypertriglyceridemia, hyperglycemia), trauma, renal failure, endocrine disorders (e.g., hyperthyroidism), pancreatic tumors, and penetrating peptic ulcer. When the pancreas is injured or the function is disrupted, pancreatic enzymes (phospholipase A, lipase, and elastase) leak into the pancreatic tissue and initiate autodigestion. Trypsin and elastase are activated proteolyses that, along with lipase, break down tissue and cell membranes resulting in edema, vascular damage, hemorrhage, and necrosis. Pancreatic tissue is replaced by fibrosis, which causes exocrine and endocrine changes and dysfunction of the islets of Langerhans.

Acute pancreatitis is considered a medical emergency (**Figure 9-17**). The mortality rate is approximately 20%, and this rate increases with advancing age and comorbidity. Serious complications can develop with acute or chronic pancreatitis. These complications include:

■ Acute respiratory distress syndrome (ARDS; see Chapter 5) (acute pancreatitis can trigger the release of chemicals that lead to this life-threatening event)

■ Diabetes mellitus (see Chapter 10) (chronic pancreatitis can damage insulin-producing cells in the pancreas)

■ Infection (acute pancreatitis can make the pancreas vulnerable to bacteria and infection; pancreatic infections are serious and require intensive treatment such as surgery to remove the infected tissue)

- Shock (see Chapter 4) (infection and the release of miscellaneous immune mediators can trigger shock in acute pancreatitis)

- Disseminated intravascular coagulation (DIC) (see Chapter 3) (can be triggered by similar pathways that trigger ARDS and shock)

- Renal failure (see Chapter 7) (shock and activation of the renin-angiotensin system leads to decreased renal perfusion)

- Malnutrition (both acute and chronic pancreatitis can decrease pancreatic enzyme production, and these enzymes are necessary for digestion and absorption; malnutrition and weight loss may occur, even when food intake remains stable)

- Pancreatic cancer (long-standing inflammation caused by chronic pancreatitis can initiate cellular mutations)

- Pseudocyst or abscess (acute pancreatitis can cause pancreatic fluids and necrotic debris to collect in cystlike pockets; a large pseudocyst or abscess that ruptures can cause complications such as internal bleeding and infection [e.g., peritonitis])

Clinical manifestations vary depending on whether the pancreatitis is acute or chronic. Manifestations of acute pancreatitis are usually sudden and severe; in contrast, manifestations of chronic pancreatitis tend to be insidious. Monitoring for the development of complications is crucial to positive patient outcomes. Clinical manifestations of acute pancreatitis include:

- Upper abdominal pain that radiates to the back, worsens after eating, and is somewhat relieved by leaning forward or pulling the knees toward the chest

- Nausea and vomiting

- Mild jaundice

- Low-grade fever

- Blood pressure and pulse changes (may be increased or decreased)

Clinical manifestations of chronic pancreatitis include:

- Upper abdominal pain

- Indigestion

- Losing weight without trying

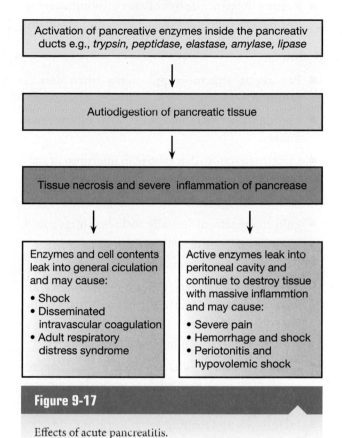

ACUTE PANCREATITIS

Precipitating factors:
alcohol consumption, biliary tract obsttruction, cancer, mumps virus

Activation of pancreative enzymes inside the pancreativ ducts e.g., *trypsin, peptidase, elastase, amylase, lipase*

↓

Autiodigestion of pancreatic tissue

↓

Tissue necrosis and severe inflammation of pancrease

↓

Enzymes and cell contents leak into general ciculation and may cause:
- Shock
- Disseminated intravascular coagulation
- Adult respiratory distress syndrome

Active enzymes leak into peritoneal cavity and continue to destroy tissue with massive inflammtion and may cause:
- Severe pain
- Hemorrhage and shock
- Periotonitis and hypovolemic shock

Figure 9-17

Effects of acute pancreatitis.

- Steatorrhea (oily, fatty, odorous stools)

- Constipation

- Flatulence

Diagnostic procedures for pancreatitis include those to verify the pancreatitis and those to identify complications. These procedures may consist of a history, physical examination, serum amylase and lipase levels, serum calcium levels, complete blood count (CBC), liver enzymes panel, serum bilirubin level, arterial blood gases (ABGs), stool analysis (lipid and trypsin levels), abdominal X-ray, abdominal computed tomography (CT), abdominal magnetic resonance imaging (MRI), abdominal ultrasound, and endoscopic retrograde cholangiopancreatography (which visualizes the duct system). Pancreatitis management requires early treatment and aggressive strategies to prevent complications. Patients with pancreatitis will likely need to be closely monitored in an intensive care unit. This monitoring should include frequent measurement of vital signs (temperature, pulse, blood pressure, and respiration) and strict measurement of intake and output (usually hourly). Treatment strategies include:

- Resting the pancreas by not eating, administering intravenous nutrition (e.g., TPN), and gradually advancing diet from clear liquids as tolerated to low fat

- Pancreatic enzyme supplements when diet is resumed

- Maintaining hydration status with intravenous fluids

- Inserting a nasogastric tube with intermittent suction for persistent nausea and vomiting

- Antiemetic agents (if vomiting is present)

- Pain management (usually includes intravenous narcotic agents and analgesics)

- Antacids and acid-reducing agents

- Anticholinergic agents (which reduce vagal stimulation, decrease GI motility, and inhibit pancreatic enzyme secretion)

- Antibiotic therapy (if infection is present)

- Insulin (which treats hyperglycemia secondary to temporary or permanent pancreatic damage and TPN)

- Identifying and treating complications early (e.g., blood transfusions for hemorrhage, dialysis for renal failure, airway management for ARDS, surgical drain for abscesses, and laparotomy for biliary obstruction)

Disorders of the Lower Gastrointestinal Tract

Disorders of the lower GI tract range from mild (e.g., diarrhea and constipation) to life threatening (e.g., appendicitis and peritonitis). These disorders can be congenital (e.g., celiac disease) or acquired (e.g., intestinal obstruction). Depending on their severity, most of these disorders can be resolved or managed with minimal residual effects.

Diarrhea

Diarrhea refers to a change in bowel pattern characterized by an increased frequency, amount, and water content of the stool. Diarrhea can result because of an increase in fluid secretion (it is secretory), a decrease in fluid absorption (it is osmotic), or an alteration in GI peristalsis (the motility is affected). Diarrhea can be acute or chronic (lasting longer than 4 weeks) and is attributed to many conditions. Acute diarrhea is often caused by viral or bacterial infections but can also be triggered by certain medications (e.g., antibiotics, antacids, and laxatives). Depending on the cause, acute diarrhea is usually self-limiting. Some causes of chronic diarrhea include inflammatory bowel diseases (e.g., Crohn's disease and ulcerative colitis), malabsorption syndromes (e.g., celiac disease), endocrine disorders (e.g., thyroid disorders), chemotherapy, and radiation.

Clinical manifestations of diarrhea vary depending on the underlying etiology. When diarrhea originates in the small intestine, stools are large, loose, and provoked by eating. Diarrhea originating in the small intestine is usually accompanied by pain in the right lower quadrant of the abdomen. When diarrhea originates in the large intestine, stools are small and frequent. Diarrhea originating in the large intestine is frequently accompanied by pain and cramping in the left lower quadrant of the abdomen. Acute diarrhea is generally infectious in origin and accompanied by cramping, fever, chills, nausea, and vomiting. Blood, pus, or mucus may be present in the stool, which can aid in diagnosis. Blood in the stool may present as frank blood (bright, red blood on the surface of the stool), occult blood (small amounts of blood hidden in the stool), or as melena (dark, tarry stool from a significant amount of bleeding higher up in the GI tract). Additionally, bowel sounds may be hyperactive. Fluid, electrolyte, and pH (usually metabolic acidosis) imbalances frequently develop regardless of whether the diarrhea is acute or chronic (see Chapter 6).

Diagnostic procedures for diarrhea focus on identifying the underlying cause and any complications. These procedures may include a history (including usual bowel pattern and completion of the Bristol Stool Chart [**Figure 9-18**]), physical examination, stool analysis (including cultures and occult blood), CBC, blood chemistry, ABGs, and abdominal ultrasound. Treatment strategies vary depending on the underlying etiology. Acute diarrhea with infectious origins usually improves with fasting. Generally, food consumption slows GI motility, allowing bacterial and viral toxins to increase. As toxin levels rise, diarrhea can become more severe. In addition to avoiding food consumption, antidiarrheal agents may be withheld for the same reason. Antibiotics may be necessary depending on the infectious agent. In noninfectious diarrhea, antidiarrheal agents slow GI motility and increase fluid absorption. Some additional medications may include anticholinergic and antispasmodic agents. When oral intake is recommended, a clear liquid diet is usually ordered until the diarrhea subsides. At that time, the diet is advanced to a regular diet as tolerated. Dietary fiber can be used to manage chronic diarrhea. The fiber acts like a sponge to absorb the excess water and increase bulk in the stool. Maintaining hydration status and correcting electrolyte and pH imbalances is crucial to managing acute or chronic diarrhea (see Chapter 6). Meticulous skin care can maintain skin integrity especially in cases of bowel incontinence.

Constipation

Constipation refers to a change in bowel pattern characterized by infrequent passage of stool. Bowel patterns vary from person to person, so the decrease in frequency is in reference to the individual's typical bowel pattern. With constipation, the stool remains in the large intestine longer than usual. The longer the stool remains in the large intestine, the more water is removed from the stool. The stool becomes hard and difficult to pass. Constipation is often caused by a

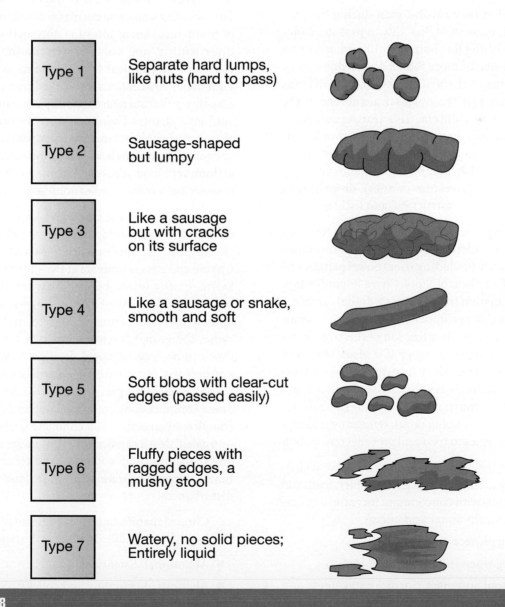

Type 1	Separate hard lumps, like nuts (hard to pass)
Type 2	Sausage-shaped but lumpy
Type 3	Like a sausage but with cracks on its surface
Type 4	Like a sausage or snake, smooth and soft
Type 5	Soft blobs with clear-cut edges (passed easily)
Type 6	Fluffy pieces with ragged edges, a mushy stool
Type 7	Watery, no solid pieces; Entirely liquid

Figure 9-18

Bristol Stool Chart.

low-fiber diet, inadequate physical activity, insufficient fluid intake, delaying the urge to defecate, or laxative abuse (which smoothes intestinal rugae). Stress (sympathetic nervous system stimulation slows GI motility) and travel can also contribute to constipation or other changes in bowel habits. Diseases of the bowel (e.g., irritable bowel syndrome), pregnancy, certain medications (e.g., narcotics, anticholinergic agents, and iron supplements), mental health problems (e.g., depression), neurologic diseases (e.g., stroke, Parkinson's disease, and spinal cord injuries), and colon cancer can cause constipation. Constipation is also common in children who are toilet training, especially if they are not ready for training or scared of toileting.

Constipation may involve pain during the passage of a bowel movement, inability to pass stool after straining or pushing for more than 10 minutes, or no bowel movements for more than 3 days. Additionally, bowel sounds may be hypoactive. The passage of large, wide stools may tear the mucosal membrane of the anus, especially in children. This tearing can cause bleeding and an anal fissure to develop. Chronic constipation can lead to pH disturbances (usually metabolic alkalosis; see Chapter 6), hemorrhoids (swollen, inflamed veins in the rectum or anus), diverticulitis, impaction, intestinal obstruction, and fistulas.

Diagnostic procedures for constipation focus on identifying the underlying cause. These procedures consist of a history (including usual bowel pattern and completion of the Bristol Stool Chart [Figure 9-18]), physical examination (may include a digital examination), abdominal X-ray, upper GI series, barium swallow, colonoscopy (for visualization of the large intestine), and proctosigmoidoscopy (for visualization of the lower bowel). Treatment strategies focus on reestablishing the individual's usual bowel pattern and preventing future constipation episodes. These strategies may involve managing or removing any underlying causes. Strategies to treat and prevent constipation may include:

- Increasing dietary fiber (e.g., vegetables, fruit, and whole grains) with concomitant increase in hydration (specifically water and juices)
- Increasing physical activity
- Defecating when initial urge is sensed
- Taking stool softeners (incorporates lipids and water into the stool)
- Limiting use of laxatives and enemas
- Digitally removing impaction (if present)

Intestinal Obstruction

An intestinal obstruction refers to blockage of intestinal contents in the small intestine (where it is most common) or large intestine. Intestinal obstructions occur because of two types of causes—mechanical and functional. Mechanical obstructions are physical barriers, and functional obstructions result from GI tract dysfunction. Mechanical obstructions can occur due to foreign bodies, tumors, adhesions, hernias, intussusception (telescoping of a portion of the intestine into another portion), volvulus (twisting of the intestine), strictures, Crohn's disease, diverticulitis, Hirschsprung's disease (also known as congenital megacolon), and fecal impaction (**Figure 9-19**). Tumors, adhesions, and hernias account for about 90% of mechanical small intestine obstructions. Tumors, diverticulitis, and volvulus are the most common causes of mechanical large intestine obstructions. Functional obstructions, also called paralytic ileuses, usually result from neurologic impairment (e.g., spinal cord injury); intra-abdominal surgery complications; chemical, electrolyte, and mineral disturbances; intra-abdominal infections (e.g., peritonitis and pancreatitis); abdominal blood supply impairment; renal and lung disease; and certain medications (e.g., narcotics).

Depending on the cause and location, intestinal obstructions can develop suddenly or gradually. Additionally, the obstruction can be partial or complete. Chyme and gas accumulate at the site of the blockage. Saliva, gastric juices, bile, and pancreatic secretions begin to collect as the blockage lingers. This GI fluid buildup increases serum electrolytes and protein and causes abdominal distension and pain. Intestinal blood flow can become impaired, leading to strangulation and necrosis. Intestinal contents will begin to seep into the abdomen as the pressure at the blockage increases. These complications are more likely to develop with a complete obstruction. If a complete obstruction goes untreated, death can occur within hours due to shock and cardiovascular collapse. Additional complications include perforation, pH imbalances, and fluid disturbances.

Clinical manifestations are a result of the GI tract blockage (**Figure 9-20**). These manifestations include:

- Abdominal distension
- Abdominal cramping and colicky pain
- Nausea and vomiting (usually gastric or bile contents)
- Constipation

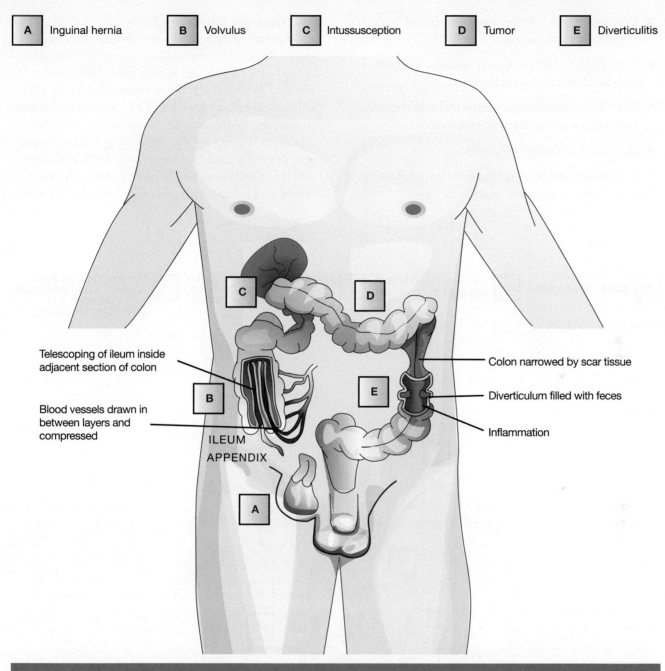

| A | Inguinal hernia | B | Volvulus | C | Intussusception | D | Tumor | E | Diverticulitis |

Telescoping of ileum inside adjacent section of colon

Blood vessels drawn in between layers and compressed

ILEUM

APPENDIX

Colon narrowed by scar tissue

Diverticulum filled with feces

Inflammation

Figure 9-19

Causes of intestinal obstruction.

- Diarrhea (some of the intestinal liquid passes around the obstruction)

- Borborygmi (audible bowel sounds; associated with mechanical obstruction)

- Intestinal rushes (forcible intestinal contractions; associated with mechanical obstruction)

- Decreased or absent bowel sounds

- Restlessness, diaphoresis, tachycardia progressing to weakness, confusion, and shock

Diagnostic procedures for intestinal obstruction are directed at identifying the obstruction, underlying etiology, and complications. These manifestations consist of a history (including usual bowel pattern), physical examination, blood chemistry, ABGs, CBC, abdominal CT, abdominal X-ray, abdominal ultrasound, sigmoidoscopy, and colonoscopy. Treatment strategies depend on the underlying causes. Strategies generally focus on correcting fluid, electrolyte, and pH imbalances (see Chapter 6); decompressing the bowel; and reestablishing bowel movements. A naso-

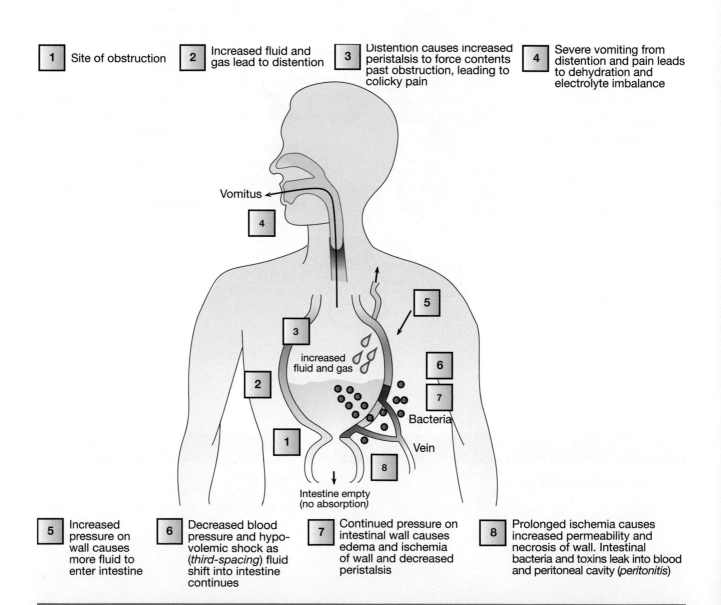

1	Site of obstruction
2	Increased fluid and gas lead to distention
3	Distention causes increased peristalsis to force contents past obstruction, leading to colicky pain
4	Severe vomiting from distention and pain leads to dehydration and electrolyte imbalance

Vomitus

increased fluid and gas

Bacteria

Vein

Intestine empty (no absorption)

5	Increased pressure on wall causes more fluid to enter intestine
6	Decreased blood pressure and hypovolemic shock as (*third-spacing*) fluid shift into intestine continues
7	Continued pressure on intestinal wall causes edema and ischemia of wall and decreased peristalsis
8	Prolonged ischemia causes increased permeability and necrosis of wall. Intestinal bacteria and toxins leak into blood and peritoneal cavity (*peritonitis*)

Figure 9-20

Effects of intestinal obstruction.

gastric tube with intermittent suctioning is inserted to decompress the bowel and relieve vomiting. The patient should fast and receive TPN until bowel function is restored. Ambulation can help restore peristalsis. Laxatives should not be used in most cases until the obstruction is resolved. Surgery is frequently necessary to relieve mechanical obstruction.

Appendicitis

Appendicitis refers to an inflammation of the vermiform appendix (**Figure 9-21**). This inflammation is most often caused by an infection. The inflammation process triggers local tissue edema, which obstructs the small structure. Fluid builds inside the appendix, and microorganisms proliferate. The appendix fills with purulent exudate, and the stretched, edematous wall compresses area blood vessels. With blood flow compromised, ischemia and necrosis develop. The pressure inside the appendix escalates, forcing bacteria and toxins out to surrounding structures. Abscesses and peritonitis can develop as bacteria escape, and gangrene can result from the worsening necrosis. The pressure inside the appendix will continue to intensify until the appendix ruptures or perforates, releasing its contents. This release can accelerate peritonitis, which can be life threatening.

Clinical manifestations reflect the pathogenesis characteristic of appendicitis. These manifestations vary significantly, from asymptomatic to sudden and severe. Sharp abdominal pain develops, gradually intensifies (over about 12–18 hours), and becomes

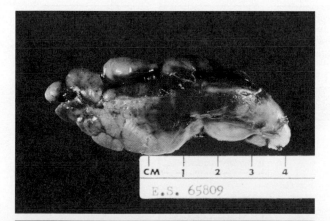

Figure 9-21

Appendicitis.

localized to the lower right quadrant of the abdomen (called McBurney point). Due to normal anatomic variations, this pain may occur anywhere in abdomen. The pain will temporarily subside if the appendix ruptures, and then the pain will return and escalate as peritonitis develops. Nausea, vomiting, and bowel pattern changes can also be associated with appendicitis. Other manifestations reflect the inflammation and infectious process (e.g., fever, chills, and leukocytosis). Additionally, the patient should be monitored for signs and symptoms of peritonitis (e.g., abdominal rigidity, tachycardia, and hypotension).

Urgent diagnosis and treatment is crucial for positive patient outcomes. Diagnostic procedures include a history, physical examination, CBC, abdominal ultrasound, abdominal X-ray, abdominal CT, and laparoscopy. Because of the life-threatening nature of appendicitis, surgery remains the cornerstone of treatment. Appendicitis is one of the most common causes for emergency surgeries in the United States. Performing the surgery prior to rupture of the appendix is paramount. Prior to rupture, the surgery can be performed through laparoscopy with minimal risk. If the appendix ruptures, an open surgical procedure is necessary to ensure that all the appendix fragments and infectious materials are removed. Extensive irrigation of the abdominal cavity is performed to flush out any remaining bacteria. The wound may be left open to heal by secondary intention (see Chapter 2) to decrease risk of infection. Tubes may be inserted to drain any abscesses. Long-term antibiotic therapy may be necessary to prevent and resolve any infections. Analgesics will be necessary to manage pain before and after surgery. Additionally, the patient should avoid activities that increase intra-abdominal pressure (e.g., straining and coughing).

Peritonitis

Peritonitis is an inflammation of the peritoneum, the membrane lining the abdominal wall and abdominal organs. Peritonitis usually presents as an acute condition, and treatment centers on resolving the underlying cause. The inflammation results from chemical irritation (e.g., ruptured gallbladder or spleen) or direct organism invasion (e.g., appendicitis and peritoneal dialysis) (**Figure 9-22**). Chemical irritation will lead to a bacterial invasion if not quickly treated. The inflammatory response triggered by the chemical increases intestinal wall permeability. The increased permeability allows passage of enteric bacteria. Necrosis or perforation of the intestinal wall also creates an opportunity for an enteric bacteria invasion.

Several protective mechanisms are activated along with the inflammatory response in an attempt to localize the problem. These mechanisms include producing a thick, sticky exudate that bonds nearby structures and temporarily seals them off. Abscesses may form in an attempt to wall off the infections. Peristalsis may slow down in a response to the inflammation, decreasing the spread of toxins and bacteria. These mechanisms only slow the progression. If the underlying cause is not treated, the condition can become critical as sepsis and shock develop.

Clinical manifestations reflect the inflammatory and infectious processes occurring. These manifesta-

tions tend to be sudden and severe. The classical manifestation of peritonitis is abdominal rigidity. The rigid, boardlike abdomen develops because of a reflexive abdominal muscle spasm that occurs in response to the peritoneal inflammation. Inflamed tissue creates abdominal tenderness and pain. Large volumes of fluid can leak into the peritoneal cavity (called third-spacing), leading to hypovolemic shock (see Chapter 4). This fluid contains protein and electrolytes, making it an optimum medium for bacterial growth. Nausea and vomiting are common responses to the intestinal irritation. Persistent inflammation impairs nerve conduction, which decreases peristalsis. This decreased peristalsis can lead to intestinal obstruction. Sepsis develops as the bacteria and toxins migrate to the circulatory system through the inflamed membranes.

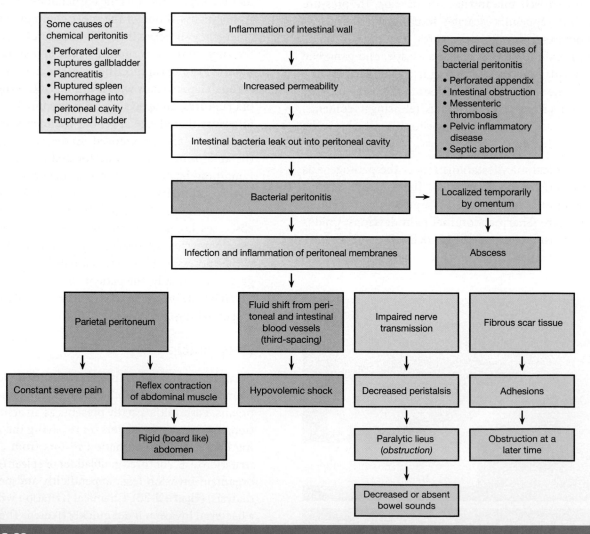

Figure 9-22

Development of peritonitis.

Fever, malaise, and leukocytosis occur because of the infectious process. Additionally, the patient should be monitored for signs of sepsis and shock (e.g., tachycardia, hypotension, restlessness, and diaphoresis).

Diagnostic procedures for peritonitis consist of a history, physical examination, CBC, abdominal X-ray, abdominal ultrasound, abdominal CT, paracentesis with peritoneal fluid analysis, and laparotomy. Treatment strategies vary based on the underlying cause. Prognosis depends on the underlying cause along with early and aggressive treatment. Management often includes surgical repair of the chemical leak and draining of the infected fluid. Long-term antibiotic therapy specific to the causative organism will be required. Correction of any fluid and electrolyte imbalance may be required. Nasogastric tube insertion with intermittent suction can relieve abdominal distention and treat intestinal obstructions. TPN will be necessary to maintain nutritional status until the peritonitis is resolved.

Celiac Disease

Celiac disease (also known as celiac sprue) is an inherited, autoimmune, malabsorption disorder. Celiac disease is considered primarily a childhood disease, but it can develop at any age. The exact cause of celiac disease is unclear, but it is most common in Caucasians and females. Tropical sprue is a related disorder that occurs in tropical regions, especially India, Southeast Asia, Central America, South America, and the Caribbean. Tropical sprue is thought to be caused by a bacterial, viral, parasitic, or amoebic infection. Unlike celiac disease that becomes a lifelong condition, tropical sprue can be resolved with antibiotic therapy. Celiac disease results from a defect in the intestinal enzymes that prevent further digestion of gliadin (a product of gluten digestion). Gluten is an ingredient of grains (e.g., wheat, barley, rye, and oats). The combination of digestive dysfunction and immune activities creates a toxic environment for the intestinal villi. The villi atrophy and flatten, resulting in decreased enzyme production and less surface area for nutrient absorption (**Figure 9-23**). Eventually, the malnutrition associated with celiac disease can cause vitamin deficiencies that deprive the brain, peripheral nervous system, bones, liver, and other organs of vital nourishment. These nutritional deficits can lead to other illnesses, including:

- Anemia
- Arthralgia (bone and joint pain)

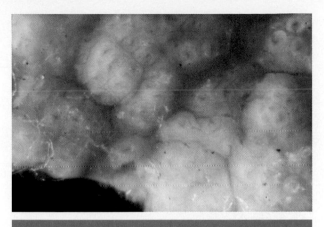

Figure 9-23

Effects of celiac disease on intestinal villi.

- Myalgia (muscle pain)
- Bone disease (e.g., osteoporosis, kyphoscoliosis, and fractures)
- Dental enamel defects and discoloration
- Intestinal cancers
- Depression
- Growth and development delays in children
- Hair loss
- Hypoglycemia
- Mouth ulcers
- Increased bleeding tendencies (e.g., bruising and nose bleeds)
- Neurologic disorders (e.g., seizures and peripheral neuropathy)
- Skin disorders (e.g., dermatitis herpetiformis and eczema)
- Vitamin or mineral deficiency, single or multiple nutrient (e.g., iron, folate, vitamin B_{12}, and vitamin K)
- Endocrine disorders (e.g., menstrual dysfunction and adrenal insufficiency)

Clinical manifestations of celiac disease vary significantly from person to person, which often delays diagnosis. In infants, clinical manifestations generally appear as cereals are added to their diet (usually around 4–6 months of age). Most of the clinical manifestations are GI in nature, but occasionally there are no GI symptoms at all. Manifestations that are not GI in nature may include irritability, lethargy, malaise, and behavioral changes. Additionally, the individual with celiac disease should be monitored for complication development. The GI clinical manifestations may include:

- Abdominal pain

- Abdominal distension, bloating, gas, and indigestion

- Constipation or diarrhea (may be chronic or occasional)

- Changes in appetite (usually decreased)

- Lactose intolerance (common upon diagnosis; usually goes away following treatment)

- Nausea and vomiting

- Steatorrhea

- Unexplained weight loss (although people can be overweight or of normal weight upon diagnosis)

Diagnostic procedures of celiac disease consist of a history, physical examination, and duodenal biopsy. There are no standardized blood tests for celiac disease, but a number of tests collectively referred to as the celiac blood panel can aid in diagnosis. This panel includes the immunoglobulin A antibody-endomysium antibodies, immunoglobulin A antigliadin antibodies, deaminated gliadin peptide antibody, immunoglobulin A antitissue transglutaminase, lactose tolerance test, and D-xylose test. Dietary management is the cornerstone of treatment. Most people (about 90%) are effectively managed by eliminating gluten from their diet. Dietary changes may also be used as a part of diagnosis—the individual is given a gluten-free diet to assess whether the symptoms improve. A gluten-free diet includes avoiding wheat and wheat products—rice and corn can be substituted. Once gluten is removed from the diet, the intestinal mucosa will return to normal after a few weeks. Even when symptoms are controlled with diet, the individual remains at risk for intestinal cancers; therefore, the individual with celiac disease should be periodically monitored for cancer development. Additionally, long-term support may be necessary for children and parents of children with celiac disease.

Inflammatory Bowel Disease

Inflammatory bowel disease (IBD) describes chronic inflammation of the GI tract, usually the intestines. IBD is chiefly seen in women, Caucasians, persons of Jewish descent, and smokers. IBD includes two disorders—Crohn's disease and ulcerative colitis. Both conditions are characterized by periods of exacerba-

tions and remissions that can vary in severity. The exact cause of IBD is unknown, but IBD is thought to be caused by a genetically associated autoimmune state that has been activated by an infection. Immune cells located in the intestinal mucosa are stimulated to release inflammatory mediators (e.g., histamine, prostaglandins, leukotrienes, and cytokines). These mediators alter the function and neural activity of the secretory and smooth muscle cells in the GI tract. Fluid, electrolyte, and pH imbalances develop. IBD can be painful, debilitating, and life threatening. Even though the two disorders are similar, some differences warrant discussion.

Crohn's Disease

Crohn's disease is an insidious, slow-developing, progressive condition that often develops in adolescence. Crohn's disease is characterized by patchy areas of inflammation involving the full thickness of the intestinal wall and ulcerations. These patchy areas and ulcerations, often called skip lesions, are separated by areas of normal tissue. The ulcers combine to form fissures divided by nodules (thickened elevations), giving the intestinal wall a cobblestone appearance. Eventually, the entire wall becomes thick and rigid, and the intestinal lumen becomes narrowed and potentially obstructed. Granulomas, nodules consisting of epithelial and immune cells, develop on the intestinal wall and nearby lymph nodes because of the chronic inflammation. The damaged intestinal wall losses the ability to process and absorb food. The inflammation also stimulates intestinal motility, decreasing digestion and absorption. Complications of Crohn's disease include:

- Malnutrition

- Anemia (especially iron deficiency because of the malnutrition)

- Fistulas

- Adhesions

- Abscesses

- Intestinal obstruction

- Perforation

- Anal fissure

- Fluid, electrolyte, and pH imbalances

- Delayed growth and development (in children)

Clinical manifestations of Crohn's disease reflect the inflammatory process and the digestive dysfunction. These manifestations intensify during exacerbations and include:

- Abdominal cramping and pain (typically in the right lower quadrant)
- Diarrhea
- Steatorrhea
- Constipation (as the intestinal lumen narrows)
- Palpable abdominal mass (thickened intestinal wall)
- Melena (if ulcers begin bleeding)
- Anorexia
- Weight loss
- Indications of inflammation (e.g., fever, fatigue, arthralgia, and malaise)

Diagnostic procedures for Crohn's disease consist of a history, physical examination, stool analysis (including cultures and occult blood), CBC, blood chemistry, abdominal X-ray, abdominal CT, abdominal MRI, barium studies (swallow and enema), sigmoidoscopy, colonoscopy, and biopsy. Treatment strategies focus on nutritional support, symptom relief, and complication minimization. Dietary management usually includes (1) a low-residue, high-calorie, high-protein diet; (2) oral nutritional supplements (e.g., Ensure and Sustacal); (3) multivitamin supplements; and (4) TPN as the disease progresses. Pharmacologic management usually includes (1) antidiarrheal agents; (2) aminosalicylates (5-ASAs) (to treat mild to moderate inflammation; (3) glucocorticoids (to treat moderate to severe inflammation); (4) immune modulators (to suppress inflammatory response); (5) biologic agents (to treat severe unresponsive Crohn's disease); (6) analgesics; and (7) antibiotics if infection is present. Surgical intestine resection may be necessary as the disease progresses and complications develop. Additional strategies involve stress management (e.g., exercise, meditation, deep breathing, biofeedback, and acupuncture) and support (e.g., group involvement and counseling).

Ulcerative Colitis

Ulcerative colitis is a progressive condition of the rectum and colon mucosa that usually develops in the 2nd or 3rd decade of life. Inflammation causes epithelium loss, surface erosion, and ulceration. The ulceration begins in the rectum and extends to involve the entire colon. Ulcerative colitis rarely affects the small intestine. The mucosa becomes inflamed, edematous, and frail. Necrosis of the epithelial tissue (specifically

at the base of the crypts of Lieberkühn) can result in abscesses, known as crypt abscesses. In an attempt to heal, granulation tissue forms, but the tissue remains fragile and bleeds easily. The ulcers combine, creating large areas of stripped mucosa. Nutritional, fluid, electrolyte, and pH imbalances develop without an adequate surface area for absorption. Complications of ulcerative colitis include:

- Malnutrition
- Anemia
- Hemorrhage
- Perforation
- Strictures
- Fistulas
- Pseudopolyps
- Toxic megacolon (life-threatening condition caused by rapid dilatation of the large intestine)
- Colorectal carcinoma
- Liver disease (because of inflammation and scarring of the bile ducts)
- Fluid, electrolyte, and pH imbalances

Clinical manifestations of ulcerative colitis reflect the inflammatory process and digestive dysfunction. Like Crohn's disease, these manifestations intensify during exacerbations. Manifestations usually include:

- Diarrhea (usually frequent [as many as 20 daily], watery stools with blood and mucus)
- Tenesmus (persistent rectal spasms associated with the need to defecate)
- Proctitis (inflammation of the rectum)
- Abdominal cramping
- Nausea and vomiting
- Weight loss
- Indications of inflammation (e.g., fever, fatigue, arthralgia, and malaise)

Diagnostic procedures for ulcerative colitis consist of a history, physical examination, stool analysis (including cultures and occult blood), CBC, blood chemistry, abdominal X-ray, abdominal CT, abdominal MRI, barium enema, colonoscopy, and biopsy. Similar to Crohn's disease, treatment strategies focus on nutritional support, symptom relief, and complication minimization. Dietary management usually includes (1) a high-fiber, high-calorie, high-protein diet; (2) oral nutritional supplements (e.g., Ensure or Sustacal); (3) multivitamin supplements; and (4) TPN as the disease progresses. Pharmacologic management usually includes (1) antidiarrheal agents; (2) antispasmodics; (3) anticholinergics; (4) aminosalicylates (5-ASAs) (to treat mild to moderate inflammation); (5) glucocorticoids (to treat moderate to severe inflammation); (6) immune modulators (to suppress inflammatory response); (7) biologic agents for severe unresponsive Crohn's disease; (8) analgesics; and (9) antibiotics if infection is present. Surgical intervention (e.g., ileostomy or colostomy) may be necessary as the disease progresses and complications develop. Additional strategies involve stress management (e.g., exercise, meditation, deep breathing, biofeedback, and acupuncture) and support (e.g., group involvement and counseling).

Irritable Bowel Syndrome

Irritable bowel syndrome (IBS) refers to a chronic GI condition characterized by exacerbations associated with stress. IBS includes alterations in bowel pattern and abdominal pain not explained by structural or biochemical abnormalities. In contrast to IBD, IBS is less serious, is noninflammatory, and does not cause permanent intestinal damage (Table 9-5). IBS is more common in women than in men. The exact cause of IBS is unknown, but IBS is thought to be triggered by stress, food (e.g., chocolate, alcohol, dairy products, carbonated beverages, vegetables, and fruits), hormone changes (e.g., menstruation), and GI infections. IBS is thought to be an intensified response to stimuli with increased intestinal motility and contractions. People

Table 9-5 Comparison of Inflammatory Bowel Disease and Irritable Bowel Syndrome

Differences Between Inflammatory Bowel Disease and Irritable Bowel Syndrome

	Inflammatory Bowel Disease		**Irritable Bowel Syndrome**
	Ulcerative colitis	*Crohn's disease*	
Epidemiology	Abrupt onset	Insidious onset	Late teens/early adulthood
	Peak ages 15 to 30/60	15 to 40	
	Caucasian > African American	Female > Male	Female > Male
	Female > Male		
Pathology	Possible autoimmune infection may precipitate familial tendency Continuous, irregular superficial inflammation of mucosal layer of colon and rectum	Possible autoimmune infection may precipitate genetic predisposition Skipping ulcerations involving mucosal and submucosal layers along the entire GI tract; 50% involve small intestine/colon Strictures/fistulas common	Cause unknown Bowel has increased response to stimuli and visceral hypersensitivity Altered perception of CNS
Signs and Symptoms			
Abdominal pain	Intermittent, mild crampy tenderness	Crampy or steady Periumbilical or right lower quadrant	Sharp, burning; may be diffuse or left lower quadrant (LLQ)
Mass present	No	Common	No
Bleeding	Common	Occasionally	No
Diarrhea	Frequent watery stools with blood and mucus	Chronic, reccurent, may have some blood	Intermittent, predominant Symptom varies with individual

Table 9-5 Comparison of Inflammatory Bowel Disease and Irritable Bowel Syndrome *(Continued)*

	Inflammatory Bowel Disease		Irritable Bowel Syndrome
	Ulcerative colitis	*Crohn's disease*	
Perianal lesions	No	One third develop perianal abscesses or fistulas	No
Weight loss	With severe diarrhea	Common	No
Fever/malaise	During severe exacerbation	With exacerbation and abscess formation	No
Psychological	As result of longstanding disease	As result of longstanding disease	Exacerbation with stressful situations
Course/prognosis	75% to 80% relapse after first attack; most have mild to moderate disease Routine colonoscopy with biopsy after having the disease for 7 to 8 years because of increased colon cancer risk	Recurrent, progressive Typically need surgery after 7 years to treat/ repair fistulas or abscesses; shortened life span	Chronic, intermittent Rare functional limitations

Source: Madara, M., & Pomarico-Denino, V. (2008). *Quick look nursing: Pathophysiology* (2nd ed.). Sudbury, MA: Jones & Bartlett Learning.

with IBS may have a low tolerance for stretching and pain in the intestinal smooth muscle, causing them to respond to stimuli to which those without IBS do not respond. Complications of IBS include hemorrhoids, nutritional deficits, social issues, and sexual discomfort.

Clinical manifestations vary from person to person. Stress and mood disorders (e.g., anxiety and depression) often worsen symptoms. These manifestations usually include:

- Abdominal distension, fullness, flatus, and bloating
- Intermittent abdominal pain exacerbated by eating and relieved by defecation
- Chronic and frequent constipation, usually accompanied by pain
- Chronic and frequent diarrhea, usually accompanied by pain
- Nonbloody stool that may contain mucus
- Bowel urgency
- Intolerance to certain foods (usually gas-forming foods and those containing sorbitol, lactose, and gluten)

- Emotional distress
- Anorexia

Diagnosis is based on clinical presentation (**Table 9-6**) and is often made by excluding other GI and psychological disorders. Diagnostic procedures consist of a history (including bowel pattern and Rome III criteria), stool analysis (including cultures and occult blood), celiac blood panel, abdominal X-ray, abdominal CT, abdominal MRI, barium studies (swallow and enema), sigmoidoscopy, colonoscopy, and biopsy. Treatment focuses on management of symptoms and may vary depending on the symptoms. Pharmacologic strategies may include antidiarrheal agents, laxatives, antispasmodics, and antidepressants. Other strategies involve avoiding triggers, maintaining adequate fiber intake, stress management (through techniques such as exercise, meditation, deep breathing, biofeedback, and acupuncture), and support (e.g., group involvement, counseling, and psychotherapy).

Diverticular Disease

Diverticular disease refers to conditions related to the development of diverticula. Diverticula (singular is diverticulum) are outwardly bulging pouches of

Table 9-6 Rome III Criteria

Twelve weeks within 12 months (need not be consecutive) of abdominal pain or discomfort that has two of three features:

1. Relieved by defecation
2. Onset associated with changes in stool frequency
3. Onset associated with changes in stool form or appearance

Symptoms that support diagnosis of IBS:

- Abnormal stool frequency (> 3/day or < 3/week)
- Abnormal stool form (lumpy and hard or watery and loose)
- Abnormal stool passage (straining, urgency, feeling of incomplete evacuation)
- Passage of mucus
- Bloating or feeling of abdominal distention

Source: Madara, M., & Pomarico-Denino, V. (2008). *Quick look nursing: Pathophysiology* (2nd ed.). Sudbury, MA: Jones & Bartlett Learning.

the intestinal wall that occur when mucosa sections or large intestine submucosa layers herniate through a weakened muscular layer (**Figure 9-24**). Diverticula may be congenital or acquired. Diverticula are thought to be caused by a low-fiber diet that results in chronic constipation. The muscular wall can become weakened from the prolonged effort of moving hard stools. Pressure increases in the intestine in an attempt to propel the stool, forcing the mucosa through areas of weakness. Diverticular disease is rare in developing countries where high-fiber diets are typical and more common in developed countries where processed foods and low-fiber diets are typical. In addition to diet, poor

bowel habits (e.g., straining and delaying the urge to defecate) can contribute to developing diverticula.

Most cases of diverticular disease are asymptomatic and are discovered incidentally. **Diverticulosis** describes asymptomatic diverticular disease. Usually there are multiple diverticula present. **Diverticulitis** refers to a state in which diverticula have become inflamed, usually because of retained fecal matter. Diverticulitis can result in potentially fatal obstructions, infection, abscess, perforation, peritonitis, hemorrhage, and shock. Diverticulitis is often asymptomatic until the condition becomes serious. When they

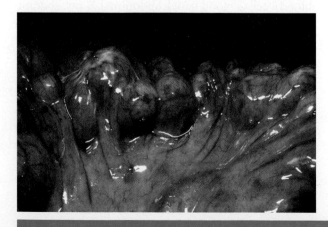 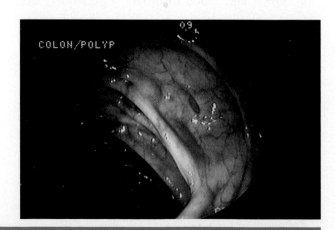

Figure 9-24

Diverticula.

appear, clinical manifestations usually include abdominal cramping followed by passing a large quantity of frank blood. Bleeding may last hours or days before spontaneously ceasing. Most people with diverticulitis (approximately 80%) will only experience a single episode of bleeding and require no further treatment. Persistent or recurrent bleeding will require further actions. In addition to bleeding, other clinical manifestations that may be present include a low-grade fever, abdominal tenderness (usually left lower quadrant), abdominal distension, constipation, obstipation (severe constipation usually caused by an intestinal obstruction), nausea, vomiting, a palpable abdominal mass, and leukocytosis.

Diagnostic procedures for diverticular disease consist of a history, physical examination, stool analysis (including that for occult blood), abdominal CT, abdominal MRI, colonoscopy, barium enema, and biopsy. Treatment strategies for diverticular disease include high-fiber diet, omitting foods with seeds or popcorn, adequate hydration, proper bowel habits (e.g., defecating when urge is sensed and not straining), stool softeners, antibiotics (if infection is present), analgesics, and colon resection. Food intake is usually decreased when active bleeding is present, and blood transfusions may be necessary depending on the amount of blood loss.

Cancers

Malignancies of the GI system originate in the GI tract or spread from other sites. Some of these cancers have moderate treatment rates (e.g., colorectal cancer), while others have high mortality rates (e.g., oral and pancreatic cancer). Typical cancer diagnosis, staging, and treatments are usually utilized (see Chapter 1).

Oral Cancer

Oral cancer can occur anywhere in the mouth, but most are squamous cell carcinomas of the tongue and mouth floor (**Figure 9-25**). Approximately 75% of cases can be attributed to smoked and smokeless tobacco. Alcohol consumption also significantly increases oral cancer risk. Additional risk factors include viral infections (especially the human papillomavirus), immuno-deficiencies, inadequate nutrition, poor dental hygiene, chronic irritation (e.g., from dentures), and exposure to ultraviolet light (as in cancer of the lips). Incidence rates of oral cancer have slightly decreased since 1980. Men are twice as likely as women to have oral cancer.

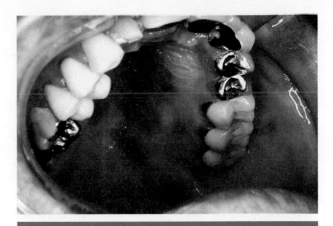

Figure 9-25

Oral cancer.

According to the American Cancer Society (2010), oral cancer is the ninth most frequent cancer in men. Prevalence and mortality rates are the highest in African American men; however, overall mortality rates have decreased since 1980. In early stages, oral cancer is very treatable. Unfortunately, most cases are advanced upon diagnosis because the cancer tends to be hidden. Oral cancer has a 5-year survival rate of 50%, which has significantly improved since 1990. Oral cancer usually appears initially as a painless, whitish thickening that develops into a nodule or an ulcerative lesion. Multiple lesions may be present. These lesions persist, do not heal, and bleed easily. Additional manifestations include a lump, thickening, or soreness in the mouth, throat, or tongue as well as difficulty chewing or swallowing food. Oral cancer often metastasizes to neck lymph nodes and esophagus. Treatment primarily consists of surgery and radiation, but surgery may be difficult depending on the location. Speech therapy is often necessary after treatment to improve chewing, swallowing, and speech.

Esophageal Cancer

Much like oral cancer, esophageal cancer is usually a squamous cell carcinoma most often affecting men. Incidence rates of esophageal cancer have remained steady, but the mortality rates have increased since 1980. According to the American Cancer Society (2010), esophageal cancer is the seventh leading cause of cancer death in men even though it did not make the list of top 10 cancers in men. The distal esophagus is the most common site. Esophageal cancer is associated with chronic irritation (e.g., GERD, achalasia, hiatal hernia, alcohol abuse, and smoked and smokeless tobacco). These tumors grow the circumference of the esophagus creating a stricture, or they can grow out into the lumen of the esophagus, creating an obstruction. Complications include esophageal obstruction, respiratory compromise, and esophageal bleeding. Esophageal cancer is usually asymptomatic in early stages, delaying diagnosis and treatment. Because of the usual late diagnosis, the prognosis is poor with esophageal cancer. Clinical manifestations, when present, typically include dysphagia, chest pain, weight loss, and hematemesis. Surgery is the treatment of choice, but chemotherapy and radiation are also frequently included in management. Speech therapy will also likely be necessary following treatment.

Gastric Cancer

Gastric cancer occurs in several forms, but adenocarcinoma (an ulcerative lesion) is the most frequent type. Incidence and mortality rates of gastric cancer in the United States have declined since 1980. However, gastric cancer is extremely prevalent worldwide (second most common type of cancer in men and third most common in women) and is the second most deadly cancer worldwide (World Health Organization, 2009). Japan has particularly high rates of gastric cancer. Gastric cancer is prevalent in men and Asians and Pacific Islanders, but mortality rates are highest among African American men. Gastric cancer has a 5-year survival rate of approximately 25%. Gastric cancer is strongly associated with increased intake of salted, cured, pickled, preserved (containing nitrates and nitrites), and smoked foods. A low-fiber diet and constipation can increase the risk because of prolonging the time the intestinal wall is exposed to these substances. Additional risk factors include family history, *H. pylori* infections, smoking, pernicious anemia, chronic atrophic gastritis, and gastric polyps.

Gastric cancer is asymptomatic in early stages, which often delays diagnosis and treatment. When present, clinical manifestations include:

- Abdominal pain and fullness
- Epigastric discomfort
- Palpable abdominal mass
- Dark stools, possibly melena
- Dysphagia that worsens over time
- Excessive belching
- Anorexia

- Nausea and vomiting
- Hematemesis
- Premature abdominal fullness after meals
- Unintentional weight loss
- Weakness and fatigue

Surgical removal of the stomach (gastrectomy) is the only curative treatment. Chemotherapy and radiation are also used as curative and palliative measures. Nutritional support (e.g., TPN) and supplements (e.g., vitamin B_{12} and iron) will be needed before, during, and after treatment.

Liver Cancer

Liver cancer most commonly occurs as a secondary tumor that has metastasized from the breast, lung, or other GI structures (**Figure 9-26**). Primary tumors are rare in the United States, but incidence and mortality rates of liver cancer have been steadily climbing since 1980. Worldwide, liver cancer is the third most common cancer in men and the fourth leading cause of cancer deaths in both sexes (WHO, 2009). Most primary tumors are caused by chronic cirrhosis or hepatitis. Liver cancer is most prevalent among men as well as Asians and Pacific Islanders. According to the American Cancer Society (2010), liver cancer is the sixth leading cause of cancer death in men and the ninth leading cause of cancer death in women. Liver cancer has a 5-year survival rate of approximately 13%. Liver cancer may be asymptomatic or mild initially. Clinical manifestations are similar to those of other liver diseases and usually include:

- Anorexia
- Fever
- Jaundice
- Nausea and vomiting
- Abdominal pain (usually in the upper right quadrant)
- Hepatomegaly
- Splenomegaly
- Portal hypertension
- Edema, third spacing (accumulation of fluid in tissue or body cavities), and ascites
- Paraneoplastic syndrome (manifestations and diseases that result from cancer)
- Diaphoresis
- Weight loss

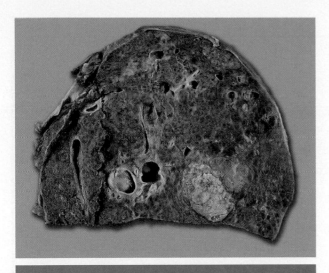

Figure 9-26

Liver cancer.

Treatment strategies vary depending on the primary site and progression of the cancer. Chemotherapy is used systemically when metastasis is evident or may be injected directly into localized tumors. If the tumor is small, a section of the liver may be surgically removed (called a hepatectomy). If the cancer is throughout the liver or has caused significant damage, a liver transplant will be the best option if metastasis has not occurred. Several nontraditional cancer treatment procedures are also available to treat liver cancer. Cryoablation is a procedure that uses extreme cold to destroy cancer cells by injecting liquid nitrogen into the tumor. Radiofrequency ablation uses electric current to heat and destroy cancer cells. Pure alcohol can be injected into the tumor to dry and eventually kill the cancer cells.

Pancreatic Cancer

Pancreatic cancer is an aggressive malignancy (most commonly adenocarcinoma) that can quickly spread to structures nearby (e.g., stomach, intestines, spleen, liver, and kidneys). The incidence and mortality rates have remained steady since 1980. According to the American Cancer Society (2010), pancreatic cancer is the 10th most common cancer in men and women, and it is the 4th leading cause for cancer death in men and women. Pancreatic cancer occurs most frequently in men and African Americans. Other risk factors include family history, obesity, chronic pancreatitis, long-standing diabetes mellitus, cirrhosis, alcohol abuse, and tobacco use. The overall 5-year survival rate is merely 5%. This

dismal prognosis is due largely to the asymptomatic nature of pancreatic cancer. Clinical manifestations do not generally develop until the cancer is well advanced and has metastasized, delaying diagnosis and treatment. These manifestations may include:

- Upper abdominal pain that may radiate to the back (pain worsens as cancer progresses)
- Jaundice
- Dark urine and clay-colored stools
- Indigestion
- Anorexia
- Weight loss
- Depression
- Malnutrition
- Hyperglycemia
- Increased clotting tendencies

No effective treatment has been developed for pancreatic cancer. Surgical removal of the tumor (called a Whipple procedure) is recommended, but few pancreatic tumors can be surgically removed. Chemotherapy and radiation are often used as palliative treatment or in combination with surgery. Any biliary blockages that develop will require repair through surgery or endoscopy.

Colorectal Cancer

Colorectal cancer most often develops from an adenomatous polyp. According to WHO (2009), colorectal cancer is the fourth most common cancer in men and women and the third most fatal worldwide. According to the American Cancer Society (2010), colorectal cancer is the third most common and most fatal cancer in men and women in the United States, but these rates have been declining since 1980. Incidence and mortality rates are the highest among men and African Americans. The 5-year survival rate for colorectal cancer is a robust 65%. Dietary factors that have been associated with colorectal cancer include excessive intake of fat, calories, red meat, processed meat, and alcohol as well as deficient intake of fiber. Other risk factors involve family history, advancing age, obesity, tobacco use, physical inactivity, and IBD. Like many other GI cancers, colorectal cancer remains asymptomatic until well advanced. When present, clinical manifestations may include:

- Lower abdominal pain and tenderness
- Blood in the stool (occult or frank)

MYTH BUSTERS

Several myths regarding the gastrointestinal system merit discussion.

MYTH 1: Smoking a cigarette helps relieve heartburn.

Actually, cigarette smoking may contribute to heartburn. Heartburn occurs when the lower esophageal sphincter (LES) relaxes, allowing the acidic contents of the stomach reflux into the esophagus. Esophagitis is more frequent in people who smoke, presumably caused by increased acid reflux. The increased reflux is thought to be because cigarette smoking relaxes the LES.

MYTH 2: After ostomy surgery, men have erectile dysfunction and women have impaired sexual function and are unable to become pregnant.

Ostomy surgery does not, in general, interfere with a person's sexual or reproductive capabilities. Ostomy surgery is a procedure in which the diseased part of the small or large intestine is removed, and the remaining intestine is attached to an opening in the abdomen. Stool is collected in a bag taped to the skin over the opening or in an internal pouch. Although some men who have had radical ostomy surgery lose the ability to achieve and sustain an erection, most men do not. Temporary erectile dysfunction may be experienced because of damage to the nerves innervating the penis. In women, ostomy surgery does not damage sexual or reproductive organs, so it is not a direct cause of sexual problems or sterility. Factors such as pain and the adjustment to a new body image may create temporary sexual problems, but these problems can usually be resolved with time and, in some cases, counseling. Unless a woman has had a hysterectomy she can still bear children.

MYTH 3: Bowel regularity means a bowel movement every day.

The frequency of bowel movements among normal, healthy people varies from three a day to three a week, and some perfectly healthy people fall outside both ends of this range. Nevertheless, even three bowel movements a day can be abnormal in someone who usually has one bowel movement a day. The key to determining normality is comparing current bowel activities to the individual's usual patterns.

- Diarrhea, constipation, or other change in bowel habits
- Intestinal obstruction
- Narrow stools
- Unexplained anemia (usually iron deficiency)
- Unintentional weight loss

Routine screening can dramatically improve prognosis. The 5-year survival rate for colorectal cancer if detected when still localized to the large intestine is approximately 90%. The CDC (2009) and American Cancer Society (2010) recommend regular colorectal screening beginning at 50 years of age for both sexes (earlier if risk factors are present). The screening tests and recommended intervals include:

- High-sensitivity fecal occult blood test (which checks for hidden blood in three consecutive stool samples) should be administered every year.
- Flexible sigmoidoscopy should be administered every 5 years.
- Colonoscopy should be administered every 10 years.

Colonoscopy also is used as a diagnostic test when symptoms are present, and it can be used as a follow-up test when the results of another colorectal cancer screening test are unclear or abnormal. Additionally, early (stage 0) cancer cells can be removed during the colonoscopy. Cancers stage I through III require extensive surgery (colon resection). Chemotherapy and radiation use varies depending on the cancer stage. The patient may require a colostomy (a colon diversionary procedure in which the colon is brought to the abdominal wall to drain into an externally attached pouch) because of the colon resection. Because colorectal cancer often reoccurs, lifestyle changes (e.g., diet and physical activity) and follow-up screenings are crucial to long-term survival.

Chapter Summary

The GI system is responsible for ingestion, absorption, and removal of food. These functions obtain essential nutrients, water, and electrolytes to maintain many physiologic activities and homeostasis. Disorders of the GI tract range from harmless to life threatening. These disorders can be congenital, infectious, structural, or cancerous in nature. Regardless of the pathogenesis, GI disorders often create short- or long-term nutritional deficits that can affect the individual's overall health. Promoting GI health focuses primarily on dietary strategies that include following a well-balanced diet.

Case Study Answers

1. D
2. B
3. C

References

American Cancer Society. (2010). Cancer facts and figures 2010. Retrieved from http://www.cancer.org/acs/groups/content/@nho/documents/document/acspc-024113.pdf

Centers for Disease Control and Prevention. (2007). Retrieved from http://www.cdc.gov/mmwr/PDF/ss/ss5803.pdf

Centers for Disease Control and Prevention. (2009). Retrieved from http://www.cdc.gov/ncbddd/bd/faq1.htm#CommonBD

Chiras, D. (2008). *Human biology* (6th ed.). Sudbury, MA: Jones and Bartlett.

Elling, B., Elling, K., & Rothenberg, M. (2004). *Anatomy and physiology*. Sudbury, MA: Jones and Bartlett.

Gould, B. (2006). *Pathophysiology for the health professions* (3rd ed.). Philadelphia, PA: Elsevier.

Madara, B., & Pomarico-Denino, V. (2008). *Pathophysiology* (2nd ed.). Sudbury, MA: Jones and Bartlett.

Professional guide to pathophysiology (2nd ed.). (2007). Philadelphia, PA: Lippincott Williams & Wilkins.

Resources

www.otolaryngology.emory.edu/GESR/1b.html (geriatric dysphagia tutorial)
www.cancer.gov
www.cancer.org
www.cdc.gov
www.mayoclinic.com
www.medlineplus.gov
www.mypyramid.gov
www.nih.gov
www.who.int

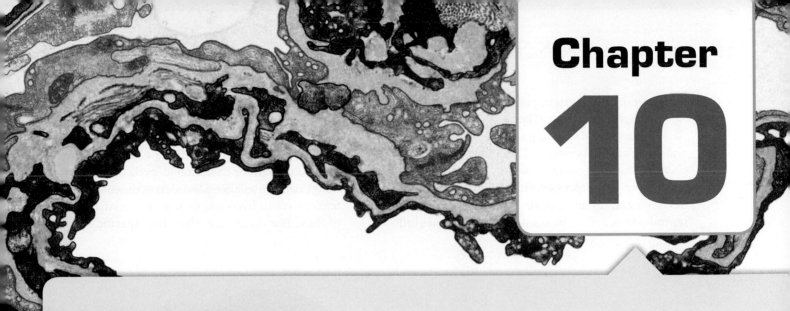

Endocrine Function

LEARNING OBJECTIVES

- Discuss normal endocrine anatomy and physiology.
- Describe and differentiate the types of diabetes mellitus.
- Compare and contrast disorders of the thyroid gland.
- Compare and contrast disorders of the parathyroid gland.
- Compare and contrast disorders of the adrenal glands.

KEY TERMS

acromegaly
Addison's disease
adrenal gland
aldosterone
alpha cell
amylin
beta cell
calcitonin
cortex
cortisol
Cushing's syndrome
delta cell
diabetes insipidus
diabetes mellitus (DM)
diabetic ketoacidosis
dwarfism
epinephrine
epsilon cell

exophthalmos
follicles
gestational diabetes
ghrelin
gigantism
glucagon
glucocorticoid
goiter
gonadocorticoid
Graves' disease
Hashimoto's thyroiditis
hyperglycemia
hyperparathyroidism
hyperpituitarism
hyperprolactinemia
hyperthyroidism
hypoglycemia
hypoparathyroidism

hypopituitarism
hypothalamic-pituitary axis
hypothalamus
hypothyroidism
insulin
islets of Langerhans
isthmus
medulla
metabolic syndrome
mineralocorticoid
myxedema
negative feedback system
norepinephrine
pancreas
pancreatic polypeptide
parathyroid gland
parathyroid hormone (PTH)
pheochromocytoma

pituitary gland
polydipsia
polyphagia
polyuria
positive feedback system
PP cell
somatostatin
syndrome of inappropriate
    antidiuretic hormone (SIADH)
T_3
T_4
thyroid gland
thyroid-stimulating hormone
    (TSH)
thyrotoxicosis
type 1 diabetes
type 2 diabetes

he endocrine system consists of glands located throughout the body (**Figure 10-1**) responsible for producing and secreting a wide range of hormones and chemical transmitters. These hormones serve as chemical messengers by traveling to various sites to regulate several processes, including (1) growth and development, (2) metabolism, (3) sexual function, (4) reproduction, and (5) mood stability. Hormones influ-ence these processes by binding to receptors on the sur-face or within their target cells. Hormones are potent substances that only require small amounts to make a significant impact at the cellular and organism level. Subtle fluctuations in hormone levels can disrupt the body's delicate balance. Disorders of the endocrine sys-tem can result from insufficient or excessive amounts of these hormones that alter their specific function.

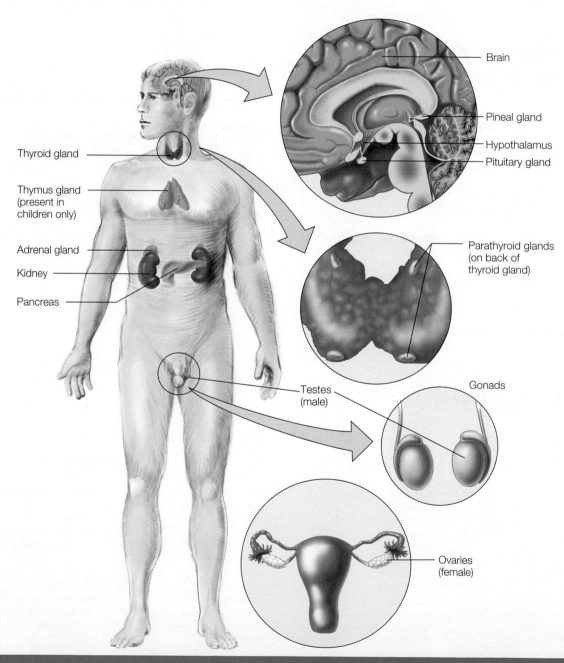

Figure 10-1

The human endocrine system.

Causes of these disorders vary and include genetic alterations, lifestyle behaviors, and tumors. Severity of these endocrine disorders can range from mild conditions that are easily managed to life-shortening or life-threatening conditions.

Anatomy and Physiology

The endocrine system is a complex messaging and control system that interfaces with several body functions. The endocrine system uses hormones to orchestrate these multifaceted communication and control operations. Endocrine glands located throughout the body produce and secrete these hormones. The term *endocrine* refers to the act of secreting substances directly into the bloodstream (**Figure 10-2**) rather than in a duct (like the exocrine glands of the gastrointestinal tract; see Chapter 9). In addition to these structures, repro-

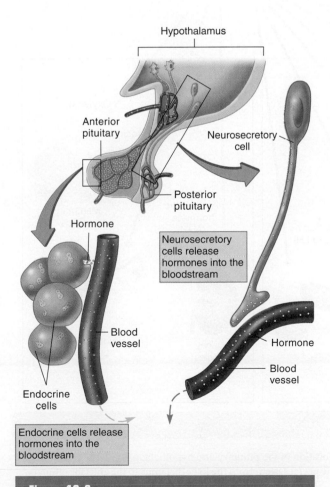

Hypothalamus

Anterior pituitary

Neurosecretory cell

Posterior pituitary

Hormone

Neurosecretory cells release hormones into the bloodstream

Blood vessel

Hormone

Blood vessel

Endocrine cells

Endocrine cells release hormones into the bloodstream

Figure 10-2

Endocrine release of hormones.

ductive glands (e.g., testes and ovaries) produce hormones (see Chapter 8). Hormones can be classified or described in regard to action (e.g., altering serum and glucose levels), source (e.g., anterior pituitary gland), or chemical structure. Hormones can be divided into four categories based on chemical composition: (1) steroids (e.g., androgens, glucocorticoids, and thyroid hormones), which are lipid soluble, (2) protein or polypeptides (e.g., insulin and growth hormone), which are water soluble, (3) amines and amino acids (e.g., epinephrine), which are water soluble, and (4) fatty acid derivatives (e.g., prostaglandins).

Release of these hormones from the gland is primarily controlled by a negative feedback system but may be controlled by a positive feedback system (see Chapter 1). The nervous system, other substances, and circadian rhythm can influence these systems. In a negative feedback loop, the end product (in this case hormones) of a biochemical process inhibits its own production—the hormone is only released when levels decline, and production stops when levels rise (e.g., insulin is released in response to serum glucose levels). In the endocrine system, a positive feedback loop is rare and occurs when one hormone product stimulates the production of another (e.g., release of oxytocin during childbirth). Tropic hormones regulate endocrine glands to produce other hormones (e.g., thyroid-stimulating hormone). Nontropic hormones directly stimulate cellular metabolism and other activities.

Once released from the gland, hormones travel through the circulatory system to their target cells in other glands and tissues. Multiple hormone signals continuously interact with these target cells, but these cells only respond to their specific hormone. This selective response is due to protein receptors located in the cell membrane or the cytoplasm. Once the hormone has acted on the target cells, the liver metabolizes and the kidneys excrete the hormone to prevent an accumulative effect.

Pituitary Gland and Hypothalamus

About the size of a pea, the pituitary gland is located at the base of the brain. The pituitary gland can be divided into two parts—the anterior and posterior pituitary gland. The pituitary gland is often referred to as the master gland. Despite its size, the pituitary gland secretes several hormones that influence many different body functions (**Figure 10-3; Table 10-1**). The hypothalamus, the basal (bottom) portion of the diencephalon, regulates the pituitary gland. The hypothal-

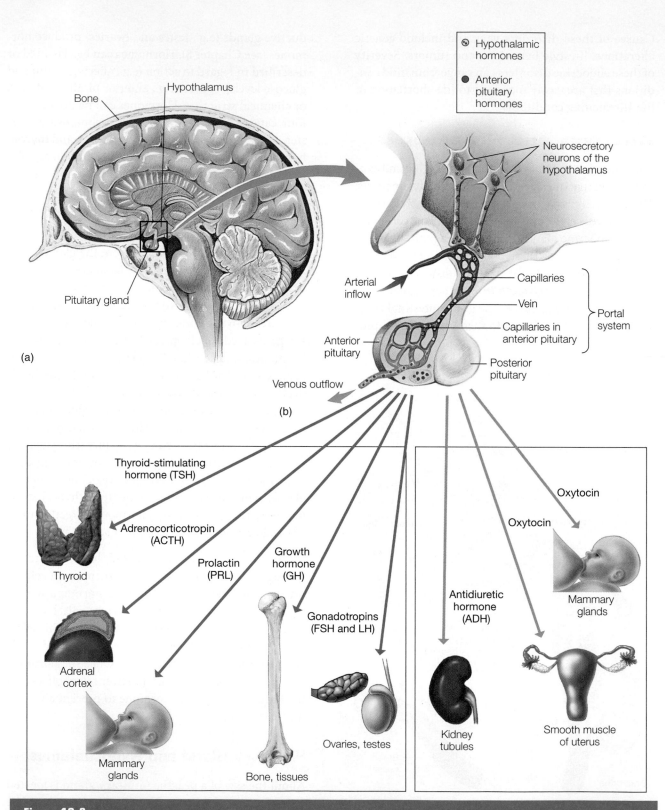

Hypothalamic hormones

Anterior pituitary hormones

Bone

Hypothalamus

Neurosecretory neurons of the hypothalamus

Arterial inflow

Capillaries

Vein

Capillaries in anterior pituitary

Portal system

Pituitary gland

Anterior pituitary

Posterior pituitary

(a)

Venous outflow

(b)

Thyroid-stimulating hormone (TSH)

Adrenocorticotropin (ACTH)

Prolactin (PRL)

Growth hormone (GH)

Gonadotropins (FSH and LH)

Antidiuretic hormone (ADH)

Oxytocin

Oxytocin

Thyroid

Adrenal cortex

Mammary glands

Bone, tissues

Ovaries, testes

Kidney tubules

Smooth muscle of uterus

Mammary glands

Figure 10-3

The pituitary gland. (a) A cross-section of the brain showing the location of the pituitary and hypothalamus. (b) The structure of the pituitary gland. Releasing and inhibiting hormones travel via the portal system from the hypothalamus to the anterior pituitary, where they affect hormone secretion.

amus connects the nervous and endocrine systems. The hypothalamus contains receptors that monitor hormone, nutrient, and ion levels. When activated, these receptors stimulate neurosecretory neurons in the hypothalamus to secrete releasing and inhibiting hormones (Figure 10-2). These hypothalamus hormones regulate the hormones produced by the anterior pituitary gland (hypothalamic-pituitary axis). In contrast to the anterior pituitary, the brain controls the posterior pituitary gland by producing neurohormones in this region.

Pancreas

The pancreas is an organ with exocrine digestive functions (see Chapter 9) and endocrine functions. The pancreas lies underneath the stomach and between the two kidneys in the retroperitoneum (space behind the peritoneum) (Figure 10-4). The endocrine functions are carried out by the islets of Langerhans, situated among the many small acini (cell clusters that produce digestive enzymes) in the pancreas. The human pancreas contains approximately 1 million islets of Langerhans, and each islet of Langerhans contains five types of cells. These cells include alpha cells that secrete glucagon, beta cells that secrete insulin, delta cells that secrete somatostatin, PP cells that secrete a pancreatic polypeptide, and epsilon cells that secrete ghrelin. Glucagon is released when serum glucose levels fall. Glucagon stimulates the breakdown of glycogen to glucose, which raises serum glucose levels. Insulin

is released when serum glucose levels increase. Insulin stimulates cellular uptake of glucose, which decreases serum glucose levels. Amylin is released from the beta cells along with insulin. Amylin has a synergistic relationship with insulin to control glucose. Somatostatin in the pancreas regulates insulin and glucagon. The pancreatic polypeptide is thought to regulate some of the other pancreatic activities. Finally, ghrelin stimulates hunger.

Thyroid Gland

The thyroid gland (Figure 10-5) is located at the base of the neck below the larynx. The thyroid gland consists of two lobes, one on either side of the trachea, connected by a thin band of tissue (isthmus) that extends across the anterior aspect of the trachea. The thyroid is a vascular gland that contains several functional units called follicles. These follicles produce three hormones: (1) thyroxine, or T_4, (2) triiodothyronine, or T_3, and (3) thyrocalcitonin, or calcitonin. T_3 and T_4 (95% of circulating thyroid hormones) regulate cellular metabolism as well as growth and development. The hypothalamus stimulates the pituitary gland to produce the thyroid-stimulating hormone (TSH) using the negative feedback system. TSH promotes the thyroid to produce T_3 and T_4. The thyroid requires iodine to synthesize these hormones. Calcitonin, along with the parathyroid hormone, regulates serum calcium levels. Calcitonin alters serum calcium levels by inhibiting osteoclast activity (which decreases calcium release from the bone) and

Table 10-1 Hormones Secreted by the Pituitary Gland

Hormone	Function
Anterior pituitary	
Growth hormone (GH)	Stimulates cell growth. Primary targets are muscle and bone, where GH stimulates amino acid uptake and protein synthesis. It also stimulates fat breakdown in the body.
Thyroid-stimulating hormone (TSH)	Stimulates release of thyroxine and triiodothyronine.
Adrenocorticotropic hormone (ACTH)	Stimulates secretion of hormones by the adrenal cortex, especially glucocorticoids.
Gonadotropins (FSH and LH)	Stimulate gamete production and hormone production by the gonads.
Prolactin	Stimulates milk production by the breast.
Melanocyte-stimulating hormone (MSH)	Function in humans is unknown.
Posterior pituitary	
Antidiuretic hormone (ADH)	Stimulates water reabsorption by nephrons of the kidney.
Oxytocin	Stimulates ejection of milk from breasts and uterine contractions during birth.

Source: Chiras, D. (2008). *Human biology* (6th ed.). Sudbury, MA: Jones & Bartlett Learning.

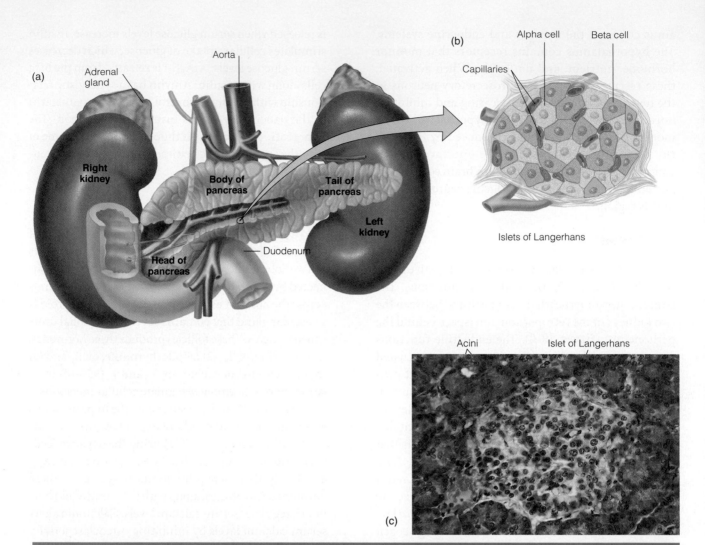

Figure 10-4

The pancreas. (a) The pancreas produces two hormones, insulin and glucagon, as well as digestive enzymes. (b) Hormones are produced by specialized cells within the islets of Langerhans. (c) The islets of Langerhans are located among the acini, very small groups of digestive-enzyme-producing cells of the pancreas.

stimulating osteoblast activity (which increases calcium deposits in the bone). Calcitonin is also regulated with a negative feedback system and is secreted when serum calcium levels are high.

Parathyroid Glands

The parathyroid glands, usually four in number, are located on the posterior surface of the thyroid. Each parathyroid gland secretes the parathyroid hormone (PTH). PTH works opposite of calcitonin to regulate serum calcium levels. PTH is secreted when serum calcium levels drop. PTH increases serum calcium lev-

els by increasing osteoclast activity (which increases calcium release from the bone) as well as increasing absorption of calcium in the gastrointestinal tract and kidneys.

Adrenal Glands

The adrenal glands are located on each kidney. Each adrenal gland has an inner portion, or medulla, and an outer portion, or cortex. The hypothalamus influences both portions of the adrenal gland but by different mechanisms. The adrenal cortex is regulated by negative feedback involving the hypothalamus and adre-

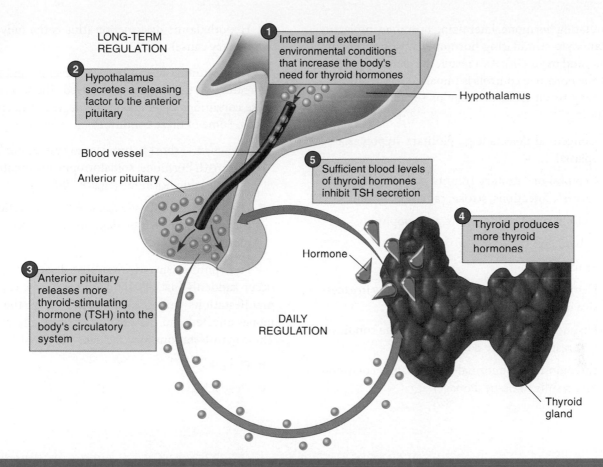

LONG-TERM
REGULATION

1 Internal and external environmental conditions that increase the body's need for thyroid hormones

Hypothalamus

2 Hypothalamus secretes a releasing factor to the anterior pituitary

Blood vessel

Anterior pituitary

5 Sufficient blood levels of thyroid hormones inhibit TSH secretion

4 Thyroid produces more thyroid hormones

Hormone

3 Anterior pituitary releases more thyroid-stimulating hormone (TSH) into the body's circulatory system

DAILY
REGULATION

Thyroid gland

Figure 10-5

The thyroid gland.

nocorticotropic hormones; the medulla is regulated by nerve impulses from the hypothalamus. The medulla produces epinephrine and norepinephrine during times of stress. Epinephrine and norepinephrine mediate the fight-or-flight response of the sympathetic nervous system (see Chapter 2). The cortex has three separate regions that produce different steroids. Mineralocorticoids are secreted by the outermost region of the adrenal cortex. The principal mineralocorticoid is aldosterone, which acts to conserve sodium and water in the body. Glucocorticoids are secreted by the middle region of the adrenal cortex. The principal glucocorticoid is cortisol, which increases serum glucose levels. Lastly, gonadocorticoids, or sex hormones, are secreted by the innermost region of the cortex. Male hormones (e.g., androgen) and female hormones (e.g., estrogen) are secreted in minimal amounts in both sexes by the adrenal cortex, but the hormones from the testes and ovaries usually mask their effect. In females, the masculinization effect of androgen secretion may become evident after menopause, when estrogen levels from the ovaries decrease.

Disorders of the Pituitary Gland

Disorders of the pituitary gland can have significant consequences because of the many hormones and processes it impacts. Like most endocrine disorders, pituitary gland disorders result in either increased or decreased levels of hormones associated with the gland (Table 10-1). These conditions can be caused by tumors (most common), infection, trauma, and necrosis.

Hypopituitarism

Hypopituitarism is a rare, complex condition in which the pituitary gland does not produce sufficient amounts of some or all of its hormones (e.g., TSH, growth hormone, adrenocorticotropic hormone [ACTH], follicle-stimulating hormone, luteinizing hormone, prolactin melanocyte-stimulating hormone, antidiuretic hormone, and oxytocin). As a result, the gland or process that the hormone controls is impaired. Hypopituitarism may result from primary or secondary causes, including:

- Congenital defects (e.g., pituitary hypoplasia or aplasia)

- Cerebral or pituitary trauma (may be a result of surgery, infections, stroke, radiation, or injury)

- Autoimmune conditions (e.g., hypophysitis)

- Tuberculosis

- Pituitary tumors

- Hemochromatosis (a condition resulting in excessive iron absorption)

- Histiocytosis X (an abnormal immune condition that results in tissue damage)

- Sarcoidosis (an abnormal inflammatory condition that results in tissue damage)

- Hypothalamic dysfunction (this is the only secondary cause)

Hypopituitarism can result in several conditions depending on the hormones involved. The severity of these conditions depends on the degree of hormone deficit. Some of these conditions include:

- **Dwarfism**—short stature caused by deficient levels of growth hormone, somatotropin, or somatotropin-releasing hormone (**Figure 10-6**)

- **Diabetes insipidus**—excessive fluid excretion in the kidneys caused by deficient antidiuretic hormone levels

Hypopituitarism is a progressive disorder that can occur suddenly but usually develops slowly. Clinical manifestations vary greatly depending on the hormones affected and the severity of those alterations. These manifestations may include:

- Fatigue

- Headache

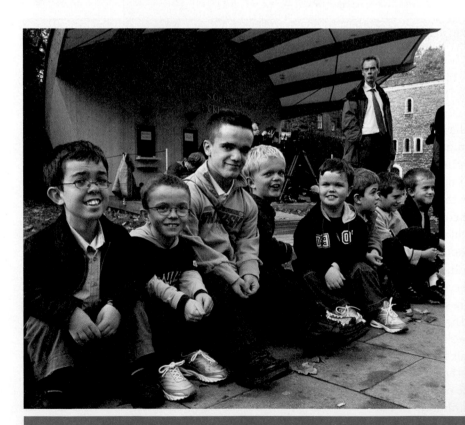
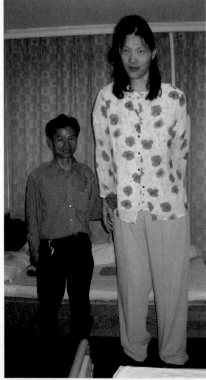

Figure 10-6

(a) Dwarfism and (b) gigantism.

- Cessation of menstruation
- Infertility (in women)
- Decreased libido
- Low tolerance for stress
- Muscle weakness
- Nausea
- Constipation
- Weight loss or gain
- Anorexia
- Abdominal discomfort
- Cold sensitivity
- Visual disturbances
- Loss of body or facial hair
- Joint stiffness
- Hoarseness
- Facial puffiness
- Thirst
- Excessive urination
- Hypotension
- Short stature
- Delayed growth and development

Diagnosis of hypopituitarism is often delayed because of the varying presentation. Diagnostic procedures usually include a history, physical examination, serum hormone levels, brain computed tomography (CT), pituitary magnetic resonance imaging (MRI), vision testing, and X-rays (to identify any bone abnormalities). Lifelong hormone replacement therapy is the cornerstone of treatment. Resolving the underlying cause is also important when possible (e.g., cancer treatment). Additional strategies depend on the specific hormones affected (e.g., infertility treatments, counseling). The patient will likely require monitoring by an endocrinologist and will need to wear a medical alert bracelet.

Hyperpituitarism

Hyperpituitarism is a condition in which the pituitary gland secretes excessive amounts of one or all of the pituitary hormones. Hyperpituitarism is most commonly caused by tumors that secrete hormone or hormone-like substances. Hyperpituitarism can result in several conditions depending on the hormones involved. The severity of these conditions depends on the degree of hormone excess. Some of these conditions include:

- Gigantism—tall stature caused by excessive growth hormone levels prior to puberty (Figure 10-6)
- Acromegaly—increased bone size caused by excessive growth hormone levels in adulthood (**Figure 10-7**)
- Syndrome of inappropriate antidiuretic hormone (SIADH)—increased renal water retention caused by excessive antidiuretic hormone levels
- Hyperprolactinemia—excessive prolactin levels that result in menstrual dysfunction and galactorrhea (inappropriate lactation)
- Cushing's syndrome—excessive cortisol levels that result from the increased ACTH levels
- Hyperthyroidism—hypermetabolic state caused by excessive thyroid hormones that result from increased TSH levels

Hyperpituitarism is a progressive disorder that can occur suddenly but usually develops slowly. Clinical manifestations vary greatly depending on the hormones affected and the severity of those alterations. These manifestations are similar to hypopituitarism and may include:

- Headache
- Visual field loss or double vision
- Excessive sweating
- Hoarseness
- Galactorrhea
- Sleep apnea
- Carpal tunnel syndrome
- Joint pain and stiffness
- Muscle weakness
- Paresthesia

Diagnosis of hyperpituitarism is often delayed because of the varying presentation. Diagnostic procedures usually include a history, physical examination, serum hormone levels, brain CT, pituitary MRI, vision testing, and X-rays (to identify any bone abnormalities). Treatment strategies depend on the underlying etiology and the hormone affected. Tumors will likely require surgery, radiation, and chemotherapy, but the tumors often reoccur. Additionally, analogues that inhibit hormone production may be given.

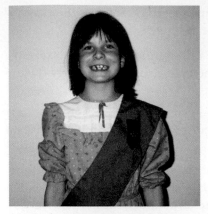

(a)

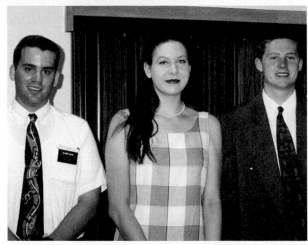

(b)

(c)

Figure 10-7

A woman with acromegaly (a) as a child, (b) as a teenager, and (c) as an adult.

Diabetes Mellitus

Diabetes mellitus (DM) refers to a group of conditions characterized by hyperglycemia (high serum glucose levels) resulting from defects in insulin production, insulin action, or both. Glucose is a vital energy source for the body, but insulin is required for glucose to travel into the cell where it can be used. Insulin acts like a key to unlock the cell membrane and allow the glucose to enter. Impaired insulin production or action results in abnormal carbohydrate, protein, and fat metabolism because of the glucose transportation issue. Some cells, such as those in the brain, digestive tract, and skeletal muscles, can use glucose without insulin to some degree. DM can occur in three forms—type 1, type 2, and gestational diabetes—each with its own pathogenesis.

DM is extremely common in the United States—24 million (7.8%) Americans have diabetes (Centers for Disease Control and Prevention, 2007). An estimated 220 million people worldwide have DM (World Health Organization, 2009). In the United States, DM prevalence rates have been climbing since 1980. DM is most common in people over 60 years of age, with nearly 25% of this population having DM. DM is most frequent among American Indians (who have the highest rates), African Americans, and Hispanics. The southeast region of the United States has the highest burden of DM. DM is a significant contributor to mortality. Although DM was only the seventh most common listed cause of death on death certificates in 2007, DM likely contributed to many more deaths. According to the CDC (2007), the risk of death for persons with DM is twice that of persons without DM. In 2007, DM cost accounted for $116 billion in direct medical costs (e.g., hospitalizations, medical care, and treatment supplies) and $58 billion in indirect costs (e.g., disability payments, time lost from work, and premature death).

DM can result in an array of acute and chronic complications. Acute complications of DM may include:

- Hyperglycemia—may be a result of excessive dietary carbohydrate intake as well as insufficient or inappropriate diabetic pharmacologic therapy.

- Diabetic ketoacidosis—pH imbalance characterized by increased ketones in the urine caused by insufficient insulin; if cells are starved for energy, the body may begin to break down fat-producing toxic acids (ketones).

- Hypoglycemia (low serum glucose level)—may result from insufficient dietary intake, increased physical activity, and excessive diabetic pharmacologic therapy.

Chronic complications are a direct result of long-term excessive glucose levels, especially when DM is not adequately managed. Over time, increased glucose levels contribute to thickening and hardening of vessel walls (much like how the sugar in icing hardens on a cake), causing diffuse ischemia and necrosis. DM complications reflect these circulatory changes. Adequate DM management can best prevent chronic complications. These complications include:

- Heart disease—heart disease death rates are 2 to 4 times higher in people with DM.

- Stroke—occurrence rates are 2 to 4 times higher in people with DM.

- Hypertension—75% of people with DM also have hypertension.

- Diabetic retinopathy.

- Blindness—DM as a result of diabetic retinopathy is the leading cause of blindness.

- Renal failure—DM is the leading cause of renal failure.

- Diabetic neuropathy—approximately 70% of people with DM have neuropathy (pain and numbness in the hands and feet).

- Amputations—approximately 60% of nontraumatic amputations occur in persons with DM.

- Periodontal disease—occurrence rates are approximately 2 times higher in people with DM.

- Pregnancy complications (e.g., birth defects and high birth weights).

- Increased susceptibility to infections and delayed healing.

- Erectile dysfunction.

Clinical manifestations of DM may vary depending on the type. These manifestations are a direct result of the excess glucose levels and include:

- Hyperglycemia

- Glucosuria (glucose is excreted in the urine in an attempt to lower serum levels)

- Polyuria (increased urine output because of the osmotic effects of the glucose in the urine)

- Polydipsia (increased thirst because of the dehydration caused by the increased urine output)

- Polyphagia (increased appetite because of the energy loss as the glucose is excreted)

- Weight loss (from increased fat catabolism)

- Blurred vision (excessive glucose changes the shape and flexibility of the lens of the eye, distorting the ability to focus and causing blurred vision)

- Fatigue (because of a lack of an energy source)

Diagnostic procedures for DM are complex. These procedures are used for diagnosing DM and complications as well as to assess DM management (**Table 10-2**). Diagnostic procedures include a history, physical examination, urinalysis (to detect the presence of

LEARNING POINTS

The classic clinical manifestations of diabetes mellitus (DM) is referred to as the *three P's*—polyuria, polydipsia, and polyphagia. As the levels of glucose increase in the bloodstream, the kidneys try to compensate by increasing urinary excretion. Normally, glucose is not found in the urine, so the presence of any glucose in the urine is an abnormal finding. Glucose has a similar relationship with water that sodium does (see Chapter 6)—*wherever glucose is, water will follow it*. Because glucose is being excreted in the urine, more water is excreted (polyuria). The excess water loss creates a fluid volume deficit, which triggers the thirst sensation in an attempt to replace the fluid (polydipsia). Additionally, the loss of glucose creates an energy deficit, which triggers the hunger sensation (polyphagia).

Table 10-2 Diagnostic Procedures for Diabetes Mellitus

Criteria for Diagnosis of Prediabetes

Impaired fasting glucose 100–125 mg/dL (fasting plasma glucose) and/or impaired glucose tolerance 140–199 mg/dL (2-hour post-75 g glucose challenge).

Criteria for Diagnosis of Diabetes

Random plasma glucose ≥ 200 mg/dL with symptoms (polyuria, polydipsia, and unexplained weight loss) and/or fasting plasma glucose ≥ 126 mg/dL[a] and/or 2-hour plasma glucose ≥ 200 mg/dL[a] post-75 g glucose challenge.

Treatment Goals for the ABCs of Diabetes

A1C
Should be < 7 % for patients in general.
Preprandial capillary plasma glucose 70–130 mg/dL.
Peak postprandial capillary plasma glucose < 180 mg/dL (usually 1–2 hours after the start of a meal). Be alert to the impact of hemoglobin variants on A1C values.
See www2.niddk.nih.gov/variants for more information.

Blood Pressure (mm Hg)

Systolic < 130
Diastolic < 80

Cholesterol—Lipid Profile (mg/dL)

LDL cholesterol < 100
HDL cholesterol
  Men > 40
  Women > 50
Triglycerides < 150

[a]Repeat to confirm on subsequent day unless symptoms are present.
Source: American Diabetes Association. (2009). American Diabetes Association standards of medical care. *Diabetes Care,* *32*(Suppl. 1): S13–S61.

glucose), fasting blood glucose test, oral glucose tolerance test, random blood glucose test, hemoglobin A1C (HgbA1C) (an average of glucose control for the previous 2–3 months), blood pressure measurement, and cholesterol panel. Treatment strategies for DM vary depending on the type, but dietary changes (American Diabetic Association recommendations) and exercise are the first line of treatment. Management also includes self-glucose monitoring, weight loss (if the patient is overweight), oral hyperglycemia medications, supplemental insulin, and complication management.

Type 1 Diabetes

Type 1 diabetes was previously called insulin-dependent DM and juvenile-onset DM. Type 1 DM develops when the body's immune system destroys pancreatic beta cells. To survive, people with type 1 DM must have insulin delivered by injection or a pump. This form of DM usually strikes children and young adults,

although disease onset can occur at any age. In adults, type 1 DM accounts for 5–10% of all diagnosed cases. The exact cause of type 1 diabetes is unknown, but most likely a viral or environmental trigger in genetically susceptible people causes an autoimmune reaction. Type 1 DM cannot be prevented.

Type 2 Diabetes

Type 2 diabetes was previously called non–insulin-dependent DM and adult-onset DM. In adults, type 2 DM accounts for about 90–95% of all newly diagnosed DM cases. Type 2 DM usually begins as insulin resistance, a disorder in which the body's cells do not use insulin properly. As the need for insulin rises, the pancreas gradually loses its ability to produce it. Type 2 DM is associated with advancing age, obesity, family history of DM, history of gestational DM, impaired glucose metabolism, and physical inactivity. African Americans, Hispanics, American Indians, Asians,

Native Hawaiians, and other Pacific Islanders are at particularly high risk for type 2 DM and its complications. Type 2 DM in children and adolescents, although still rare, is being diagnosed more frequently among American Indians, African Americans, Hispanics, Asians, and Pacific Islanders. Type 2 DM is usually managed initially with oral antidiabetic medications that increase insulin production and action. As the condition progresses, supplemental insulin is often necessary as pancreatic production declines.

Gestational Diabetes

Gestational diabetes is a form of glucose intolerance diagnosed during pregnancy. Gestational DM occurs most frequently among African Americans, Hispanics, and American Indians. Other risk factors include obesity and a family history of DM. During pregnancy, gestational DM requires treatment (usually lifestyle changes and insulin) to normalize maternal blood glucose levels to avoid fetal complications. Immediately after pregnancy, 5–10% of women with gestational DM are diagnosed with DM, usually type 2. Women who have had gestational DM have a 40–60% chance of developing DM within 5–10 years.

Metabolic Syndrome

Metabolic syndrome is a cluster of risk factors occurring together—hyperglycemia, high blood pressure, hypercholesterolemia, and increased waist circumference. Metabolic syndrome is not a form of DM, but it is related because metabolic syndrome increases the risk of cardiovascular disease, DM, and stroke. Diagnostic

MYTH BUSTERS

There are several myths regarding diabetes mellitus (DM) in the community that merit discussion.

MYTH 1: **People with diabetes cannot eat sweets or chocolate.**

If chocolate and other sweets are eaten as part of a healthy meal plan, or combined with exercise, people with DM can eat them. They are no more off-limit foods for people with DM than they are for people without DM.

MYTH 2: **Eating too much sugar causes diabetes.**

DM is caused by a combination of genetic and lifestyle factors, not from eating too much sugar. However, being overweight does increase your risk for developing type 2 DM. If there is a family history of DM, following a healthy meal plan and getting regular exercise are recommended to manage weight.

MYTH 3: **Pills for DM are oral insulin.**

Oral medications for DM work to affect the ability of the body to produce insulin and use insulin better—they are not oral insulin. Going through the gastrointestinal system would destroy the insulin; therefore, insulin is injected.

MYTH 4: **Drinking water can excrete the extra sugar in the blood.**

Extra glucose in the blood cannot be excreted by drinking extra water. However, DM can be controlled by eating healthy food, being physically active, controlling weight, routine examinations, taking prescribed medications, and monitoring blood glucose often.

MYTH 5: **Fruit is a healthy food. Therefore, it is acceptable to eat large quantities of fruit.**

Fruit is a healthy food, containing fiber and lots of vitamins and minerals. Because fruit contains carbohydrates that break down quickly into simple sugars, it needs to be included in a healthy meal plan, but amounts should be controlled because fruit will raise blood glucose levels.

MYTH 6: **When taking oral diabetic medications or insulin, people with DM can eat anything they want.**

The oral medications or insulin taken for DM are more effective when they do not have to work as hard to lower blood glucose. Combining medicines with a healthy meal plan and physical activity gives better glucose control.

MYTH 7: **Once one begins taking oral diabetic medications or insulin for type 2 diabetes, they must be taken for life.**

Sometimes, there are temporary circumstances that cause elevated glucose levels (e.g., glucocorticoid therapy, total parental nutrition administration), and diabetic medications will only be needed during those events. With weight loss, exercise, and healthy dieting, some people who have been started on oral diabetic medications and/or insulin find that they can control their blood glucose without medications.

criteria of metabolic syndrome include the presence of more than one of those risk factors. Treatment strategies focus on lifestyle changes (e.g., weight loss, dietary changes, and physical activity) to prevent complication development.

Disorders of the Thyroid

Because of the thyroid hormone's responsibilities, disorders of the thyroid have a significant impact on metabolic activities. These disorders result in an increase or decrease in the thyroid hormones. Several etiologies can result in these conditions, including tumors, congenital defects, damage (from surgery, radiation, infections, etc.), and aging. These conditions are usually easily managed with medications and surgery.

Goiter

A goiter refers to a visible enlargement of the thyroid gland (**Figure 10-8**). This enlargement is usually painless but may affect the respiratory and gastrointestinal systems. The enlargement is not necessarily malignant.

Goiters can occur in hyperthyroidism, hypothyroidism, and normal thyroid states. Iodine deficiency is the most common cause of goiters in the United States. Iodine deficiency leads to decreased T_3 and T_4 production. TSH production increases in an attempt to compensate for the low levels of thyroid hormones. Increased levels of TSH produce thyroid hyperplasia and hypertrophy. This similar reaction occurs in both hyperthyroidism and hypothyroidism states.

Hypothyroidism

Hypothyroidism refers to a condition in which the thyroid does not produce sufficient amounts of the thyroid hormones. Hypothyroidism is relatively common (1 out of 500 Americans has the condition) and may be a result of hypothalamus, pituitary, or thyroid (the most common) dysfunction. Several conditions can result in hypothyroidism. Hypothyroidism risk increases with age (especially for those over 50 years old). First, a previous or currently ongoing inflammation of the thyroid gland can leave a large percentage of thyroid cells damaged and incapable of producing

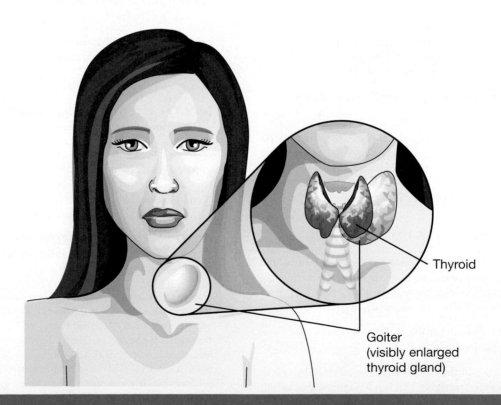

Thyroid

Goiter
(visibly enlarged
thyroid gland)

Figure 10-8

Goiter.

sufficient hormone amounts. The most common cause of thyroid gland failure is called autoimmune thyroiditis (also called **Hashimoto's thyroiditis**). The second major cause is iatrogenic (resulting from medical treatments). The treatment of many thyroid conditions, such as hyperthyroidism, warrants partial or complete surgical removal of the thyroid gland. If the total remaining thyroid-producing cells are not enough to meet the needs of the body, hypothyroidism develops. This result is often the goal of the surgery for thyroid cancer. Similarly, goiters and some other thyroid conditions can be treated with radioactive iodine therapy. The aim of the radioactive iodine therapy (for benign conditions) is to kill a portion of the thyroid to prevent goiters from growing larger or developing into hyperthyroidism. Occasionally, the radioactive iodine treatment can damage too many cells, but this consequence is usually preferred over the original problem.

The clinical manifestations of hypothyroidism vary widely, depending on the severity of the hormone deficiency. Generally, clinical manifestations tend to be insidious and develop slowly, often over a number of years. These clinical manifestations reflect decreased thyroid activity (e.g., metabolism) and usually include:

- Fatigue
- Sluggishness
- Increased sensitivity to cold
- Constipation
- Pale, dry skin
- Facial edema
- Hoarseness
- Hypercholesterolemia
- Unexplained weight gain
- Myalgia
- Arthralgia
- Muscle weakness
- Heavier than normal menstrual periods
- Brittle fingernails
- Hair loss or thinning
- Bradycardia
- Hypotension
- Constipation
- Depression
- Goiter

Advanced hypothyroidism, known as **myxedema**, is rare, but when it occurs, myxedema can be life threatening. Clinical manifestations include marked hypotension, respiratory depression, hypothermia, lethargy, and coma.

Diagnostic procedures for hypothyroidism include a history, physical examination, serum thyroid hormone levels, serum TSH, and cholesterol panel. Hypothyroidism is easily managed with thyroid hormone replacement. Additional strategies are implemented to manage symptoms and may include weight management (e.g., low-calorie diet and increased physical activity), constipation measures (e.g., stool softener and increase in dietary fiber and fluid intake), and avoidance of cold temperatures.

Hyperthyroidism

Hyperthyroidism refers to a condition of excessive levels of thyroid hormones. This overabundance of thyroid hormones results in a hypermetabolic state. Hyperthyroidism can result from a variety of conditions including:

- Excessive iodine
- **Graves' disease** (autoimmune condition that stimulates thyroid hormone production)
- Nonmalignant thyroid tumors (which produce thyroid or thyroidlike hormones)
- Thyroid inflammation (increased capillary permeability resulting from the inflammatory process leads to additional thyroid hormones to be released in the bloodstream)
- Taking large amounts of thyroid hormone replacement

Hyperthyroidism can mimic other health problems, and clinical manifestations can vary, making diagnosis difficult. Clinical manifestations reflect increased thyroid activity and may include:

- Sudden weight loss
- Tachycardia
- Hypertension
- Increased appetite
- Nervousness, anxiety or anxiety attacks, and irritability
- Tremor (usually a fine trembling in the hands)
- Diaphoresis
- Changes in menstrual patterns

- Increased sensitivity to heat
- Diarrhea
- Goiter
- Difficulty sleeping
- **Exophthalmos** (protruding eyes with decreased blinking and movement) (**Figure 10-9**)

Thyroid crisis (storm), also called **thyrotoxicosis**, is a sudden worsening of hyperthyroidism symptoms that may occur with infection or stress. Fever, decreased mental alertness, and abdominal pain may occur. Thyrotoxicosis is a medical emergency. Additional complications of hyperthyroidism include dysrhythmias, heart failure, and osteoporosis.

Diagnostic procedures for hyperthyroidism include a history, physical examination, serum thyroid hormone levels, serum TSH, radioactive iodine uptake test, and thyroid scan. Hyperthyroidism can usually be easily managed with medication and surgery. Pharmacologic treatment usually includes radioactive iodine (which shrinks the gland), antithyroid agents (to decrease hormone production), and beta blockers

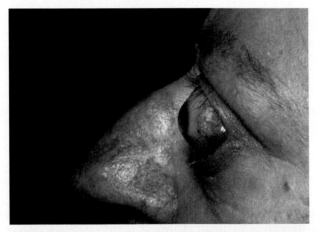
(a)

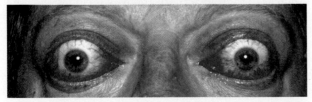
(b)

Figure 10-9

Exophthalmos.

LEARNING POINTS

Hypothyroidism and hyperthyroidism present very differently. When considering the clinical manifestations of these disorders, think about what increasing or decreasing thyroid hormones would do in the body. With hypothyroidism, the hormone levels are decreased and so are all the clinical manifestations (e.g., bradycardia, hypotension, depression, and constipation), with the exception of weight. With hyperthyroidism, the hormone levels are increased and so are all the clinical manifestations (e.g., tachycardia, hypertension, anxiety, and diarrhea) with the exception of weight.

(to treat cardiac symptoms). Surgical removal of the thyroid (thyroidectomy) with subsequent hormone replacement is warranted when the patient does not respond to or tolerate medications. Even with treatment, exophthalmus usually remains. Strategies to improve discomfort associated with exophthalmus include cool compresses, wearing sunglasses, eye lubricants, and elevating the head of the bed. Increasing caloric and calcium intake is crucial to maintain weight and prevent bone loss.

Disorders of the Parathyroid

Parathyroid disorders result in an increase or decrease in PTH. Because of PTH's responsibilities, disorders of the parathyroid have a significant impact on calcium balance that has a domino effect on other electrolytes (phosphorus and magnesium; see Chapter 6). Several etiologies can result in these conditions, including tumors, congenital defects, damage (from surgery, radiation, infections, etc.), and renal failure. These conditions are usually easily managed with medications and surgery.

Hypoparathyroidism

Hypoparathyroidism refers to a condition in which the parathyroid gland does not produce sufficient amounts of PTH. Hypoparathyroidism can be caused by congenital defects (a lack of one or more of the four parathyroid glands) as well as by damage following surgery, radiation, or autoimmune conditions. Hypoparathyroidism results in hypocalcemia and a subsequent increase in phosphorus. Additionally, hypomagnesemia and metabolic alkalosis can develop. The clinical manifestations reflect these electrolyte and pH imbalances. These manifestations include:

- Paresthesias of the fingertips, toes, and lips
- Muscle twitching or spasms (tetany)
- Fatigue or weakness
- Dysrhythmias
- Hypotension
- Abdominal cramping
- Diarrhea
- Painful menstruation
- Patchy hair loss
- Dry, coarse skin
- Brittle nails
- Anxiety or nervousness
- Headaches
- Depression or mood swings
- Memory loss

Diagnostic procedures for hypoparathyroidism include a history, physical examination, serum PTH check, blood chemistry, electrocardiogram (EKG), X-rays, and bone density studies. Treatment regimens rarely include PTH replacement. Strategies are generally focused on correcting electrolyte and pH imbalances (see Chapter 6).

Hyperparathyroidism

Hyperparathyroidism refers to a condition of excessive PTH production by the parathyroid glands. Hyperparathyroidism may be caused by tumors, hyperplasia, or chronic hypocalcemia (renal failure). Hyperparathyroidism will result in hypercalcemia. The excessive calcium levels can lead to decreases in phosphorus, increases in magnesium, and metabolic acidosis (see Chapter 6). Clinical manifestations reflect these electrolyte and pH imbalances and may include:

- Osteoporosis
- Renal calculi
- Polyuria
- Abdominal pain
- Constipation
- Fatigue or weakness
- Flaccid muscles

- Dysrhythmias
- Hypertension
- Depression or forgetfulness
- Bone and joint pain
- Nausea and vomiting
- Anorexia

Diagnostic procedures for hyperparathyroidism include a history, physical examination, serum PTH check, blood chemistry, EKG, X-rays, and bone density studies. Treatment varies depending on the underlying etiology. Tumors will likely require surgery and radiation. Calcitonin may be administered to shift the calcium from the bloodstream to the bones. Phosphates may be administered to correct phosphorus deficits, which will decrease calcium levels (see Chapter 6). Increasing fluid intake (either oral or intravenous) will increase renal excretion of calcium. Additionally, magnesium and pH imbalances may need correcting (see Chapter 6).

Disorders of the Adrenal Glands

Adrenal gland disorders may affect one or both areas of the adrenal gland. These disorders result in an increase or decrease in one or more adrenal hormones. Depending on the hormone affected and the severity, these disorders can have serious consequences. Several etiologies can result in these conditions including tumors, congenital defects, medications (e.g., corticosteroids), and damage (from surgery, radiation, infections, etc.). These conditions are usually easily managed with medications and surgery, but they can become life threatening if not managed promptly.

Pheochromocytoma

Pheochromocytoma is a rare tumor of the adrenal medulla. The tumor excretes epinephrine and norepinephrine and can be life threatening because of the effects of epinephrine and norepinephrine (e.g., increased blood pressure and tachycardia). Pheochromocytoma can occur as a single tumor or multiple tumors in one or both adrenal glands, but the tumor is rarely malignant (10% of cases). Clinical manifestations reflect the fight-or-flight response and include:

- Hypertension
- Tachycardia

- Forceful heartbeat
- Profound diaphoresis
- Abdominal pain
- Sudden onset of severe headaches
- Anxiety
- Feeling of extreme fright
- Pallor
- Weight loss

Diagnostic procedures for pheochromocytoma include a history, physical examination, serum levels of epinephrine and norepinephrine, abdominal CT, abdominal MRI, m-iodobenzylguanidine scintiscan (a nuclear scan to confirm pheochromocytoma), and biopsy. If not promptly treated, pheochromocytoma can lead to hypertensive crisis, stroke, renal failure, psychosis, and seizures. Surgical removal of the tumor or adrenal gland is the cornerstone of treatment. Antihypertensive medications are often necessary until surgery can be performed.

Cushing's Syndrome

Cushing's syndrome is a condition of excessive amounts of glucocorticoids. The most common cause of this excess is iatrogenic, resulting from ingestion of glucocorticoid medications. When these medications are ingested, they mimic the body's own hormones. This condition can also be caused by adrenal tumors that secrete glucocorticoids or pituitary tumors that secrete ACTH and cortisol. Paraneoplastic syndrome resulting from cancers outside the endocrine system can also cause Cushing's syndrome by increasing production of ACTH and cortisol. Glucocorticoids are essential for life but can produce serious effects in excessive amounts (**Figure 10-10**). Clinical manifestations are a direct result of the excessive amounts of glucocorticoids and include:

- Obesity (especially around the trunk)
- Round, full, red face ("moon" face)
- Fatty pad between shoulders ("buffalo hump")
- Muscle weakness
- Delayed growth and development
- Acne
- Broad purple striae (marks) on abdomen, thighs, and breast

CASE STUDY

A 68-year-old woman with an 8-year history of diabetes mellitus (DM) presents to the clinic for worsening dyspnea and cough. She has had chronic obstructive pulmonary disease (COPD) (see Chapter 5) since age 55. She now has dyspnea from walking one third of a block, as well as a persistent cough. She has managed her type 2 DM with diet and exercise. Her last glycosylated hemoglobin (HgbA1C) measured 1 month ago was 6.8% (a normal range is 4–6%). Physical examination reveals an anxious woman with blood pressure of 134/70 mm Hg, pulse of 116, respiratory rate of 24 breaths per minute, and weight of 190 pounds. Expiratory wheezing is present bilaterally. No accessory muscles are being used. No cyanosis is present. The lab evaluation results are: arterial blood gas (ABG) 7.46; PaO_2 60; $PaCO_2$ 40; O_2 Sat 88% (see Chapter 6). She is started on albuterol (bronchodilator) and a course of prednisone (glucocorticoid) at 40 mg/day for 3 days, and then tapering over 2 weeks. On day 3, she calls back to the clinic to report that her blood glucose level is 358 mg/dL at 4:00 p.m.

1. Which of the following is the most likely cause of this patient's acute loss of glucose control?

   A. An acid–base imbalance

   B. Prednisone therapy

   C. COPD exacerbation

   D. Albuterol

2. All of the following are important for this patient to learn regarding glucocorticoid therapy, but which is the most important?

   A. Monitor cuts for healing.

   B. Take the medication with food.

   C. Do not stop taking the medication abruptly.

   D. Contact her healthcare provider if she has any manifestations of infection.

3. Which of the following endocrine conditions is this patient at risk of developing?

   A. Hyperthyroidism

   B. Pheochromocytoma

   C. Addison's disease

   D. Cushing's syndrome

4. Given this patient's acute loss of glucose control, which of the following interventions would the nurse expect to be ordered for this patient?

   A. Insulin as needed per routine sliding scale (dosing based on blood glucose levels)

   B. Increase exercise

   C. Decrease caloric intake

   D. Decrease prednisone dose

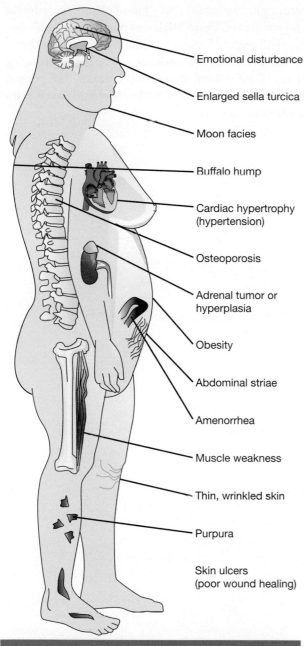

- Emotional disturbance
- Enlarged sella turcica
- Moon facies
- Buffalo hump
- Cardiac hypertrophy (hypertension)
- Osteoporosis
- Adrenal tumor or hyperplasia
- Obesity
- Abdominal striae
- Amenorrhea
- Muscle weakness
- Thin, wrinkled skin
- Purpura
- Skin ulcers (poor wound healing)

Figure 10-10

Signs and symptoms of Cushing's syndrome.

- Thin skin that bruises easily
- Delayed wound healing
- Osteoporosis
- Hirsutism (abnormal hair growth)
- Insulin resistance
- Hypertension

- Edema
- Hypokalemia
- Mood changes and psychosis

Diagnostic procedures for Cushing's syndrome include a history, physical examination, serum hormone levels (e.g., cortisol and ACTH), serum glucose, complete blood count (CBC), blood chemistry, bone density studies, adrenal and pituitary CT and MRI, and biopsy. Treatment varies depending on the underlying cause. Gradual tapering of any glucocorticoids being administered is crucial. If these medications are suddenly discontinued, the adrenal gland does not have the opportunity to initiate production, leading to an adrenal crisis. Tumors will likely require surgical removal and radiation. Interventions may be necessary to manage specific complications as they develop (e.g., osteoporosis, DM, and hypertension).

Addison's Disease

Addison's disease refers to a deficiency of adrenal cortex hormones (glucocorticoids, mineralocorticoids, and androgens). Addison's disease can be caused by damage resulting from autoimmune conditions (the most common cause), infections (e.g., tuberculosis, human immunodeficiency virus, fungal infections, and meningitis), hemorrhage, and tumors. Additionally, Addison's disease may result from pituitary dysfunction that results in insufficient ACTH levels. Clinical manifestations reflect the deficiency of the hormones and usually develop slowly over weeks to months. These manifestations include:

- Hypotension
- Changes in heart rate
- Hypoglycemia
- Chronic diarrhea
- Hyperpigmentation
- Pallor
- Extreme weakness and fatigue
- Anorexia
- Mouth lesions on the inside of a cheek (buccal mucosa)
- Nausea and vomiting
- Salt craving
- Slow, sluggish movement

- Unintentional weight loss
- Mood changes and depression
- Hyperkalemia

Diagnostic procedures for Addison's disease include a history, physical examination, serum hormone levels (e.g., cortisol, ACTH, and androgens), serum glucose levels, CBC, blood chemistry, adrenal and pituitary CT and MRI, and biopsy. Addison's disease will require lifelong hormone replacement therapy. Increases in hormone doses may be required during times of infections, stress, and trauma. The patient should wear a medical alert bracelet and carry extra medication at all times.

Chapter Summary

The endocrine system is responsible for producing a wide range of hormones that are necessary for a variety of processes. Endocrine disorders are often caused by congenital defects, tumors, or gland damage. These conditions vary from harmless to life threatening, and most of these disorders are managed easily with medications and surgery. Clinical manifestations of these conditions reflect the hormones affected and the degree of deviation. Regardless of the disorder and the severity, lifelong management is necessary to prevent significant complications or death.

Case Study Answers

1. B
2. C
3. D
4. A

References

Centers for Disease Control and Prevention. (2007). Retrieved from http://www.cdc.gov/diabetes/pubs/pdf/ndfs_2007.pdf

Chiras, D. (2008). *Human biology* (6th ed.). Sudbury, MA: Jones and Bartlett.

Elling, B., Elling, K., & Rothenberg, M. (2004). *Anatomy and physiology.* Sudbury, MA: Jones and Bartlett.

Gould, B. (2006). *Pathophysiology for the health professions* (3rd ed.). Philadelphia, PA: Elsevier.

Madara, B., & Pomarico-Denino, V. (2008). *Pathophysiology* (2nd ed.). Sudbury, MA: Jones and Bartlett.

Professional guide to pathophysiology (2nd ed.). (2007). Philadelphia, PA: Lippincott Williams & Wilkins.

World Health Organization. (2009). Retrieved from http://www.who.int/mediacentre/factsheets/fs312/en/index.html

Resources

www.cancer.gov

www.cancer.org

www.cdc.gov

www.diabetes.org

www.mayoclinic.com

www.medlineplus.gov

www.nih.gov

www.who.int

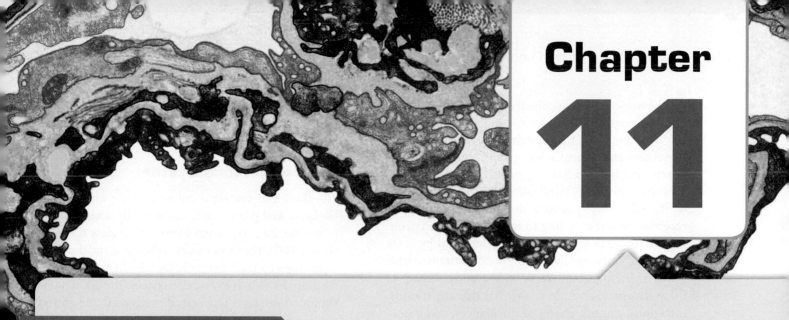

Neural Function

LEARNING OBJECTIVES

- Discuss normal neural anatomy and physiology.
- Describe and compare congenital neurologic disorders.
- Compare and contrast traumatic neurologic disorders.
- Compare and contrast infectious neurologic disorders.
- Describe and compare vascular neurologic disorders.
- Compare and contrast types of seizure disorders.
- Compare and contrast chronic degenerative neurologic disorders.
- Compare and contrast types of dementia.
- Describe and compare cancers of the nervous system.

KEY TERMS

action potential
afferent nerve
afferent tracts
AIDS dementia
  complex
Alzheimer's disease
  (AD)
amyotrophic lateral
  sclerosis (ALS)
arachnoid layer
ascending fibers
aura
automatism
autonomic
  hyperreflexia
autonomic nervous
  system
autoregulation
axon
basal ganglia
basilar skull fracture
brain
brain stem
cauda equina
cauda equina
  syndrome
central nervous
  system (CNS)

cerebellum
cerebral aneurysm
cerebral contusion
cerebral palsy (CP)
cerebral vascular
  accident (CVA)
cerebrospinal fluid
  (CSF)
cerebrum
chorea
comminuted skull
  fracture
communicating
  cerebrospinal fluid
  flow
compound skull
  fracture
concussion
countercoup
coup
cranial nerves
Creutzfeldt-Jakob
  disease (CJD)
Cushing's reflex
Cushing's triad
dementia
dendrite
depolarization

depressed skull
  fracture
dermatome
descending fibers
diencephalon
dorsal root
dura mater
efferent nerve
efferent tracts
encephalitis
epidural hematoma
epilepsy
epithalamus
flexor reflex
focal seizure
foramen magnum
frontal lobe
generalized seizure
gyrus
hematoma
hemorrhagic stroke
herniation
Huntington's disease
hydrocephalus
hypothalamus
increased intracranial
  pressure
interneuron

intracerebral
  hematoma
ischemic stroke
linear skull fracture
lobe
longitudinal fissure
medulla
meninges
meningitis
meningocele
midbrain
Monro-Kellie
  hypothesis
motor nerve
multiple sclerosis (MS)
myasthenia gravis
myasthenic crisis
myelin sheath
myelomeningocele
nerve
neuroglia
neuromelanin
neuron
neurotransmitter
node of Ranvier
noncommunicating
  cerebrospinal fluid
  flow

obstructive
  cerebrospinal fluid
  flow
occipital lobe
parasympathetic
  nervous system
parietal lobe
Parkinson's disease
peripheral nerve
peripheral nervous
  system (PNS)
pia mater
plexus
pons
postictal period
postsynaptic cell
  membrane
presynaptic terminal
prion
resting potential
reticular activation
  system
reticular formation
rootlet
Schwann cell
seizure
sensory nerve
spina bifida

spina bifida occulta
spinal cord
spinal cord injury (SCI)
spinal reflex arc
spinal shock
status epilepticus
subarachnoid
  hemorrhage
subdural hematoma
substantia nigra
subthalamus
sulcus
sympathetic nervous
  system (SNS)
synapse
synaptic cleft
temporal lobe
terminal bouton
thalamus
transient ischemic
  attack (TIA)
traumatic brain injury
  (TBI)
ventral root
ventricle
vertebral canal
white matter

he nervous system consists of complex structures that control many body functions and cognition. The functions this system manages include (1) structures such as muscles, glands, and organs; (2) heartbeat; (3) blood flow; (4) breathing; (5) digestion; (6) urination; and (7) defecation. The nervous system works with other systems to maintain homeostasis by receiving and responding to input from the environment. Disorders of the nervous system may be acute or chronic, but regardless, these conditions often have grave or life-altering effects on the body. Causes of these disorders include congenital defects, trauma, infections, tumors, chemical imbalances, and vascular changes.

Anatomy and Physiology

The nervous system is an intricate network of specialized cells and tissue that receive and react to environmental stimuli on a physiologic and cognitive level. To communicate this input, these structures conduct electric impulses between the brain and the rest of the body. The nervous system consists of three main components—brain, spinal cord, and nerves. The brain and spinal cord make up the central nervous system (CNS), and the nerves make up the peripheral nervous system (PNS).

Central Nervous System

The skull and vertebral column house and protect the brain and spinal cord. Additionally, a set of three tough membranes, called meninges, encase the CNS (Figure 11-1). The dura mater is the outer and toughest layer. The arachnoid layer is the middle layer, named for its spider web–like vascular system. The pia mater is the innermost layer that rests directly on the brain and spinal cord. Cerebrospinal fluid (CSF) is a plasmalike liquid that fills the space between the arachnoid and the pia mater layers to provide additional cushion and support to the CNS. The choroid plexus cells in the brain's ventricles continuously produce the CSF. The ventricles are interconnected, hollow areas of the brain where CSF fills and flows freely between them. Excess CSF drains into the bloodstream.

The brain is located within the skull and contains billions of neurons. Neural tissue contains two basic types of cells—neuroglia and neurons. Neuroglia cells

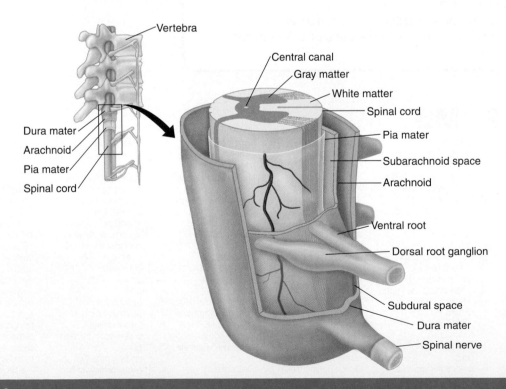

Figure 11-1

The meninges enclose the brain and the spinal cord.

provide several important supportive roles in the nervous system. Neuroglia cells scaffold neural tissue as well as isolate and protect neuron cell membranes. Additionally, neuroglia cells regulate interstitial fluid, defend the neuron against pathogens, and assist with neural repair.

Neurons are the fundamental unit of the nervous system that generate bioelectrical impulses and transmit them from one area of the body to another. Neurons occur in several sizes and shapes, but all neurons share similar characteristics. Neurons do not have the ability to divide; therefore, when neurons are lost due to aging or injury, they cannot be replaced. Not all cell death results in loss of functioning. For example, if neurons are damaged in one area of the brain, neurons in other areas can eventually assume those functions. In the PNS, severed nerves can regenerate to a point to reestablish connections with the tissue it once supplied. In the brain or spinal cord, severed axons cannot be repaired. Severed spinal cord nerves result in paralysis and loss of sensation below the area of damage. In addition to being unable to divide, nerve cells require a constant supply of oxygen and glucose. This characteristic makes neurons vulnerable to the effects of hypoxia and hypoglycemia. Neurons can begin dying within minutes of these events.

Most neurons have a spherical cell body that houses the nucleus, most of the cytoplasm, and organelles. Neurons contain projections called **axons** and **dendrites** that make connections with nearby cells (**Figure 11-2**). Axons transmit impulses away from the cell body, and dendrites transmit impulses toward the

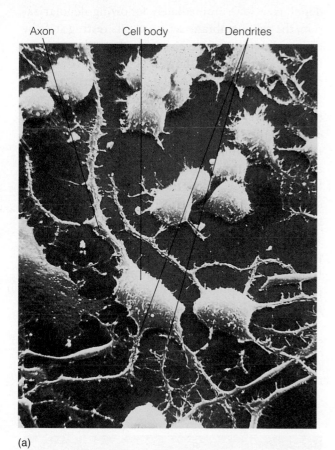

Axon   Cell body   Dendrites

(a)

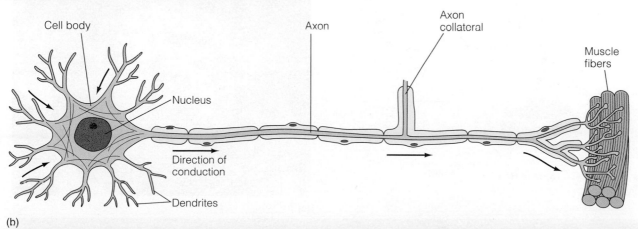

Cell body

Axon

Axon collateral

Muscle fibers

Nucleus

Direction of conduction

Dendrites

(b)

Figure 11-2

A neuron. (a) A scanning electron micrograph of the cell body and dendrites. (b) Collateral branches may occur along the length of the axon. In motor neurons, when the axon terminates, it branches many times, ending in individual muscle fibers.

cell body. When the axon reaches its destination, it often branches into several small fibers that terminate into miniscule bulges, called **terminal boutons**. These terminal boutons communicate with neurons, muscle fibers, or glands. Axons may be surrounded by a **myelin sheath** that increases the rate of impulse transmission approximately 400 times faster than unmyelinated nerves (**Figure 11-3**). **Schwann cells** produce the myelin sheath, and these Schwann cells are separated by **nodes of Ranvier**. Because of the myelin, the impulses move at greater speeds down the axon, jumping from one node to the next (like stones skipping across water). Bundles of these myelinated nerves are referred to as **white matter**. Impulses move in a slow, wavelike pattern in unmyelinated nerves. A **synapse** refers to the gap between the neurons. This gap includes the **presynaptic terminal** (e.g., terminal bouton or some similar structure), the **synaptic cleft** (space between neurons), and a **postsynaptic cell membrane** (**Figure 11-4**). The presynaptic and postsynaptic terminals are opposite ends of the nerve.

Electrical impulses of the nervous system are not like the electrical current that powers appliances, which is formed by the flow of electrons. Small ionic changes (e.g., potassium and sodium moving across cell membranes) generate neural impulses. Creating this charge is referred to as **action potential** (**Figure 11-5**). The plasma side of the neuron membrane has a slight charge at rest, or **resting potential**, because of the sodium ions concentrated on the outside of the cell. When the neuron is stimulated, protein gates open and sodium flows into the cell. The rapid inflow of positively charged sodium ions increases the charge (this is called **depolarization**). Immediately following depolarization, the cell membrane returns to its resting state by the rapid outflow of the positively charged potassium ions. When generated, these impulses travel down the nerve to trigger the release of **neurotransmitters** from the presynaptic terminal. The neurotransmitters cross the synaptic cleft, only in one direction, to stimulate an electrical reaction in nearby neurons. Synaptic transmission of the impulse takes a mere millisecond. This electrical reaction passes through those neurons to the next synapse, where the process repeats. At each synaptic transmission, a small burst of neurotransmitters is released and then removed. Neurotransmitters are either destroyed by enzymes or reabsorbed by the postsynaptic membrane to be recycled for the next transmission. In addition to stimulating the action potential of neurons, some neurotransmitters inhibit action potential.

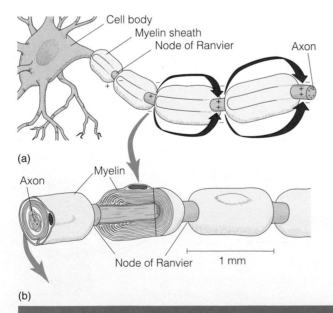

(a)

(b)

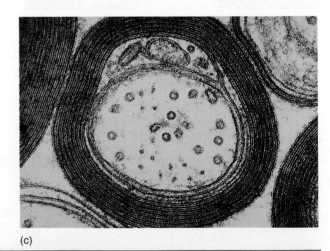

(c)

Figure 11-3

A myelinated nerve. (a) The myelin sheath allows impulses to "jump" from node to node, greatly accelerating the rate of transmission. (b) The node of Ranvier. (c) A transmission electron micrograph of an axon in the cross section, showing a myelin sheath.

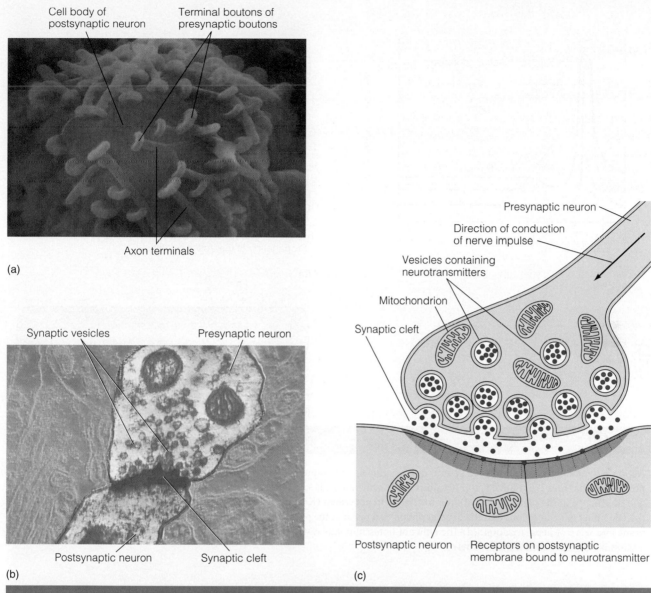

Cell body of postsynaptic neuron

Terminal boutons of presynaptic boutons

Axon terminals

(a)

Synaptic vesicles

Presynaptic neuron

Postsynaptic neuron

Synaptic cleft

(b)

Presynaptic neuron

Direction of conduction of nerve impulse

Vesicles containing neurotransmitters

Mitochondrion

Synaptic cleft

Postsynaptic neuron

Receptors on postsynaptic membrane bound to neurotransmitter

(c)

Figure 11-4

The function of neurotransmitters in the synaptic cleft. (a) A scanning electron micrograph showing the terminal boutons of an axon ending on the cell body of another neuron. (b) A transmission electron micrograph showing the details of the synapse. (c) The arrival of the impulse stimulates the release of neurotransmitters held in synaptic vesicles in the axon terminals. Neurotransmitter diffuses across the synaptic cleft and binds to the postsynaptic membrane, where it elicits another action potential that travels down the dendrite to the cell body.

The brain is responsible for a variety of physiologically vital functions and cognitive activities. The brain accomplishes these functions in part through a set of cranial nerves. Twelve pairs of cranial nerves branch directly from the base of the brain (Figure 11-6). Some of the cranial nerves only carry sensory fibers (I, II, and VIII), others only carry motor fibers (III, IV, VI, XI,

and XII), and few carry both (V, VII, IX, and X). Each nerve travels from the brain through the foramen to its destination.

The major regions of the brain include the cerebrum (including cerebral cortex), diencephalon (thalamus and hypothalamus), brain stem (pons, midbrain,

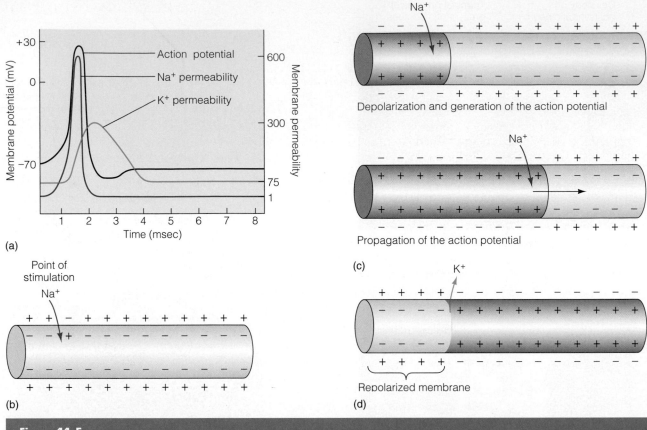

Figure 11-5

Action potential. (a) Stimulating the neuron creates a bioelectric impulse, which is recorded as an action potential. The resulting potential shifts from 270 millivolts to 130 millivolts. The membrane is said to be depolarized. This graph shows the shift in potential and the change in the permeability of sodium (Na⁺) and potassium (K⁺) ions, which is largely responsible for the action potential. (b) The influx of sodium ions and the depolarization that occur at the point of stimulation. (c) The impulse travels along the membrane as a wave of depolarization. (d) The efflux of potassium ions restores the resting potential, allowing the neuron to transmit additional impulses almost immediately.

and medulla), and cerebellum (**Figure 11-7**). The **cerebrum** is the largest of the regions (80% of total mass) and controls the higher thought processes. A thin layer of gray matter, referred to as cerebral cortex, surrounds the cerebrum (**Figure 11-8**). A thick central core of white matter lies beneath the gray matter. This white matter contains bundles of axons that transmit impulses from the cerebral cortex to the spinal cord, enhancing communication and coordination of activities. The cerebrum is divided into right and left hemispheres by a **longitudinal fissure**. Although minor shifts of one hemisphere into the other may occur, impinging of one hemisphere on the other can have significant and life-threatening effects. Numerous folds, or **gyri**, increase the surface area of the cerebrum. **Sulci** refer to the grooves in between the gyri. At birth, these folds are minimal, but they increase as the brain develops into adulthood. Within each hemisphere are subdivisions

called **lobes** named for the bone of the skull that covers it (**Figure 11-9**). The **frontal lobe** facilitates voluntary motor activity and plays a role in personality traits. The **parietal lobe** receives and interprets sensory input with the exception of smell, hearing, and vision. The **occipital lobe** processes visual information. The **temporal lobe** plays an essential role in hearing and memory. Areas within and across these lobes can be classified as three types—motor (which stimulates muscle activity), sensory (which receives sensory information), and association (which integrates information and initiates coordinated responses).

The **diencephalon** includes the thalamus and hypothalamus (**Figure 11-10**). The **thalamus** receives and relays most of the sensory input, affects mood, and initiates body movements (especially those associated with fear or anger). The **subthalamus** participates in

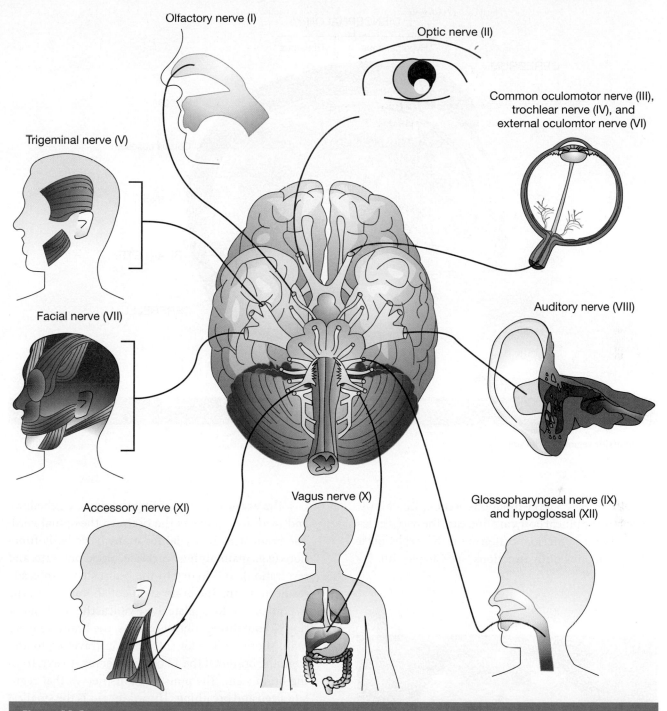

Olfactory nerve (I)

Optic nerve (II)

Common oculomotor nerve (III),
trochlear nerve (IV), and
external oculomtor nerve (VI)

Trigeminal nerve (V)

Facial nerve (VII)

Auditory nerve (VIII)

Accessory nerve (XI)

Vagus nerve (X)

Glossopharyngeal nerve (IX)
and hypoglossal (XII)

Figure 11-6

The cranial nerves.

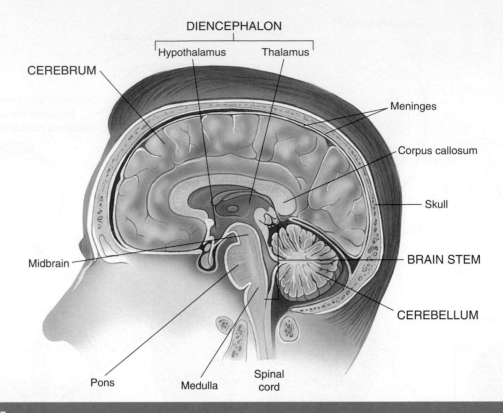

DIENCEPHALON

Hypothalamus   Thalamus

CEREBRUM

Meninges

Corpus callosum

Skull

Midbrain

BRAIN STEM

CEREBELLUM

Pons   Medulla   Spinal cord

Figure 11-7

The major regions of the brain.

motor activities, but the functions of the **epithalamus**, especially the pineal body, are unclear. The **hypothalamus** is the most inferior portion of the diencephalon; it regulates many bodily functions (see Chapter 10).

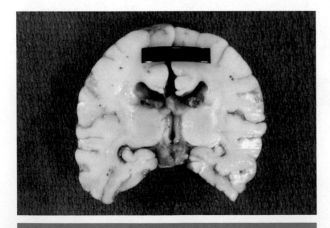

Figure 11-8

The cerebrum.

The **brain stem** (including the pons, cerebellum, and medulla) connects the brain to the spinal cord. The brain stem is crucial for many basic body functions (e.g., maintaining heart rate, blood pressure, and respiration), and injury to the brain stem can easily result in death. The brain stem collaborates with the hypothalamus to regulate these vital activities. In addition to containing control regions, the brain stem is a main thoroughfare for information traveling to and from the brain. Of the 12 cranial nerves, 10 exit from the brain stem. The **pons** contains nerves that regulate sleep and breathing. The **midbrain** is the smallest region of the brain, and it acts as a sort of relay station for auditory and visual information. The midbrain controls the visual and auditory systems as well as eye movement. The **medulla** is a conduction pathway for ascending and descending nerve tracts. The medulla coordinates heart rate, peripheral vascular resistance, breathing, swallowing, vomiting, coughing, and sneezing. Most of the many nerve fibers passing through the brain stem have branches that terminate in a region of the brain stem called the **reticular formation**. The reticular formation acts like a gatekeeper, receiving all incoming and outgoing information. The reticu-

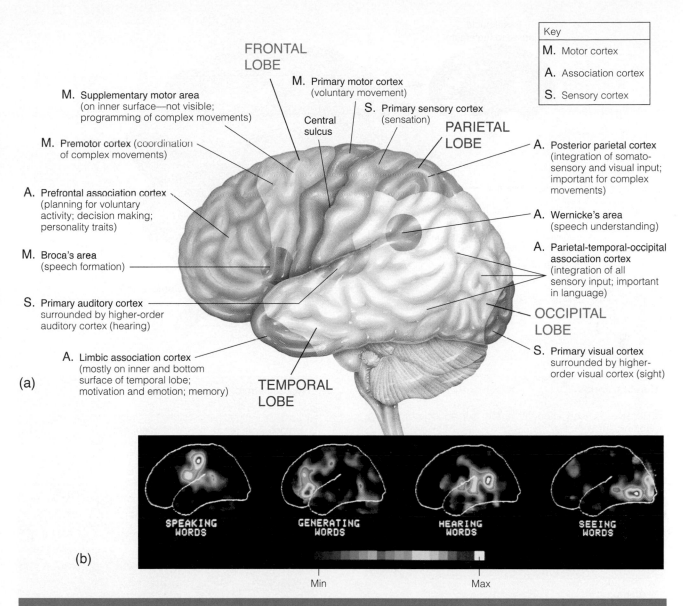

FRONTAL LOBE

M. Supplementary motor area (on inner surface—not visible; programming of complex movements)

M. Premotor cortex (coordination of complex movements)

A. Prefrontal association cortex (planning for voluntary activity; decision making; personality traits)

M. Broca's area (speech formation)

S. Primary auditory cortex surrounded by higher-order auditory cortex (hearing)

A. Limbic association cortex (mostly on inner and bottom surface of temporal lobe; motivation and emotion; memory)

(a)

TEMPORAL LOBE

M. Primary motor cortex (voluntary movement)

Central sulcus

S. Primary sensory cortex (sensation)

PARIETAL LOBE

Key

M. Motor cortex

A. Association cortex

S. Sensory cortex

A. Posterior parietal cortex (integration of somato-sensory and visual input; important for complex movements)

A. Wernicke's area (speech understanding)

A. Parietal-temporal-occipital association cortex (integration of all sensory input; important in language)

OCCIPITAL LOBE

S. Primary visual cortex surrounded by higher-order visual cortex (sight)

SPEAKING WORDS   GENERATING WORDS   HEARING WORDS   SEEING WORDS

(b)

Min   Max

Figure 11-9

The lobes of the cerebrum. (a) The cerebral cortex has three principal functions: receiving sensory input, integrating sensory information, and generating motor responses. Special sensory areas handle vision, smell, taste, and hearing. (b) A PET scan reveals the locations of increased blood flow in the brain during performance of certain tasks.

lar formation sends impulses to the cerebral cortex through specialized nerve fibers. These fibers make up the reticular activation system (**Figure 11-11**). The reticular formation and reticular activation system are responsible for alertness during the day and can prevent sleeping at night.

The cerebellum communicates with other regions of the brain to coordinate the synergistic motion of muscle movement and balance as well as cognition. Deep within the cerebrum, diencephalon, and mid-

brain is a set of key structures called the basal ganglia. The basal ganglia play a pivotal role in coordination, motor movement, and posture. Portions of the cerebrum and diencephalon comprise the limbic system (**Figure 11-12**). The limbic system works in conjunction with the hypothalamus to influence instinctive behavior, emotions, motivation, mood, pain, and pleasure.

The spinal cord exits the skull through the large and only opening in the skull, called the foramen magnum. The spinal cord extends through the vertebral

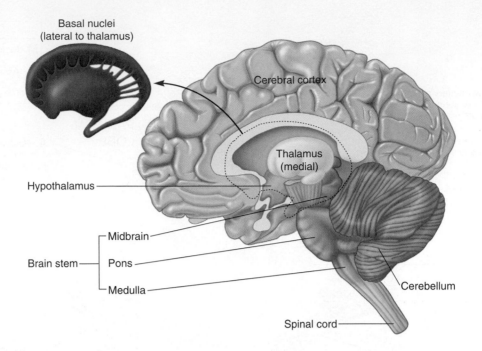

Basal nuclei
(lateral to thalamus)

Cerebral cortex

Thalamus
(medial)

Hypothalamus

Midbrain

Brain stem — Pons

Medulla

Cerebellum

Spinal cord

Cerebral cortex

- Receives sensory information from skin, muscles, glands, and organs
- Sends messages to move skeletal muscles
- Integrates incoming and outgoing nerve impulses
- Performs associative activities such as thinking, learning, and remembering

Basal nuclei

- Play a role in the coordination of slow, sustained movements
- Suppress useless patterns of movement

Thalamus

- Relays most sensory information from the spinal cord and certain parts of the brain to the cerebral cortex
- Interprets certain sensory messages such as those of pain, temperature, and pressure

Hypothalamus

- Controls various homeostatic functions such as body temperature, respiration, and heartbeat
- Directs hormone secretions of the pituitary

Cerebellum

- Coordinates subconscious movements of skeletal muscles
- Contributes to muscle tone, posture, balance, and equilibrium

Brain stem

- Origin of many cranial nerves
- Reflex center for movements of eyeballs, head, and trunk
- Regulates heartbeat and breathing
- Plays a role in consciousness
- Transmits impulses between brain and spinal cord

Figure 11-10

The regions of the brain and their functions.

canal to the second lumbar vertebra. At this point, the spinal cord transitions into individual nerve roots referred to as the cauda equina. The spinal cord consists of 31 pairs of spinal nerves that branch off at regular intervals (**Figure 11-13**).

The central portion of the spinal cord is an H-shaped area of gray matter, which contains nerve cell bodies. White matter comprised of nerve fiber tracts, or pathways, surround the gray matter (**Figure 11-14**). Ascending fibers, or afferent tracts, carry sensory

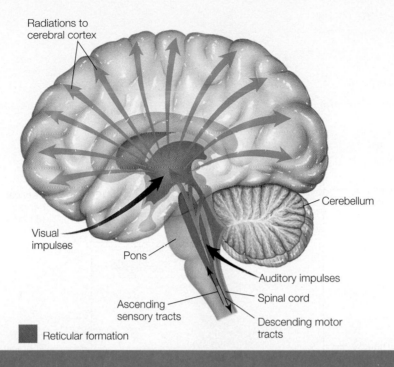

Radiations to
cerebral cortex

Cerebellum

Visual
impulses

Pons

Auditory impulses

Spinal cord

Ascending
sensory tracts

Descending motor
tracts

Reticular formation

Figure 11-11

The reticular activation system.

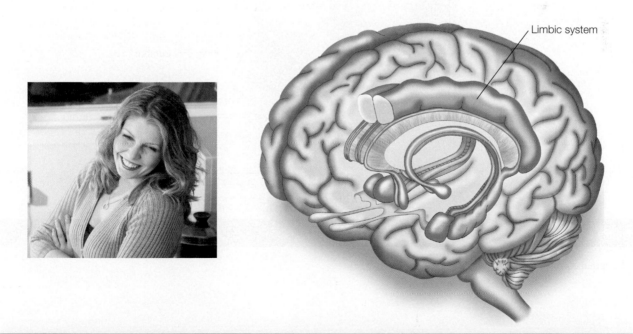

Limbic system

Figure 11-12

The limbic system. The odd assortment of structures shown in green is the limbic system. The limbic system is the seat of emotions such as joy and instincts and is home to other functions as well.

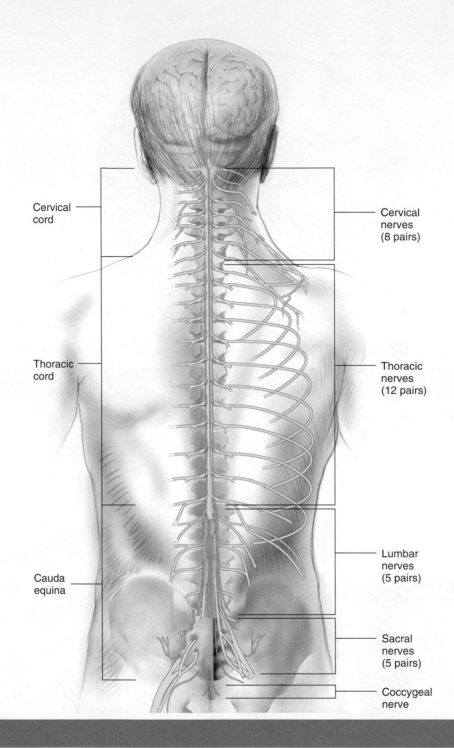

Cervical cord

Cervical nerves (8 pairs)

Thoracic cord

Thoracic nerves (12 pairs)

Lumbar nerves (5 pairs)

Cauda equina

Sacral nerves (5 pairs)

Coccygeal nerve

Figure 11-13

The spinal cord.

information in the form of action potentials from the periphery back to the brain. **Descending fibers**, or **efferent tracts**, carry motor impulses in the form of action potentials from the brain to the fibers of the PNS. The ascending fibers have a variety of tracts that communicate specific sensory input. These pathways include anterior spinothalamic tracts (which permit sensations of light touch, pressure, tickling, and itching), lateral spinothalamic tracts (which allow the sensations of pain and temperature), spinocerebellar tracts (which establish the body's position in relation to the cerebellum), corticospinal tracts (which coordinate movements, especially in the hands), vestibulospinal tracts (which are responsible for involuntary movements), and reticulospinal tracts (also responsible for involuntary movements).

The **spinal reflex arcs** refer to the process that creates an unconscious response to stimuli (**Figure 11-15**). An example of this arc can be seen when the patella is gently tapped with a reflex hammer. The tendon stretch reflex is elicited when the patella is tapped, causing the lower leg to sharply move forward (called extension) and then backward (called flexion). **Flexor reflex** refers to a withdrawal reflex in response to touching an unpleasant stimulus (e.g., extreme heat). The flexor reflex causes the muscles of a limb to withdraw the limb from the source of the stimulus without any conscious action. The tracts of the spinal cord and brain regulate these impulses.

Peripheral Nervous System

The **nerves** of the PNS consist of bundles of nerve fibers, and each fiber is part of the neuron. These nerves trans-port messages to and from the CNS. These nerves end on receptors that respond to a variety of internal and external stimuli. The 31 spinal nerve pairs (8 cervical, 12 thoracic, 5 lumbar, 5 sacral, and 1 coccygeal) branch directly off the spinal cord to make up the PNS. Each spinal nerve pair is named for the vertebral level at which it exits the spinal cord (e.g., C3 is the 3rd cervical nerve and T12 is the 12th thoracic nerve) and innervates specific areas of the body (**Figure 11-16**). Ganglia refer to collections of nerve cell bodies outside the CNS. Spinal nerves arise from several small nerves called **rootlets** along the dorsal and ventral surfaces of the spinal cord (**Figure 11-17**). Approximately 6–8 rootlets combine to form each **dorsal root** and **ventral root**. These roots come together to form the spinal nerve.

Each spinal nerve of the PNS is comprised of two types of nerves—sensory and motor. The **sensory nerves**, or **afferent nerves**, carry impulses (regarding information) from the body to the brain. A **dermatome** is the area of the skin innervated by a given pair of spinal sensory nerves. Each spinal nerve, with the exception of C1, has a specific body surface area

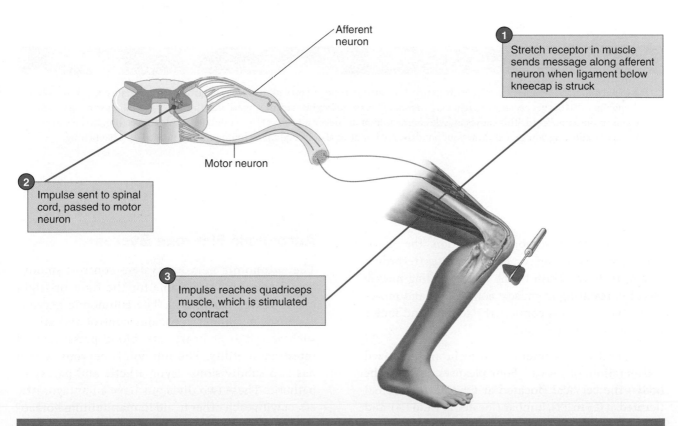

Afferent neuron

1 Stretch receptor in muscle sends message along afferent neuron when ligament below kneecap is struck

Motor neuron

2 Impulse sent to spinal cord, passed to motor neuron

3 Impulse reaches quadriceps muscle, which is stimulated to contract

Figure 11-14

Spinal cord nerve tracts.

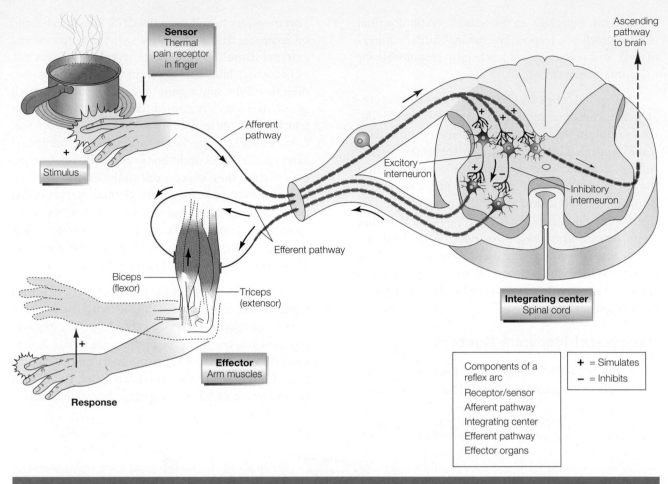

Sensor
Thermal pain receptor in finger

Stimulus

Afferent pathway

Excitory interneuron

Inhibitory interneuron

+ = Simulates

Ascending pathway to brain

Biceps (flexor)

Triceps (extensor)

Efferent pathway

Integrating center
Spinal cord

Effector
Arm muscles

Response

Components of a reflex arc
Receptor/sensor
Afferent pathway
Integrating center
Efferent pathway
Effector organs

+ = Simulates
− = Inhibits

Figure 11-15

The spinal reflex arc. When you accidentally touch a hot pan on the stove, you withdraw your hand before your brain even knows what is happening. This occurs because of a reflex arc. Sensory fibers send impulses to the spinal cord. The sensory impulses stimulate motor neurons in the spinal cord. This causes muscle contraction in the flexor muscles (1) and inhibits muscle contraction in the extensor muscles (2), allowing you to withdraw your hand. Nerve impulses also ascend to the brain to let it know what is happening.

to which it obtains sensory information. The **motor nerves,** or **efferent nerves,** carry impulses (regarding action) from the brain to the corresponding muscle receptor, resulting in muscle contraction and movement. **Interneurons** connect the sensory and motor neurons in the spinal cord.

Several nerves intersect to form an organized collaboration, or **plexus.** Four plexuses occur in the body—the cervical (located at C1 to C4), brachial (located at C5 to T1), lumbar (located at L1 to L4), and sacral (located at L4 to S4). These plexuses branch into the **peripheral nerves** that supply sensory and motor functions to many areas of the body.

Autonomic Nervous System

The **autonomic nervous system** controls smooth muscles and is responsible for the fight-or-flight response (see Chapter 2). The autonomic nervous system is not under conscious control and affects such activities as heart rate, blood pressure, and intestinal motility. The autonomic nervous system has two subdivisions—sympathetic and parasympathetic. These two divisions have an antagonistic effect with each other to aid in maintaining homeostasis (**Figure 11-18**). The **sympathetic nervous system (SNS)** is responsible for the fight-or-flight response. This response is initiated when a person

MYTH BUSTERS

Some myths surrounding the brain warrant discussion.

MYTH 1: The brain is gray.

The living, pulsing brain currently residing in your skull is not just a dull, bland gray organ like often depicted in movies; the brain is also white, black, and red. Like many myths, this one has a grain of truth, because much of the brain is gray. Sometimes the entire brain is referred to as gray matter. However, the brain also contains white matter, which comprises nerve fibers that connect the gray matter. The black component is called substantia nigra, which is Latin for "black substance." The substantia nigra is black because of neuromelanin, a specialized type of pigment. Finally, we have red because of the many blood vessels in the brain.

MYTH 2: Listening to classical music, especially by Mozart, increases intelligence.

How did this myth get started? In the 1950s, a physician named Albert Tomatis began the trend, claiming success using Mozart's music to help people with speech and auditory disorders. In the 1990s, 36 students in a study at the University of California at Irvine listened to 10 minutes of a Mozart sonata before taking an IQ test. The study reported that the students' IQ scores went up by about 8 points, and the Mozart effect was born. Multiple products have been sold based on this assumption. However, the original University of California at Irvine study has been controversial in the scientific community. Other scientists have been unable to replicate the original results, and current scientific evidence does not support that listening to Mozart, or any other classical music, increases intelligence. However, some evidence indicates that learning an instrument improves concentration, self-confidence, and coordination. Mozart certainly cannot hurt you, and you might even enjoy it if you try it, but you will not get any smarter.

MYTH 3: You only use 10% of your brain.

This myth is probably one of the most well-known myths about the brain. This assumption seems puzzling at first glance. We have the biggest brain in proportion to our bodies of any animal, so why would we not use all of it? Many people have jumped on the idea, writing books and selling products that claim to tap into the other 90%. Believers in psychic abilities point to this ability as proof, saying that people with these abilities have tapped into the rest of their brains. This myth is false. In addition to 100 billion neurons, the brain is also full of other types of cells that are continually in use. Significant neurologic deficits can occur from even minor damage depending on the location, so it is highly unlikely that we could function with only 10% of our brain in use. Brain scans have shown that no matter what we are doing, our brains are always active. Some areas are more active at any one time than others, but unless we have brain damage, no one part of the brain is completely turned off. So, there is no hidden, extra potential you can tap into, in terms of actual brain space.

MYTH 4: Games like sudoku and Brain Age keep your brain young.

There is some truth to this myth! Continued mental engagement has benefits, and puzzles can help you get good at a specific skill, like memorizing grocery lists or hand–eye coordination. But most evidence suggests that practicing a task only helps you get better at that particular task. Far better for mental function is physical exercise. Regular fitness exercise is especially effective in the elderly, who may suffer from gradual problems with cognitive function such as planning ahead and abstract thinking.

LEARNING POINTS

How do we learn and store memories? Learning is the acquisition and retention of new information, and memory is the storage and recall of information. Both are dependent on proper nutrition and adequate sleep. Newly acquired memory is first stored in the short-term memory, where it is held for seconds to hours. Cramming for tests puts most of the information into short-term memory. Unfortunately, soon after the test, the information fades—a good reason not to cram! Long-term memory holds information for days to years. Transferring information from short- to long-term requires special efforts such as repetition, mnemonics, and rhymes. Recalling information in short term is often faster than recalling information in long-term memory. When information is lost from short-term memory, it is usually lost forever. Information you cannot recall from long-term memory, on the other hand, is often still there; it just requires time or stimuli to extract it. However, not all information in long-term memory is stored forever. Memories are stored in neurons throughout the cerebral cortex (especially the temporal lobe), cerebellum, and the limbic system. The hippocampus seems to be crucial in transferring information from short- to long-term memory. So, use this knowledge to help you study by not cramming and moving information from short- to long-term memory by paying attention, making the information memorable, and relating new information with facts you already know. But do not forget that you still have to get plenty of rest and eat a balanced diet to optimize your learning potential!

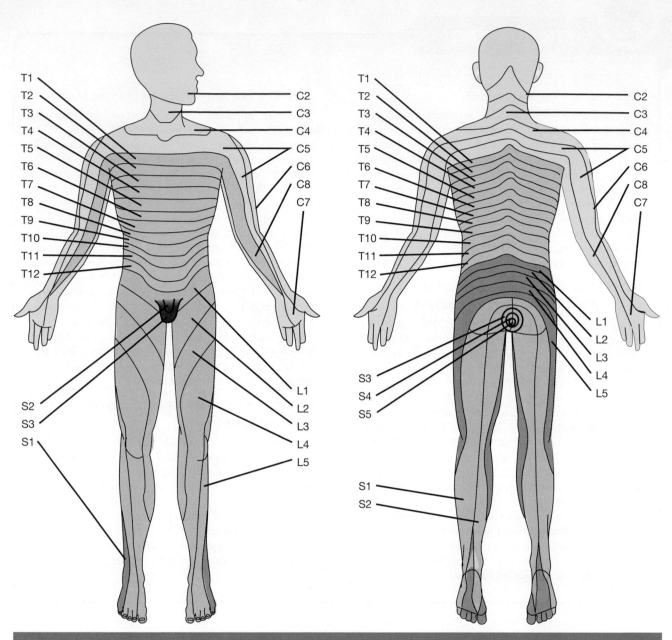

Figure 11-16

Spinal nerve innervation.

is startled or faced with danger and is augmented by secretions of the adrenal medulla. The **parasympathetic nervous system** is responsible for the rest-and-digest response. Neurotransmitters and receptors are important in the autonomic nervous system because the SNS and the parasympathetic nervous system will stimulate or inhibit these sites, leading to the physiologic response (**Table 11-1**). The SNS stimulates the adrenergic receptors while the parasympathetic nervous system stimulates the cholinergic receptors. Medications can be given that can stimulate or inhibit these receptors as well.

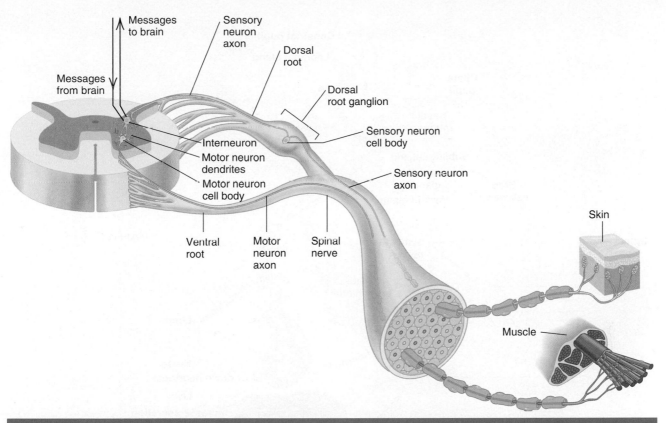

Figure 11-17

The dorsal root ganglion.

Table 11-1 Types of Autonomic Receptors

Neurotransmitter	Receptor	Primary Locations	Responses
Acetylcholine (cholinergic)	Nicotinic	Postganglionic neurons	Stimulation of smooth muscle and gland secretions
	Muscarinic	Parasympathetic target: organs other than the heart	Stimulation of smooth muscle and gland secretions
		Heart	Decreased heart rate and force of contraction
Norepinephrine (adrenergic)	Alpha$_1$	All sympathetic target organs except the heart	Constriction of blood vessels, dilation of pupils
	Alpha$_2$	Presynaptic adrenergic nerve terminals	Inhibition of release of norepinephrine
	Beta$_1$	Heart and kidneys	Increased heart rate and force of contraction; release of renin
	Beta$_2$	All sympathetic target organs except the heart	

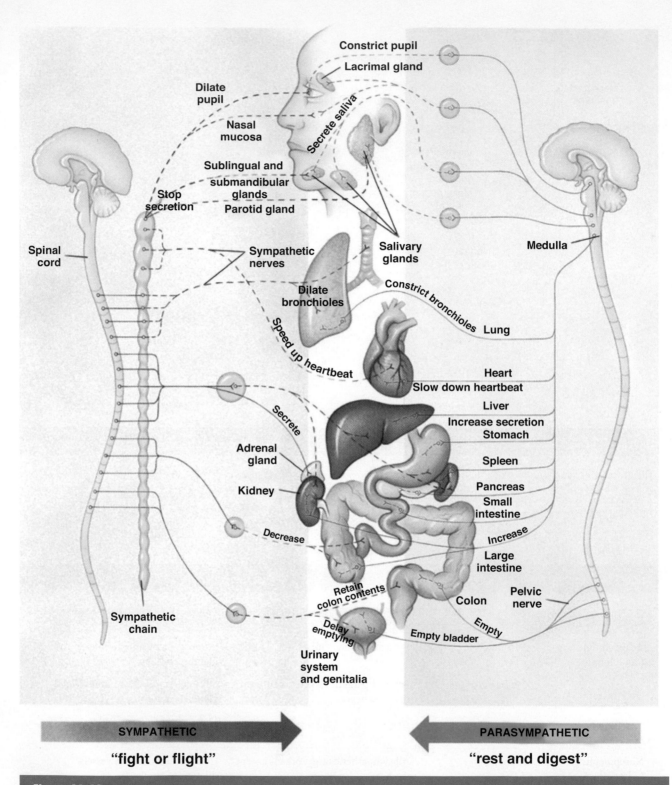

Constrict pupil

Lacrimal gland

Dilate pupil

Nasal mucosa

Secrete saliva

Sublingual and submandibular glands

Stop secretion

Parotid gland

Spinal cord

Sympathetic nerves

Salivary glands

Medulla

Dilate bronchioles

Constrict bronchioles

Lung

Speed up heartbeat

Heart

Slow down heartbeat

Secrete

Liver

Increase secretion
Stomach

Adrenal gland

Spleen

Kidney

Pancreas

Small intestine

Decrease

Increase

Large intestine

Retain colon contents

Colon

Pelvic nerve

Sympathetic chain

Delay emptying

Empty

Empty bladder

Urinary system and genitalia

SYMPATHETIC

"fight or flight"

PARASYMPATHETIC

"rest and digest"

Figure 11-18

Comparison of the two divisions of the autonomic nervous system.

Congenital Neurologic Disorders

Congenital defects of the nervous system are often serious with lifelong consequences. These disorders often have limited treatment options and require long-term management of complications.

Hydrocephalus

Hydrocephalus is a condition in which excess CSF accumulates within the skull, which dilates the ventricles and compresses the brain and blood vessels (**Figure 11-19**). The pressure from the excess CSF thins the cortex, causing severe brain damage. The CSF accumulates when the CSF flow is disrupted (referred to as noncommunicating or an obstructive hydrocephalus) or when it is not properly absorbed by the bloodstream (referred to as communicating hydrocephalus). Hydrocephalus is a common condition (affecting 1 out of 500 children), which may be present at birth or develop later in life. Risk factors for hydrocephalus at any age include prematurity, pregnancy complications, other congenital defects (especially nervous system defects), nervous system tumors, CNS infections, cerebral hemorrhage, and severe head injuries. If left untreated, hydrocephalus is often fatal (50–60% mortality rate). Prognosis depends on early treatment and comorbidity.

Clinical manifestations of hydrocephalus reflect the increased intracranial pressure (ICP). These mani-

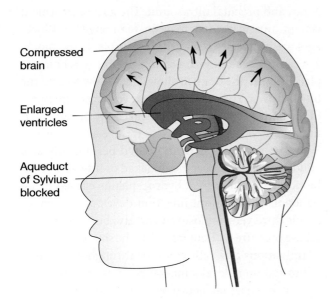

Compressed brain

Enlarged ventricles

Aqueduct of Sylvius blocked

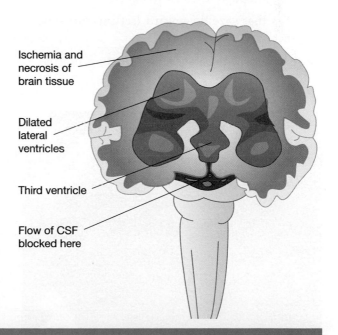

Ischemia and necrosis of brain tissue

Dilated lateral ventricles

Third ventricle

Flow of CSF blocked here

Figure 11-19

Hydrocephalus development.

festations vary by age group, underlying etiology, and disease progression. In infants, clinical manifestations often include:

- An unusually large head (**Figure 11-20**)
- A rapid increase in the head size
- A bulging fontanelle, or soft spot, on the top of the head
- Vomiting (often projectile)
- Lethargy
- Irritability
- High-pitched cry
- Feeding difficulties
- Seizures
- Eyes that gaze downward (setting-sun appearance)
- Development delay

In older children and adults, the head cannot enlarge because the sutures have closed. Clinical manifestations in these groups may include:

- Headache followed by vomiting
- Nausea
- Blurred vision or diplopia (double vision)
- Sluggish pupil response to light
- Eyes that gaze downward (setting-sun appearance)
- Problems with balance, coordination, or gait

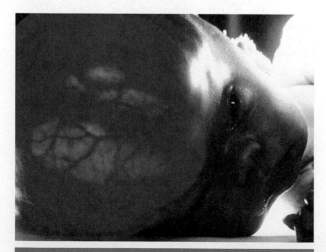

Figure 11-20

Hydrocephalus.

- Extreme fatigue
- Slowing or regression of development
- Memory loss
- Confusion
- Urinary incontinence
- Irritability
- Personality changes
- Impaired performance in school or work

Diagnostic procedures for hydrocephalus may be conducted during pregnancy or after birth. These procedures consist of a history, physical examination (including head circumference measurement and a neurologic assessment), head computed tomography (CT), head magnetic resonance imaging (MRI), head X-ray, and prenatal ultrasound. The goal of treatment is to minimize brain damage by reducing CSF. Blockages are surgically removed, if possible. If the blockage cannot be removed, a shunt (flexible tube) may be placed within the brain to allow CSF to flow around the blocked area. The shunt tubing travels to another part of the body, such as the peritoneal cavity or right atrium, where the extra CSF can be drained and absorbed. Shunt replacement may be needed periodically as a child grows or if it becomes blocked or infected. Antibiotic therapy will treat hydrocephalus caused by an infection or if a shunt infection develops. An endoscopic third ventriculostomy can also be performed to relieve pressure without replacing the shunt. Follow-up examinations generally continue throughout a child's life to monitor developmental progress and to manage any intellectual, neurologic, or physical problems. A multidisciplinary team (e.g., nurses, occupational therapists, educational specialists, social services personnel, and support groups) can provide emotional support and assistance with the care of those patients who have significant brain damage.

Spina Bifida

Spina bifida is the most common birth defect in the United States, affecting approximately 1 child of every 1,500 births each year (Centers for Disease Control and Prevention, 2010a). Spina bifida is a neural tube defect that can vary in severity from mild to debilitating. Neural tube development begins early in pregnancy, starting at the cervical area and progressing toward the lumbar area, and the neural tube usually closes by the 4th week of gestation. In spina bifida, the posterior spinous processes on the vertebrae fail to fuse. This opening permits the meninges and spinal cord to herniate, resulting in neurologic impairment. The lumbar area of the vertebrae is most commonly the site of the defect. The exact cause of spina bifida is unknown, but it is thought to be a result of genetic and environmental influences. Spina bifida is most common in Caucasian and Hispanic populations. Additional maternal risk factors for developing this defect include family history of neural defects, folate deficiency, certain medications (e.g., antiseizure agents), diabetes mellitus, prepregnancy obesity, and increased body temperature (e.g., from hot tubs, saunas, and tanning beds). Complications of spina bifida include physical and neurologic impairments as well as hydrocephalus and meningitis. Children with spina bifida are usually of normal intelligence, but they may have learning problems because of the chronic nature of the condition.

Spina bifida occurs in three forms, each varying in severity (**Figure 11-21**). These types include:

- **Spina bifida occulta** is the mildest form. It results in a small gap in one or more of the vertebrae. The spinal nerves and meninges do not usually protrude through the opening, so most children with this form have no clinical manifestations and experience no neurologic deficits. The defect may not be evident other than a dimple, birthmark, or tuft of hair over the site.

- **Meningocele** is a rare form that involves the same bony defect as in spina bifida occulta, but the meninges protrude through the vertebral opening. The meninges and CSF form a sac on the surface of the infant's back. Transillumination (shining light through the tissue) can confirm the absence of nerve tissue in the sac. Because the spinal cord develops normally, neurologic impairment is usually not present, and these membranes can be removed by surgery with little or no damage to nerve pathways. However, infection or rupture of the sac can lead to neurologic impairment.

- **Myelomeningocele**, also known as open spina bifida, is the most severe form. In this form, the spinal canal remains open along several vertebrae in the lower or middle back. The meninges, spinal cord, spinal nerves, and CSF protrude through this large opening at birth and form a sac on the infant's back (**Figure 11-22**). Skin covers the sac in some cases. However, tissues and nerves are exposed in most cases, making the infant vulnerable to life-threatening infections. Neurologic impairment (often including paralysis), bowel and bladder problems (e.g., incontinence, urinary tract infections, and constipation), seizures, and other medical complications (e.g., skin conditions and latex allergies) are common.

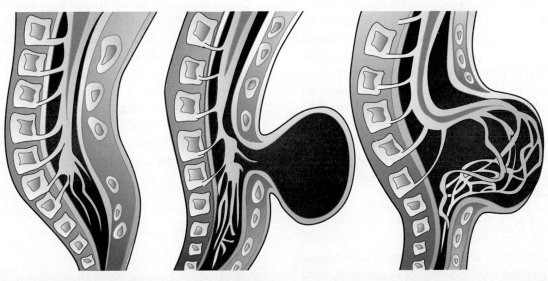

Spina bifida occulta   Meningocele   Myelomeningocele

Figure 11-21

Most common types of spina bifida.

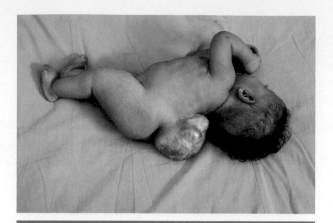

Figure 11-22

Meningomyocele.

CASE STUDY

M.S. is a 26-year-old woman pregnant with her first child. Her husband accompanied her to all her prenatal visits. An ultrasound during a routine visit at 34 weeks' gestation revealed that the baby had hydrocephalus and a myelomeningocele. The parents were initially devastated but remained very excited about the birth of their first child. M.S. was scheduled for a cesarean section at 38 weeks' gestation, and the couple was anxious about their child's condition and care following birth.

M.S. delivered a baby boy by caesarean section; he was transferred to the pediatric intensive care unit. On admission to the nursery, the baby's vital signs and weight were within normal limits, but the head circumference was large. He had bulging fontanelles and a high-pitched cry. The nurse noted a saclike projection in the lumbar region of his spine.

1. Discuss the rationale for delivering the infant by cesarean section.

2. Discuss the significance of the infant's clinical manifestations.

3. Discuss the complications associated with myelomeningocele.

Clinical manifestations depend on the type and severity of spina bifida. Diagnostic procedures may be performed during pregnancy or after birth. These procedures may include a history, physical examination, check of maternal serum and amniotic fluid alpha-fetoprotein levels, prenatal ultrasound, spinal X-ray, spinal CT, and spinal MRI. Treatment strategies vary depending on the type and severity. For instance, spina bifida occulta often requires no treatment. Surgery is the mainstay of treatment for the other two types; however, suggested timing of the surgery (in utero, immediately after birth, or delayed) remains debated. Surgery usually includes replacing meninges and closing the vertebral opening. A shunt may be placed during surgery to control hydrocephalus. Performing the surgical repair in utero may enhance outcomes but will not restore lost neurologic functioning. Additional risk may be incurred with this procedure including premature delivery and death. If spina bifida is diagnosed before birth, cesarean delivery is preferred to prevent rupture of the sac or damage to any exposed nerves. Long-term support of a multidisciplinary team (e.g., a nurse, physical therapist, social worker, and an education specialist) will be necessary to limit complications and promote positive outcomes.

Cerebral Palsy

Cerebral palsy (CP) refers to a group of nonprogressive disorders that appear in infancy or early childhood and permanently affect motor movement and muscle coordination. In addition to motor dysfunction, other cerebral functioning may be affected (e.g., cognition and communication). CP usually results from damage to the cerebellum during the prenatal period (often

during childbirth), but it can occur any time during the first 3 years of life, when the brain is developing. CP can also occur because of brain abnormalities. In the United States, CP occurs in approximately 3–4 out of 1,000 births. CP is not curable, but the right treatment can make a significant impact on the child's prognosis. These therapies are costly. According to the CDC (2004), the average lifetime cost (direct and indirect) for one person with CP is estimated to be $921,000 (in 2003 dollars). The estimated lifetime costs (direct and indirect) for all people with CP who were born in 2000 will total $11.5 billion (in 2003 dollars). Contributing factors to developing CP include:

- Prematurity
- Breech births (feet first rather than head first)
- Multiple fetuses
- Hypoxia
- Hypoglycemia (in either the mother or the child)
- Cerebral hemorrhage
- Neurologic infections (e.g., meningitis and encephalitis)
- Head injury

- Maternal infections during pregnancy (e.g., rubella and varicella)

- Maternal exposure of toxins during pregnancy (e.g., mercury)

- Severe jaundice

Clinical manifestations of CP may or may not be evident at birth. These manifestations vary in severity from mild to severe. CP may affect the entire body (resulting in quadriplegia) or one area (resulting in diplegia); CP may affect one side or both sides of the body. Manifestations may include:

- Persistence of early reflexes (e.g., Moro reflex)

- Development delays

- Ataxia (lack of muscle coordination when performing voluntary movements)

- Spasticity (stiff muscles)

- Hyperreflexia (exaggerated reflexes)

- Asymmetrical walking gait, with one foot or leg dragging

- Unusual positioning of limbs when resting or when held up (e.g., scissor position of the legs)

- Excessive drooling

- Difficulties swallowing, sucking, or speaking

- Facial grimaces

- Tremors

- Difficulty with precise motions (e.g., writing and buttoning a shirt)

Complications of CP result because of these clinical manifestations and may include:

- Balance and coordination issues

- Contractures (shortening of a muscle causing severe limitation in movement)

- Malnutrition

- Communication issues and speech delays

- Learning or cognition difficulties

- Seizures

- Visual issues

- Urinary incontinence

- Chronic pain

Diagnostic procedures for CP include a history, physical examination, head CT, head MRI, and electroencephalogram (EEG) as well as hearing and vision screening. Treatment strategies focus on maximizing functioning and minimizing complications. Management is long term and requires a multidisciplinary team (e.g., the primary care provider, nurses, a social worker, a physical therapist, an occupational therapist, a speech therapist, a dietician, and education specialists). Strategies often include:

- Muscle relaxants

- Botulinum toxin type A (Botox) injections directly into spastic muscles

- Antiseizure medications

- Pain management (e.g., massage therapy and analgesics)

- Physical therapy

- Occupational therapy

- Speech therapy

- Braces and orthopedic devices (e.g., splints)

- Ambulation devices (e.g., walker and wheelchair)

- Surgical procedures to relieve contractures or to sever nerves of spastic muscles

- Support groups

- Individualized education program

Infectious Neurologic Disorders

Nervous system infections can have serious effects because of initiating the infectious and inflammatory response (see Chapter 2). These infections can be caused by a number of bacterial, viral, and fungal pathogens. Regardless of the causative agent, neurologic compromise (either temporary or permanent) can result. Early diagnosis and treatment is imperative for positive outcomes.

Meningitis

Meningitis refers to an inflammation of the meninges, usually resulting from an infection. The CSF may also become affected. Any number of bacteria (e.g., *Neisseria meningitidis*, *Streptococcus pneumoniae*, and *Haemophilus influenzae*) and viruses (e.g., enterovirus, measles, influenza, and herpes) can cause this infection. The infectious agents invade the meninges through the blood or nearby structures or by direct access (e.g., wounds). Additional causes of meningitis include tumors and allergens. The infection or irritant triggers the inflammatory process, leading to swelling of the meninges and increased ICP. Risk factors for developing meningitis include being less than 25 years of age, living in a community setting (e.g., a college dormitory), pregnancy, working with animals, and immunodeficiency. Depending on the cause of the infection, meningitis can be self-limiting (as with viral) or life-threatening (as with acute bacterial). Complications of meningitis include permanent neurologic damage, seizures, hearing loss, blindness, speech difficulties, learning disabilities, behavior problems, paralysis, renal failure, adrenal gland failure, shock, and death.

Clinical manifestations of meningitis result from the inflammation of the meninges. Initially, these manifestations mimic an influenza infection (e.g., fever, chills, and malaise). Clinical manifestations usually develop over a couple of days and include:

- Fever and chills
- Mental status changes (e.g., confusion and lethargy)
- Nausea and vomiting
- Photophobia
- Severe headache
- Stiff neck (meningismus)
- Agitation
- Bulging fontanelle
- Decreased consciousness
- Opisthotonos (abnormal positioning that involves rigidity and severe arching of the back with the head thrown backward)
- Poor feeding or irritability in children
- Tachypnea (increased breathing)
- Rash

Diagnostic procedures of meningitis include a history, physical examination, throat cultures, lumbar puncture with CSF analysis, polymerase chain reaction test, and head CT. Treatment varies depending on the underlying etiology. Strategies may include antibiotics (if bacterial), hydration, and fever management. Vaccinations, including those for *Haemophilus influenzae*, pneumococcal, and meningococcal, are the cornerstone of meningitis prevention.

Encephalitis

Encephalitis refers to an inflammation of the brain and spinal cord, usually resulting from an infection.

A virus (e.g., coxsackievirus, echovirus, poliovirus, adenovirus, herpes virus, cytomegalovirus, Eastern equine encephalitis virus, West Nile virus, St. Louis virus, measles, and mumps) most frequently causes this infection. Viral exposure occurs through respiratory inhalation of droplets, ingestion of contaminated food or beverages, insect bites (especially mosquitoes and parasites), and skin contact. Encephalitis can also result from bacterial infections such as Lyme disease, tuberculosis, and syphilis. The infection triggers the inflammatory response that causes vasodilatation, increased capillary permeability, and leukocyte infiltration. The inflammatory process can cause nerve cell degeneration and diffuse brain destruction. Encephalitis may be primary or secondary. Primary encephalitis involves direct viral infection of the brain and spinal cord. In secondary encephalitis, a viral infection first occurs elsewhere in the body and then travels to the brain.

Most cases of encephalitis are mild and self-limiting, but in rare cases, encephalitis can be severe and life threatening. Those particularly vulnerable to more severe progression of encephalitis include immune compromised persons (e.g., those with AIDS), young children, older adults, those living in high-incidence areas, and those frequently outdoors. Complications of encephalitis include cerebral edema, cerebral hemorrhage, and brain damage.

Clinical manifestations of encephalitis result from meningeal irritation and neurologic damage. These manifestations are similar to meningitis but with a more gradual onset. In most cases, clinical manifestations are mild and go undetected. When present, manifestations of encephalitis may include:

- Flulike symptoms (e.g., fever, lethargy, and joint pain)
- Headache
- Neck rigidity
- Confusion and hallucinations
- Personality changes (e.g., flat affect, impaired judgment, and withdrawal from social interactions)
- Diplopia
- Seizures
- Muscle weakness
- Paresthesia or paralysis
- Loss of consciousness
- Tremors
- Abnormal deep tendon reflexes

- Rash
- Bulging fontanelle (in infants)

Diagnostic procedures for encephalitis include a history, physical examination, head CT, head MRI, EEG, lumbar puncture with CSF analysis, polymerase chain reaction test, and serum viral antibodies. Encephalitis is usually self-limiting, so treatment is largely supportive. Treatment strategies often include:

- Rest
- Adequate nutrition, including plenty of liquids
- Reorientation and emotional support
- Analgesics and antipyretics to relieve headaches and fever
- Antiviral agents (if viral)
- Antibiotic therapy (if bacterial)
- Corticosteroids to reduce cerebral edema
- Antiseizure agents
- Sedatives to treat irritability and restlessness
- Physical, speech, and occupational therapy as necessary for any residual neurologic dysfunction

Many of the encephalitis causative organisms can be prevented. Prevention strategies include vaccinations, wearing protective clothing when outside (e.g., long-sleeve shirts), using mosquito repellant, and eliminating water sources around the home (e.g., standing water in containers).

Traumatic Neurologic Disorders

Traumatic neurologic disorders vary significantly in severity and presentation depending on the location and extent of damage. Even minor injuries can have substantial effects on neurologic functioning. Traumatic injuries to the nervous system can result from a number of events that cause physical damage (e.g., motor vehicle accidents, gunshot wounds, and falls). Commonly, a number of these traumatic conditions overlap and occur concurrently (e.g., subdural hematoma and increased intracranial pressure).

Brain Injuries

A **traumatic brain injury (TBI)** is usually caused by a sudden and violent blow or jolt to the head (called a closed injury) or a penetrating (known as an open injury) head wound that disrupts the normal brain function. However, not all blows or jolts to the head result in a TBI. With TBIs, the brain collides with the skull (**Figure 11-23**) and any penetrating objects (**Figure 11-24**). These events can bruise the brain, damage nerve fibers, and cause hemorrhaging. According to the CDC (2010c), the main sources of TBI are falls (25%), motor vehicle accidents (17%), penetration of an object (17%), and assaults (10%). TBIs vary from mild (e.g., a brief change in mental status or consciousness) to severe (e.g., an extended period of unconsciousness or amnesia after the injury). TBIs contribute to a substantial number of deaths and cases of permanent disability annually. According to the CDC (2010d), 1.7 million Americans sustain a TBI each year—50,000 of those die. Persons at highest risk for experiencing a TBI include:

- Males (twice as likely as females)
- Young children 0–4-year-olds and 15–19-year-olds
- Adults 75 years of age or older
- Certain military personnel (e.g., paratroopers)
- African Americans (highest death rates)

Many TBIs will result in a wide range of long-term and potentially life-altering complications such as changes in thinking, sensation, language, or emotions. TBIs can increase the risk for seizures, Alzheimer's disease, and Parkinson's disease. Multiple mild TBIs can have an accumulative effect and result in neurologic dysfunction, cognitive deficits, and death. This damage can be seen in the recent study regarding professional football players (Schwenk et al., 2007) and a growing number of evidence. These players, especially those who encounter routine impacts (e.g., linemen), had higher rates of cognitive deficits (e.g., memory impairment) and neurologic diseases (e.g., Alzheimer's disease, Parkinson's disease, and depression).

Closed TBIs often result in a couple of conditions. **Concussion** describes a momentary interruption of brain function. Concussions usually result from a mild blow to the head that causes sudden movement of the brain, disrupting neurologic functioning. Concussions may or may not lead to a loss of consciousness. Amnesia, confusion, sleep disturbances, and headaches may follow a concussion for weeks or months. **Cerebral contusion** refers to a bruising of the brain with rupture of small blood vessels and edema. Most contusions result from a blunt blow to the head that causes the brain to make sudden impact with the skull. The initial area the brain impacts with the skull is

FORWARD/BACKWARD CLOSED HEAD INJURY   **SIDE-TO-SIDE CLOSED HEAD INJURY**

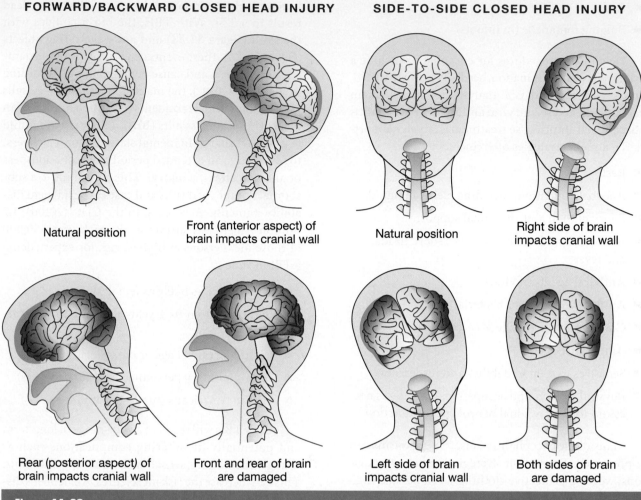

Natural position

Front (anterior aspect) of brain impacts cranial wall

Natural position

Right side of brain impacts cranial wall

Rear (posterior aspect) of brain impacts cranial wall

Front and rear of brain are damaged

Left side of brain impacts cranial wall

Both sides of brain are damaged

Figure 11-23

Closed traumatic brain injury.

referred to as the coup. The brain then rebounds and impacts with the opposite side of the skull, causing another area of damage referred to as the countercoup (Figure 11-25). Contusions vary in severity depending on the extent of damage and the amount of bleeding. The presence and severity of residual effects depend on that severity.

Open TBIs can result in serious issues. In addition to the tissue damage from the impact of the brain with the skull, open TBIs can cause damage from the penetrating object and skull fragments. The skull fractures as the object breaches it. Much like when an egg is broken, the skull usually ends up in multiple pieces when encountering an external force. A fracture may be a linear skull fracture (a simple crack), a comminuted skull fracture (several fracture lines), a compound skull fracture (a fracture where the brain

tissue is exposed), a depressed skull fracture (the bone fragments are displaced into the brain), or a basilar skull fracture (located at the base of the skull and usually accompanied by CSF leakage). In addition to the brain damage from impact and penetrating objects, open TBIs are at higher risk for developing infections because of a break in the first line of defense (see Chapter 2). As discussed in previous sections, infections of the nervous system can have serious consequences.

Clinical manifestations of TBIs may be vague and develop slowly, or they may be sudden and severe. Symptoms may improve and then suddenly worsen. The outward appearance of the head is not an indication of the injury severity—serious injuries can occur with the skin and the skull intact. When a TBI is suspected, the individual should be asked to give an

(a) Closed injury—direct and contrecoup injury

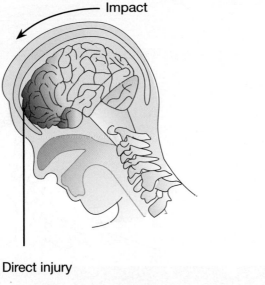

Impact — Direct injury

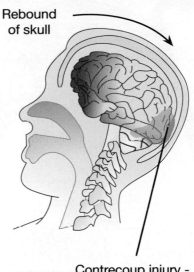

Rebound of skull — Contrecoup injury - brain hits skull

(b) Open injury

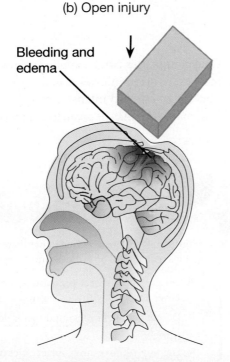

Bleeding and edema

Depressed fracture

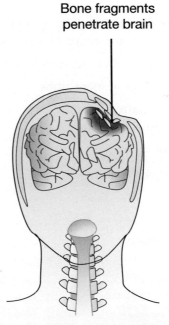

Bone fragments penetrate brain

Figure 11-24

Open traumatic brain injury.

account of the accident. Not being able to recall details is an indication of a TBI. Additional clinical manifestations may include:

- Indications of a concussion (e.g., amnesia, confusion, and headache)

- Changes in or unequal size of pupils
- Seizures
- Asymmetrical facial features
- Fluid draining from the nose, mouth, or ears (may be clear or bloody; likely CSF)

(a) Primary impact

Coup

(b) Secondary impact

Contrecoup

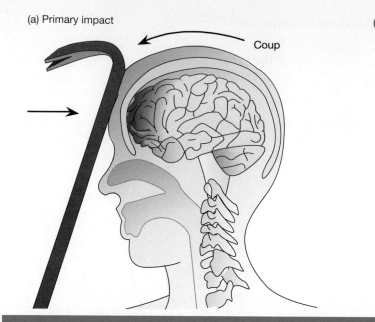
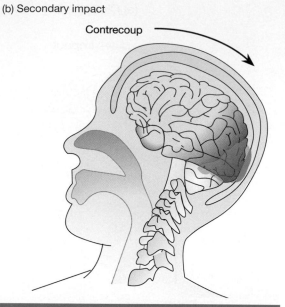

Figure 11-25

Coup and contracoup injuries.

- Fracture in the skull or face, bruising of the face, swelling at the site of the injury, or scalp wound
- Impaired hearing, smell, taste, speech, or vision
- Inability to move one or more limbs
- Irritability (especially in children), personality changes, or unusual behavior
- Loss of consciousness
- Bradypnea (slowed breathing)
- Hypotension
- Restlessness
- Lack of coordination
- Lethargy
- Stiff neck
- Vomiting

Diagnostic procedures for TBI consist of a history, physical examination (including using the Glasgow Coma Scale [Figure 11-26]), head CT, head MRI, and ICP monitoring. Treatment strategies vary depending on the severity and time since injury. Immediate emergency care for TBI focuses on limiting brain damage. Mild TBIs usually require no treatment other than rest and analgesics (specifically acetaminophen [Tylenol]) if headache is present. Nonsteroidal anti-inflammatory drugs, such as aspirin and ibuprofen (Motrin), should be avoided because they can increase bleeding risk.

Cold compresses can be applied to any outward edema. Severe brain injuries usually require hospitalization and often need intensive care. Osmotic diuretics (e.g., mannitol) may be given to reduce cerebral edema.

LEARNING POINTS

Immediately following a head injury there are some key actions that should be avoided, including:

- Do *not* apply direct pressure to a bleeding site; cover a wound with sterile gauze.
- Do *not* wash a head wound that is deep or bleeding a lot.
- Do *not* remove any object sticking out of a wound.
- Do *not* move the person unless it is absolutely necessary.
- Do *not* shake the person if he or she seems dazed.
- Do *not* remove a helmet if you suspect a serious head injury.
- Do *not* pick up a fallen child with any sign of a head injury.
- Do *not* drink alcohol within 48 hours of a serious head injury

Parameter	Score	Response
Eye opening	Spontaneous	4
	To voice	3
	To pain	2
	No response	1
Best verbal response	Oriented, converses	5
	Disoriented, converses	4
	Inappropriate words	3
	Incomprehensible sounds	2
	No response or intubated	1
Best motor response	Follows commands	6
	Localizes response (pushes away stimulus)	5
	Withdraws	4
	Abnormal flexion (decorticate)	3
	Abnormal extension (decerebrate)	2
	No response	1

Highest score = 15; lowest score = 3
Terms and Descriptive Behaviors for Levels of Consciousness
- Alert—Fully awake; aware of self and environment; appropriate, spontaneous response to stimuli.
- Confusion—Disoriented to person, time, and place (progresses from time to person to place); has difficulty following commands; may be agitated or irritable; may hallucinate.
- Delirium—disoriented to person, place and time; often agitated and uncooperative.
- Lethargy—Orientated to time, person, and place but somnolent; speech and thought processes slowed.
- Obtundation—decreased alertness accompanied by psychomotor retardation; can be aroused only with repeated verbal or tactile stimulation.
- Stupor—Awakens only to vigorous stimulation such as shaking; responds appropriately to painful stimuli; verbal responses are incomprehensible.
- Coma—Cannot be aroused; does not respond to verbal or tactile stimulation; brain stem reflexes may or may not be intact; may exhibit decerebrate or decorticate posturing.
- Light coma—Can be aroused; no spontaneous movement; withdraws appropriately to painful stimuli; brain stem reflexes (pupillary responses, gag, and corneal reflexes) are intact.
- Deep coma—Cannot be aroused; unresponsive to painful stimuli; absent brain stem reflexes; decerebrate posturing.

Figure 11-26

Glasgow Coma Scale.

Additionally, antiseizure agents and sedatives may be needed. Surgery can be performed to remove blood or repair fractures. Physical, speech, and occupational therapy may be required after the acute injury phase to minimize residual neurologic dysfunction. Prevention strategies for TBIs include wearing a seat belt when driving or riding in a motor vehicle, using appropriate child safety seats, wearing a helmet when appropriate (e.g., when playing sports, riding a bicycle, or skating), making the home safe (e.g., removing tripping hazards, having adequate lighting, using safety gates), storing firearms in locked cabinets, never driving impaired, and supervising children when playing.

Increased Intracranial Pressure

Increased intracranial pressure describes increased volume in the limited space of the cranial cavity. Increased ICP may occur because of a TBI as well as other conditions that would increase the volume in the skull (e.g., tumor, hydrocephalus, cerebral edema, and hemorrhage). The delicate pressure–volume relationship between ICP; volume of CSF, blood, and brain tissue; and cerebral perfusion is explained by the **Monro-Kellie hypothesis**. The Monro-Kellie hypothesis states that the cranial cavity cannot be compressed, and the volume inside the cavity is fixed (normal ICP is 60–200 mm H_2O or 4–15 mm Hg). The skull and its components (blood, CSF, and brain tissue) create a state of volume equilibrium, such that any increase in volume of one component must be compensated by a decrease in volume of another. This compensation is primarily accomplished by shifts in the CSF and, to a lesser extent, blood volume. These fluids respond to increases in volume of the remaining components. For example, an area of bleeding into the brain tissue (e.g., epidural hematoma) will be compensated by the downward displacement of CSF and venous blood. Transient increases in ICP routinely occur with position changes, coughing, or sneezing. These compensatory mechanisms are able to maintain a normal ICP for changes in volume up to a point (approximately 100–120 mL of volume increases).

In addition to shifting volumes, the brain has two other compensatory mechanisms to maintain tissue perfusion—autoregulation and the Cushing's reflex. With autoregulation, the blood vessels dilate to increase blood flow and constrict if the ICP is increased. The Cushing's reflex is a complex cascade of events that results in increased blood pressure. When the mean arterial pressure (average blood pressure) drops below the ICP, the hypothalamus increases sympathetic stimulation. This stimulation causes vasoconstriction, increased cardiac contractility, and increased cardiac output. If unresolved, the increased ICP eventually leads to what is described as the Cushing's triad—increased blood pressure, bradycardia, and changes in respiratory pattern (Figure 11-27). Baroreceptors in the carotid arteries detect the increase in blood pressure, triggering a parasympathetic response through vagal stimulation that induces bradycardia. Bradycardia may also be stimulated by the increased ICP impinging on the vagal nerve, causing a parasympathetic response. As pressure escalates inside the skull, space becomes limited and the brain tissue shifts downward. An irregular respiratory pattern, called Cheyne-Stokes, and bradypnea typically result from increased pressure on the brain stem due to swelling, or from a brain stem herniation.

Herniation is a feared complication of increased ICP. Herniation refers to the displacement of brain tissue. There are several types of herniation (Figure 11-28). The cerebral hemispheres, diencephalon, and midbran displace downward in transtentorial (central) herniation. The pressure created by this herniation impairs the cerebral blood flow, CSF, reticular activation system, and respirations. Uncal (uncinate) herniation occurs when the uncus (a hooklike anterior end of the hippocampal gyrus) of the temporal lobe shifts downward past the tentorium cerebelli (the extension of the dura mater that separates the cerebellum from the inferior portion of the occipital lobes). This herniation creates pressure on cranial nerve III, the posterior cerebral artery, and the reticular activation system. Cerebellar, or tonsillar (intrafratentorial), herniation occurs when the cerebellar tonsils (rounded lobules on the undersurface of each cerebellar hemisphere) are pushed downward through the foramen magnum. This herniation compresses the brain stem and vital centers, causing death.

Regardless of the cause, increased ICP past the point of compensation compresses cerebral blood

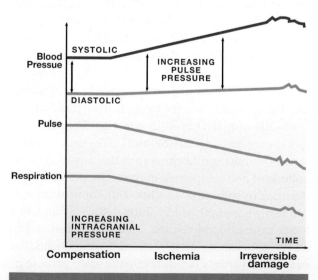

Figure 11-27

Vital sign changes with increased intracranial pressure.

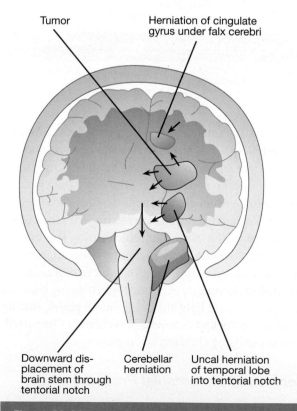

Figure 11-28

Types of herniation.

vessels and other structures as well as shifts content (**Figure 11-29**). Eventually, brain tissue dies. Increased ICP is a life-threatening situation that requires prompt treatment. If left untreated, increased ICP causes declining neurologic function, leading to death.

Clinical manifestations of increased ICP vary depending on age and reflect the effects of the rising pressures. These manifestations generally include:

- Decreasing level of consciousness (this results from pressure on the brain stem and cerebral cortex)
- Vomiting, often projectile (results from pressure on the medulla)
- Increasing blood pressure with increasing pulse pressure (the difference between systolic and diastolic pressure) (results of Cushing's reflex)

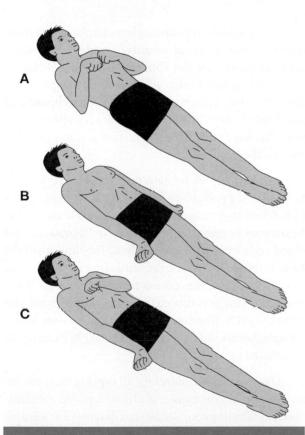

Figure 11-29

Decorticate and decerebrate posturing. (a) Decorticate response. Flexion of arms, wrists, and fingers with adduction in upper extremities. Extension, internal rotation, and plantar flexion in lower extremities. (b) Decerebrate response. All four extremities in rigid extension with hyperpronation of forearms and plantar extension of feet. (c) Decorticate response on the left side of the body and decerebrate response on the right side of the body.

- Bradycardia (response to the increasing blood pressure)
- Papilledema (results from increased pressure of CSF, which causes swelling around the optic disk)
- Fixed and dilated pupils (which results from pressure on cranial nerve III)
- Posturing

Manifestations in infants include:

- Separated sutures
- Bulging fontanelle

Manifestations in older children and adults include:

- Behavior changes
- Severe headache (results from stretching of the dura and walls of the large blood vessels)
- Lethargy
- Neurologic deficits
- Seizures

Diagnostic procedures for increased ICP consist of a history, physical examination (including completing the Glasgow Coma Scale), head CT, head MRI, and ICP monitoring. Increased ICP requires prompt diagnosis and treatment for optimal patient outcomes. Treatment strategies vary depending on the underlying etiology, and attempts should be made to resolve the source of pressure if possible (e.g., remove tumor or blood). Additional strategies are similar to those for TBIs and may include respiratory support (e.g., oxygen therapy or endotracheal intubation with mechanical ventilation), semi-Fowler's positioning, draining excess CSF, osmotic diuretics, corticosteriods, seizure precautions (e.g., low lighting and minimal stimulation), antiseizure agents, sedatives, stool softeners (because straining increases ICP), antiulcer agents (for those at high risk for stress ulcers), thermoregulation, and glucose management. Rarely, surgical removal of a skull segment may be performed.

Hematomas

Secondary brain damage can be caused by additional injurious factors such as hemorrhaging. A **hematoma** is a collection of blood in the tissue that develops from ruptured blood vessels. Hematomas can develop immediately or slowly because of a TBI or surgery. Hematomas are classified by their location (**Figure 11-30**).

TYPES OF INTRACRANIAL HEMATOMAS

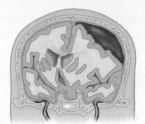

(a) Subdural

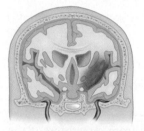

(b) Intracerebral

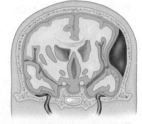

(c) Epidural

Figure 11-30

Types of hematomas. (a) Beneath the dura but outside the brain (subdural hematoma). (b) Within the substance of the brain tissue (intracerebral hematoma). (c) Outside the dura and under the skull (epidural hematoma).

Epidural hematomas result from bleeding between the dura and skull, usually caused by an arterial tear. Clinical manifestations of epidural hematomas include marked neurologic dysfunction that usually develops within a few hours of injury. The typical symptom pattern of an epidural hematoma is a brief loss of consciousness, followed by a short period of alertness, then loss of consciousness again. This pattern may not appear in all people. **Subdural hematomas** develop between the dura and arachnoid, frequently caused by a small venous tear (**Figure 11-31**). Because it is a result of a venous tear, subdural hematomas generally develop slowly. Subdural hematomas follow several patterns. With acute subdural hematomas, manifestations of neurologic deficits are present within 24 hours of an injury. This type progresses rapidly and has a high mortality. With subacute subdural hematomas, ICP increases over a period of about a week after the injury. With chronic subdural hematomas, manifestations develop several weeks after the injury because of a slow leak. Chronic subdural hematomas are more common in elderly adults because of brain atrophy, giving the hematoma more space to develop. **Intracerebral hematomas** result from bleeding in the brain tissue itself. Intracerebral hematomas are caused by

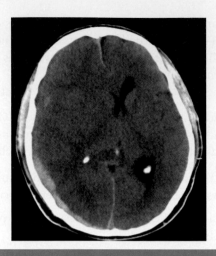

Figure 11-31

Midline shift associated with right-sided subdural hematoma.

contusion or shearing injuries but can also result from hypertension, cerebral vascular accidents (strokes), aneurysms, or vascular abnormalities. In addition to these hematomas, a subarachnoid hemorrhage results from bleeding in the space between the arachnoid and pia. The primary clinical presentation is a severe headache that has a sudden onset and that is worse near the back of the head.

In all types of hematomas, the bleeding leads to localized pressure on nearby tissue and increases ICP. Blood may coagulate and form a solid mass. The hematoma becomes encapsulated by fibroblasts, and blood cells within the capsule lyse. The fluid from the hemolysis exerts osmotic pressure, drawing more fluid into the capsule. This edema increases the size of the mass, applying pressure on the surrounding tissue and increasing ICP. Bleeding can trigger vasospasms, worsening ischemia. Additionally, increasing ICP can result in herniation.

Diagnostic procedures for all types of hematomas and hemorrhaging consist of a history, physical examination (including completing the Glasgow Coma Scale), head CT, head MRI, cerebral angiogram, and intracranial pressure monitor. Treatment strategies depend on the location and bleeding severity. No treatment may be required in mild cases in which the volume is small and the bleeding has ceased. Surgical removal of the blood through a burr hole or a craniotomy is often required. In some cases, removal of the blood may not be possible. In these cases, significant residual neurologic deficits that require physical, speech, and occupational therapy may remain. Additionally, strategies similar to those for TBIs and increased ICP (e.g., respiratory management, seizure precautions, and thermoregulation) may be required.

Spinal Cord Injuries

Spinal cord injuries (SCIs) result from direct injury to the spinal cord or indirectly from damage to surrounding bones, tissues, or blood vessels. SCIs are often caused by motor vehicle accidents, falls, violence, and sports injuries. Minor injuries to the spinal cord can occur because of weakening vertebral structures (e.g., rheumatoid arthritis or osteoporosis). Direct damage can occur if the spinal cord is pulled, pressed sideways, or compressed (**Figure 11-32**). This damage may occur if the head, neck, or back twists abnormally during an accident or injury. Hemorrhage, fluid accumulation, and edema can occur inside or outside the spinal cord (but within the spinal canal). The accumulation of blood or fluid can compress the spinal cord and damage it. Spinal shock refers to a temporary suppression of neurologic function because of spinal cord compression. In spinal shock, neurologic function gradually returns. SCIs are most common in Caucasians and males, with 40.2 years being the average age at injury.

SCIs result in a significant loss of neurologic functioning, often requiring extensive, long-term management. SCIs can also result in death, either immediately or because of complications (e.g., pneumonia, embolism, or septicemia). The degree of dysfunction depends on the severity of the injury and the location (Figure 11-16). The injury may result in a partial or complete disruption of the neurons and neural tracts anywhere along the spinal cord. SCIs are classified based on the location of damage (e.g., C4, T12) and degree of function. An injury to one of the eight cervical segments of the spinal cord causes quadriplegia (tetraplegia)—loss of all or most function in all four limbs. Injury to the thoracic, lumbar, or sacral regions causes paraplegia—loss of lower extremity function. The individual may experience complete paralysis (no voluntary use of the affected limbs) or incomplete paralysis (some voluntary use of the affected limbs). Incomplete quadriplegia is the most frequently occurring injury (approximately 30%). The spinal cord does not extend beyond the first lumbar vertebra, so injuries at and below this level do not cause SCIs. However, they may cause cauda equina syndrome (injury to the nerve roots in the area of the cauda equina). Complications of SCIs are numerous and can contribute to mortality associated with SCIs. These complications may include:

- Autonomic hyperreflexia (a massive sympathetic response that can cause headaches, hypertension, tachycardia, seizures, stroke, and death; most commonly associated with injuries above T6)

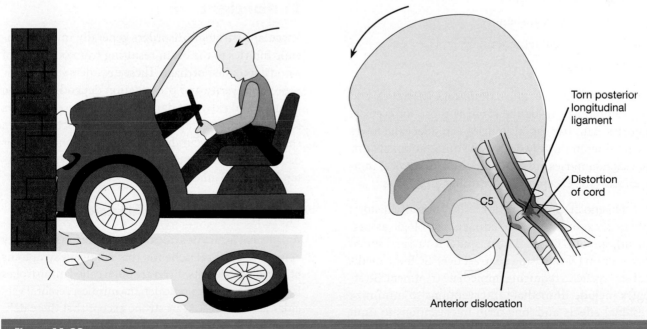

Figure 11-32

Spinal cord injuries.

- Neurogenic shock (an abnormal vasomotor response secondary to disruption of sympathetic impulses)
- Respiratory failure (caused by paralysis of the respiratory muscles)
- Effects of immobility (e.g., constipation, pulmonary infections, urinary infections, thrombus, impaired skin integrity, contractures)
- Changes in bowel and bladder function (e.g., urinary retention, incontinence, and constipation)
- Sexual dysfunction (e.g., erectile dysfunction)
- Chronic pain

Clinical manifestations of SCIs depend on the level of injury. Cervical injuries can affect both the upper and lower extremities. Manifestations of cervical injuries include:

- Breathing difficulties resulting from paralysis of the respiratory muscles
- Loss of normal bowel and bladder control (e.g., constipation, incontinence, and bladder spasms)
- Paresthesia
- Sensory changes
- Spasticity (increased muscle tone)
- Pain
- Weakness or paralysis
- Blood pressure instability
- Temperature fluctuations
- Diaphoresis

Thoracic injuries affect the lower extremities, and the symptoms can be the same as those for cervical injuries. Lumbar sacral injuries can affect the lower extremities in varying degrees. Manifestations of lumbar sacral injuries are similar to those of cervical injuries, with the exception of breathing difficulties.

Diagnostic procedures for SCIs consist of a history, physical examination (including a neurologic assessment), spinal CT, spinal MRI, spinal X-ray, and spinal myelogram (X-ray using contrast dye). SCIs are medical emergencies requiring immediate treatment. Strategies include immediate interventions to minimize residual effects and long-term interventions to limit complications. Immediate strategies may include:

- Immobilization of the spine
- Corticosteroid agents to reduce swelling

- Spinal traction to reduce the fracture and immobilize the spine
- Surgical repair of vertebral fractures or surgical removal of the fluid compressing the spinal cord (this is called decompression laminectomy)
- Respiratory management (e.g., oxygen therapy and endotracheal intubation with mechanical ventilation)
- Bed rest

Long-term strategies may include:

- Physical, occupational, and speech therapy
- Mobility assistive devices (e.g., a wheelchair)
- Long-term respiratory management (e.g., mechanical ventilation)
- Meticulous skin care
- Bowel and bladder training or management (e.g., catheterization and stool softeners)
- Antispasmotic agents and botulinum toxin type A (Botox) injections to treat muscle spasms
- Pain management
- Nutritional support
- Prompt treatment of infections (pneumonia is the leading cause of death)

Vascular Neurologic Disorders

Vascular neurologic disorders generally involve ischemic injuries to the brain resulting from occlusion of blood flow or hemorrhage. These disorders vary significantly in severity and presentation depending on the location and extent of damage. Often these disorders result in some degree of neurologic dysfunction. These conditions may occur due to congenital abnormalities or chronic diseases such as hypertension, hypercholesterolemia, and atherosclerosis.

Transient Ischemic Attack

A transient ischemic attack (TIA) refers to a temporary episode of cerebral ischemia that results in symptoms of neurologic deficits. TIAs are often called ministrokes because these neurologic deficits mimic a cerebral vascular accident (CVA) or stroke except that these deficits resolve within 24 hours (1–2 hours in most cases). TIAs may occur singly or in a series. TIAs are warning signs that a CVA may be impending; however, not all CVAs are preceded by a TIA. This ischemia can occur because of a cerebral artery occlusion (e.g., thrombus, embolus, or plaque), cerebral arteries narrowing (e.g., atherosclerosis or spasms), or cerebral artery injury (e.g., inflammation or hypertension). Additional risk factors of TIAs include migraines, smoking, diabetes mellitus, advancing age, inadequate nutrition, hypercholesterolemia, oral contraceptive usage, excessive alcohol consumption, and illicit drug use. Complications of TIAs include permanent brain damage from the lack of oxygen and glucose, injury from falls, and CVA from the ischemia.

Clinical manifestations of TIAs begin suddenly and last for a short period. Within 24 hours, symptoms disappear completely. TIAs are not strokes, but the manifestations are the same. These manifestations reflect the location of the ischemia and may include:

- Muscle weakness or paralysis of the face, arm, or leg (usually unilateral)
- Paresthesia on one side of the body
- Aphasia (difficulty speaking) or receptive aphasia (difficulty understanding spoken language)
- Dysphagia (difficulty swallowing)
- Dysgraphia (difficulty writing)
- Difficulty reading
- Vision issues (e.g., diplopia, nystagmus, and partial or complete loss of vision)
- Changes in sensation (e.g., touch, pain, temperature, pressure, hearing, and taste)
- Change in levels of consciousness (e.g., lethargy, unconscious, or coma)
- Personality, mood, or emotional changes
- Confusion
- Agnosia (inability to recognize or identify sensory stimuli)
- Ataxia
- Vertigo (abnormal sensation of movement) or dizziness
- Incontinence of bowel or bladder

Because clinical manifestations often resolve prior reaching a healthcare facility, diagnosis may be made based on a history alone. Additional diagnostic procedures consist of a physical examination (including a neurologic assessment and blood pressure), head CT, head MRI, carotid ultrasound, cerebral arteriogram, EEG, serum clotting studies, blood chemistry, complete blood count, erythrocyte sedimentation rate test (can identify inflammatory process), and serum lipids test. Treatment strategies for TIAs focus on preventing the occurrence of a CVA. These strategies typically include managing any underlying conditions (e.g., hypertension, atherosclerosis, and diabetes mellitus). Medications, such as antiplatelet aggregation agents (e.g., aspirin and clopidogrel [Plavix]) or anticoagulants (e.g., warfarin [Coumadin]), may be used to prevent clotting. Angioplasty (balloon dilatation) can open narrowed arteries, or a carotid endarterectomy (surgical removal of plaque) can increase cerebral blood flow. Lifestyle management includes smoking cessation, minimizing dietary cholesterol and fat, increasing dietary fruits and vegetables, exercising regularly, limiting alcohol consumption, and eliminating illicit drug use.

Cerebral Vascular Accident

Much like a TIA, a cerebral vascular accident (CVA), or stroke, refers to an interruption of cerebral blood supply (**Figure 11-33**). The chief difference between a CVA and TIA is that CVA damage is permanent. A CVA is an infarction of the brain, so it is often referred to as a brain attack. This interruption of blood flow may result from a total vessel occlusion (e.g., thrombus, embolus, or plaque) or cerebral vessel rupture (e.g., cerebral aneurysm, arteriovenous malformation, or hypertension); therefore, there are two major types of CVA—ischemic and hemorrhagic. Ischemic strokes are the most common (80%), and hemorrhagic strokes are the most deadly. Five minutes (sometimes less) of altered tissue perfusion can lead to irreversible cell damage from the lack of oxygen and glucose. CVA can result in significant neurologic dysfunction and death. CVA is the chief cause of long-term disability

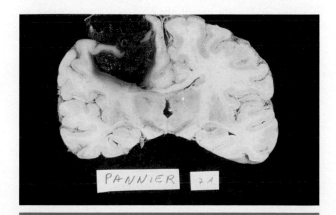

Figure 11-33

Cerebral vascular accident (CVA).

and third leading cause of death in the United States (CDC, 2009b). In the United States, someone experiences a CVA every 40 seconds. In 2009, the cost associated with this widespread problem with extensive consequences in the United States reached nearly $69 billion. CVA prevalence and mortality in the United States is highest among African Americans and those living in the Southeast. Additional risk factors include physical inactivity, obesity, hypertension, smoking, hypercholesterolemia, diabetes mellitus, atherosclerosis, oral contraceptive usage, excessive alcohol consumption, and illicit drug use.

Clinical manifestations of CVA are similar to those of a TIA except that CVA symptoms do not resolve. These manifestations may improve with time and therapy, but these manifestations can remain, creating complications. In addition to the manifestations of neurologic impairment associated with TIAs, headaches may be present with hemorrhagic strokes because of increasing ICP.

Diagnostic procedures for CVA consist of a history, physical examination (including a neurologic assessment), head CT, head MRI, carotid ultrasound, cerebral arteriogram, serum clotting studies, blood chemistry, and complete blood count. A CVA is a medical emergency that requires prompt treatment to minimize brain damage. Determining whether the CVA is ischemic or hemorrhagic in origin prior to treatment is crucial because the interventions vary depending on the type. Additionally, some interventions for ischemic strokes can worsen hemorrhagic strokes (e.g., thrombolytic agents). The differential diagnosis should be made as soon as possible because early treatment will improve outcomes. Optimally, treatment should be delivered within 3 hours of symptom onset; therefore, persons or family members of persons who seem to be experiencing a CVA should make note of when the symptoms began. Ischemic strokes are treated with thrombolytic agents (to dissolve any clots) and aspirin (to limit platelet activity). This treatment is contraindicated in persons with a recent history of bleeding issues. Additionally, procedures such as angioplasty or carotid endarterectomy may be necessary for ischemic strokes. Surgical repair of aneurysms or arteriovenous malformations as well as blood removal may be required for hemorrhagic strokes. Corticosteroids may also be administered with either type to reduce cerebral edema, and antihypertensive agents may be used to reduce blood pressure. A multidisciplinary approach (using a team made up of a nurse, physical therapist, speech therapist, occupational therapist, dietician, and social worker) should be initiated as soon as the patient is stable and may be required long term to minimize or prevent complications. Depending on the degree of dysfunction, strategies may be necessary to prevent complications of immobility (e.g., constipation, impaired skin integrity, contractures, and infections).

Cerebral Aneurysm

A **cerebral aneurysm** is a localized outpouching of a cerebral artery (see Chapter 4). This weakening of the artery may occur as a congenital defect or develop later in life because of conditions such as hypertension, connective tissue diseases (e.g., Marfan syndrome), TBIs, and arterial wall infections (**Figure 11-34; Figure 11-35**). This bulging artery segment can put pressure on surrounding tissue. Additionally, the aneurysm may leak or rupture, causing a CVA or death. There are several types of aneurysm, but most cerebral aneurysms are berry or saccular. Cerebral aneurysms most frequently occur in multiples on the circle of Willis.

Many cerebral aneurysms are asymptomatic until they grow large enough to compress surrounding structures or ruptures. Clinical manifestations that may appear as the aneurysm compresses nearby structures include vision issues (e.g., diplopia and loss of vision), headache, eye pain, or neck pain. A sudden, severe headache is an indication that the aneurysm has ruptured. Additional manifestations resemble those of increased ICP and CVA.

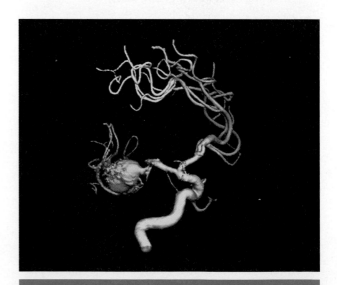

Figure 11-34

Cerebral aneurysm.

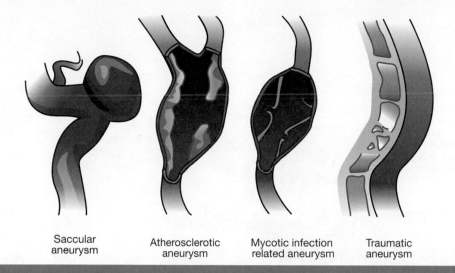

Saccular aneurysm   Atherosclerotic aneurysm   Mycotic infection related aneurysm   Traumatic aneurysm

Figure 11-35

Types of cerebral aneurysms.

Often diagnosis occurs inadvertently with a head CT or MRI. Additional diagnostic procedures include a history, physical examination, cerebral arteriography, and EEG. If discovered prior to rupture, treatment strategies include surgical repair (if possible) and managing contributing factors (e.g., hypertension). Rupture is a medical emergency that requires immediate surgical repair. Additional strategies are similar to those for a CVA and subarachnoid hemorrhage.

Seizure Disorders

A seizure is a transient physical or behavior alteration that results from an abnormal electrical activity in the brain. Mechanisms that may be responsible for this abnormal electrical activity include altered membrane ion channels, altered extracellular electrolytes, and imbalanced excitatory and inhibitory neurotransmitters. Some neurons are hypersensitive or remain in a partial state of depolarization, increasing excitability. Seizures can occur secondary to trauma, hypoglycemia, electrolyte disorders, acidosis, infection, tumors, or chemical ingestion (e.g., medications, illicit drugs, and alcohol). Additionally, seizures can occur as a disorder referred to as epilepsy. Epilepsy results from spontaneous firing of abnormal neurons and is characterized by recurrent seizures for which there is no underlying or correctable cause. According to the CDC (2010b), epilepsy affects about 2 million Americans. About 10% of people will experience a seizure sometime during their lifetime, and about 3% will have had a diagnosis of epilepsy by age 80. Complications of seizures include brain damage, TBIs, aspiration, mood disorders, and status epilepticus (seizures that last longer than 20 minutes or subsequent seizures occur before the individual has fully regained consciousness).

Seizures can be classified into two broad categories—focal and generalized. Focal seizures, also called partial seizures, occur in just one part of the brain. About 60% of people with epilepsy have focal seizures. These seizures vary depending on the area of the brain affected, and they are frequently described by the area of the brain in which they originate (**Figure 11-36**). In a simple focal seizure, the individual having the seizure remains conscious but experiences unusual feelings or sensations that can take many forms. The individual may experience sudden and unexplainable feelings of joy, anger, sadness, or nausea. Additionally, the individual may hear, smell, taste, see, or feel things that are not real. In a complex focal seizure, the individual has changes in or loss of consciousness, producing a dreamlike experience. People having a complex focal seizure may display strange, repetitive behaviors (e.g., blinking, twitching, moving one's mouth, walking in a circle) called automatisms. These seizures usually last just a few seconds. Some people with focal seizures, especially complex focal seizures, may experience auras (unusual sensations just prior to an impending seizure). These auras are actually simple focal seizures in which the person maintains consciousness. The symptoms an individual has and the progression of those symptoms tend to be similar with every seizure. The symptoms of focal seizures can easily be confused

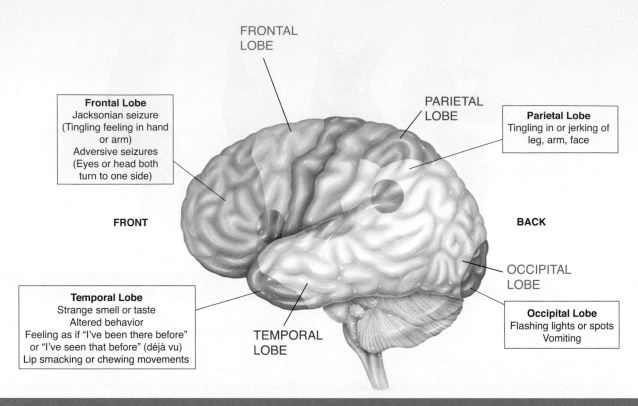

FRONTAL
LOBE

PARIETAL
LOBE

Frontal Lobe
Jacksonian seizure
(Tingling feeling in hand
or arm)
Adversive seizures
(Eyes or head both
turn to one side)

Parietal Lobe
Tingling in or jerking of
leg, arm, face

FRONT

BACK

OCCIPITAL
LOBE

Temporal Lobe
Strange smell or taste
Altered behavior
Feeling as if "I've been there before"
or "I've seen that before" (déjà vu)
Lip smacking or chewing movements

TEMPORAL
LOBE

Occipital Lobe
Flashing lights or spots
Vomiting

Figure 11-36

Manifestations of focal seizures depending on the regions of the brain.

with other disorders (e.g., migraine headaches, narcolepsy, syncope, and psychiatric disorders), so those disorders should be ruled out.

Generalized seizures are a result of abnormal neuronal activity on both sides of the brain. These seizures may cause loss of consciousness, falls, or massive muscle spasms. There are many kinds of generalized seizures. A person having an absence seizure (previously called a petit mal seizure) may appear to be staring into space and/or have jerking or twitching muscles (Figure 11-37). Tonic seizures cause stiffening of muscles of the body, generally those in the back and extremities. Clonic seizures cause repeated jerking movements of muscles on both sides of the body. Myoclonic seizures cause jerks or twitches of the upper body, arms, or legs (Figure 11-38). Atonic seizures cause a loss of normal muscle tone. The affected person will fall down or may drop his or her head involuntarily. Tonic-clonic seizures (previously called grand mal seizures) cause a mixture of symptoms, including stiffening of the body and repeated jerks of the arms and/or legs as well as loss of consciousness (Figure 11-39). The individual having a generalized seizure may be confused, fatigued, and fall into a deep sleep following the seizure; the time

during which these manifestations occur is referred to as the postictal period. Not all seizures can be easily defined as either focal or generalized. Some people have seizures that begin as focal seizures but then spread to the entire brain. Other people may have both types of seizures but with no clear pattern.

Diagnostic procedures for seizure disorders consist of a history (including a description of the seizure activity if possible), physical examination, head CT, head MRI, head positron emission tomography (PET), and EEG. Treatment focuses on preventing the occurrence and limiting the duration of the seizure activity. Treatment strategies can be grouped into two categories—those to manage acute seizures and those to prevent seizures. Most seizures resolve spontaneously within a few minutes, but employing safety precautions can prevent injury. During a seizure, positioning the individual on his or her side can prevent aspiration (vomiting is common). Additionally, the head should be protected. Items should not be forced in between the individual's teeth; it is more likely to cause harm than to help. Attempts should not be made to restrain the individual; this also is more likely to cause injury. Airway management and oxygen therapy may also be

BETWEEN SEIZURES:
Normal appearance

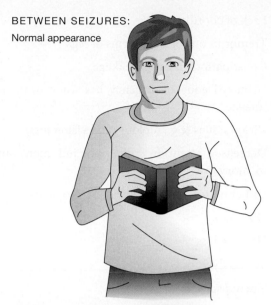

DURING SEIZURE:
Vacant stare
Eyes roll upward
Lack of response

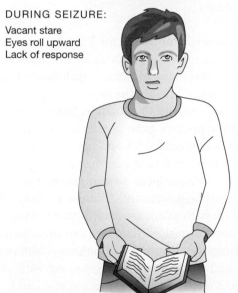

Figure 11-37

Absence seizures.

Jerking of arms,
shoulder, and head

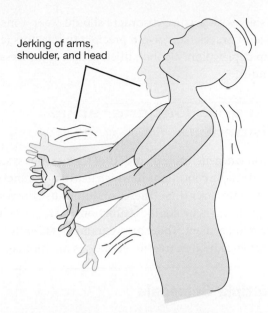

Episodes typically occur soon after awakening

Figure 11-38

Myoclonic seizures.

necessary to minimize hypoxia. If status epilepticus develops, medication (e.g., muscle relaxants, antiseizure agents) will often be administered intravenously to stop the seizure. Following a seizure, the individual should be allowed to sleep as desired. For epilepsy, antiseizure agents will be administered daily to minimize the frequency and duration of seizure activity. These medications require close monitoring and accurate administration to ensure therapeutic dosing and limit side effects. If medications are not successful in controlling seizure activity, surgical resection or transaction of the region in which the abnormal electrical activity originates might be necessary. Additionally,

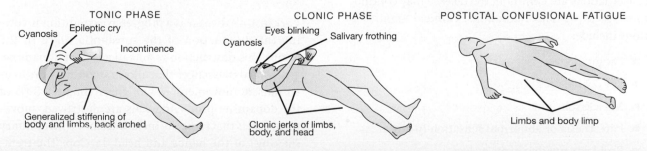

TONIC PHASE

Cyanosis   Epileptic cry
                        Incontinence

Generalized stiffening of
body and limbs, back arched

CLONIC PHASE

            Eyes blinking
Cyanosis   Salivary frothing

Clonic jerks of limbs,
body, and head

POSTICTAL CONFUSIONAL FATIGUE

Limbs and body limp

Figure 11-39

Tonic-clonic seizures.

persons with seizure disorders should wear a medical-alert bracelet and avoid precipitating factors (e.g., sleep deprivation, alcohol, illicit drugs, and excessive stimuli).

Chronic Degenerative Disorders

Chronic degenerative disorders of the nervous system include those conditions in which neurologic function deteriorates over time. These conditions usually result in significant neurologic dysfunction that requires lifelong management. These disorders are not usually preventable, and often treatment options are limited.

Multiple Sclerosis

Multiple sclerosis (MS) is a debilitating autoimmune condition that involves a progressive and irreversible demyelination of brain, spinal cord, and cranial nerves neurons. This damage occurs in diffuse patches throughout the nervous system and slows or stops nerve impulses. The progression of this damage varies from person to person. Like most autoimmune disorders, the underlying cause is unknown. According to the National Institutes of Health (2010b), approximately 300,000 Americans have MS. The prevalence rates are the highest among women, Caucasians, and those living in temperate climates. The onset of symptoms usually occurs between 20 and 40 years of age. Complications of MS include epilepsy, paralysis (most often the legs), and depression.

Clinical manifestations of MS vary depending on the degree of damage and the specific nerves affected; however, MS is characterized by remissions and exacerbations. Exacerbations may last for days to months. Fever, hot baths, sun exposure, and stress can trigger or worsen these episodes. Although remissions and exacerbations are common, the disease may continue to progress without remissions. Clinical manifestations include:

- Fatigue
- Loss of balance
- Muscle spasms
- Paresthesia or abnormal sensation in any area
- Problems moving arms or legs
- Weakness in one or more arms or legs
- Unsteady gait

- Lack of coordination
- Tremor in one or more arms or legs
- Constipation and stool leakage
- Urinary frequency, urgency, hesitancy, or incontinence
- Vision issues (e.g., diplopia and vision loss)
- Decreased attention span, poor judgment, and memory loss
- Difficulty reasoning and solving problems
- Dizziness
- Hearing loss
- Sexual dysfunction
- Slurred speech
- Dysphagia

There is no definitive test for MS, which can delay diagnosis. Diagnostic procedures for MS may consist of a history, physical examination (including a neurologic assessment), MRI studies (brain and spinal cord), lumbar puncture with CSF analysis (this often shows high levels of protein, gamma globulin, and lymphocytes), and nerve conduction studies. No cure for MS exists; however, treatment can slow the progression. Treatment strategies focus on minimizing symptoms and maximizing quality of life. These strategies include medications such as corticosteroids (treats exacerbations), interferons (slows damage), and immunemodulators (suppresses immune response). Additionally, physical and occupational therapy along with assistive devices (e.g., wheelchair, walkers, and handrails) can maximize functioning. Coping strategies, support, proper nutrition, and adequate rest can promote and maintain overall health.

Parkinson's Disease

Parkinson's disease is a progressive condition involving the destruction of the substantia nigra in the brain. This destruction results in a lack of dopamine, a chemical messenger that allows smooth, coordinated muscle movement. When approximately 80% of the dopamine-producing cells are destroyed, movement issues that typically include tremors (involuntary shaking) of the hands and head develop. The tremors may disappear or decrease when the body part is moved intentionally. The cause of Parkinson's disease is unknown. According to the NIH (2010c), approximately 500,000 Americans have been diagnosed with Parkinson's disease, and prevalence rates are evenly distributed across gender, social, ethnic, geographic, and economic groups.

Clinical manifestations of Parkinson's disease vary depending on the degree of dopamine deficit. These manifestations often include (**Figure 11-40**):

- Slowing or stopping of automatic movements (e.g., blinking)
- Constipation
- Dysphagia

- Drooling
- Unsteady gait
- Masklike appearance to face
- Myalgia
- Problems with movement, including the following:
  - Difficulty initiating or continuing movement (e.g., walking or getting out of a chair)
  - Loss of fine hand movements (writing may become small and difficult to read; eating can become more difficult)
  - Shuffling gait
  - Slowed movements
- Rigid or stiff muscles (often beginning in the legs)
- Tremors
  - Tremors usually occur in the limbs at rest or when the arm or leg is held out
  - Tremors go away during purposeful movement
  - Eventually, tremors can be seen in the head, lips, tongue, and feet
  - Tremors may be worse when the affected individual is tired, excited, or stressed
  - Finger-thumb rubbing (called "pill-rolling" tremor) may be present
- Slowed, quieter speech with monotone voice
- Stooped position
- Anxiety, stress, and tension
- Confusion
- Dementia
- Depression
- Syncope
- Hallucinations
- Memory loss
- Seborrhea (oily skin)

Much like MS, Parkinson's disease does not have a definitive test. Diagnostic procedures consist of a history, physical examination (including neurologic assessment), and other tests to rule out other conditions. There is no cure for Parkinson's disease. The goal of treatment is to control symptoms. Medications (e.g., levadopa and dopamine agonists) can increase the levels of dopamine, but the effects of the medications often diminish over time, requiring dose increases.

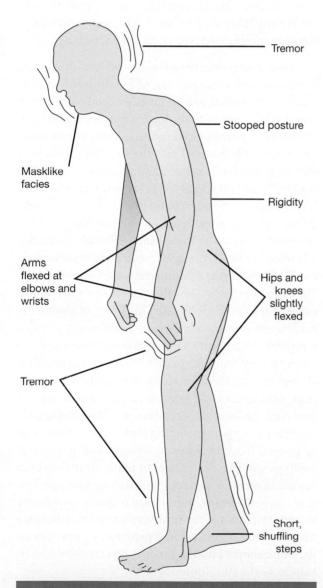

Tremor
Stooped posture
Masklike facies
Rigidity
Arms flexed at elbows and wrists
Hips and knees slightly flexed
Tremor
Short, shuffling steps

Figure 11-40

Clinical presentation of Parkinson's disease.

Medications may reach maximum dosing, and symptom control will be lost. Deep brain stimulation is a common surgical treatment for Parkinson's disease. Additionally, physical and occupational therapy along with assistive devices (e.g., wheelchair, walkers, and handrails) can maximize functioning. Coping strategies, support, proper nutrition, and adequate rest can promote and maintain overall health.

Amyotrophic Lateral Sclerosis

Amyotrophic lateral sclerosis (ALS), also called Lou Gehrig's disease after the famous baseball player who died of it, is a disease that involves damage of the upper motor neurons of the cerebral cortex and lower motor neurons of the brain stem and spinal cord. Sensory neurons, cognitive function, and cranial nerves III, IV, and VI are not affected. The nerves lose their ability to trigger muscle movement, resulting in muscle weakness, disability, paralysis, and eventually death (usually within 5 years of onset of symptoms). ALS may also increase the risk for dementia. In most cases, the cause of ALS is undetermined, but genetics plays a role in 10% of cases. Researchers are exploring several possible causes of ALS. The first possible cause is free radical damage (see Chapter 1). The inherited form of ALS often involves a mutation in a gene responsible for producing a strong antioxidant enzyme that protects cells from damage caused by free radicals. The second possible cause being explored is glutamate's influence. People who have ALS typically have higher than normal levels of glutamate, a chemical messenger in the brain, in their CSF. Too much glutamate is toxic to some nerve cells. Finally, possible autoimmune responses are being studied as a possible trigger for ALS.

The exact number of cases in the United States is unknown, but the NIH (2010a) estimates that 20,000 Americans have ALS. Though this condition is not necessarily common, ALS is a public concern because there is no means to preventing the continuous and rapid decline in motor function. In 2010, a National ALS registry was launched to collect, manage, and analyze information about people with ALS. This registry will provide information that will illuminate the scope and epidemiology of the problem as well as guide practice and research.

Clinical manifestations of ALS become progressively worse as more motor neurons are damaged. The loss of upper motor neurons results in spastic paralysis and hyperreflexia, and the loss of lower motor neurons results in flaccid paralysis. Early manifestations of ALS include:

- Footdrop (difficulty lifting the front of the foot and toes)
- Lower extremities weakness
- Hand weakness or clumsiness
- Slurred speech or dysphagia
- Muscle cramps and twitching in upper extremities and the tongue

The disease frequently begins in the upper or lower extremities and then spreads to other parts of the body. As the disease advances, muscles become progressively weaker until they are paralyzed. ALS eventually affects chewing, swallowing, speaking, and breathing.

Like other degenerative neurologic disorders, there is no definitive test for ALS. Diagnostic procedures are often used to rule out other conditions. These procedures consist of a history, physical examination (including a neurologic assessment), electromyogram (an electrode is inserted into the muscles to measure electrical activity), nerve conduction studies, MRI studies (head and spinal cord), lumbar puncture with CSF analysis, and muscle biopsy. ALS has no cure. Treatment strategies focus on slowing the progression and controlling symptoms. Riluzole (Rilutek), a benzothiazole, is the only medication approved by the Food and Drug Administration for slowing ALS. The drug appears to slow the disease's progression in some people, perhaps by reducing levels of glutamate. Additionally, stem cell therapy is being explored as a possible treatment. Antispasmodic agents may be given to treat muscle spasms. Physical, occupational, and speech therapy, along with assistive devices (e.g., wheelchairs and braces) can maximize muscle function. Because of aspiration and dysphagia risk, nutritional support including high-caloric foods, soft or pureed foods, thickened liquids, and parenteral feedings will become critical to maintaining optimal health as muscles weaken. Respiratory management (e.g., oxygen therapy, pulmonary hygiene, respiratory treatments, and mechanical ventilation) will become necessary as muscle weakness progresses. Coping strategies and support for the patient and caregivers can be helpful as the condition worsens.

Myasthenia Gravis

Myasthenia gravis is an autoimmune condition in which acetylcholine receptors are impaired or destroyed by IgG autoantibodies. This acetylcholine receptor compromise leads to a disruption of normal communication between the nerve and muscle at the neuromuscular junction. This disruption causes weakness of the voluntary skeletal muscles because of inadequate nerve stimulation. Muscle weakness typically increases during periods of activity and improves after periods of rest. Muscles that control eye and eyelid movement, facial expression, chewing, talking, and swallowing are often, but not always, involved in the disorder. The muscles that control breathing and neck and limb movements may also be affected. Myasthenia gravis is common (2–3 cases per 10,000 people) and affects gender, ethnic, and age groups equally. The exact trigger for the autoimmune response is unclear, but the thymus gland is thought to play a role. Persons with myasthenia gravis often have a thymus gland abnormality (e.g., hyperplasia and tumors). Some factors can worsen myasthenia gravis and cause a **myasthenic crisis**, including fatigue, illness, stress, extreme heat, alcohol consumption, and certain medications (e.g., beta blockers, calcium channel blockers, quinine, and some antibiotics). Myasthenic crisis is a potentially life-threatening complication, which occurs when the muscles become too weak to maintain adequate ventilation.

Clinical manifestations of myasthenia gravis reflect the muscle weakness. These manifestations may include:

- Breathing difficulty
- Dysphagia
- Difficulty climbing stairs, lifting objects, or rising from a seated position
- Dysarthria
- Drooping head
- Facial paralysis or weakness
- Fatigue
- Hoarseness or changing voice
- Eye and vision issues (e.g., diplopia, ptosis, blurred vision, and difficulty maintaining gaze)

Diagnosis of myasthenia gravis is primarily made on clinical presentation. Diagnostic procedures consist of a history, physical examination (including a neurologic assessment), edrophonium test (a short-acting anticholinesterase inhibitor called edrophonium is injected and a sudden, although temporary, improvement in muscle strength indicates possible myasthenia gravis), serum antibody levels, nerve conduction study, electromyogram, and thymus CT or MRI. Myasthenia gravis has no cure, but treatment strategies can manage symptoms. Medications used to treat the disorder include anticholinesterase agents, which help improve neuromuscular transmission and increase muscle strength. Immunosuppressive drugs may also be used; these medications improve muscle strength by suppressing the production of abnormal antibodies. Other therapies include a thymectomy, plasmapheresis (removal of abnormal antibodies from the blood), and high doses of immunoglobulins. Additional self-care strategies to maximize health and functioning include proper nutrition, adequate rest, assistive devices, coping strategies, and support.

Huntington's Disease

Huntington's disease (HD), or Huntington's chorea, is a condition caused by a genetically programmed degeneration of neurons in the brain. HD is an autosomal dominant disorder (see Chapter 1) involving a defect on chromosome 4. The defect causes a segment of DNA, called a CAG repeat, to occur many more times than usual. Normally, this section of DNA is repeated 10–35 times within the DNA coding sequence, but it is repeated 36–120 times in persons with HD. This defect leads to progressive atrophy of the brain, particularly in the basal ganglia and the frontal cortex (**Figure 11-41**). The ventricles dilate, gamma-aminobutyric acid levels diminish, and acetylcholine levels fall. As the gene is transmitted from one generation to the next, the number of repeats (called CAG repeat expansion) tends to increase. With a larger number of repeats, the chance of developing symptoms at an earlier age increases. Therefore, as the disease is transmitted in families, it becomes evident at younger and younger ages. The

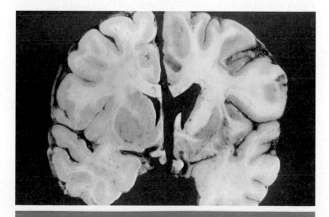

Figure 11-41

Neurologic changes of Huntington's disease.

earlier HD symptoms appear, the faster it progresses. Most cases of HD appear between 30 and 40 years of age, but HD may appear in childhood or adolescence in a small number of cases. In general, the duration of the illness ranges from 10 to 30 years. The most common causes of death are infection (most often pneumonia), injuries related to a fall, or other complications (e.g., suicide). According to the NIH (2009), more than 15,000 Americans have HD. At least 150,000 others have a 50% risk of developing the disease, and thousands more of their relatives live with the possibility of developing HD.

Clinical manifestations of HD reflect the cerebral atrophy caused by the neural degeneration. Initially, manifestations are insidious and vary from person to person. Family members may first notice that the individual experiences mood swings or becomes uncharacteristically irritable, apathetic, passive, depressed, or angry. Other behavioral symptoms may include antisocial behavior, hallucinations, paranoia, and psychosis. These symptoms may lessen as the disease progresses or, in some individuals, may continue and include aggression or severe depression. HD may produce a dementia as the individual's judgment, memory, and other cognitive functions become affected. Early signs often include having trouble driving, learning new things, remembering facts, answering questions, or making decisions. Some people may even display changes in handwriting. As the disease progresses, concentration on intellectual tasks becomes increasingly difficult. In some people, the disease may begin with uncontrolled, rapid, jerky movements (chorea) (e.g., tremors, grimaces, and twitching) in the fingers, feet, face, or trunk. These movements often intensify when the person is anxious. HD can also begin with mild clumsiness, unsteady gait, and rigidity. Some people develop chorea manifestations later, after the disease has progressed. Chorea often creates serious problems with ambulation, increasing the likelihood of falls. As the disease progresses, speech becomes slurred and other functions (e.g., swallowing, eating, speaking, and walking) continue to decline. Many people with HD remain aware of their environment and are able to express emotions, but some cannot recognize their family members.

Because of its psychologic manifestations, HD is often mistaken for psychiatric disorders. Diagnostic procedures of HD include a history, physical examination, psychiatric evaluation, genetic testing for the defective gene (either before or after the onset of symptoms), head CT, head MRI, and head PET. There is no cure and no treatment to stop the progression. Treatment strategies focus on slowing the progression and managing symptoms to maximize functioning. Tetrabenazine (Xenazine) is the first medication specifically approved by the Food and Drug Administration for the treatment of HD signs and symptoms. Xenazine reduces the jerky, involuntary movements of HD by increasing the amount of dopamine available in the brain. Tranquilizers and antipsychotic agents can control movements, violent outbursts, and hallucinations. Antidepressant agents can control depression and the obsessive-compulsive rituals that some people with HD develop. Some evidence suggests that coenzyme Q10 may also slow the course of the disease. Physical, occupational, and speech therapy can maximize function. Coping strategies, support, adequate hydration, proper nutrition, and regular exercise for both the patient and caregivers can support optimal health. New therapies are currently under investigation, including stem cell therapy, new medications, and new combinations of existing medications.

Dementia

Dementia refers to a group of conditions in which cortical function is decreased, impairing cognitive skills (e.g., language, logical thinking, judgment, and learning) and motor coordination. Issues with memory are common with dementia and include short-term memory losses as well as confusion of historical events. Behavioral and personality changes interfere with relationships, work, and activities of daily living. Vascular disease (e.g., atherosclerosis), infections, toxins, and genetic conditions may cause dementia. There are several types of dementia, each with limited treatment options. Although great strides have been made in recent years, most types of dementia remain poorly understood.

Alzheimer's Disease

Alzheimer's disease (AD) is the most common form of dementia. In AD, healthy brain tissue degenerates and atrophies (**Figure 11-42**). This atrophy causes a steady decline in memory and mental abilities. The exact etiology of AD is unknown, but three pathologic characteristics are associated with AD. Amyloid plaques, which contain fragments of a protein called beta-amyloid peptide, mix with a collection of additional proteins, neuron remnants, and other nerve cell pieces. Neurofibrillary tangles, found inside neurons, are abnormal collections of a protein called tau. Normal tau is required for healthy neurons; however, in

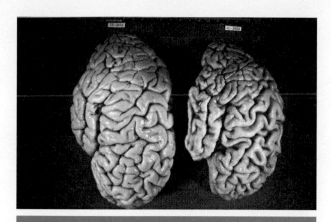

Figure 11-42

Alzheimer's disease.

AD, tau clumps together. As a result, neurons fail to function normally and eventually die. Finally, connections between neurons responsible for memory and learning are lost. Neurons cannot survive when their connections to other neurons are lost. As neurons die throughout the brain, the affected regions begin to atrophy, or shrink. By the final stage of AD, damage is widespread and brain tissue has shrunk significantly.

AD is not a part of normal aging, but risk does increase with age (onset is usually after 60 years of age). Prevalence rates are higher in women, in part because of a longer life expectancy. Some evidence suggests that AD rates are higher in those persons with less education, but the precise reason why this occurs is unknown. Some researchers theorize that the more the brain is used, the more synapses are created, which provides a greater reserve with aging. Additional risk factors include family history, hypertension, hypercholesterolemia, diabetes mellitus, and history of TBI. According to the NIH (2008), as many as 5 million Americans suffer from AD; this number is double what it was in 1980. AD has recently surpassed diabetes mellitus as the sixth leading cause of death among American adults. Notably, mortality rates for AD are on the rise, unlike heart disease and cancer death rates, which are continuing to decline. Complications such as infections (primarily pneumonia and urinary tract infections), injuries related to falls, malnutrition, dehydration, and decubitus ulcers contribute to the mortality associated with AD.

The onset of AD tends to be insidious. Clinical manifestations may start with mild memory loss and confusion, but AD eventually leads to irreversible mental impairment that destroys a person's ability to remember, reason, learn, and imagine. This course may extend 10–20 years. Clinical manifestations may include:

- Memory loss (e.g., one might repeat things, forget conversations or appointments, misplace things, and eventually forget the names of family members and everyday objects)

- Problems with abstract thinking (e.g., trouble balancing a checkbook, a problem that progresses to trouble recognizing and dealing with numbers)

- Difficulty finding the right word to express thoughts or even follow conversations

- Difficulty reading and writing

- Disorientation, even in familiar surroundings

- Loss of judgment (e.g., not knowing what to do if food on the stove is burning)

- Difficulty performing familiar tasks (e.g., driving, cooking, bathing, dressing, and eating)

- Personality changes (e.g., mood swings, paranoia, stubbornness, withdrawal, depression, anxiety, and aggression)

- Hallucinations

- Incontinence of bowel or bladder

Diagnosis of AD is often difficult and often involves ruling out other conditions. Diagnostic procedures consist of a history, physical examination (including a neurologic assessment and mental status evaluation), head CT, head MRI, and head PET. There is no cure for AD, nor are there any therapies that will slow the progression. Medications can manage symptoms and maximize functioning. Cholinesterase inhibitors (e.g., donepezil [Aricept], rivastigmine [Exelon], and galantamine [Razadyne]) can improve neurotransmitter levels in the brain in some cases. Memantine (Namenda) is the newest drug approved specifically to treat AD. Memantine blocks N-methyl-D-aspartic acid receptors, which are glutamate receptors. Memantine may be given in combination with a cholinesterase inhibitor. Other medications may be given to control aggression. Alternative therapies that may improve symptoms include vitamin E, ginkgo, and Huperzine A, but the research evidence is mixed regarding the efficacy of these therapies. Other strategies may include memory aids (e.g., calendars), nutritional support, physical exercise, cognitive activities, safety precautions (e.g., supervision and removing clutter), maintaining a calm environment, and social interactions (e.g., adult day care).

Coping strategies and support for both the patient and the caregiver can decrease stress and anxiety.

Creutzfeldt-Jakob Disease

Creutzfeldt-Jakob disease (CJD) is a rare, but rapidly progressive form of dementia caused by an infectious prion. A prion is an abnormal protein particle that causes proteins to fold abnormally, especially in nervous tissue. The prion renders the protein dysfunctional, creating plaques and vacuoles (empty spaces) (Figure 11-43). CJD occurs in two types (classic and variant) and three main categories (sporadic, hereditary, and acquired). Although also caused by a prion, classic CJD is *not* related to bovine spongiform encephalopathy, or mad cow disease. However, the new variant *is* related to bovine spongiform encephalopathy. The most common form of classic CJD occurs sporadically, caused by the spontaneous transformation of normal prion proteins into abnormal prions. This sporadic disease occurs worldwide, including the United States, at an annual rate of approximately 1 case per 1 million people (CDC, 2009a). Hereditary CJD is rare and occurs when the abnormal protein is inherited. Finally, acquired CJD is rare (accounting for fewer than 1% of cases worldwide) and occurs when the individual is exposed to infected materials (e.g., via tissue transplants and ingestion). The prion is resistant to common methods of sterilization and disinfection. CJD has a long incubation period (up to 40 years) after being introduced into the brain; however, CJD is rapidly progressing and always fatal (usually within 1 year of onset).

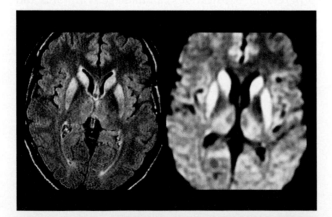

Figure 11-43

Creutzfeldt-Jakob disease.

Clinical manifestations of CJD develop rapidly and include:

- Blurred vision
- Ataxia
- Hallucinations
- Lack of coordination
- Muscle twitching
- Myoclonic jerks or seizures
- Spasticity
- Anxiety
- Personality changes
- Profound confusion or disorientation
- Lethargy
- Speech impairment

Diagnostic procedures for CJD consist of a history, physical examination (including a neurologic assessment and mental status evaluation), EEG, head MRI, and other tests to rule out other forms of dementia (e.g., lumbar puncture, serum tests). There is no known cure for CJD. Interleukins and other immunomodulator agents may slow the progression of the disease. Custodial care (nonmedical care that assists with activities of daily living) may be required early in the course of the disease. Medications may be needed to control aggressive behaviors, spasticity, pain, and seizure activity. Providing a safe environment, controlling aggressive or agitated behavior, and meeting physiologic needs may require monitoring and assistance in the home or in an institutionalized setting. Family counseling may help in coping with the changes required for home care.

AIDS Dementia Complex

Dementia is common in later stages of AIDS (see Chapter 2) and is referred to as AIDS dementia complex, or human immunodeficiency virus– (HIV–) associated encephalopathy. The HIV invades the brain tissue and may be exacerbated by other infections and tumors that are frequently associated with AIDS. Clinical manifestations include encephalitis, behavioral changes, and a gradual decline in cognitive function (e.g., trouble with concentration, memory, and attention). Persons with AIDS dementia complex also show progressive slowing of motor function with a loss of dexterity and coordination. In children with congenital HIV, the brain is often affected, causing mental retardation and delayed motor development. A staging system is used to describe the condition's progression. The staging system ranges from 0 (normal) to 4 (nearly vegetative). Diagnostic procedures of AIDS dementia complex consist of a history, physical examination (including a neurologic assessment and mental status evaluation), head CT, head MRI, and biopsy. When left untreated, AIDS dementia complex can be fatal. Aggressive antiretroviral therapy is the cornerstone of treatment.

Cancers of the Nervous System

Nervous system malignancies can originate in the brain or spinal cord, and they may spread from other sites. Regardless of the etiology, these cancers can result in significant neurologic dysfunction and death. Typical cancer diagnosis, staging, and treatments are usually utilized (see Chapter 1).

Brain Tumors

Brain tumors, whether malignant or benign, can be life threatening because they often increase ICP and are difficult to access (**Figure 11-44**). Brain tumors may be primary, but most are secondary tumors. Any cancer can spread to the brain, but the most common types that do so include breast cancer, colon cancer, kidney cancer, lung cancer, melanoma, and sarcoma. Primary tumors are thought to arise from genetic mutations. The risk for this mutation increases with age and exposure to radiation and occupational chemicals. In the United States, prevalence and mortality rates of brain tumors are highest among Caucasians and males (National Cancer Institute, 2009). Complications of brain tumors include neurologic deficits, seizures, personality changes, and death. The 5-year survival rate for brain tumors is nearly 35%. Clinical manifestations of brain tumors vary depending on size and location. These manifestations reflect the increase in ICP and may include:

- New onset or change in pattern of headaches
- Headaches that gradually become more frequent and more severe

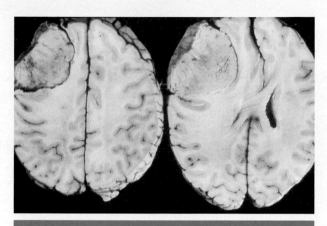

Figure 11-44

Brain tumor.

- Unexplained nausea or vomiting
- Vision problems (e.g., blurred vision, diplopia, or loss of peripheral vision)
- Gradual loss of sensation or movement in an extremity
- Balance difficulties
- Speech difficulties
- Confusion
- Hearing problems
- Hormonal (endocrine) disorders

Diagnostic procedures consist of a history, physical examination (including a neurologic assessment), head MRI, biopsy, and other tests to determine cancer histology. Treatment of brain tumors depends on the size and location of the originating cancer, if any. If possible, surgical removal of the tumor is recommended. Additional treatment options include radiation and chemotherapy. Regardless of the strategy, rehabilitation will be necessary to minimize residual neurologic dysfunction. Rehabilitation will likely require physical, occupational, and speech therapy.

Chapter Summary

The nervous system is a complex network that receives, organizes, and responds to internal and external stimuli, which is vital for homeostasis. The nervous system controls all sensory and motor functions. Damage to this system, even minor, can result in significant neurologic deficits. The nature and severity of those deficits depends on the location and extent of damage. This damage can result from trauma, infections, tumors, chemical imbalances, or genetic conditions. Regardless of the neurologic disorder, the individual may face significant neurologic dysfunction and even death. Supporting neurologic health involves strategies such as observing safety precautions (e.g., wearing safety equipment), avoiding illicit drug use, minimizing alcohol consumption, getting vaccinations, and maintaining adequate nutrition.

Case Study Answers

1. Delivering the child by cesarean section prevents damage to the fragile myelomeningocele, which could worsen neurologic complications.

2. Classic manifestations of hydrocephalus include bulging fontanelles, a high-pitched cry, and a large head circumference. A neonate's fontanelles should be flat; bulging indicates increased pressure within the brain. A high-pitched cry also is a sign of ICP. The saclike projection in his lumbar region is consistent with spina bifida.

3. Myelomeningoceles can cause life-threatening infections in the neonate if the sac loses its integrity prior to surgical closure. In addition, myelomeningocele leads to neurologic deficits similar to a spinal cord injury including neurogenic bladder and bowel, weakness of the lower extremities, and paralysis when located in the lumbar region. Defects located higher than the thoracic level result in more severe neurologic damage; those in the thoracic level and above may cause preterm or neonatal death. Because the central nervous system, including all of its components, develops early, hydrocephalus most commonly occurs in conjunction with neural tube defects. Latex allergies are common in children with neural tube defects because of the need for daily intermittent urinary catheterization.

References

Centers for Disease Control and Prevention. (2004). Retrieved from http://www.cdc.gov/ncbddd/dd/cp3.htm#cost

Centers for Disease Control and Prevention. (2009a). Retrieved from http://www.cdc.gov/ncidod/dvrd/cjd

Centers for Disease Control and Prevention. (2009b). Retrieved from http://www.cdc.gov/stroke/facts.htm

Centers for Disease Control and Prevention. (2010a). Retrieved from http://www.cdc.gov/ncbddd/spinabifida/data.html

Centers for Disease Control and Prevention. (2010b). Retrieved from http://www.cdc.gov/Epilepsy

Centers for Disease Control and Prevention. (2010c). Retrieved from http://www.cdc.gov/traumaticbrain-injury/causes.html

Centers for Disease Control and Prevention. (2010d). Retrieved from http://www.cdc.gov/TraumaticBrain-Injury/index.html

Chiras, D. (2008). *Human biology* (6th ed.). Sudbury, MA: Jones and Bartlett.

Elling, B., Elling, K., & Rothenberg, M. (2004). *Anatomy and physiology.* Sudbury, MA: Jones and Bartlett.

Gould, B. (2006). *Pathophysiology for the health professions* (3rd ed.). Philadelphia, PA: Elsevier.

Madara, B., & Pomarico-Denino, V. (2008). *Pathophysiology* (2nd ed.). Sudbury, MA: Jones and Bartlett.

National Cancer Institute. (2009). Retrieved from http://seer.cancer.gov/statfacts/html/brain.html

National Institutes of Health. (2008). Retrieved from http://www.nia.nih.gov/NR/rdonlyres/7DCA00DB-1362-4755-9E87-96DF669EAE20/13991/ADFactSheetFINAL2510.pdf

National Institutes of Health. (2009). Retrieved from http://www.ninds.nih.gov/disorders/huntington/detail_huntington.htm

National Institutes of Health. (2010a). Retrieved from http://www.ninds.nih.gov/disorders/amyotrophiclateralsclerosis/detail_amyotrophiclateralsclerosis.htm

National Institutes of Health. (2010b). Retrieved from http://www.ninds.nih.gov/disorders/multiple_sclerosis/detail_multiple_sclerosis.htm#158953215

National Institutes of Health. (2010c). Retrieved from http://www.ninds.nih.gov/disorders/parkinsons_disease/detail_parkinsons_disease.htm

Professional guide to pathophysiology (2nd ed.). (2007). Philadelphia, PA: Lippincott Williams & Wilkins.

Schwenk, T., Gorenflo, D., Dopp, R., and Hipple, E. (2007), Depression and pain in retired professional football players. *Medicine & Science in Sports & Exercise, 39*(4), 599-605.

Resources

www.alsa.org

www.americanheartassociation.org

www.cancer.gov

www.cancer.org

www.cdc.gov

www.epilepsyfoundation.org

www.mayoclinic.com

www.medlineplus.gov

www.michaeljfox.com

www.nih.gov

www.ninds.nih.gov

www.parkinson.org

www.spinalcord.org

www.strokeassociation.org

www.who.int

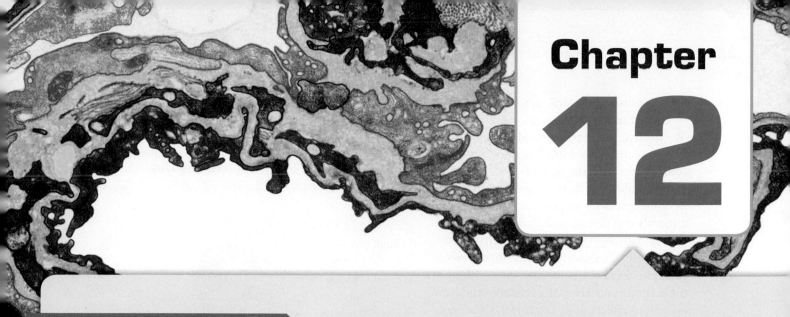

Musculoskeletal Function

LEARNING OBJECTIVES

- Discuss normal musculoskeletal anatomy and physiology.
- Compare and contrast congenital musculoskeletal disorders.
- Compare and contrast traumatic musculoskeletal disorders.
- Compare and contrast metabolic bone disorders.
- Compare and contrast inflammatory joint disorders.
- Describe and discuss chronic muscle disorders.
- Describe and discuss bone cancers.

KEY TERMS

actin	Ewing's sarcoma	myofibril	sciatica
amphiarthrose	fascia	myofilament	scoliosis
ankylosing spondylitis	fat embolism	myosin	sesamoid bone
ankylosis	fibromyalgia	oblique fracture	short bone
appendicular skeleton	flat bone	open fracture	simple fracture
axial skeleton	fracture	osteoarthritis (OA)	skeletal muscle
bone	gout	osteoblast	skeleton
bone marrow	greenstick fracture	osteoclast	smooth muscle
callus	herniated intervertebral disk	osteocyte	spiral fracture
cardiac muscle	hyaline cartilage	osteomalacia	spongy bone
cartilage	impacted fracture	osteomyelitis	sprain
chondrosarcoma	incomplete fracture	osteonecrosis	strain
closed fracture	irregular bone	osteopenia	stress fracture
comminuted fracture	joint capsule	osteoporosis	suture
compact bone	joint	osteosarcoma	synarthrose
compartment syndrome	kyphosis	Paget's disease	synovial fluid
complete fracture	lamella	pathologic fracture	synovial joint
compression fracture	ligament	periosteum	tendon
crepitus	long bone	red marrow	tophus
depressed fracture	lordosis	reduce	transverse fracture
diaphysis	matrix	rheumatoid arthritis (RA)	yellow marrow
dislocation	muscle fiber	rickets	
epiphysis	muscular dystrophy (MD)	sarcomere	

The musculoskeletal system consists of bones, joints, muscles, ligaments, tendons, and other connective tissue that provide support for the body and protection of organs. The musculoskeletal system collaborates with the nervous system to make movement possible. The musculoskeletal system plays a role in homeostasis by storing calcium and other minerals that can be mobilized when needed. Additionally, hematopoiesis occurs in the bone (see Chapter 3). Disorders of the musculoskeletal system may be acute or chronic. Many of these conditions are easily treatable and leave no lasting effects (e.g., fractures). Other conditions can leave the individual with chronic pain or significant disability (e.g., fibromyalgia). These disorders may have congenital, genetic, autoimmune, trauma, nutritional deficits, and excessive use causes.

Anatomy and Physiology

The structures of the musculoskeletal system are essential for standing erect and locomotion. This system also gives the human body form and stability while protecting the body's vital organs. The musculoskeletal system plays a role in homeostasis and is the site for hematopoiesis. The musculoskeletal system consists of bones, joints, muscles, ligaments, tendons, and other connective tissue that work together to accomplish these functions. Connective tissue describes biologic material that supports and binds tissues and organs together. Chief components of connective tissue include elastic fibers and collagen (a protein substance).

Bones

Bone is a specialized form of connective tissue. At first glance, the bone appears to be a dry, dead material, and, in fact, the word *skeleton* is derived from a Greek word that means "dried-up body." Looks can be deceiving because this could not be farther from the truth. Bone is a living, metabolically active tissue. This tissue is the site of fat and mineral storage (especially calcium) as well as hematopoiesis. The human body contains 206 bones of varying shapes and sizes that make up the skeleton (**Figure 12-1**). This skeleton provides support and protection for vital organs such as the heart, lungs, and

brain. The skeleton is divided into two divisions—axial and appendicular. The axial skeleton forms the long axis of the body and includes the skull, vertebral column, and rib cage. The appendicular skeleton consists of bones that form the arms, shoulders, pelvis, and legs.

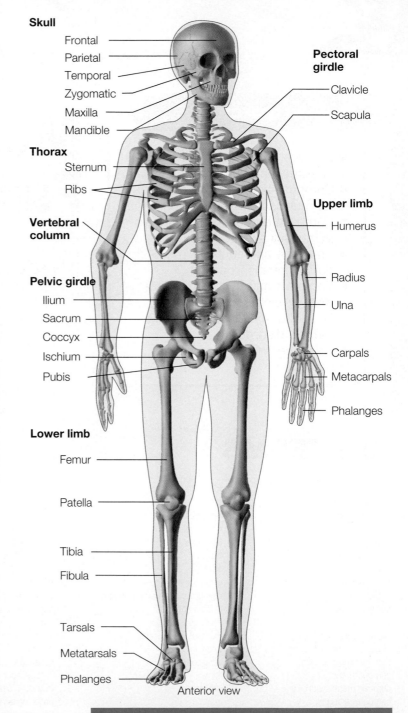

Skull
Frontal
Parietal
Temporal
Zygomatic
Maxilla
Mandible

Pectoral girdle
Clavicle
Scapula

Thorax
Sternum
Ribs

Vertebral column

Upper limb
Humerus
Radius
Ulna
Carpals
Metacarpals
Phalanges

Pelvic girdle
Ilium
Sacrum
Coccyx
Ischium
Pubis

Lower limb
Femur
Patella
Tibia
Fibula
Tarsals
Metatarsals
Phalanges

Anterior view

Figure 12-1

The human skeleton.

Five types of bone are found within the skeleton—long, short, flat, irregular, and sesamoid bones (**Figure 12-2**). **Long bones** (**Figure 12-3**) are bones that have bodies (**diaphyses**) that are longer than they are wide, growth plates (**epiphyses**) at either end, hard out-

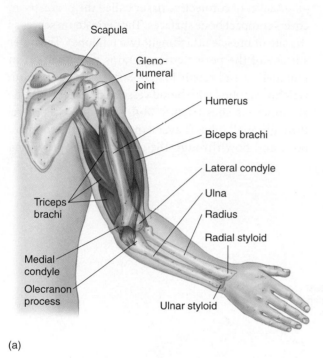

(a)

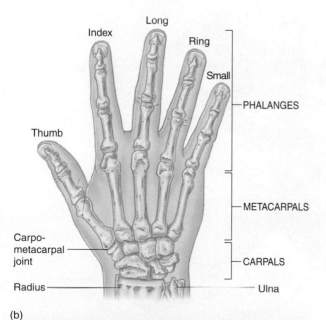

(b)

Figure 12-2

Classifications of bones. (a) The scapula is a flat bone, and the humerus, ulna, and radius are long bones. (b) The carpals, or wrist bones, are short bones.

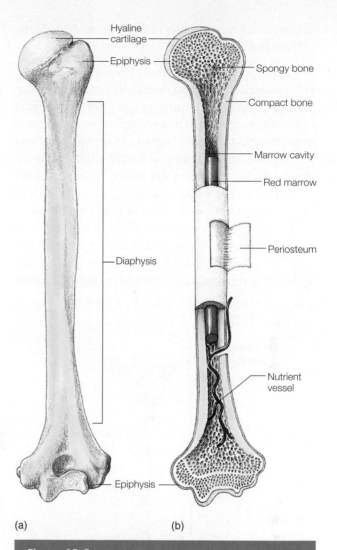

(a)   (b)

Figure 12-3

Long bones. (a) Drawing of the humerus. Notice the long shaft and dilated ends. (b) Longitudinal section of the humerus showing compact bone, spongy bone, and marrow.

er surfaces (**compact bone**), and inner regions (**spongy bone**) that are less dense than the outer regions and contain bone marrow. Both ends of long bones are covered in hyaline cartilage to help protect the bone by reducing friction and absorbing shock. Long bones include some of the longest bones in the body (e.g., femur, humerus, and tibia) as well as some of the smallest (e.g., metacarpals, metatarsals, and phalanges). **Short bones** are bones that are approximately as wide as they are long, and their primary function is providing support and stability with little movement. Short bones contain only a thin layer of compact bone along with spongy bone and relatively large amounts of bone marrow. Examples of short bones include the carpals and tarsals.

Flat bones are strong, level plates of bone that provide protection to the body's vital organs and a base for muscular attachment. Anterior and posterior surfaces of flat bones are formed from compact bone to provide strength, and the center consists of spongy bone and varying amounts of bone marrow. In adults, most red blood cells are formed in flat bones. Examples of flat bones include the scapula, sternum, skull, pelvis, and ribs. **Irregular bones** do not fall into any other category, due to their nonuniform shape. Irregular bones primarily consist of spongy bone, with a thin outer layer of compact bone. Examples of irregular bones include the vertebrae, sacrum, and mandible. **Sesam-**

oid bones are usually short or irregular bones embedded in a tendon. Sesamoid bones are often present in a tendon where it passes over a joint and serve to protect the tendon. Examples of sesamoid bones include the patella, pisiform (smallest of the carpals), and the two small bones at the base of the first metatarsal.

A layer of connective tissue called the **periosteum** covers compact bone surfaces. The periosteum serves as the site of muscle attachment (via tendons). The outer surface of the periosteum contains cells that aid in remodeling and repair (**osteoblasts**). The periosteum is richly supplied with blood vessels that enter the bone at numerous sites (**Figure 12-4**). These vessels travel through small tubes (haversian canals) in the compact bone and flow through the spongy bone, providing

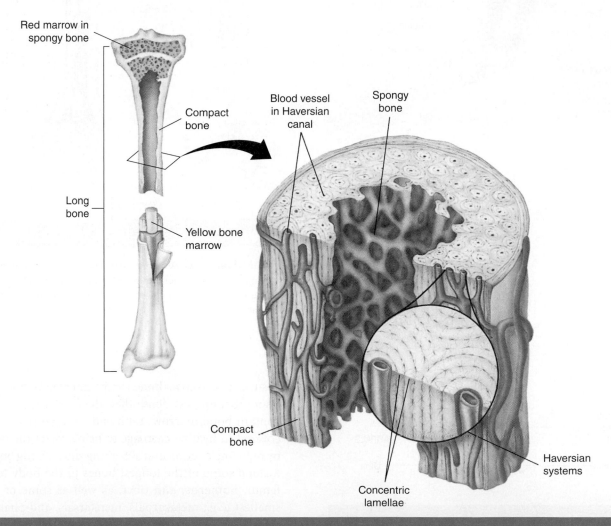

Figure 12-4

Shaft of the bone.

Table 12-1 Structural Elements of Bone

Bone Cells	Function
Osteoblasts	Builds bone through collagen
Osteoclasts	Cells of the bone that enable matrix to be absorbed and assist with release of calcium and phosphate
Osteocytes	Mature bone cells that help maintain bone matrix; also play a major role in release of calcium into blood

Source: Madara, M., & Pomarico-Denino, V. (2008). *Quick look nursing: Pathophysiology* (2nd ed.). Sudbury, MA: Jones & Bartlett Learning.

nutrients and oxygen while removing waste products. The periosteum is also richly supplied with nerve fibers. Inside the shaft of long bones is a large cavity for **bone marrow**. Marrow cavities in most bones of a fetus or newborn contain red marrow. **Red marrow**, so named because of its color, serves as the blood-cell factory (hematopoiesis). As humans age, this red marrow is slowly replaced by fat, creating **yellow marrow**. Yellow marrow begins to form during adolescence and is present in most bones by adulthood. At this point, hematopoiesis continues in the vertebrae, pelvis, and a few other sites. The yellow marrow can be reactivated to produce blood cells under certain circumstances (e.g., after an injury).

The bone is a dynamic tissue that is constantly undergoing remodeling to repair aging bone or to adjust for things such as changes in activity. For example, spongy bone is remodeled to increase bone strength when a person's activity level increases after periods of inactivity. During remodeling, cells called **osteoclasts** break down some spongy bone while osteoblasts rebuild new compact bone to increase bone strength (**Table 12-1**). Osteoblasts lay down new bone during the remodeling, and when osteoblasts become surrounded by calcified extracellular material, it is referred to as an **osteocyte**. Bone tissue contains many of these osteocytes organized in thin layers called **lamellae** (**Figure 12-5**). The osteocytes are embedded in extracellular material, referred to as the **matrix**. The matrix consists of calcium phosphate crystals (hydroxyapatite) that make the bones hard and strong. The matrix also contains collagen fibers that reinforce the bone, giving

it flexible strength. Balance between the mineral and collagen is necessary for optimal bone function. Bone without adequate mineral quantities is too flexible; bone without adequate collagen amounts is extremely brittle.

Several hormones influence bone structure. Growth hormone produced by the anterior pituitary gland works with thyroid hormones to control normal bone growth (see Chapter 10). Growth hormone increases the rate of growth by causing cartilage and bone cells to reproduce and lay down their intercellular matrix as well as stimulating mineralization within the matrix. Bones grow in two ways—appositional growth and endochondral growth. In appositional growth, new bone forms on the surface of a bone. In endochondral growth, bone eventually replaces new cartilage growth in the epiphyseal plate. Calcitonin and parathyroid hormone regulate bone remodeling and mineralization of calcium (see Chapter 10). Estrogen inhibits formation of osteoclasts in women, whereas testosterone increases bone length and density in men. Vitamin D also plays a critical role in bone metabolism. Vitamin D is a fat-soluble vitamin that controls the absorption of calcium from the intestine and increases calcium and phosphate reabsorption in the kidneys. Proper nutrition (including adequate intake of dietary calcium and vitamin D) and physical activity from childhood onward are essential for the development and maintenance of healthy bone.

During fetal development, the skeleton forms from hyaline cartilage. **Cartilage** is a shiny connective tissue that is tough and flexible. Several types of cartilage can be found throughout the body in the ears, nose, and joints, but **hyaline cartilage** is the type most associated with bone. This cartilage is often found in **joints**—structures that connect bones of the skeleton. Joints are classified by their degree of movement—moveable, slightly moveable, and immoveable. The most common type of joint is the freely moveable, or synovial, joint (**Figure 12-6**). **Synovial joints** are complex and vary significantly, but they all have similar features. Synovial joints contain cartilage that is lubricated by a transparent viscous fluid (**synovial fluid**) secreted by the synovial membrane (soft tissue that lines the noncartilaginous surfaces within joints). This lubricated cartilage reduces friction by providing a slippery surface for bones to move freely. In addition to lubrication, synovial fluid contains leukocytes to fight infections in the joints and provides nutrients to the cartilage. The second commonality is the presence of a **joint capsule**,

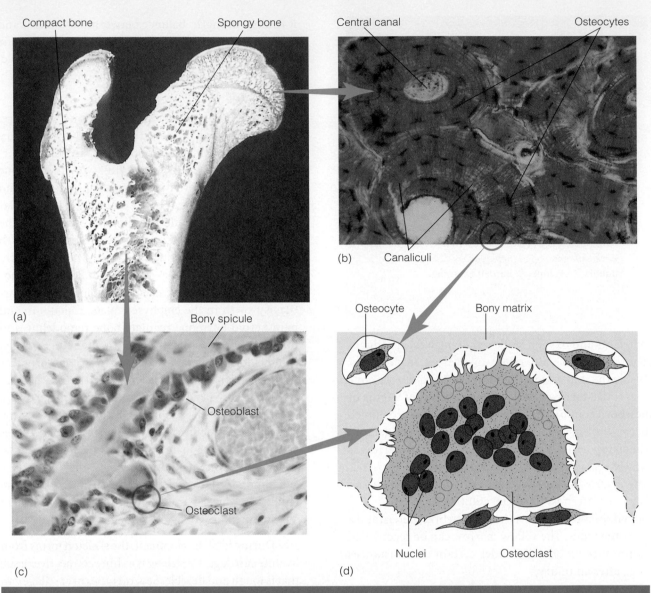

Figure 12-5

Bone. (a) Compact and spongy bone of the humerus. (b) Light micrograph of the lamella (concentric circles) showing the osteocytes and canaliculi. (c) Photomicrograph of spongy bone showing osteoblasts and osteoclasts. (d) An osteoclast digesting the surface of a bony spicule (sharp body or spike).

a structure that joins one bone to another. The outer layer of the synovial joint capsule consists of dense connective tissue that attaches to the periosteum of adjacent bones. Many of these joints contain parallel bundles of dense connective tissue called **ligaments**. Ligaments connect bones to bones in a joint and provide support to the joint.

Slightly moveable joints, or **amphiarthroses**, can be seen in the vertebral column (**Figure 12-7**). An intervertebral disk unites each vertebra. The inner portion of the disk serves as a cushion, absorbing the impact of walking and running. The outer, fibrous portion holds the disk in place and joins one vertebra to the next.

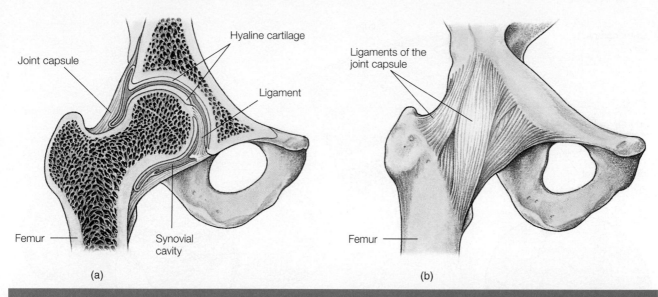

Hyaline cartilage

Joint capsule

Ligament

Femur

Synovial
cavity

(a)

Ligaments of the
joint capsule

Femur

(b)

Figure 12-6

A synovial joint. (a) A cross section through the hip joint (a ball-and-socket joint) showing the structures of the synovial joint. (b) Ligaments in the outer portion of the joint capsule help support the joint.

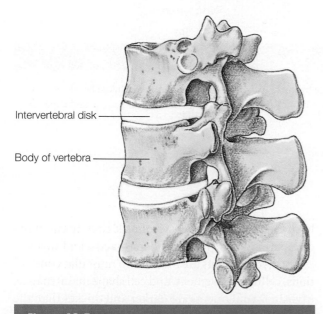

Intervertebral disk

Body of vertebra

Figure 12-7

A slightly movable joint. The intervertebral disks allow for some movement, giving the vertebral column flexibility.

The skull is an example of immoveable joints, or synarthroses (**Figure 12-8**). In the skull, the bones interlock together to form immoveable joints called sutures. Fibrous connective tissue extends the space between the interlocking bones, holding them together.

Another immoveable joint is the pubic symphysis. The two pubic bones come together to form the pubic symphysis. Fibrocartilage holds these bones together.

Muscles

Locomotion requires a skeleton with moveable joints as well as muscles acting on the bones. Skeletal muscles refer to muscles that connect to bone. Other forms of muscles include smooth and cardiac muscles. Smooth muscles line walls of hollow organs and tubes and are found in the eyes, skin, and glands. Smooth muscles are involuntary, meaning they work without conscious control by the brain. Cardiac muscle comprises the heart and is under involuntary control. Skeletal muscles are the most frequently occurring muscle type, making up approximately 40% of the body's weight. The more than 350 skeletal muscles are under voluntary control of the brain (**Figure 12-9**). Virtually every muscle in the body attaches to bones through structures like tendons. Tendons are specialized tough cords or bands of dense connective tissue that are continuous extensions of the periosteum. Most muscles cross one or more joints. Muscles contract to produce movement of the bones at the joints. Muscles work in groups to collaborate smooth movements (**Figure 12-10**). When one muscle contracts to produce a movement, the antagonistic (opposing) muscles relax to allow the

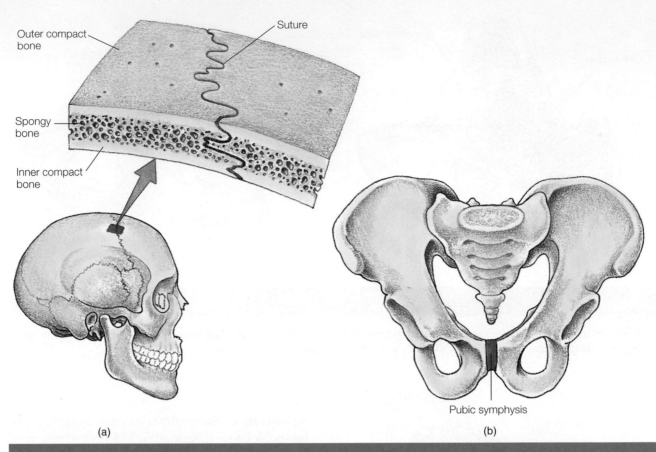

Figure 12-8

Immovable joints. (a) Many of the bones of the skull are held in place by joints called *sutures*. The bones are linked by fibrous tissue, and the joints are immovable. (b) The pubic symphysis is another immovable joint. During childbirth it softens and expands to permit delivery.

movement. Muscles contract in response to nerve stimulation (see Chapter 11). Because muscle fibers are elastic, the fibers return to their normal length after contracting. Not all skeletal muscles make bones move. Some muscles steady joints, allowing other muscles to act. These muscles assist with posture, permitting the body to sit or stand upright against gravitational pull. Like nerve cells, muscle fibers are excitable cells with high action potential, allowing them to respond to stimulation faster.

Skeletal muscles are comprised of muscle fibers, connective tissue, blood vessels, and nerves (**Figure 12-11**). Each skeletal **muscle fiber** or cell is a cylinder with multiple nuclei. Within each fiber are **myofibrils**, threadlike structures that extend the entire

length of the muscle fiber. Myofibrils contain two types of **myofilaments** (protein fibers)—actin and myosin. **Actin** myofilaments are involved in muscular contractions, cellular movement, and cell shape maintenance. **Myosin** myofilaments are darker and thicker than the actin. Myosin myofilaments are fibrous globulins (type of protein) that work with actin to form actomyosin. The alignment of these two kinds of myofilaments gives the skeletal muscle its striated appearance (alternating light and dark bands) (**Figure 12-12**). Myofilaments are organized into repeated structural units called **sarcomeres** (**Figure 12-13**). Muscle fibers contract by sliding actin filaments over myosin filaments. This sliding occurs by the myosin filament pulling the actin filament. The myosin attaches to the actin when calcium is released from inside the muscle fibers. Calcium is stored

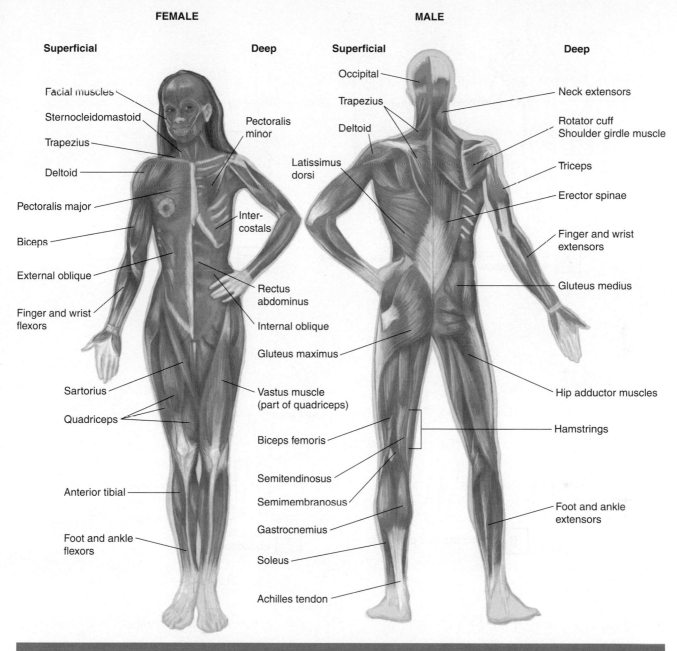

FEMALE

Superficial   Deep

Facial muscles

Sternocleidomastoid
Pectoralis
minor

Trapezius

Deltoid

Pectoralis major

Inter-
costals

Biceps

External oblique

Rectus
abdominus

Finger and wrist
flexors
Internal oblique

Gluteus maximus

Sartorius
Vastus muscle
(part of quadriceps)

Quadriceps

Biceps femoris

Semitendinosus

Anterior tibial
Semimembranosus

Gastrocnemius

Foot and ankle
flexors
Soleus

Achilles tendon

MALE

Superficial   Deep

Occipital
Neck extensors

Trapezius
Rotator cuff
Shoulder girdle muscle
Deltoid

Latissimus
dorsi
Triceps

Erector spinae

Finger and wrist
extensors

Gluteus medius

Hip adductor muscles

Hamstrings

Foot and ankle
extensors

Figure 12-9

Skeletal muscles.

in the smooth endoplasmic reticulum (see Chapter 2), which forms an extensive network inside muscle fibers. Impulses from nerve cells, specifically motor neurons, trigger this release of calcium. Once the calcium causes the head of the myosin to attach to the actin filament, adenosine triphosphate in the muscle provides the energy to pull the actin filament inward. In order to meet the muscle cell's high energy needs, adenosine triphosphate is recycled repeatedly in rapid succession. During vigorous activity, adenosine triphosphate stores deplete, oxygen levels drop sharply, glucose production ceases, and lactic acid accumulates.

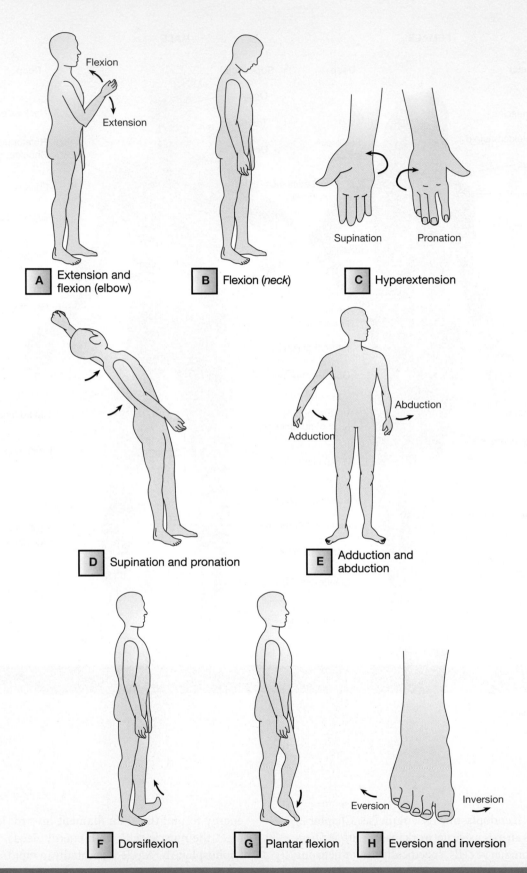

Figure 12-10

Common body movements.

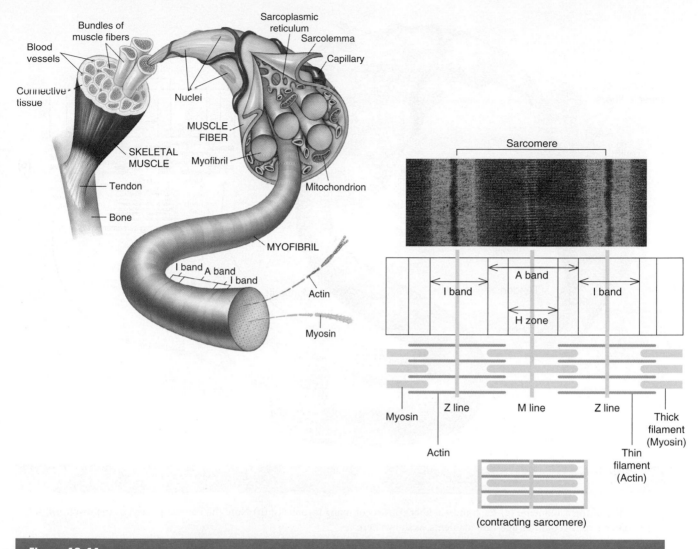

Figure 12-11

Structure of a skeletal muscle.

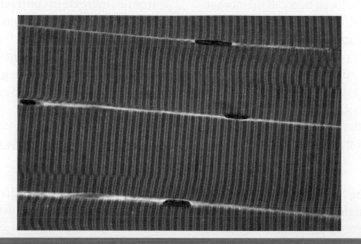

Figure 12-12

Striated pattern of skeletal muscle.

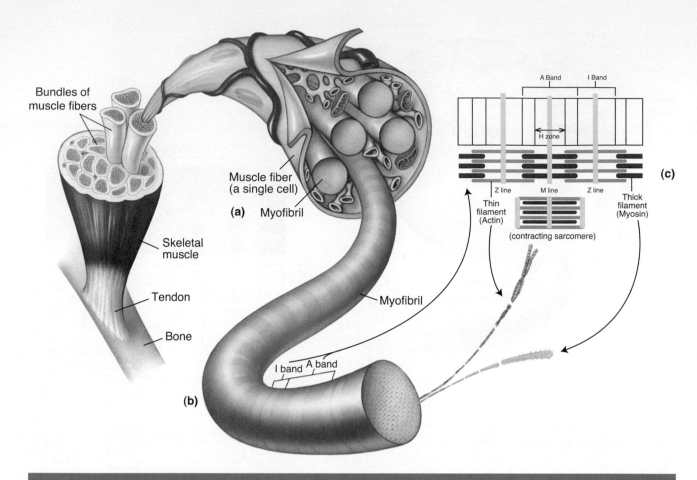

Bundles of muscle fibers

Muscle fiber (a single cell)

(a) Myofibril

Skeletal muscle

Tendon

Bone

Myofibril

I band A band

(b)

A Band I Band

H zone

Z line M line Z line

Thin filament (Actin)

Thick filament (Myosin)

(contracting sarcomere)

(c)

Figure 12-13

Structure of the sarcomere. (a) Each muscle fiber consists of many myofibrils. (b) Note the banded pattern of the myofibril. (c) Sarcomeres consist of thick and thin filaments, as shown here.

Each muscle fiber is enclosed by a cell membrane (sarcolemma) (**Figure 12-14**). Numerous muscle fibers are bundled together and surrounded by connective tissue called endomysium. Additional connective tissue called perimysium surrounds several of these bundles, grouping them together to form a muscle. Yet another layer of connective tissue called epimysium and fibrous connective tissue (**fascia**) surround these muscles. This fascia may also surround muscle groups.

Along with stimulating bone growth, growth hormone causes muscle growth. The number of muscle fibers or cells in a muscle remains relatively constant throughout the life span. Increases in muscle sizes reflect increases in individual muscle fibers. When muscles work harder, they respond by becoming larger and stronger. The increase in size and strength results

from an increase in contractile protein inside the muscle fiber. Unfortunately, muscle protein is produced and destroyed quickly. In fact, approximately half of the muscle gained in a weight-lifting program is broken down 2 weeks after ceasing the activity. The only way to maintain the muscle gain is to continue the weight-lifting program.

Congenital Musculoskeletal Disorders

Some musculoskeletal disorders are congenital in nature and primarily affect posture. These conditions may be apparent at birth or materialize as the child grows. During growth spurts, muscular development lags behind skeletal growth; this lag results in inadequate skeletal support. Additionally, conditions with developmental abnormalities (e.g., Down

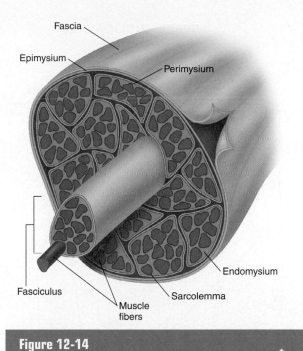

Figure 12-14

Muscle group.

syndrome and cerebral palsy) may become aggravated during these growth periods. These postural deformities require early treatment to prevent progression and complications.

Kyphosis

Kyphosis refers to an increase in the curvature of the thoracic spine outward (**Figure 12-15**). Often called hunchback, kyphosis can develop during the adolescent growth spurts because of poor posture or secondary to osteoporosis. Severe kyphosis can impair lung expansion and ventilation. Exercises (including back strengthening) and proper posture can usually reverse mild deformities. Bracing and surgical correction may be necessary for more severe cases.

Lordosis

Lordosis refers to an exaggerated concave of the lumbar spine (Figure 12-15). Often called swayback, lordosis may develop during adolescent growth spurts or because of poor posture. Obesity can increase the tendency toward this posture because of an altered center of gravity and postural compensation. Much like kyphosis, treatment for lordosis also includes exercises, proper posture, bracing, and surgery.

Scoliosis

Scoliosis refers to a lateral deviation of the spine (**Figure 12-16**). This lateral curvature may affect the thoracic or lumbar area or both. Scoliosis may also

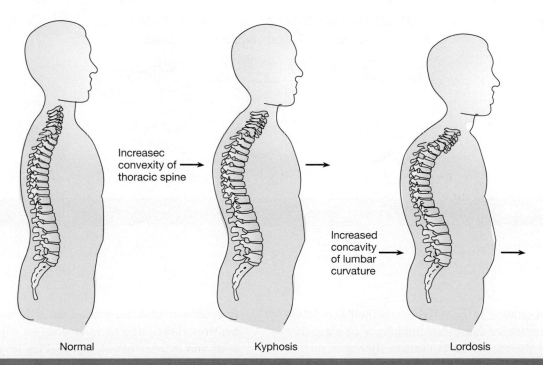

Figure 12-15

Kyphosis and lordosis.

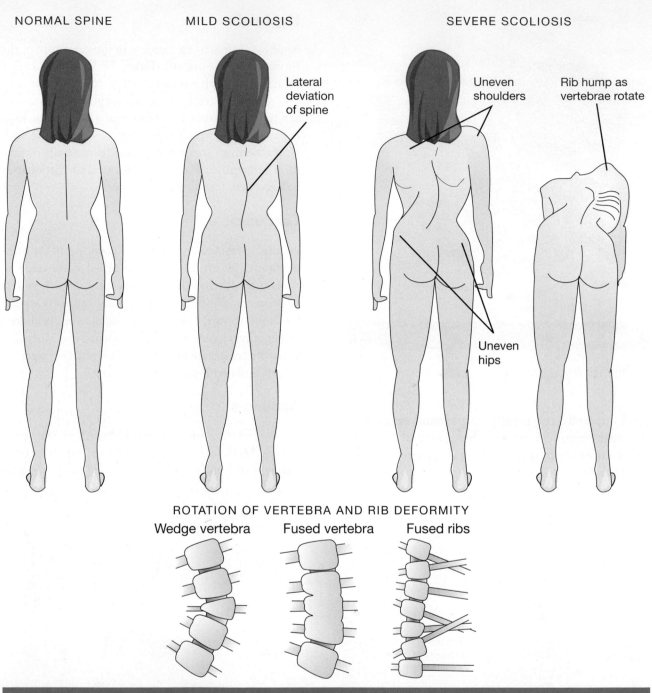

NORMAL SPINE   MILD SCOLIOSIS   SEVERE SCOLIOSIS

Lateral deviation of spine

Uneven shoulders

Rib hump as vertebrae rotate

Uneven hips

ROTATION OF VERTEBRA AND RIB DEFORMITY

Wedge vertebra   Fused vertebra   Fused ribs

Figure 12-16

Scoliosis.

include a rotation of the vertebrae on their axis. Stress on the vertebrae causes an imbalance in osteoclast activity; therefore, the curvature increases during growth spurts. Scoliosis may also be associated with kyphosis and lordosis. Scoliosis varies in severity and is more common in females. Most cases are idiopathic, but causes may include genetic influences, embryon-ic developmental deformities (usually involving the hemivertebrae), degenerative diseases (e.g., osteoporosis and osteoarthritis), unequal leg lengths, spinal nerve compression, and asymmetrical muscle support (e.g., partial paralysis, muscular dystrophy, cerebral palsy, poliomyelitis, trauma, or spinal tumors). Complications of scoliosis include pulmonary compromise, chronic pain, degenerative arthritis of the spine, intervertebral disk disease, and sciatica.

Clinical manifestations vary depending on the degree of curvature and are exaggerated when an affected person bends over. These manifestations may include:

- Asymmetrical hip and shoulder alignment
- Asymmetrical thoracic cage
- Asymmetrical gait
- Back pain or discomfort
- Fatigue
- Indications of respiratory compromise (e.g., dyspnea and reduced chest expansion)

Because of the prevalence of scoliosis in adolescent females, schools often conduct periodic scoliosis screening. Diagnostic procedures consist of a history, physical examination, spinal X-rays, and a scoliometer (which measures the angle of trunk rotation). Without treatment, the curvature often progresses into adulthood. Patient outcomes improve with early treatment. Treatment strategies may include exercises (including back strengthening), bracing, and surgical correction (with instrumentation or fusion).

Traumatic Musculoskeletal Disorders

Traumatic musculoskeletal disorders are usually mild and easily treated; however, occasionally these conditions can result in life-threatening complications (e.g., fat embolism and osteomyelitis). Many of these conditions are caused by similar events that lead to traumatic neurologic disorders (e.g., falls, motor vehicle accidents, and sports-related injuries). Additionally, neurologic dysfunction may result in conjunction with the musculoskeletal injury. These traumatic conditions are on the rise because of increasing numbers of children and adults participating in fitness, recreation, and sport activities. Some contributing factors to these injuries include inappropriate or inadequate equipment, training, or warm-up techniques; more aggressive approaches to sports; and failure to allow minor injuries to heal.

Fractures

A fracture is a break in the rigid structure of the bone (**Figure 12-17**). Fractures are the most common type of traumatic musculoskeletal disorders. Fractures mainly occur as a primary condition because of falls, motor vehicle accidents, and sports-related injuries. Additionally, fractures can occur secondary to conditions that weaken the bone (e.g., osteoporosis, Paget's disease, and bone cancer). Fractures are classified depending on characteristics such as the direction of fracture line, number of fracture lines, or other characteristics (**Figure 12-18**). Fracture types include:

- Simple fracture—a fracture with a single break in the bone and bone ends maintain their alignment and position, including the following types:
  - Transverse fracture—a fracture straight across the bone shaft

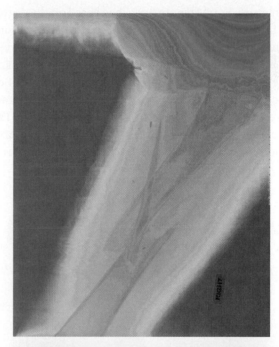
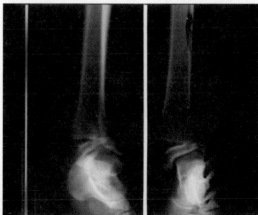

Figure 12-17

Fractures.

- Oblique fracture—a fracture at an angle to the bone shaft
- Spiral fracture—a fracture that twists around the bone shaft
- Comminuted fracture—a fracture with multiple fracture lines and bone pieces
- Greenstick fracture—an incomplete fracture in which the bone is bent and only the outer curve of the bend is broken; commonly occurs in children because of minimal calcification and often heals quickly
- Compression fracture—a fracture in which the bone is crushed or collapses into small pieces

Multiple other terms may also be used to describe a fracture. Fractures are described based on the degree of break. Complete fractures occur when the bone is broken into two or more separate pieces; however, in incomplete fractures, the bone is partially broken (e.g., greenstick). Additionally, fractures are described as open or closed. Open fractures, or compound fractures, result when the skin is broken (**Figure 12-19**). The bone fragments or edges may be angled and protrude out of the skin. Open fractures have more dam-

age to soft tissue and are at risk for infection. In closed fractures, the skin is intact. Impacted fractures occur when one end of the bone is forced into the adjacent bone. Pathologic fractures refer to fractures that result from a weakness in the bone structure secondary to conditions such as tumors or osteoporosis. Stress fractures, or fatigue fractures, occur from repeated excessive stress. These fractures are common in the tibia, femur, and metatarsals. Finally, depressed fractures occur in the skull when the broken piece is forced inward on the brain.

When the bone breaks, blood from damaged vessels in the periosteum and bone marrow pours into the fracture and forms a hematoma, or blood clot (**Figure 12-20**). Necrosis occurs to the broken ends of the bone because of the blood vessel damage. The necrotic tissue is reabsorbed and eventually replaced by new bone. Within a few days of the fracture, fibroblasts (connective tissue from the periosteum) invade the clot. These fibroblasts secrete collagen fibers, which form a mass of cells and fibers called a callus. The callus bridges the broken bone ends together inside and outside. The callus takes 2–6 weeks to form. Then, osteoblasts from the periosteum invade the callus, which

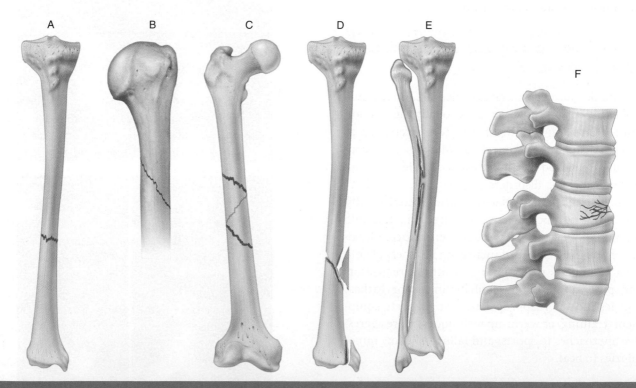

Figure 12-18

Classifications of fractures. (a) Transverse fracture of the tibia. (b) Oblique fracture of the humerus. (c) Spiral fracture of the femur. (d) Comminuted fracture of the tibia. (e) Greenstick fracture of the fibula. (f) Compression fracture of a vertebral body.

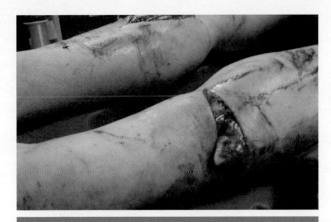

Figure 12-19

Open fracture.

slowly converts the callus to bone. This ossification process can take 3 weeks to several months (usually 4–6 weeks). Healing time can vary depending on age, nutritional status, blood supply, and fracture type and location. The callus begins large and is often palpable, but osteoclasts gradually remodel the bone by removing the excess bone. This remodeling process leaves little to no evidence that the fracture occurred and may take as long as a year.

Multiple complications can result from fractures. Delayed union, malunion, or nonunion may occur due to poor nutrition, inadequate blood supply, malalignment, and premature weight bearing. Additional fracture complications include compartment syndrome, fat embolism, osteomyelitis, and osteonecrosis. Compartment syndrome is a serious condition that results from pressure increases in a compartment, usually the muscle fascia in the case of fractures. The pressure impinges on the nerves and blood vessels contained within the compartment, potentially compromising the distal extremity. Compartment syndrome requires prompt identification and treatment to prevent permanent tissue damage. Clinical manifestations usually include excruciating pain that is beyond what would be expected given the injury. Compartment syndrome can be diagnosed by measuring pressures inside the muscle fascia. Treatment usually includes removing the cast (if present) and an immediate fasciotomy to relieve the pressure. A fat embolism occurs when there is an opportunity for fat to enter the bloodstream (e.g., surgery). Fatty marrow can enter the bloodstream after a fracture to one of the long bones. The emboli can travel to vital organs such as the lungs, brain, or heart, which can be fatal. Fat embolism can be prevented with early

immobilization of the fracture. Osteomyelitis refers to an infection of the bone tissue. Osteomyelitis is a serious complication because it often goes undetected, can take months to resolve, and can result in bone or tissue necrosis. Osteomyelitis is treated with potent antibiotic therapy (often long-term) and surgery (e.g., debridement). Osteonecrosis, or avascular necrosis, is death of bone tissue due to a loss of blood supply. Osteonecrosis can result from displaced fractures or dislocations. Osteonecrosis often requires surgical replacement of the necrotic bone and/or joint.

Clinical manifestations of a fracture reflect the tissue trauma caused by the bone fragments as well as the disruption of function. These manifestations may include:

- Deformity (e.g., angulation, shortening, and rotation)
- Swelling and tenderness at the site (due to inflammatory process triggered by the tissue trauma)
- Inability to move the affected limb
- Crepitus (grating sound or sensation)
- Pain (results from tissue trauma and muscle spasms triggered by the bone fragments)
- Paresthesia
- Muscle flaccidity progressing to spasms

Diagnostic procedures of fractures consist of a history, physical examination, and X-rays. Treatment strategies include immediate immobilization with devices such as splints or traction (application of a force or weight pulling a limb). The fracture is reduced to restore the bone's normal positioning. Reduction can be accomplished with closed manipulation by applying pressure or traction or open manipulation with surgery. During surgery, devices such as pins, plates, rods, or screws may be placed to secure the bone fragments in position. Any necrotic tissue or foreign material is also removed in a process called debridement. When a fracture is suspected, do not give the individual with the injury anything by mouth in the event that surgery is necessary to repair the fracture. Surgical repair may be delayed up to a few days after the injury to allow the edema secondary to the inflammatory response to resolve. Immobilization of the fracture during that time is crucial to prevent complications. Long-term immobilization for bone healing to occur is accomplished with casts, splints, or traction. Traction maintains bone alignment and prevents muscle spasms. As the fracture is healing, exercise is helpful to limit mus-

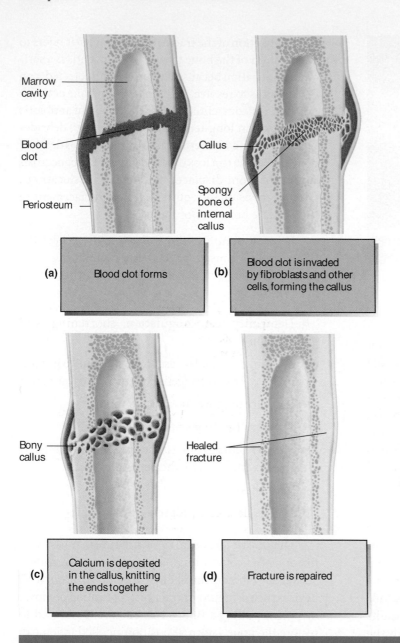

Marrow cavity

Blood clot

Periosteum

(a) Blood clot forms

Callus

Spongy bone of internal callus

(b) Blood clot is invaded by fibroblasts and other cells, forming the callus

Bony callus

Healed fracture

(c) Calcium is deposited in the callus, knitting the ends together

(d) Fracture is repaired

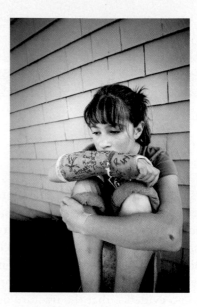

Figure 12-20

Stages of fracture repair.

cle atrophy, joint stiffness, and contracture formation as well as to maintain adequate circulation.

Dislocation

Dislocation refers to the separation of two bones where they meet at a joint (**Figure 12-21**). The two bones are no longer in their normal position. The dislocation may involve a complete or partial (subluxation) loss of contact. The injury causes deformity and immobility of the joints, and it may cause damage to the nearby ligaments and nerves. Dislocations usually result from a sudden impact to the joint (e.g., blow, fall, or other trauma), but they may be congenital (e.g., congenital hip dysplasia) or pathologic (e.g., arthritis, ligament injuries, paralysis, or neuromuscular disease). Any joint can be affected, but dislocations are especially common in the shoulder and clavicle joints.

Clinical manifestations of a dislocated joint may include:

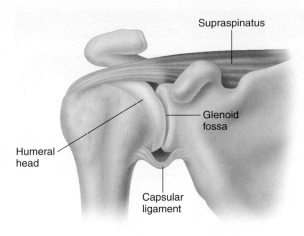

Normal

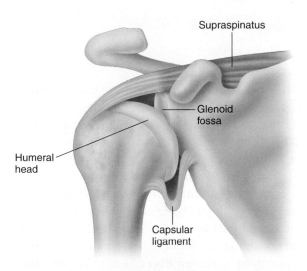

Anterior dislocation

Figure 12-21

Anterior dislocation of the shoulder.

- Visibly out-of-place, discolored, or deformed joint
- Limited movement
- Swelling or bruising
- Intense pain, especially with movement or weight bearing
- Paresthesia near the injury (often distal to the injury)

Diagnostic procedures for dislocations consist of a history, physical examination, X-rays, and magnetic

CASE STUDY

T.J. is a 34-year-old woman who is being admitted to the orthopedic unit following a motor vehicle accident. She was driving her car through an intersection when someone ran a stop sign and hit her. She was diagnosed in the emergency room with a compound fracture of the left femur and a comminuted fracture of the left ankle.

When she arrived in the orthopedic unit at 1600, her left leg was immobilized with an air cast and ice bags were applied. She was medicated in the emergency room with morphine sulfate, 2 mg intravenously at 1200. The nursing admission assessment data revealed that T.J. had no significant medical problems. Her vital signs on admission to the unit were: temperature 99.2°F, pulse 90 beats per minute, respirations 24 breaths per minute, oxygen saturation at 95% on room air, and blood pressure 140/80. She was scheduled for surgery in the morning to repair both fractures.

1. Explain the type of fractures this patient has incurred.
2. List the top three priority nursing interventions for this patient upon admission.
3. What are some complications this patient is at high risk for developing?
4. What is the significance of the patient's vital signs?

resonance imaging (MRI). Immediately following the injury, treatment strategies focus on limiting tissue damage. These immediate strategies include:

- Immobilize the area above and below the joint with a splint or sling in the position the joint was found.
- Do not attempt to straighten or move the joint.
- Assess for tissue perfusion (e.g., blanch test on skin in the affected area) and report any suspected tissue perfusion impairment immediately.
- Apply ice to ease pain and swelling.
- Do not move the person unless the injury has been completely immobilized.
- Do not move a person with an injury to weight-bearing joints (e.g., hip, pelvis, or knees) unless it is absolutely necessary.
- Do not give the person anything by mouth (in case surgery is needed).

Table 12-2 Sprain Grading System

Grade	Degree of Damage	Clinical Findings and Implications
Grade I	Minimal damage or disruption	Prognosis is variable (injury may require surgery) Requires a prolonged healing/rehabilitation period
Grade II	Moderate damage	Tender without swelling No bruising Active and passive range of motion are painful Prognosis is good with no expectation of instability or functional loss
Grade III	Complete disruption of the ligament	Moderate swelling and bruising Very tender with more diffuse tenderness than grade I Range of motion is very painful and restricted Joint may be unstable, and functional loss may result

Source: AAOS. (2004). *Paramedic: Anatomy & physiology.* Sudbury, MA: Jones & Bartlett Learning.

After stabilization of the injury, treatment depends on the site and severity of the injury. Reduction may occur spontaneously, or gentle manipulation may be used to return the bones to their usual position (closed reduction). Depending on the amount of pain and swelling, a local anesthetic or even a general anesthetic may be administered before a closed reduction. Pain usually subsides after the joint is reduced. Surgical reduction (open reduction) may be necessary if blood vessels or nerves are damaged or if the dislocation is reoccurring (common with dislocations of the shoulder). After the reduction, the joint will need to be immobilized with a splint or sling for several weeks. Analgesics and muscle relaxants may be required during this recovery period. After the splint or sling is removed, a gradual rehabilitation program (primarily physical therapy) designed to restore the joint's range of motion and strength is often needed. Strenuous activity with the injured joint should be avoided until full movement, normal strength, and stability have been regained. Some dislocations, such as with the hip, may need up to several months to heal. Healing of dislocations is slowed when ligament damage or soft tissue damage is also present. Preinjury function is usually restored, but some residual deficits may occur in more severe injuries.

Sprains

A **sprain** is an injury to a ligament that often involves stretching or tearing of the ligament. Sprains are caused when a joint is forced to move into an unnatural position (e.g., twisting one's ankle). The severity of the sprain is described using a grading scale (**Table 12-2; Figure 12-22**). Of all sprains, ankle and knee sprains occur most often. The injury triggers the inflammatory process resulting in edema and pain at the site. Additionally, blood vessels may be damaged, resulting in bleeding and bruising. Bleeding into the joint capsule can delay healing. If a tear occurs, granulation tissue develops along with the inflammation. Collagen fibers form to create a link between the torn ligament fragments, and eventually, fibrous tissue binds them together. Sprained ligaments swell rapidly and are painful. Generally, the degree of pain reflects the severity of injury. Other clinical manifestations may include joint stiffness, limited function, disability, and discoloration (usually bruising). Diagnostic procedures of sprains may consist of a history, physical examination, X-rays, and MRIs. Most sprains can be managed at home. Treatment strategies include:

- Apply ice immediately to reduce pain and swelling; wrap the ice in a cloth—do not place ice directly on the skin because it can worsen tissue damage.
- Immobilize joint with a splint or an elastic wrap or bandage (e.g., ACE bandage).
- Elevate the swollen joint above the level of the heart.
- Rest the affected joint for several days and gradually increase activity.

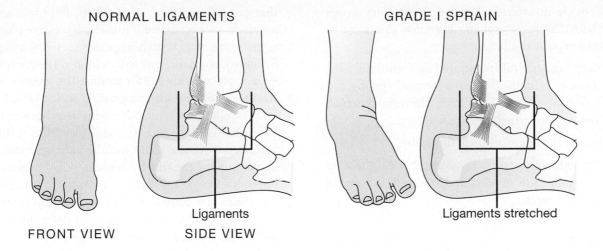

NORMAL LIGAMENTS

GRADE I SPRAIN

Ligaments

FRONT VIEW   SIDE VIEW

Ligaments stretched

GRADE I SPRAIN

GRADE III SPRAIN

Ligaments slightly
torn

Ligaments torn
completely

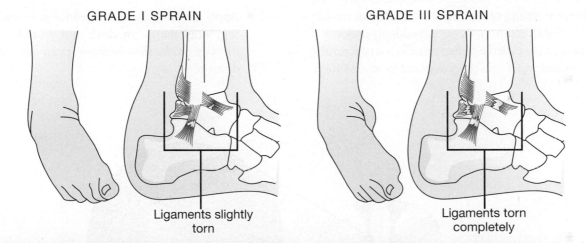

Figure 12-22

Sprain grading system.

LEARNING POINTS

The treatment strategies for soft tissue injuries such as sprains and strains can be remembered using the acronym PRICE.

P = Protect the injured limb from further injury by not using the joint. The patient may need crutches or splints to accomplish this.

R = Rest the injured limb, but do not avoid all activity; exercise other muscles to minimize deconditioning.

I = Ice the area (e.g., cold pack, a slush bath, a compression sleeve filled with cold water) as soon as possible after the injury to limit swelling and continue to ice the area for 10–15 minutes (any longer than that may cause tissue damage) four times a day for 48 hours.

C = Compress the area with an elastic wrap or bandage; compressive wraps or sleeves made from elastic or neoprene are best.

E = Elevate the injured limb above the level of the heart whenever possible to help prevent or limit swelling.

- Provide nonsteroidal anti-inflammatory drugs (NSAIDs) (e.g., aspirin, ibuprofen [Motrin]) to relieve pain and inflammation.

- Keep pressure off the injured area until the pain subsides (usually 7–10 days for mild sprains and 3–5 weeks for severe sprains). The injured person may require crutches when walking.

- Repair the ligament tears surgically.

- Rehabilitate (usually including physical therapy) to regain joint motion and strength, beginning within 1 week.

Strains

A **strain** is an injury to a muscle or tendon that often involves stretching or tearing of the muscle or tendon (**Figure 12-23**). Strains may occur suddenly or develop over time. Also called a pulled muscle, a strain results from an awkward muscle movement or excess force that can be caused by an accident, improper use of a muscle, or overuse of a muscle. Excessive physical activity, improper stretching prior to activity, and poor flexibility can contribute to this injury. The lower back is the most common site for strains. The severity of the strain is described using a grading scale (Table 12-2). Strains follow the same pathogenesis as sprains (e.g., inflammation, granulation, and bleeding). Clinical manifestations of a strain include pain, stiffness, difficulty moving the affected muscle, skin discoloration (often bruising), and edema. Diagnostic procedures for strains may consist of a history, physical examination, X-rays, and MRIs. Treatment strategies for strains are similar to those for sprains. These strategies may include:

- Apply ice immediately to reduce pain and swelling; wrap the ice in cloth and do not place ice directly on the skin because it can worsen tissue damage.

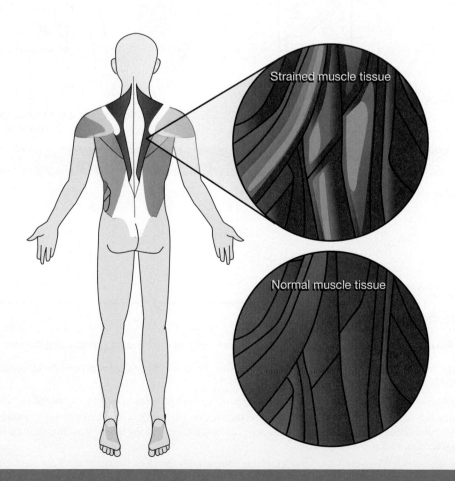

Figure 12-23

Strained muscle tissue.

- Use ice for the first 3 days, and then, either heat or ice may be helpful.
- Rest the affected muscle for at least a day.
- Keep the affected muscle elevated above the level of the heart (if possible).
- Avoid using the affected muscle until pain subsides; then, advance activity slowly and in moderation.
- Use NSAIDs to relieve pain and inflammation.
- Use muscle relaxants to relieve muscle stiffness.
- Repair severe tendon tears surgically.
- Rehabilitate (usually including physical therapy) to regain muscle movement and strength as necessary.

Herniated Intervertebral Disk

A **herniated intervertebral disk** describes a state in which the nucleus pulposus (inner gelatinous component of the intervertebral disk) protrudes through the annulus fibrosus (the tough outer covering of the disk) (**Figure 12-24**). This condition may also be called

a slipped disk and ruptured disk. The tear in the capsule may occur suddenly or gradually. This condition may be considered an orthopedic or neurologic problem because protrusions into the extradural space can exert pressure on the spinal cord, interfering with nerve conduction (**Figure 12-25**). Sensory, motor, or autonomic function may be impaired depending on the location. The most frequently involved vertebrae are in the lumbosacral region, but some may involve the cervical disks. If pressure on nerve tissue or blood supply is prolonged or severe, permanent neurologic damage may result. A herniated intervertebral disk often occurs due to improper body mechanics, lifting heavy objects, or trauma (e.g., a fall or a blow to the back). Additional contributing factors include degenerative changes secondary to aging and demineralization secondary to metabolic conditions (e.g., osteoporosis).

Herniated intervertebral disks may be asymptomatic. When present, manifestations may include:

- **Sciatica** (a radiating, aching pain, sometimes with tingling and numbness, that starts in the buttock and extends down the back or side of one leg)
- Pain, paresthesia, or weakness in the lower back and one leg, or in the neck, shoulder, chest, or arm

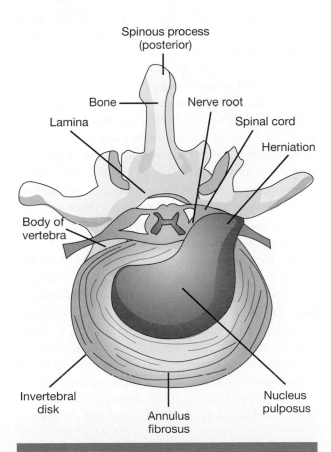

Figure 12-24

Herniated vertebral disc.

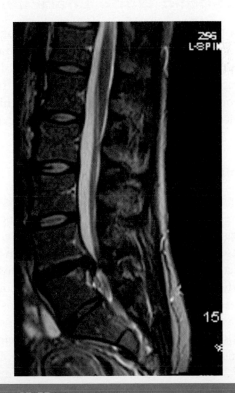

Figure 12-25

Spinal cord compression by a herniated disk.

- Low back pain or leg pain that worsens by sitting, coughing, sneezing, laughing, bending, or walking
- Limited mobility

Spinal tumors and herniated intervertebral disks may present similarly, so a differential diagnosis should be made. Diagnostic procedures may consist of a history, physical examination (including neurologic assessment), spinal X-rays, spinal computerized tomography (CT), spinal MRI, nerve conduction study, myelogram (injection of contrast medium into the spinal fluid, followed by X-rays), and electromyography. Immediate treatment for herniated intervertebral disks may include a short period of rest, analgesics, NSAIDs, muscle relaxants, physical therapy (including back-strengthening exercises), heat/cold application, and traction. Most people will recover and return to their normal functioning. A small number of people will need further treatment such as injections (e.g., corticosteroid and chemonucleolysis) into the site or surgical repair (e.g., diskectomy, laminectomy, and spinal fusion). Weight loss may be beneficial if the patient is overweight.

Metabolic Bone Disorders

Metabolic bone disorders refer to a variety of bone conditions caused by mineral abnormalities. These abnormalities may be caused by genetic factors or dietary deficits. Metabolic bone disorders are usually treated easily once identified, but they can lead to significant complications if left untreated (e.g., electrolyte disturbances and fractures).

Osteoporosis

Osteoporosis is a condition characterized by a progressive loss of bone calcium that leaves the bones brittle (**Figure 12-26**). This loss can occur due to either a decrease in osteoblast activity or an increase in osteoclast activity. The spongy bone becomes porous, particularly in the vertebrae and wrist, and the compact bone becomes thin (**Figure 12-27**). Osteoporosis can occur as a primary or secondary condition. This common disease occurs because of several factors including genetic, dietary, and hormonal influences. By the age of 20, the average woman has acquired most of her skeletal mass. A large decline in bone mass occurs with advanced age, increasing the risk of osteoporosis. For women this occurs around the time of menopause

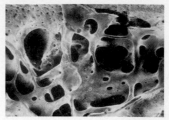

(a)

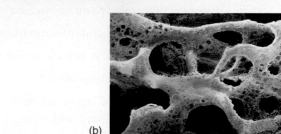

(b)

Figure 12-26

Osteoporosis. The loss of estrogen or prolonged immobilization weakens bone. In these situations, bone is dissolved and becomes brittle and easily breakable. (a) Normal bone. (b) Bone weakened by osteoporosis.

because of hormonal changes. A person with high bone mass as a young adult will be more likely to have a higher bone mass later in life; therefore, achieving maximum bone mass in young adulthood is important for maintaining bone health throughout the life span. Adequate calcium consumption and physical activity (including weight-bearing exercises) early is vital to achieve maximum bone mass in adulthood. In addition to calcium, deficient intake of protein, vitamin C, and vitamin D as well as excessive intake of phosphorus (high levels in soda) increase the risk of osteoporosis. Caucasians (especially those with fair skin tone) and Asians are at higher risk for developing osteoporosis because of genetically smaller bones. Other risk factors include smoking, excessive alcohol or caffeine consumption, using certain medications (e.g., corticosteriods, chemotherapy, thyroid replacements, heparin, and antacids), having specific health conditions (e.g., Cushing's disease, thyroid dysfunction, bone tumors, malabsorption, and anorexia nervosa), and being underweight. Osteoporosis leads to an increased risk of bone fractures typically in the wrist, hip, and spine. A recent report by the surgeon general estimated that by 2020, one in two Americans aged 50 years or older will be at risk for fractures from osteoporosis or low bone mass. This risk for fractures significantly increases mortality rates in the elderly, particularly with hip fractures.

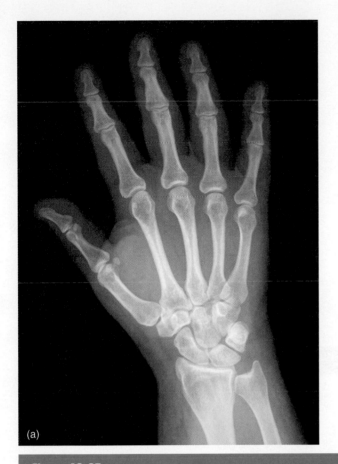
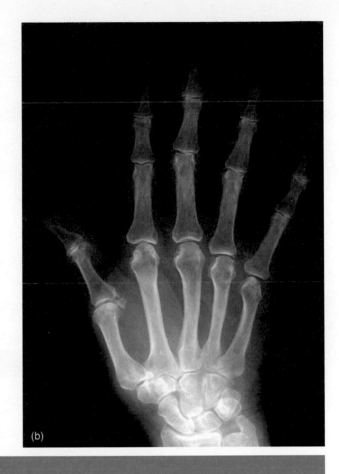

(a)

(b)

Figure 12-27

Bone changes of osteoporosis. (a) An X-ray of normal bones. (b) An X-ray of bones affected by osteoporosis.

Osteoporosis is often asymptomatic in early stages. As the disease progresses, clinical manifestations may include:

- Osteopenia (bone mass that is less than expected for age, ethnicity, or gender)
- Bone pain or tenderness
- Fractures with little or no trauma
- Low back and neck pain
- Kyphosis (**Figure 12-28**)
- Height reduction (as much as 6 inches) over time

Because of its prevalence rates, screening for osteoporosis should be conducted periodically on those persons at risk. Diagnostic procedures include a history, physical examinations, bone density scans (e.g., dual energy X-ray absorptiometry), X-rays, and spinal CT. Treatment strategies focus on impeding further bone loss and, in some cases, restoring bone density. These strategies may include:

- Proper nutrition (especially increasing dietary calcium and vitamin D)
- Increasing physical activity (including weight-bearing activities)
- Eliminating modifiable risk factors (e.g., smoking cessation and limited alcohol and caffeine consumption)
- Pharmacologic therapies, including the following:
  - Bisphosphonates (which inhibit bone breakdown, preserve bone mass, and increases bone density)
  - Estrogen receptor modulators (which mimic estrogen)
  - Calcitonin

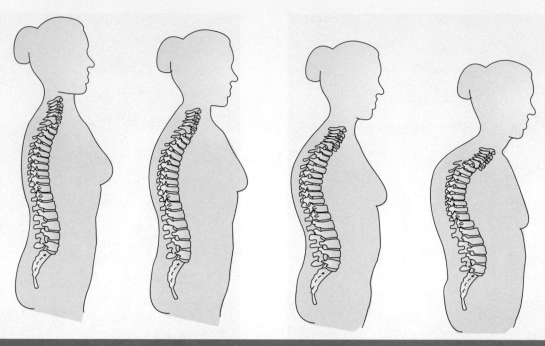

Kyphosis and height changes associated with osteoporosis.

- - Parathyroid hormone
- Safety measures (e.g., assistive devices, handrails, removing clutter)
- Pain management (e.g., analgesics, heat and cold application, relaxation techniques)
- Surgical repair of fractures or weakened bones

Rickets and Osteomalacia

Rickets is a softening and weakening of bones in children, usually because of an extreme and prolonged vitamin D, calcium, or phosphate deficiency. When this condition occurs in adults, it is called osteomalacia. If the blood levels of these minerals become too low, calcium and phosphate are released from the bones to maintain homeostasis. This shift of minerals out of the bone leads to weak and soft bones. Vitamin D is essential in promoting absorption of calcium and phosphorus from the gastrointestinal tract, which is necessary to build bone density. Vitamin D is absorbed from food or produced by the skin when exposed to sunlight. Lack of vitamin D production by the skin may occur in people who live in climates with little exposure to sunlight, must stay indoors (e.g., bedbound or institutionalized persons), or work indoors during the daylight hours. Dietary deficiency

may occur with persons who are lactose intolerant, do not drink milk products, or follow a vegetarian diet. Infants who are only breastfed may also develop vitamin D deficiency because human milk does not supply the proper amount of vitamin D. Using very strong sunscreen and limiting sun exposure to minimize skin cancer risk may also increase the risk for vitamin D deficiency. Conditions that reduce the digestion or absorption of fats will make it more difficult for vitamin D to be absorbed into the body (e.g., celiac disease and having had a gastrectomy). Insufficient dietary calcium and phosphorus intake can also lead to rickets, but it is rare in developed countries because calcium and phosphorous are found in milk and green vegetables. Rickets may also occur because of genetic influences. Hereditary rickets occurs when the kidneys are unable to reabsorb phosphate. For this reason, rickets may also occur in renal disease. Occasionally, rickets may occur in children who have liver disorders or who cannot convert vitamin D to its active form.

Clinical manifestations of rickets and osteomalacia develop slowly as the bones weaken. Rickets (**Figure 12-29**) may become apparent as the soft bones cannot support the growing child. Manifestations in adults and children usually include:

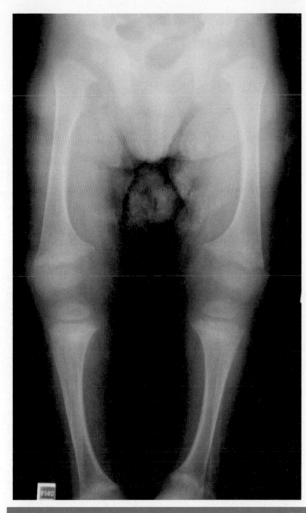

Figure 12-29

Rickets.

- Skeletal deformities (e.g., bowed legs, asymmetrical skull, scoliosis, kyphosis, pelvic deformities, sternum projection)

- Fractures

- Delayed growth in height or limbs

- Dental problems (e.g., defects in tooth structure, dental caries, poor enamel, delayed teeth formation)

- Bone pain (usually a dull, aching pain or tenderness in the spine, pelvis, and legs)

- Muscle cramps or weakness

Diagnostic procedures for rickets and osteomalacia include a history, physical examination, serum mineral levels, serum parathyroid hormone levels, serum alkaline phosphatase, X-rays, and bone density study. Treatment focuses on correcting or managing the underlying cause. Providing calcium, phosphorus, or vitamin D that is lacking will eliminate most symptoms. Vitamin D levels can be increased through dietary intake (e.g., fish, liver, and processed milk), exposure to moderate amounts of sunlight, or vitamin D supplements. Calcium levels can be increased through dietary intake (e.g., dairy products; dark green, leafy vegetables; and nuts). Positioning or bracing may be used to reduce or prevent deformities. Some skeletal deformities may require corrective surgery.

Paget's Disease

Paget's disease is a progressive condition characterized by abnormal bone destruction and remodeling, which results in bone deformities (**Figure 12-30**). Usual bone

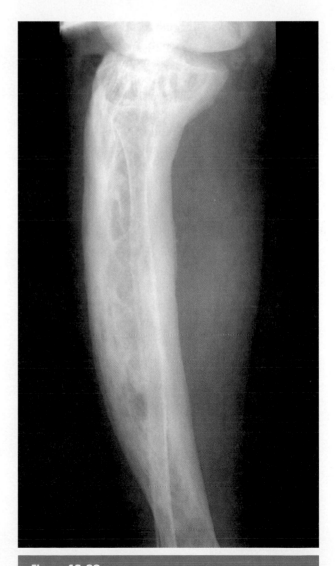

Figure 12-30

Paget's disease.

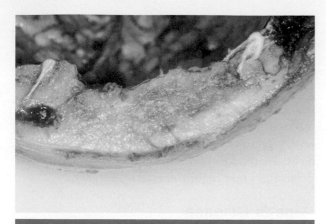

Figure 12-31

Paget's disease.

metabolism allows old bone to be recycled into new bone throughout the life span. In Paget's disease, the rate at which old bone is broken down and new bone is formed is distorted. Excessive bone destruction occurs along with the replacement of bone by fibrous tissue and abnormal bone. The new bone is bigger but weakened and filled with new blood vessels (**Figure 12-31**). Over time, Paget's disease results in fragile, misshapen bones. The disease may only be in one or two areas of the skeleton or throughout the body. This condition often involves long bones, skull, pelvis, and vertebrae. The exact cause of Paget's disease is unknown, but it is thought be caused by a virus capable of increasing osteoclast activity or genetic defects that produces an increase in interferon-6. Paget's disease is more common with age. Complications of Paget's disease include pathologic fractures, osteoarthritis, heart failure (related hypercalcemia and increased cardiac workload to pump blood to the affected areas), osteosarcoma (bone cancer), and nerve compression.

The clinical manifestations of Paget's disease vary depending on the area affected. The condition is often insidious in onset and may be asymptomatic early. When present, clinical manifestations may include:

- Bone pain (may be severe and persistent)
- Skeletal deformities (e.g., bowing of the legs, asymmetrical skull, and enlarged head)
- Fractures
- Headache
- Hearing and vision loss
- Joint pain or stiffness
- Neck pain
- Reduced height
- Warmth over the affected bone
- Paresthesia or radiating pain in the affected region (due to nerve compression)
- Hypercalcemia

Diagnostic procedures for Paget's disease consist of a history, physical examination, bone scan, X-rays, serum alkaline phosphatase, and serum calcium. Mild cases may only require periodic monitoring and no treatment. Treatment strategies focus on reducing fractures and deformities. Pharmacologic therapies may include bisphosphonates (which increase bone density), calcitonin (which increases bone density), NSAIDs (to alleviate pain and inflammation), and analgesics (to relieve pain). Surgery may be required to correct severe bone deformities.

Inflammatory Joint Disorders

Inflammatory joint disorders involve a group of arthritic conditions that are often degenerative in nature. These conditions involve inflammation that can be triggered by an autoimmune response, excessive use, increased physical stress, or injury. Complications of these conditions often include chronic pain and disability. Treatment strategies focus on slowing the progression, managing pain, and promoting independence.

Osteoarthritis

Osteoarthritis (OA), also known as the wear-and-tear arthritis and degenerative joint disease, is a localized joint disease characterized by deterioration of articulating cartilage and its underlying bone as well as bony overgrowth (**Figure 12-32**). The surface of the cartilage becomes rough and worn, interfering with joint movement. Tissue damage triggers the release of enzymes from local cells that accelerate cartilage disintegration. Eventually, the subchondral bone is exposed and damaged, and cysts and osteophytes (bone spurs) develop as the bone attempts to remold itself. Pieces of the osteophytes and cartilage break off into the synovial cavity, which further increases irritation. Additionally, nearby muscles and ligaments may become weakened and loose. All these changes cause narrowing of the joint space, joint instability, stiffness, and pain. The joints most commonly affected by OA are the knees, hips, and those in the hands and spine. OA is not inflammatory in origin, but inflammation results from the tissue irritation. Erosion of the cartilage is usually secondary to excessive mechanical stress on the joint (e.g., obesity, overuse, injury, and congenital musculoskeletal conditions). Additionally, OA may occur as a primary condition in which the cause is idiopathic. The Centers for Disease Control and Prevention (CDC) (2009b) estimates that nearly 27 million Americans have OA, with women having higher prevalence rates than men. OA is a significant contributor of disability, healthcare cost, and job loss in the United States.

Disease onset is gradual and usually begins after the age of 40. Clinical manifestations often develop slowly and worsen over time. These manifestations include:

- Joint pain that worsens during or after movement or weight bearing
- Joint tenderness with light pressure
- Joint stiffness, especially upon rising in the morning or after a period of inactivity
- Enlarged, hard joints
- Joint swelling
- Limited joint range of motion

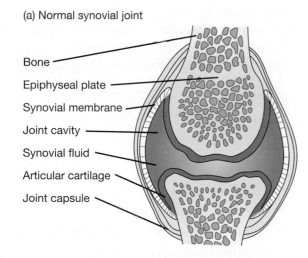

(a) Normal synovial joint

Bone
Epiphyseal plate
Synovial membrane
Joint cavity
Synovial fluid
Articular cartilage
Joint capsule

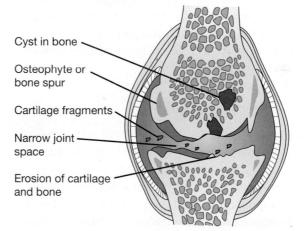

(b) Pathalogic changes in osteoarthritis

Cyst in bone
Osteophyte or bone spur
Cartilage fragments
Narrow joint space
Erosion of cartilage and bone

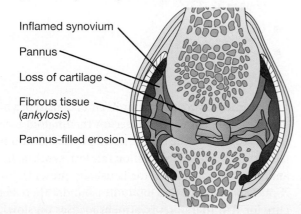

(c) Pathologic changes in rheumatoid arthritis

Inflamed synovium
Pannus
Loss of cartilage
Fibrous tissue (*ankylosis*)
Pannus-filled erosion

Figure 12-32

Pathological changes associated with osteoarthritis and rheumatoid arthritis.

- Crepitus
- Hard nodules around the affected joint (bone spurs)

Diagnostic procedures for OA consist of a history, physical examination, X-rays, and MRIs. There is currently no cure for OA. The goals of treatment are to increase joint strength, maintain joint mobility, reduce disability, and relieve pain. Treatment strategies may include a combination of physical therapy, weight loss/management, ambulatory aids (e.g., walkers and canes), orthopedic devices (e.g., braces and splints), pharmacologic agents, and surgery. Pharmacologic therapies may involve oral analgesics, NSAIDs, and corticosteroids. Additionally, synthetic synovial fluid and corticosteroids may be injected directly into the joint. Herbal therapies that may be helpful include glucosamine, chondroitin, and ginger, although research evidence is mixed regarding their efficacy. Pain management may consist of adequate rest, heat/cold application, topical agents that create a cool or hot sensation, water therapy (e.g., whirlpool, water aerobics), acupuncture, tai chi, and yoga. Surgery may be necessary to repair or replace damaged joints. These procedures may include arthroscopy to trim torn and damaged cartilage, osteotomy to change the alignment of a bone and relieve stress on the bone or joint, surgical fusion, and arthroplasty to completely or partially replace the damaged joint with an artificial joint.

Rheumatoid Arthritis

Rheumatoid arthritis (RA) is a systemic, autoimmune condition involving multiple joints. In RA, the inflammatory process primarily affects the synovial membrane, but it can also affect other organs (e.g., heart, skin, and eyes). Most cases of RA follow a typical autoimmune pattern of remissions and exacerbations. RA usually starts with an initial acute inflammatory episode after which the joint may appear to recover. The process continues with each exacerbation. This repeated process includes synovitis, pannus formation (granulation tissue), cartilage erosion (due to enzymes from the pannus), fibrosis, and ankylosis (joint fixation and deformity) (Figure 12-32). The recurring inflammation has a cumulative effect as it thickens the synovium, which can eventually invade and destroy the cartilage and bone within the joint. The muscles, tendons, and ligaments that hold the joint together weaken and stretch. The course and the severity of the illness can vary considerably. RA usually affects joints on both sides of the body equally. Wrists, fingers, knees, feet,

and ankles are the most commonly affected. Gradually, the joint loses its shape and alignment.

The exact cause of RA is unknown, but it is thought to be caused by a genetic vulnerability that permits a virus or bacteria to trigger the disease. Risk factors include family history, advancing age (however, there is a juvenile form), and smoking. RA is more common in women, and research is being conducted to explore the potential role hormones play. RA rates in the United States have declined since 1990. According to the CDC (2009c), an estimated 1.3 million Americans have RA.

Like other autoimmune disorders, RA is usually characterized by remissions and exacerbations. The disease onset is usually insidious with vague manifestations that can mimic other conditions. Clinical manifestations are progressive and may include:

- Fatigue
- Anorexia
- Low-grade fever
- Lymphadenopathy
- Malaise
- Muscle spasms
- Morning stiffness, which lasts more than 1 hour
- Warmth, tenderness, and stiffness in the joints when not used for as little as an hour
- Bilateral joint pain
- Swollen and boggy joints
- Limited joint range of motion
- Contractures and joint deformity (e.g., boutonniere deformity and swan neck deformity) (**Figure 12-33**)
- Unsteady gait
- Depression
- Anemia

Diagnostic procedures for RA may consist of a history, physical examination, serum rheumatoid factor test, serum anticyclic citrullinated peptide antibodies test, erythrocyte sedimentation rate test, synovial fluid analysis (rheumatoid factor is usually present), joint X-rays, joint MRIs, and joint ultrasounds. There is no cure for RA; therefore, treatment focuses on slowing the progression, managing the pain, and promoting independence. Early, aggressive treatment for RA can delay joint destruction. Treatment strategies are complex and often require a multidisciplinary team (made

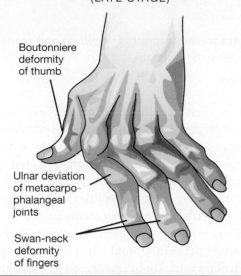

Boutonniere
deformity
of thumb

Ulnar deviation
of metacarpo-
phalangeal
joints

Swan-neck
deformity
of fingers

Figure 12-33

Joint deformities associated with rheumatoid arthritis.

up of a rheumatologist, nurse, and a wide range of therapists). Strategies may include:

- Adequate rest and pace activities

- Physical and occupational therapy (including that for range of motion)

- Regular exercise

- Pharmacologic therapies, including the following:

  - NSAIDs (to relieve pain and inflammation)
  - Corticosteroids (either orally or as an intra-articular injection to decrease inflammation)
  - Disease-modifying antirheumatic drugs (to decrease inflammatory response), including the following:
    - Gold compounds
    - Immunosuppressant agents (e.g., methotrexate)
    - Antimalarial agents
  - Biologic response-modifying agents (e.g., infliximab [Remicade]) (which blocks the tumor necrosis factor, an inflammatory cytokine associated with RA)
  - Herbal therapies including thunder god vine, plant oils, and fish oil

- Nonpharmacologic pain management (e.g., relaxation techniques, tai chi)

- Application of heat and cold

- Splint and braces (to support joints, maintain proper alignment, and prevent deformities)

- Assistive devices (e.g., walkers and rails)

- Coping strategies and support

- Surgical repair (e.g., synovectomy and arthroplasty)

Gout

Gout is an inflammatory disease resulting from deposits of uric acid crystals (monosodium urate) in tissues and fluids within the body (**Figure 12-34**). The body produces uric acid when it breaks down purines, a substance naturally found in the body as well as in certain foods (e.g., organ meats, shellfish, anchovies, herring, asparagus, and mushrooms). Normally, uric acid dissolves in the blood and is excreted by the kidneys. Gout is caused by an overproduction or underexcretion (most common) of uric acid (urate), but not all people with hyperuricemia have gout. Gout is most common in males and African Americans. Gout may occur as a primary inborn error in metabolism or secondary to some contributing factor. The contributing factors include being overweight or obese, having certain diseases (e.g., hypertension, diabetes mellitus, renal disease, and sickle cell anemia), consuming alcohol (beer and spirits more so than wine), using certain medication (e.g., diuretics), and eating a diet rich in meat and seafood.

Gout typically follows four phases. Initially, the individual with gout is asymptomatic as uric levels climb in the bloodstream and uric acid crystals deposit in the tissue (**Figure 12-35**). Crystals accumulate, damaging tissue. This damage triggers an acute inflammation that characterizes the second phase, referred to as acute flares or attacks. A flare is distinguished by pain, burning, redness, swelling, and warmth at the affected

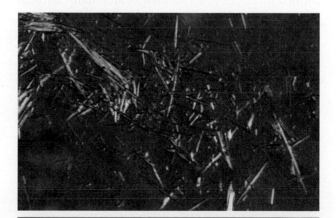

Figure 12-34

Uric acid crystals in the synovial fluid.

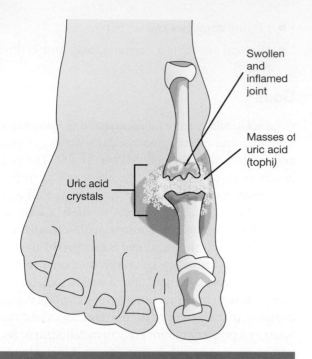

Uric acid crystals

Swollen and inflamed joint

Masses of uric acid (tophi)

Figure 12-35

Gout.

joint lasting days to weeks. Pain may be mild or excruciating. Most initial attacks occur in the lower extremities. The metatarsophalangeal joint of the big toe is the presenting joint for 50% of people with gout. After the acute attack subsides, the person may enter intercritical periods in which the disease is clinically inactive until the next flare. The person with gout continues to have hyperuricemia, which results in continued deposits of uric acid crystals in tissues that causes damage. These intercritical periods become shorter as the disease progresses. Reoccurring attacks are often precipitated by sudden increases in serum uric acid. Finally, chronic gout is characterized by chronic arthritis, with soreness and aching of joints. People with gout may also develop **tophi** (large, hard nodules comprised of uric acid crystals deposited in soft tissue) usually in cooler areas of the body (e.g., toes, elbows, ears, and distal finger joints). Because some renal calculi (kidney stones) are comprised of uric acid, renal calculi may also be associated with gout (see Chapter 7).

Clinical manifestations of gout vary depending on the phases the individual is experiencing. Manifestations of acute gout attacks include:

- Intense pain at the affected joint (usually the big toe) that frequently starts during the night and is often described as throbbing, crushing, burning, or excruciating

- Joint warmth, redness, swelling, and tenderness (even to light touch)
- Fever

After a first gout attack, people will have no symptoms for varying lengths of time. Some people will go months or even years between gout attacks. A number of people develop chronic gouty arthritis, but others have no further attacks. Those people with chronic arthritis develop joint deformities and limited joint mobility. With chronic gout, joint pain and other symptoms will be present most of the time. Tophi may form below the skin around joints or in other places with chronic gout. Tophi can cause a local inflammatory response and may drain a chalky material.

Diagnostic procedures for gout include a history, physical examination, serum uric acid levels, urine uric acid levels (will be low in those with gout caused by underexcretion), synovial fluid analysis (presence of uric acid crystals), and joint X-rays. Treatment strate-

MYTH BUSTERS

Arthritis is a common condition with several myths that should be dispelled.

MYTH 1: Cracking your joints causes arthritis.

As arthritis myths go, this one is a biggie. When you crack a joint you are actually either snapping the ligament over the joint or pulling on the joint, which causes a negative nitrogen bubble. You are not cracking the bone, just manipulating the joint to make it feel better, so cracking your joints does *not* cause arthritis.

MYTH 2: Being double-jointed increases your risk for arthritis.

The term *double-jointed* is actually a misnomer. Nobody has two joints where there should be one. Some people have hypermobility (or extra flexibility) in their joints, but there is no evidence to suggest this causes arthritis. However, hypermobility could cause other injuries such as sprains, strains, and tears.

MYTH 3: Vaccinations can cause arthritis.

This notion is a hot issue, but the Arthritis Foundation's position is that immunizations (particularly rubella) do not cause arthritis. No research evidence has supported this myth. Some immunizations can cause some short-term joint aching, but this is not the same as arthritis.

gies focus on lowering uric acid levels, usually with medications and dietary changes. Medications often vary depending on the current phase of gout the patient is experiencing. These strategies may include:

- Pharmacologic therapy for acute gout attacks, including the following:
  - NSAIDs to control inflammation and pain; higher doses may be used to stop an acute attack
  - Colchicine, an analgesic that is particularly effective in reducing gout pain
  - Corticosteroids to relieve inflammation and pain
- Pharmacologic therapies to prevent the complications associated with frequent gout attacks, including the following:
  - Xanthine oxidase inhibitors (e.g., allopurinol [Zyloprim]) to block uric acid production

  - Probenecid (Probalan) to improve renal excretion of uric acid
- Avoiding triggers (e.g., stress, high protein intake, and alcohol)

Ankylosing Spondylitis

Ankylosing spondylitis is a progressive inflammatory disorder affecting the sacroiliac joints, intervertebral spaces, and costovertebral joints. The inflammation starts in the vertebral joints. As the inflammation persists, new bone forms in an attempt to remodel the damage. Fibrosis and calcification, or fusion, of the joints follows. The vertebral joints become fixed, or ankylosed, and lose mobility. Inflammation begins in the lower back at the sacroiliac joints and progresses up the spine. The vertebrae appear square, and the vertebral column becomes rigid and loses curvature (**Figure 12-36**). The exact cause of ankylosing spon-

NORMAL ANATOMY

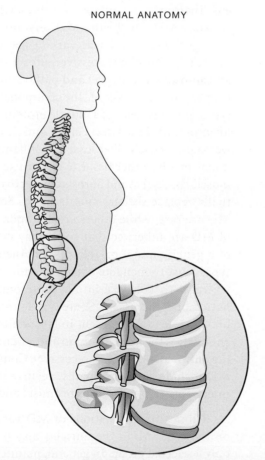

Normal S-curve of spine

ANKYLOSING SPONDYLITIS

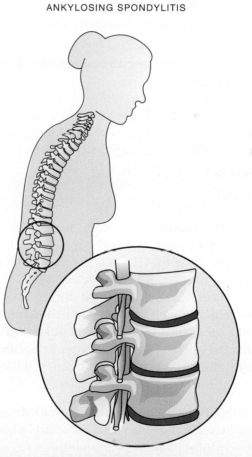

Loss of normal curvature

Figure 12-36

Ankylosing spondylitis.

dylitis is unknown, though genetic factors seem to be involved. In particular, people who have a gene called HLA-B27 are at significantly increased risk of developing ankylosing spondylitis. Ankylosing spondylitis is more common in males than in females and typically appears between 20 and 40 years of age. Complications include kyphosis, osteoporosis, respiratory compromise (due to reduced lung expansion resulting from fusion of the rib cage), endocarditis (inflammation of the internal cardiac structures), and uveitis (inflammation of the eye).

Clinical manifestations of ankylosing spondylitis reflect the decreased joint mobility. The individual may experience periods of remission and exacerbation. Manifestations worsen as the disease progresses and may include:

- Intermittent lower back pain (early)
- Pain and stiffness that typically worsens with inactivity (e.g., when sleeping) and improves after activity
- Lower back pain that evolves to include the entire back
- Pain in other joints (especially the shoulders, hips, or lower extremities)
- Muscle spasms
- Fatigue
- Low-grade fever
- Weight loss
- Kyphosis

Diagnostic procedures of ankylosing spondylitis may consist of a history, physical examination, test for serum presence of the HLA-B27 gene, erythrocyte sedimentation rate test, X-rays, CTs, and MRIs. The goal of treatment is to relieve pain and stiffness as well as prevent or delay complications and spinal deformity. Ankylosing spondylitis treatment is most successful when initiated before the disease causes irreversible damage (e.g., fusion), especially in positions that limit function. Treatment strategies may include:

- NSAIDs, disease-modifying antirheumatic drugs, corticosteroids, and tumor necrosis factor blockers to relieve inflammation, pain, and stiffness
- Muscle relaxants to treat muscle spasms
- Physical therapy (including range of motion exercises and positioning)
- Surgical repair

- Health-promoting lifestyle behaviors (e.g., proper nutrition, adequate rest, stress management, and smoking cessation)
- Coping strategies and support

Chronic Muscle Disorders

Chronic muscle disorders include conditions that result from a wide range of causes (e.g., genetic predisposition, trauma, and infection). These conditions may lead to chronic pain, weakness, and paralysis. Chronic muscle disorders may be progressive, requiring lifelong treatment. Because most of these conditions have no known cure, treatment often aims to manage symptoms.

Muscular Dystrophy

Muscular dystrophy (MD) refers to a group of inherited disorders characterized by degeneration of skeletal muscle. Muscles become weaker as damage worsens. There are nine different forms of MD (including Becker's MD, Duchenne MD, myotonic MD, and limb-girdle MD), each with varying patterns of inheritance (e.g., X-linked recessive, autosomal dominant, and autosomal recessive) and pathogenesis (e.g., age of onset and progression). The commonality across all types is the presence of a muscle protein abnormality (dystrophin). This defect causes muscle dysfunction, weakness, muscle fiber loss, and inflammation, and it may involve other tissue (e.g., cardiac and smooth muscle tissue). Fat and fibrosis connective tissue eventually replace skeletal muscle fibers. Some types of MD are rare, while others are common. Most types of MD are inherited, but some may occur because of a genetic mutation (often spontaneously). Some types cause tremendous disability and rapidly decline whereas others have minimal symptoms and hardly noticeable progression. Some types present in childhood, while others present in late adulthood. Duchenne MD is the most common and severe type, affecting only males (X-linked recessive). Complications of MD include cardiomyopathy, recurrent respiratory infections, respiratory compromise, and death.

Clinical manifestations of MD vary depending on the type. All of the muscles may be affected or only a selected group. In general, manifestations may include:

- Mental retardation (in some types)
- Muscle weakness that slowly worsens to hypotonia

- Muscle spasms
- Delayed development of muscle motor skills
- Difficulty using one or more muscle groups
- Poor coordination
- Drooling
- Ptosis (eyelid drooping)
- Frequent falls
- Problems walking (e.g., delayed walking)
- Gower's maneuver (an affected child pushes to an erect position by using his or her hands to climb the legs)
- Progressive loss of joint mobility and contractures (e.g., clubfoot and foot drop)
- Unilateral calf hypertrophy
- Scoliosis or lordosis

Diagnostic procedures for MD may consist of a history, physical examination, muscle biopsy, electromyelography, electrocardiogram, serum creatine kinase levels, test for serum presence of defective dystrophin, and genetic testing. Additionally, fetal chorionic villus testing can be performed prenatally at 12 weeks' gestation. There is no cure for MD; however, gene therapy may potentially be the answer. Currently, the goal of treatment is to maintain motor function and prevent deformities as long as possible. Treatment strategies may include physical therapy, muscle relaxants, immunosuppressant agents, assistive devices (e.g., walker, braces, and splints), and surgical contracture release. Additionally, coping strategies and support for the patient and caregivers may be beneficial.

Fibromyalgia

Fibromyalgia is a syndrome predominately characterized by widespread muscular pains and fatigue. Fibromyalgia affects muscles, tendons, and surrounding tissue, but it does not affect the joints. Eighteen fibromyalgia-specific pressure points, where pain or tenderness may be stimulated, have been identified in the neck, shoulder, trunk, and limbs. No apparent inflammation or degeneration is associated with fibromyalgia. The cause remains uncertain, but fibromyalgia may be related to an altered central neurotransmission that results in sensitivity to substance P (a neurotransmitter responsible for pain sensation). In fibromyalgia, the brain's pain receptors seem to develop a sort of pain memory and become more sensitive to pain signals. Additional postulated causes include physical or

MYTH BUSTERS

Fibromyalgia remains a mysterious condition, and two myths about fibromyalgia deserve discussion.

MYTH 1: **Fibromyalgia is an autoimmune disease.**

Fibromyalgia is *not* an autoimmune disease. Autoimmune disease is the result of a body's overactive and inappropriate immune response. There is no evidence that fibromyalgia is an autoimmune disease. However, people with fibromyalgia also commonly have one or more autoimmune diseases.

MYTH 2: **Fibromyalgia is a psychologic problem.**

Fibromyalgia is a physical disorder with real, measurable, biologic abnormalities. This myth probably causes the most frustration to fibromyalgia patients. After years of being told, "It is all in your head," patients finally have proof that fibromyalgia is a very real, physical illness. Research studies have revealed a number of biologic abnormalities, but despite the scientific evidence, fibromyalgia continues to be dismissed as a psychologic problem by many in the medical community who continue to insist that the symptoms are caused by depression.

emotional trauma, sleep disturbances, altered skeletal muscle metabolism, infections, and genetic predisposition. The CDC (2009a) estimates that approximately 5 million Americans have fibromyalgia, with the prevalence rates being highest among women.

Clinical manifestations may vary depending on the weather, stress, fatigue, physical activity, and time of day. Fibromyalgia is characterized by widespread pain, typically described as a constant, dull muscle ache. Fatigue, sleep disturbances, depression, irritable bowel syndrome, headaches, and memory problems may also occur with fibromyalgia. Conditions often associated with fibromyalgia include RA, systemic lupus erythematosus, and ankylosing spondylitis.

Diagnostic procedures for fibromyalgia center on the 18 identified pressure points. Diagnosis is based on the presence of widespread pain (at least 3 months' duration) and tenderness on 11 of 18 pressure points. Additional diagnostic procedures consist of a history, physical examination, and other tests to rule out other conditions. Treatment strategies focus on minimizing symptoms and improving overall health. These strategies may include stress reduction, regular exercise, adequate rest, proper nutrition, heat application, massage therapy, acupuncture, physical therapy, analgesics, NSAIDs, antidepressant agents, and antiseizure agents (specifically pregabalin [Lyrica]). Coping strategies, counseling, and support may also be helpful.

Bone Tumors

Tumors of the musculoskeletal system typically arise from the bone. The majority of bone tumors are malignant and occur as secondary tumors from other cancers (e.g., breast, lung, and prostate cancers). Bone tumors rarely occur as primary tumors. The exact cause of these primary tumors is unknown, but it is slightly more common in men and Caucasians than in women and other races. The overall 5-year survival rate is approximately 68%. Paget's disease increases the risk of developing primary bone cancer.

Bone cancer is described based on the type of cell in which the cancer originates. Bone cancer types include:

■ Osteosarcoma—Osteosarcoma is an aggressive tumor that begins in the bone cells, usually in the femur, tibia, or fibula (**Figure 12-37**). Osteosarcoma occurs most often in children and young adults.

■ Chondrosarcoma—Chondrosarcoma is a slow-growing tumor that begins in cartilage cells that are commonly found on the ends of bones. Chondrosarcoma most frequently affects older adults.

■ Ewing's sarcoma—Ewing's sarcoma is an aggressive tumor in which the origin is unknown. Ewing's sarcoma may begin in nerve tissue within the bone.

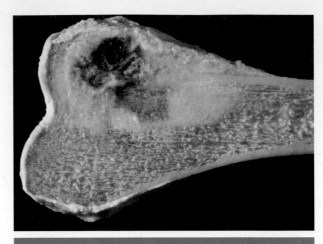

Figure 12-37

Osteosarcoma.

Ewing's sarcoma occurs most frequently in children and young adults.

Bone tumors are often asymptomatic in early stages. When present, clinical manifestations usually include pathologic fractures, bone pain, and a palpable mass. Diagnostic procedures for bone tumors may consist of a history, physical examination, X-rays, CTs, MRIs, positron emission tomography, bone scan, and biopsy. Treatment varies depending on the type and stage of the cancer. Surgical excision or amputation is often the treatment of choice. Radiation and chemotherapy may be used following surgery or if the tumor is inoperable.

Chapter Summary

The musculoskeletal system forms the framework for the body, provides support and protection, and allows for movement. Damage to this system is likely to cause issues with mobility. Musculoskeletal disorders vary from short-lived and mild to long-term and debilitating. Although most are not life threatening, many of these disorders can result in life-altering effects. Musculoskeletal damage may be caused by trauma, genetic defects, metabolic imbalances, as well as daily wear and tear. Supporting musculoskeletal health involves strategies such as weight management, proper nutrition, regular exercise, abstaining from smoking, and observing safety precautions (e.g., wearing safety equipment).

Case Study Answers

1. A compound fracture is a fracture in which the skin has been broken, and comminuted fractures are those fractures in which the bone is in multiple pieces.

2. Keep the left leg immobilized and the wound covered until surgery. Do not give the patient anything by mouth until the surgery, and manage pain.

3. The patient is at high risk for infection, especially osteomyletis, because of a break in the first line of defense. The patient is also at high risk for fat embolism because the fracture involved the femur. Finally, the patient is at high risk for compartment syndrome because of the multiple fractures, especially since one is a comminuted fracture.

4. The low-grade fever is likely a result of injury and inflammation, not infection. An infectious process will likely take 24–48 hours to develop. The elevation in the blood pressure along with the pulse being on the high end of normal may be a result of acute pain.

References

Centers for Disease Control and Prevention. (2009a). Retrieved from http://www.cdc.gov/arthritis/basics/fibromyalgia.htm

Centers for Disease Control and Prevention. (2009b). Retrieved from http://www.cdc.gov/arthritis/basics/osteoarthritis.htm

Centers for Disease Control and Prevention. (2009c). Retrieved from http://www.cdc.gov/arthritis/basics/rheumatoid.htm

Chiras, D. (2008). *Human biology* (6th ed.). Sudbury, MA: Jones and Bartlett.

Elling, B., Elling, K., & Rothenberg, M. (2004). *Anatomy and physiology*. Sudbury, MA: Jones and Bartlett.

Gould, B. (2006). *Pathophysiology for the health professions* (3rd ed.). Philadelphia, PA: Elsevier.

Madara, B., & Pomarico-Denino, V. (2008). *Pathophysiology* (2nd ed.). Sudbury, MA: Jones and Bartlett.

Professional guide to pathophysiology (2nd ed.). (2007). Philadelphia, PA: Lippincott Williams & Wilkins.

Resources

www.cancer.gov

www.cancer.org

www.cdc.gov

www.mayoclinic.com

www.medlineplus.gov

www.nih.gov

www.nof.org

www.osteo.org

www.who.int

go.jblearning.com/story

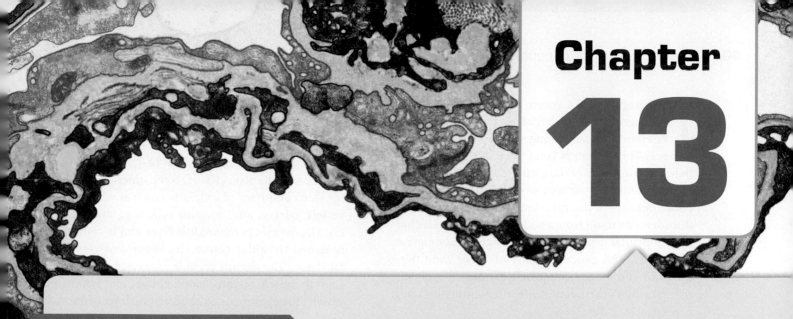

Integumentary Function

LEARNING OBJECTIVES

- Discuss normal integumentary anatomy and physiology.
- Compare and contrast congenital integumentary disorders.
- Describe and discuss integumentary changes and conditions associated with aging.
- Compare and contrast inflammatory integumentary disorders.
- Compare and contrast infectious integumentary disorders.
- Describe and discuss traumatic integumentary disorders.
- Describe and discuss chronic integumentary disorders.
- Describe and discuss integumentary cancers.

KEY TERMS

acne vulgaris
albinism
apocrine gland
atopic eczema
birthmark
burn
café au lait spot
carbuncle
cellulitis
contact dermatitis
dermis
eccrine gland

epidermis
folliculitis
furuncle
hemangioma
herpes simplex type 1
herpes zoster
hypodermis
impetigo
keratin
lentigo
macular stain
melanin

mole
Mongolian spot
necrotizing fasciitis
papule
pediculosis
pigmented birthmark
port-wine stain
psoriasis
rosacea
scabies
sebaceous gland
sebum

skin
skin cancer
skin tag
tinea
urticaria
vascular birthmark
verruca
vesicle
vitiligo
welt

The integumentary system protects the body from pathogen invasions, regulates temperature, senses environmental changes, and maintains water balance. This system is comprised of the skin, nails, hair, mucous membranes, and glands. Disorders of the integumentary structures can result in numerous issues because of the functions of this system. These disorders can result from a wide range of causes including congenital defects, advancing age, inflammation, infections, and cancers. Many of these conditions are mild and may not require treatment (e.g., birthmarks) while others can be life threatening (e.g., skin cancer).

Anatomy and Physiology

The **skin**, along with the nails, hair, mucous membranes, and glands, constitutes the integumentary system. Along with participating with sensory functions, the integumentary system has a key role in immunity (see Chapter 2), temperature regulation, and water balance. Additionally, this system excretes a small amount of waste products. The integumentary system is the body's largest organ system, covering all external sur-

faces and accounting for approximately 15% of the body's weight.

The skin consists of three layers—hypodermis, dermis, and epidermis (**Figure 13-1**). The **hypodermis**, or subcutaneous tissue, is the innermost layer of the skin comprised of soft, fatty tissue as well as blood vessels, nerves, and immune cells (e.g., macrophages). The **dermis** is the middle layer and is comprised of dense, irregular connective tissue and very little fat tissue. The dermis includes nerves, hair follicles, smooth muscle, glands, blood vessels, and lymphatic vessels. The **epidermis** is the outermost layer of the skin and is comprised of squamous epithelia, or flat sheets of cells. The epidermis consists of five distinct layers (**Figure 13-2**). New cells proliferate from the innermost layer and push upward. The outer layers often contain 25 sheets of dead cells that continuously shed. Most of these cells produce **keratin**, a protein that strengthens skin, and **melanin**, a pigment that protects the skin from ultraviolet (UV) rays.

Sebaceous glands produce **sebum**, which moisturizes and protects the skin. Two types of sweat glands are located throughout the skin—eccrine and apocrine

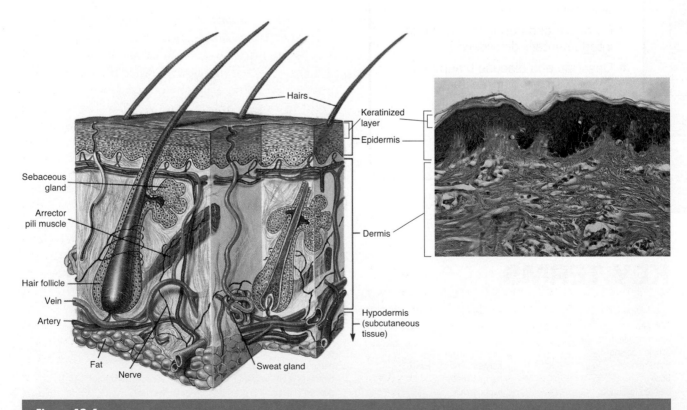

Figure 13-1

The layers of the skin.

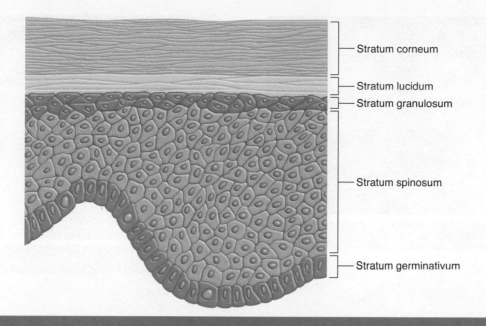

Labels:
- Stratum corneum
- Stratum lucidum
- Stratum granulosum
- Stratum spinosum
- Stratum germinativum

Figure 13-2

The layers of the epidermis.

glands. **Eccrine glands**, or merocrine glands, secrete sweat through skin pores in response to the sympathetic nervous system. **Apocrine glands** open into hair follicles in the axillae, scalp, face, and external genitalia.

Additionally, the skin has a complex mixture of normal flora that varies depending on the area of the body. This normal flora consists mostly of bacteria and fungi and can create an opportunistic infection when there is a skin injury. These superficial opportunistic infections can develop into a severe systemic infection if not managed appropriately.

Congenital Integumentary Disorders

Congenital disorders of the integumentary system can vary widely in severity. Many conditions occur because of an error during embryonic development. These errors may occur randomly, due to environmental influences, or because of genetic abnormalities. These errors may cause minor conditions with only aesthetic problems (e.g., birthmarks) or life-altering states (e.g., albinism). Occasionally, these seemingly benign conditions may be associated with other more serious problems that warrant further investigation. Treatment is often unnecessary, but when needed, treatment options are usually limited.

Birthmarks

Birthmarks are skin anomalies that are present at birth or shortly after. Most birthmarks are harmless and may even shrink or disappear with age. Birthmarks vary from barely noticeable to disfiguring. These abnormalities may be flat or raised, have regular or irregular borders, and have different shades of coloring including brown, tan, black, pale blue, pink, red, or purple. Birthmarks cannot be prevented and are not the result of anything done or not done during pregnancy. There are two types of birthmarks—vascular and pigmented.

Vascular birthmarks consist of blood vessels that have not formed correctly; therefore, these birthmarks are generally red. The types of vascular birthmarks include macular stains, hemangiomas, and port-wine stains. **Macular stains** are also called salmon patches, angel kisses, and stork bites (**Figure 13-3**). These abnormalities are the most common type of vascular birthmark. These birthmarks are faint red marks often occurring on the forehead, eyelids, posterior neck, nose, upper lip, or posterior head. On a baby, these birthmarks may be more noticeable when crying. Most often these marks fade on their own by 2 years of age, although they may last into adulthood. **Hemangiomas**, also referred to as strawberries, are birthmarks that appear as a bright red patch or a nodule of extra blood vessels in the skin (**Figure 13-4**). These birthmarks may

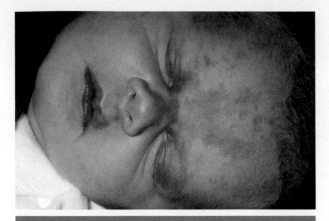

Figure 13-3

Macular stain.

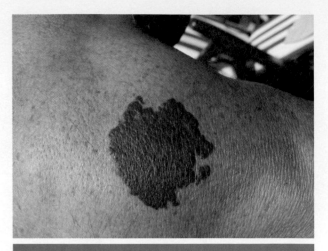

Figure 13-5

Port-wine stain.

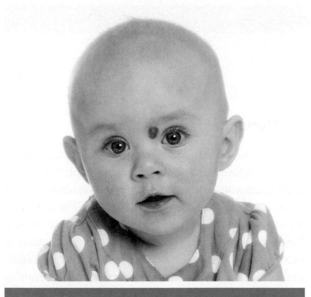

Figure 13-4

Hemangioma.

be superficial or deep. The deep hemangiomas may be bluish because they involve deeper blood vessels. Hemangiomas grow during the first year of life and then usually recede over time. Some hemangiomas, particularly larger ones, may leave scars as they regress; these scars can be corrected by minor plastic surgery. Many hemangiomas are on the head or neck, although they can be anywhere on the body. Most hemangiomas are benign and not associated with other medical conditions, but they can cause complications if their location interferes with sight, feeding, breathing, or other bodily functions. **Port-wine stains** are discolorations that look like wine was spilled on an area of the body,

hence their name (**Figure 13-5**). These birthmarks most often occur on the face, neck, arms, and legs. Port-wine stains can be any size, but they grow only as the child grows. They tend to darken over time and can thicken and have a cobblestone texture in mid-adulthood unless treated. Port-wine stains will not resolve spontaneously, and those occurring near the eye should be assessed for possible complications.

Pigmented birthmarks are made of a cluster of pigment cells, which cause color in skin. These birthmarks can be many different colors, from tan to brown, gray to black, or even blue. The most common pigmented birthmarks are café au lait spots, Mongolian spots, and moles. **Café au lait spots** are very common birthmarks that are the color of coffee with milk, hence their name (**Figure 13-6**). These birthmarks can be any-

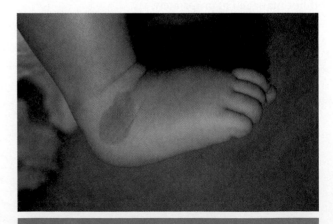

Figure 13-6

Café au lait spot.

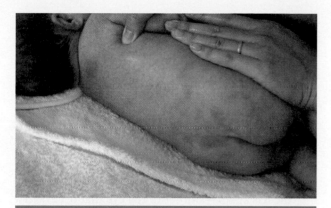

Figure 13-7

Mongolian spot.

MYTH BUSTERS

A myth about birthmarks warrants discussion—*Birthmarks are a result of something the mother did or ate while pregnant.* There is no truth to old wives' tales about stains being caused by something the mother did or ate. The cause of most birthmarks is unknown. Birthmarks can be inherited, but usually are not, and they typically are unrelated to trauma to the skin during childbirth.

where on the body and sometimes increase in number as a child gets older. One café au lait spot alone is not usually a concern, but the child should be further evaluated if there are several spots larger than a quarter, which can be a sign of neurofibromatosis (see Chapter 1). **Mongolian spots** are flat, bluish-gray patches often found on the lower back or buttocks (**Figure 13-7**). These birthmarks are most common on those with darker complexions, such as on children of Asian, American Indian, African, Hispanic, and Southern European descent. They usually fade, often completely, by school age without treatment.

Mole (congenital nevi, hairy nevi) is a general term for brown nevi (the singular is nevus). Most people get moles at some point in life. When present at birth, the mole is called a congenital nevus and will last a lifetime. Large or giant congenital nevi are more likely to develop into skin cancer (melanoma) later in life; however, all moles should be monitored for cancerous changes. Moles can be tan, brown, or black; can be flat or raised; and may have hair growth.

Diagnosis of birthmarks is often made during a physical examination. Treatment strategies vary depending on the type of birthmark, some of which cannot be treated. With the exception of macular stains, which usually fade away on their own, vascular birthmarks are treatable. Hemangiomas are usually left untreated, as they typically shrink back into themselves by age 9. Larger or more serious hemangiomas often are treated with steroids. Lasers are the treatment of choice for port-wine stains. Most port-wine stains lighten significantly after several laser treatments, although some return and need retreatment. Laser treatment is typically started in infancy when the stain and the blood vessels are smaller. Marks on the head and neck are the

most responsive to laser treatment. Pigmented birthmarks are usually left untreated, with the exception of moles and, occasionally, café au lait spots. Moles (particularly large or giant congenital nevi) are surgically removed. Café au lait spots can be removed with laser treatment but often return. Some birthmarks can be disfiguring and embarrassing for children. Special opaque makeup can be used to conceal or minimize the appearance of some birthmarks. Additionally, support and coping strategies can be helpful.

Disorders of Melanin

Melanin is a pigment that provides color and protection. Disorders involving melanin result in alterations in skin coloring and can leave the skin vulnerable to the harmful effects of UV light. Melanin disorders include albinism and vitiligo. **Albinism** is a recessive condition that results in little or no melanin production. Melanin deficits cause a lack of pigment in the skin, hair, and iris of the eye (**Figure 13-8**). In addition to coloring

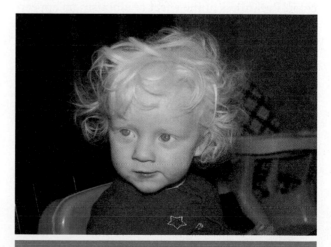

Figure 13-8

Albinism.

and protection, melanin also plays a role in the development of certain optical nerves. Therefore, all forms of albinism cause problems with eye development and function. There are two main types of albinism:

1. Type 1 albinism—caused by defects that affect melanin production.

2. Type 2 albinism—caused by a defect in the P gene; people with this type have slight coloring at birth.

The most severe form of albinism is oculocutaneous albinism. People with this form of albinism appear to have white or pink hair, skin, and iris color, as well as have vision problems. Another form of albism, called ocular albinism type 1, affects only the eyes. The affected person's skin and eye colors are usually in the normal range; however, an eye exam will reveal no coloring of the retina. Hermansky-Pudlak syndrome is a form of albinism caused by a single gene. Hermansky-Pudlak syndrome can occur with a bleeding disorder as well as with lung and bowel diseases. Other complex diseases may lead to color loss in only a certain area (localized albinism). These conditions include:

■ Chédiak-Higashi syndrome—lack of coloring all over the skin, but not complete

■ Tuberous sclerosis—small areas without skin coloring

■ Waardenburg's syndrome—often a lock of hair that grows on the forehead is affected, or no coloring in one or both irises

Clinical manifestations of albinism are usually, but not always, apparent in a person's skin, hair, and eye color. Regardless of the effect of albinism on appearance, all people with the disorder experience vision impairments. Manifestations may include:

■ Skin changes—Although the most recognizable form of albinism results in milky white skin, skin pigmentation can range from white to nearly the same as relatives without albinism. For some people with albinism, skin pigmentation never changes. For others, melanin production may begin or increase during childhood and adolescence, resulting in slight increases in pigmentation. Some people may develop freckles, moles (with or without pigment), or lentigines (large frecklelike spots) with exposure to the sun.

■ Hair changes—Hair color can range from very white to brown. People of African or Asian descent who have albinism may have hair color that is yel-

low, reddish, or brown. Hair color may also change by early adulthood.

■ Eye changes—Eye color can range from very light blue to brown and may change with age. The lack of pigment in the irises makes them somewhat translucent, meaning they cannot completely block light from entering the eye. This translucence can cause very light-colored eyes to appear red in some lighting because of light reflecting off the back of the eye and passing back out through the iris again—similar to red eye that occurs in a flash photograph.

■ Vision changes—Multiple vision issues can result from the lack of melanin, including:

  ▪ Nystagmus (rapid, involuntary back-and-forth eye movement)
  ▪ Strabismus (inability of both eyes to stay directed at the same point or to move in unison, or crossed eyes)
  ▪ Extreme nearsightedness or farsightedness
  ▪ Photophobia (sensitivity to light)
  ▪ Astigmatism (abnormally shaped cornea)
  ▪ Functional blindness

Diagnostic procedures for albinism consist of a history, physical examination (including a thorough ophthalmology exam), and genetic testing (most accurate). Although there is no cure for albinism, people with the disorder can take steps to improve vision and avoid damage from sun exposure. These strategies often include:

■ Using sunscreen with a high sun protection factor against UVA and UVB rays

■ Wearing protective clothing (e.g., long-sleeved shirts, long pants, and hats)

■ Limiting time outdoors, especially between 10:00 a.m. and 4:00 p.m., when UV rays are the most intense

■ Wearing sunglasses (UV protected), which may relieve light sensitivity

■ Wearing glasses to correct vision problems and eye position

■ Having eye muscle surgery to correct abnormal eye movements (i.e., nystagmus)

Albinism does not impair intellectual development, although people with albinism often feel socially isolated and may experience discrimination. Coping strategies and support may be beneficial in addressing these issues. The visual issues may become educational challenges. Educational strategies may include sitting at the front of the classroom, using large-print books and notes, and printing materials with high-contrast colors (e.g., black and white).

Vitiligo refers to a rare condition characterized by small patchy areas of hypopigmentation (**Figure 13-9**). Vitiligo occurs when the cells that produce melanin die or no longer form melanin, causing slowly enlarging white patches of irregular shapes on the skin. Vitiligo affects all races but may be more noticeable and disfiguring in people with dark skin tones. The exact cause of vitiligo is unknown, but potential causes include an autoimmune condition, genetic influences, sunburn, and emotional stress. Vitiligo has also been associated with pernicious anemia, hypothyroidism, and Addison's disease. Although any area of the body may be affected, depigmentation usually develops first on sun-exposed areas (e.g., hands, feet, arms, face, and lips). While it can start at any age, vitiligo often first appears between 10 and 30 years of age. Vitiligo generally appears in one of three patterns—focal (depigmentation is limited to one or a few areas of the body), segmental (loss of skin color occurs on only one side of the body), and generalized (pigment loss is widespread across many parts of the body, often symmetrically).

The natural course of vitiligo is difficult to predict. Sometimes the patches stop forming without treatment. In most cases, pigment loss spreads and can eventually involve most of the skin's surface. In addition to patchy skin depigmentation, clinical manifestations may include depigmentation of the hair, mucous membranes, and retina.

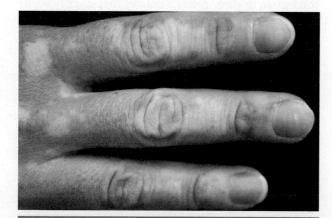

Figure 13-9

Vitiligo.

Diagnosis of vitiligo includes a history, physical examination, skin biopsy, serum autoantibody level measurements, serum thyroid hormone level measurements, and serum B_{12} level measurements. There is no cure for vitiligo. The goal of treatment is to stop or slow the progression of pigment loss and attempt to return some pigment. Treatment and coping strategies may include:

- Light therapy (exposure to controlled intense UV light in a clinic or hospital)
- Pharmacotherapy, including the following:
  - Oral synthetic melanizing agent (e.g., trimethylpsoralen [Trisoralen])
  - Topical corticosteroid agents
  - Topical immunosuppressants (e.g., pimecrolimus [Elidel] and tacrolimus [Protopic])
  - Topical repigmenting agents (e.g., methoxsalen [Oxsoralen])
  - Oral or topical photochemotherapy (e.g., psoralen plus UV-A)
- Skin graft
- Autologous melancyte transplant (still experimental)
- Permanent depigmentation of the remaining skin (a last resort reserved for extreme cases)
- Sun safeguards (e.g., sunscreen and protective clothing)
- Coping strategies and support, which may include:
  - Makeup or skin dyes
  - Tattooing (most effective around the lips)

Integumentary Changes Associated With Aging

The skin undergoes several changes with aging. Sensations of pain, vibration, cold, heat, pressure, and touch usually decrease. These changes may be related to decreases in blood flow to touch receptors or the brain that can occur with age. Decreases in these sensations can increase the risk of injury including falls, decubitus ulcers, burns, and hypothermia.

In addition to sensory changes, the skin also undergoes other changes. The skin loses elasticity, integrity, and moisture over time. Environmental factors, genetic makeup, and nutrition contribute to these changes. The greatest single contributing factor is sun exposure. Natural pigments seem to provide some protection against sun-induced skin damage. Blue-eyed, fair-skinned people show more of these aging skin changes than people with darker, more heavily pigmented skin. With aging, the epidermis thins even though the number of cell layers remains unchanged. The number of melanocytes decreases, but the remaining melanocytes increase in size. Aging skin thus appears thin, pale, and translucent. Large pigmented spots (called age spots, liver spots, or lentigos) may appear in sun-exposed areas (**Figure 13-10**). Changes in the connective tissue reduce the skin's strength and elasticity, especially in sun-exposed areas. Dermis blood vessels become fragile, which can lead to bruising, cherry angiomas, and other similar conditions. Sebaceous glands produce less sebum over time. Men experience a minimal decrease, usually after the age of 80. Women gradually produce less sebum beginning after menopause. This decrease in sebum can make it difficult to maintain skin moisture, resulting in dryness and itching. The subcutaneous fat layer, which provides insulation and padding, thins. This waning subcutaneous layer

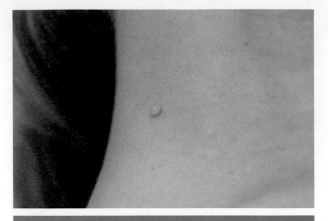

Figure 13-11

Skin tags.

increases risk of skin injury and reduces the ability to maintain body temperature. Additionally, this fat layer absorbs some medications, and loss of this layer changes the actions of these medications. The sweat glands produce less sweat with aging. This decrease in perspiration contributes to the difficulty in controlling body temperature. Aging skin repairs itself more slowly than younger skin. Wound healing may be up to four times longer. This sluggish repair contributes to decubitus ulcer formation and infections. The presence of chronic diseases (e.g., diabetes mellitus and arteriosclerosis) along with other changes with aging (e.g., impaired immunity and circulatory changes) further delay healing.

Other skin abnormalities may develop over time. Abnormalities such as skin tags and other blemishes are more common in older people. Skin tags are benign, soft brown or flesh-colored masses that usually occur on the neck (**Figure 13-11**). Most skin tags are painless, but they can become inflamed in the presence of constant friction (e.g., from clothing). Skin tags are more common in persons who are obese or have diabetes mellitus. Skin tags can be removed with surgery, cryotherapy, and cautery.

Inflammatory Integumentary Disorders

Inflammatory skin diseases include a broad group of conditions, ranging in severity from mild itching to serious medical complications. These noncontagious conditions may occur in isolation or in conjunction with other conditions. Most of these disorders can be resolved or managed easily with treatment.

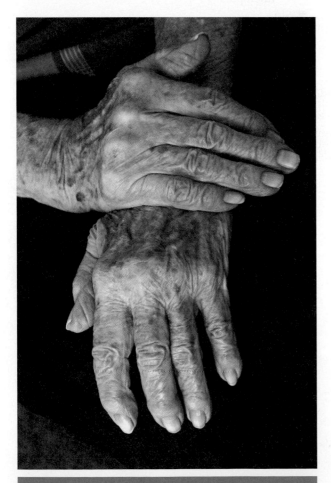

Figure 13-10

Lentigo.

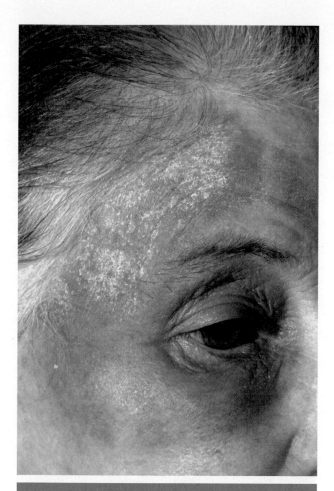

Figure 13-12

Contact dermatitis.

Contact Dermatitis

Contact dermatitis is an acute inflammatory reaction triggered by direct exposure to an irritant or allergen-producing substance (**Figure 13-12**). Contact dermatitis is not contagious or life threatening. Contact dermatitis varies in severity depending on the substance, area affected, exposure extent, and individual sensitivity. Chemicals, acids, and soaps may cause irritant contact dermatitis. This type of contact dermatitis does not involve the immune system, just the inflammatory response. Irritant contact dermatitis produces a reaction similar to a burn. Manifestations of irritant contact dermatitis typically include erythema and edema but may also include pain, pruritus, and vesicles (blisters). Allergic contact dermatitis results from substances such as metals, chemicals, cosmetics, and plants. Sensitization occurs on the first exposure to the substance, and subsequent exposures to the substance produce manifestations, which is a type IV cell-medi-

ated hypersensitivity (see Chapter 2). The reaction is usually delayed, with manifestations appearing 24–48 hours after exposure. Typically, manifestations of allergic contact dermatitis include pruritus, erythema, and edema at the site, but small vesicles may also be present. Diagnostic procedures include a history, physical examination, and allergy testing. Treatment of contact dermatitis centers on identifying and removing the causative agent. If the offending agent can be avoided, the rash usually resolves in 2–4 weeks. Self-care measures, such as wet compresses and anti-inflammatory creams (e.g., corticosteroid agents), can help soothe skin and reduce inflammation. Systemic anti-inflammatory agents may be used in severe cases.

Atopic Eczema

Atopic eczema is a chronic inflammatory condition triggered by an allergen (**Figure 13-13**). This condition has an inherited tendency and may be accompanied by asthma and allergic rhinitis. Atopic eczema

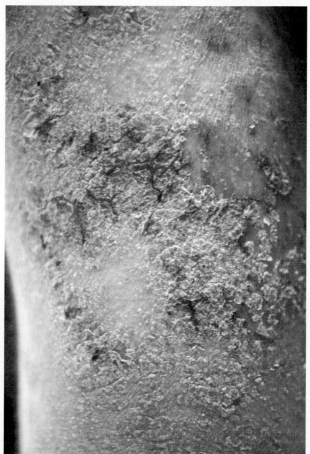

Figure 13-13

Atopic dermatitis.

is most common in infants and usually resolves by early adulthood. Atopic eczema tends to be characterized by remissions and exacerbations. The exact cause is unknown, but atopic eczema may result from an immune system malfunction. Complications include secondary bacterial skin infections, neurodermatitis (permanent scarring and discoloration from chronic scratching), and eye problems (e.g., conjunctivitis). Atopic eczema may affect any area, but it typically appears on the arms and behind the knees. Clinical manifestations may include:

- Red to brownish-gray colored skin patches
- Pruritus, which may be severe, especially at night
- Vesicles
- Thickened (lichenified), cracked, or scaly skin
- Irritated, sensitive skin from scratching

Diagnostic procedures for atopic eczema include a history, physical examination, allergy testing, and skin biopsy (to rule out other causes). Treatment focuses on decreasing the inflammatory process. These strategies may include:

- Avoiding factors that can worsen manifestations, such as:
  - Long, hot baths or showers
  - Dry skin
  - Stress
  - Sweating
  - Rapid changes in temperature
  - Low humidity
  - Solvents, cleaners, soaps, or detergents
  - Wool or synthetic fabrics or clothing
  - Dust or sand
  - Cigarette smoke
  - Certain foods (e.g., eggs, milk, fish, soy, and wheat)
- Avoiding scratching
- Moisturizing the skin by applying ointments (e.g., petroleum jelly) 2–3 times a day
- Using a humidifier
- Employing the following strategies when washing or bathing:
  - Keep water contact brief and use little soap.
  - Do not excessively scrub or dry the skin.
  - After bathing, apply lubricating creams, lotions, or ointment on the skin while it is damp to trap moisture in the skin.

- Using the following pharmacologic agents:
  - Antihistamine agents (may be topical or oral)
  - Corticosteroid agents (may be topical or oral)
  - Immunomodulators (may be topical or oral)
  - Antibiotics (may be topical or oral if infection is present)
  - Allergen desensitizing injections
- Receiving phototherapy

Urticaria

Urticaria, or hives, are raised erythematous skin lesions (welts) (**Figure 13-14**). These lesions are a result of a type I hypersensitivity reaction (see Chapter 2). This reaction is often triggered by food (e.g., shellfish and nuts) and medicine (e.g., antibiotics) ingestion. Urticaria may also be a result of emotional stress, excessive perspiration, diseases (e.g., autoimmune conditions and leukemia), and infections (e.g., mononucleosis). Urticaria results from histamine release initiated

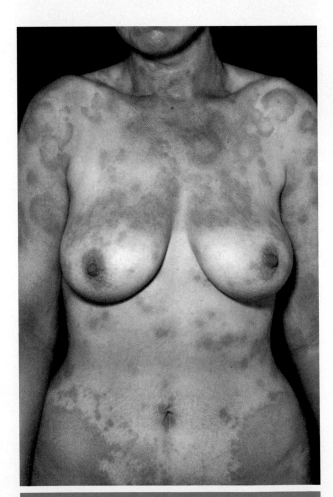

Figure 13-14

Urticaria.

by these substances or conditions. Urticaria are usually short-lived and harmless, but breathing can be impaired when the swelling occurs around the face (angioedema). Additionally, the type I hypersensitivity reaction can progress to an anaphylactic reaction (see Chapter 2) and shock (see Chapter 4). The diffuse welts may grow large, spread, and fuse together. These welts turn white when pressure is applied (called blanching). In addition to patchy welts, pruritus may also be present. Diagnostic procedures for urticaria include a history, physical examination, and allergy testing. Treatment focuses on ceasing the inflammatory reaction and maintaining respiratory status (if appropriate). Mild urticaria may disappear without any treatment. Treatment strategies to reduce itching and swelling include:

- Avoiding hot baths or showers
- Avoiding irritating the area (e.g., with tight-fitting clothing or rubbing)
- Taking antihistamines (e.g., diphenhydramine [Benadryl])

Severe reactions, especially if angioedema is present, may require epinephrine (adrenaline) or corticosteroid injections. Additionally, airway maintenance may be necessary, including an artificial airway, oxygen therapy, and mechanical ventilation. Epinephrine (adrenaline) and other bronchodilator agents can also be administered directly into the respiratory tract to improve ventilation.

Psoriasis

Psoriasis is a common chronic inflammatory condition that affects the life cycle of the skin cells (**Figure 13-15**). Cellular proliferation is significantly increased, causing cells to build up too rapidly on the skin's surface (**Figure 13-16**). The process of skin cells growing in the innermost layers of the skin and then rising to the surface normally takes weeks, but with psoriasis, this process occurs over 3–4 days. This buildup leads to thickening of the dermis and epidermis because dead cells cannot shed fast enough. The exact cause of psoriasis is unknown, but it does have a familial tendency. Psoriasis is thought to be a result of an autoimmune process in which the body, specifically T lymphocytes, mistakes normal skin cells as foreign. Psoriasis can affect people of any age, but the onset is most frequently between 15 and 35 years of age. The onset may be sudden or gradual, and many sufferers will experience remissions and exacerbations. The following may

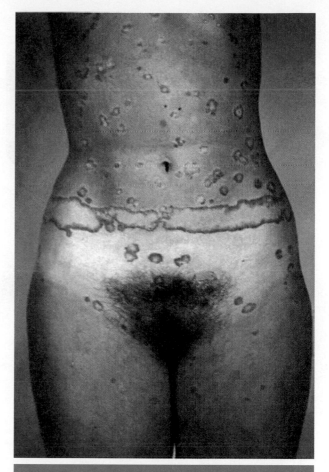

Figure 13-15

Psoriasis.

trigger a psoriasis exacerbation or make the condition more difficult to treat:

- Bacterial or viral infections in any location
- Dry air or dry skin
- Skin injuries (e.g., cuts, burns, and insect bites)
- Certain medicines (e.g., antimalaria agents, beta blockers, and lithium)
- Stress
- Too little or too much sunlight
- Excessive alcohol consumption

Severity varies widely from being a mere nuisance to being disabling; as many as 30% of persons with psoriasis also have arthritis, referred to as a psoriatic arthritis. In general, psoriasis may be severe in persons who have a weakened immune system (e.g., those with AIDS, those with autoimmune conditions, or those who are receiving chemotherapy). Psoriatic lesions

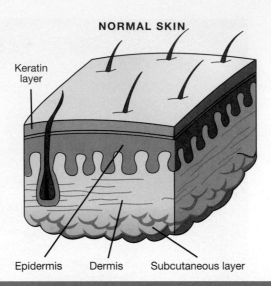

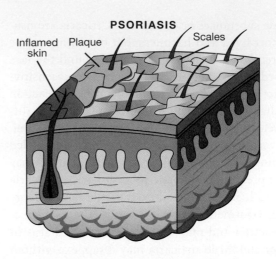

Figure 13-16

Psoriasis development.

begin as a small, red papule (firm and solid elevation) that enlarges. These lesions most often occur on the elbows, knees, and trunk, but they can appear anywhere on the body. The psoriatic lesions can progress into one of the following types of psoriatic lesions:

- Erythrodermic—intense erythema that covers a large area
- Guttate—small, pink-red spots
- Inverse—erythema and irritation that occur in the armpits, groin, and skin folds
- Plaque—thick, red patches covered by flaky, silver-white scales (the most common type)
- Pustular—white blisters surrounded by red, irritated skin

Other manifestations may include:

- Genital lesions in males
- Joint pain or aching (psoriatic arthritis)
- Nail changes such as thickening, yellow-brown spots, dents (pits) on the nail surface, and separation of the nail from the base
- Severe dandruff on the scalp

Diagnostic procedures for psoriasis include a history, physical examination, and skin biopsy. Other tests may be conducted to rule out other conditions that mimic psoriasis (e.g., seborrheic dermatitis and tinea corporis). No cure exists for psoriasis, but treatment

can improve symptoms significantly in most cases. The goal of psoriasis treatment is to interrupt the increased cell cycle and improve manifestations. Psoriasis treatment usually requires a multiprong approach and includes three main approaches—topical treatments, phototherapy, and systemic medications. These strategies may include:

- Topical treatments, including the following:
  - Corticosteroid agents (to slow cell turnover by suppressing the immune system)
  - Vitamin D analogues (to slow down the skin cell growth)
  - Anthralin (Dritho-Scalp) (to normalize DNA activity in skin cells, remove scales, and smooth skin)
  - Retinoids (to normalize DNA activity in skin cells and possibly decrease inflammation)
  - Calcineurin inhibitors (to disrupt the activation of T lymphocytes in order to reduce inflammation and plaque buildup)
  - Salicylic acid (to promote shedding of dead skin cells and reduce scaling)
  - Coal tar (to reduce scaling, itching, and inflammation, but the action is unknown)
  - Moisturizers (to reduce dryness, itching, and scaling; ointment-based moisturizers are the most effective)
- Phototherapy, including the following:
  - Sunlight (UV light, whether natural or artificial, causes activated T lymphocytes in the

skin to die, which slows cell turnover, reduces scaling, and decreases inflammation)
- Broadband ultraviolet B (UVB) phototherapy
- Narrowband UVB phototherapy (which is a newer treatment and more effective than broad band UVB treatment)
- Photochemotherapy, or psoralen plus ultraviolet A (administering psoralen, a light-sensitizing medication before exposure to UVA light to increase the response to the light)
- Excimer laser (a controlled beam of UVB light of a specific wavelength is directed to only the involved skin)

- Systemic pharmacotherapy (primarily reserved for severe or resistant cases and used for brief periods because of the potential of serious side effects), including the following:
  - Retinoids (which are related to vitamin A; this group of drugs may reduce the production of skin cells)
  - Methotrexate (which decreases the production of skin cells and suppresses inflammation)
  - Cyclosporine (which suppresses the immune system similarly to methotrexate)
  - Hydroxyurea (which suppresses the immune system but not as effectively as methotrexate and cyclosporine)
  - Immunomodulator drugs (which block interactions between certain immune system cells)

In addition to these main strategies, stress management (e.g., coping strategies and support) and avoiding psoriasis triggers may be beneficial.

Infectious Integumentary Disorders

Skin infections are common and frequently caused by a number of pathogens (e.g., bacteria, viruses, and parasites). These organisms usually gain access through a break in this first line of defense. These agents often trigger the inflammatory response as well. These infections can occur in any of the skin layers or structures (e.g., hair follicles). These conditions may be acute or chronic and vary widely in severity. In most cases, infectious integumentary disorders resolve easily with treatment.

Bacterial Infections

Any number of bacteria that the body has as normal flora or that it encounters may cause bacterial skin infections. These infections can vary from mild to life

threatening. Bacteria in the *Staphylococcus* and *Streptococcus* genera are common culprits. These infections can result in numerous conditions including:

- **Folliculitis**—Folliculitis refers to infections involving the hair follicles. Folliculitis is characterized by tender, swollen areas that form around hair follicles, often on the neck, breasts, buttocks, and face.
- **Furuncles**—Furuncles, or boils, refers to an infection that begins in the hair follicles and then spreads into the surrounding dermis. Furuncles most commonly occur on the face, neck, axillae, groin, buttocks, and back. A furuncle lesion starts as a firm, red, painful nodule that develops into a large, painful mass, which frequently drains large amounts of purulent exudate. **Carbuncles** refer to clusters of furuncles.
- **Impetigo**—Impetigo is a common and highly contagious skin infection. Although it can occur without an apparent break, impetigo typically arises from a break in the skin (especially from animal bites, human bites, insect bites, and trauma). Impetigo spreads easily to others by direct contact with skin or contaminated objects (e.g., eating utensils, towels, clothing, and toys). Lesions usually begin as small vesicles that enlarge and rupture, forming the characteristic honey-colored crust (**Figure 13-17**). These lesions can spread throughout the body through self-transfer of the exudate. Impetigo is typically caused by a staphylococcal infection. These bacteria produce a toxin that causes impetigo to spread to nearby skin. The toxin attacks collagen, a protein that helps bind skin cells together. Once this protein is damaged,

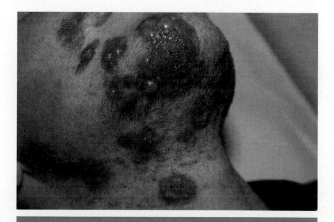

Figure 13-17

Impetigo.

bacteria can spread quickly. Pruritus is common, and lymphadenopathy (swollen lymph nodes) can occur near the lesions.

- **Cellulitis**—Cellulitis refers to an infection deep in the dermis and subcutaneous tissue. Cellulitis usually results from a direct invasion through a break in the skin, especially those breaks where contamination is likely (e.g., intravenous drug use and bites), or spreads from an existing skin infection. Cellulitis appears as a swollen, warm, tender area of erythema (**Figure 13-18**). Additionally, systemic manifestations of infection are usually present (e.g., fever, leukocytosis, malaise, and arthralgia). If left untreated, cellulitis can lead to necrotizing fasciitis, septicemia, and septic shock.

- **Necrotizing fasciitis**—Necrotizing fasciitis is a rare, serious infection, but rates are rising. One out of four people with this infection will die because of it. Also known as the flesh-eating bacteria, necrotizing fasciitis can aggressively destroy skin, fat, muscle, and other tissue (**Figure 13-19**). This infection is typically a result of a highly virulent strain of gram-positive, group A, beta-hemolytic *Streptococcus* that invade through a minor cut or scrape. The bacterium begins to grow and release harmful toxins that directly destroy the tissue, disrupt blood flow, and break down material in the tissue. The first sign of infection may be a small, reddish, painful area on the skin. This area quickly changes to a painful bronze- or purple-colored patch that grows rapidly. The center of the lesion may become black and necrotic. Exudate is often present. The wound may quickly grow in less than an hour. Systemic manifestations may include

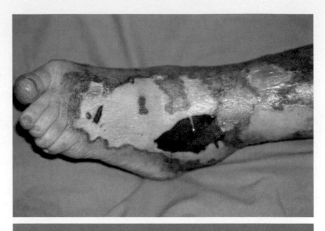

Figure 13-19

Necrotizing fasciitis.

fever, tachycardia, hypotension, and confusion. Complications of necrotizing fasciitis include gangrene and shock.

Diagnostic procedures for all bacterial skin infections center on the identification of the causative organism, usually through cultures. Once the organism is identified, treatment focuses on eradicating the organism with appropriate antibiotic therapy (either systemic or topical). Care should be taken with draining any wounds because it can spread the infection. Additionally, strategies may include maintaining adequate hydration, wound care, surgical debridement, drainage, antipyretic agents, and analgesic agents.

Viral Infections

A number of viruses can cause a multitude of skin issues, each with its own manifestations and treatments. These infections can result in numerous conditions, including:

- **Herpes simplex type 1**—Herpes simplex (HSV) type 1, or cold sore, is a viral infection typically affecting the lips, mouth, and face. The common infection usually begins in childhood. HSV type 1 can involve the eyes, leading to conjunctivitis. Additionally, HSV type 1 can result in meningoencephalitis. The virus is transmitted by contact with infected saliva. The primary infection may be asymptomatic. After the primary infection, the virus remains dormant in the sensory nerve ganglion to the trigeminal nerve until it is reactivated, similar to the pathogenesis of HSV type 2 (see Chapter 8). Reactivation may be a result of

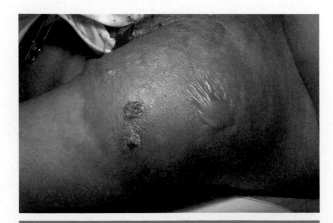

Figure 13-18

Cellulitis.

an infection, stress, or sun exposure. When reactivated, HSV type 1 causes painful blisters or ulcerations that are preceded by a burning or tingling sensation. The lesions will resolve spontaneously within 3 weeks, but healing can be accelerated with oral or topical antiviral agents.

- **Herpes zoster**—Herpes zoster, or shingles, is caused by the varicella-zoster virus. The condition appears in adulthood years after a primary infection of varicella (chickenpox) in childhood. The virus lies dormant on a cranial nerve or a spinal nerve dermatome until it is activated years later. The virus affects this nerve only, giving the condition its typical unilateral manifestations. These manifestations include pain, paresthesia, and a vesicular rash that develops in a line over the area innervated by the affected nerve (**Figure 13-20**). This rash may appear red or silvery, and it occurs on one side of the head or torso depending on the nerve affected. The skin often becomes extremely sensitive, and pruritus may be present. The rash may persist for weeks to months. In some cases, especially in older persons, neuralgia or pain may continue long after the rash disappears. Blindness may result if the eye is affected. Antiviral agents can limit the condition's duration and severity. Antidepressant and anticonvulsant agents have been beneficial in relieving the neuralgia.

- **Verrucae**—Verrucae, or warts, are caused by a number of the human papillomaviruses. Verrucae can develop at any age and often resolve spontaneously. They can be transmitted through direct skin contact between people or within the same person. The human papillomavirus replicates in the

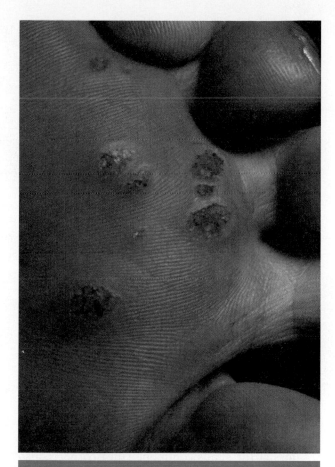

Figure 13-21

Verrucae.

skin cells, causing irregular thickening. Lesions can appear, varying in color, shape, and texture depending on the type (**Figure 13-21**). Treatment includes a wide range of local applications of laser treatments, cryotherapy with liquid nitrogen, electrocautery, and topical medications (e.g., keralytic, cytotoxic, and antiviral agents), but the verrucae may return after treatment.

Parasitic Infections

A number of parasitic infections can occur on the skin, including those caused by fungi and other organisms. These conditions are usually diagnosed through microscopic examination of skin scrapings processed with potassium hydroxide. Many of these organisms feed off the dead skin cells of the host and may use the host as a breeding ground. Some of the numerous parasitic skin infections include:

- **Tinea**—Tinea causes several types of superficial fungal infections described by the area of the body

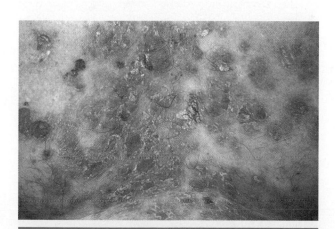

Figure 13-20

Herpes zoster.

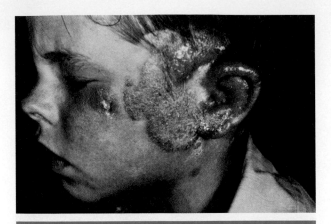

Figure 13-22

Tinea.

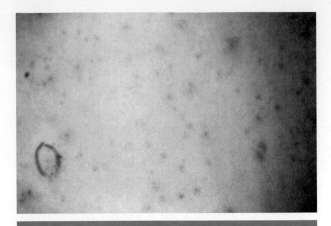

Figure 13-23

Scabies.

affected. These fungi typically grow in warm, moist places (e.g., showers). Tinea typically manifests as a circular, erythematous rash (**Figure 13-22**). This rash is typically associated with pruritus and burning. Tinea capitis is an infection of the scalp that is common in school-aged children. Along with the typical rash associated with tinea, hair loss at the site is common. Tinea corporis, also called ringworm, is an infection of the body. Tinea pedis, also called athlete's foot, involves the feet, especially the toes. Tinea unguium is an infection of the nails, typically the toenails. The infection begins at the tip of one or two nails and then usually spreads to other nails. The nail initially turns white and then brown, causing it to thicken and crack. Several topical and systemic antifungal agents are available to treat tinea infections, but several weeks of treatment may be necessary to resolve the infection.

■ Scabies—Scabies is a result of a mite infestation. The male mites fertilize the females and then die. The female mites burrow into the epidermis, laying eggs over a period of several weeks through tracks. After laying the eggs, the female mites die. The larvae hatch from the eggs and then migrate to the skin's surface. The larvae burrow in search of nutrients and mature to repeat the cycle. This burrowing appears as small, light brown streaks on the skin (**Figure 13-23**). The burrowing and fecal matter left by the mites triggers the inflammatory process, leading to erythema and pruritus. The mites can only survive for short periods without a host, so transmission usually results from close

contact. Several topical treatments are available, but multiple applications are usually needed to successfully eradicate the infestation. Clothing, linens, and other fabrics will likely require treatment as well.

■ Pediculosis—Pediculosis refers to a lice infestation that can take three forms—*Pediculus humanus corpus* (body louse), *Pediculus pubic* (pubic louse), and *Pediculus humanus capitis* (head louse). Lice are small, brown, parasitic insects that feed off human blood and cannot survive for long without the human host (**Figure 13-24**). The female lice lay eggs (nits) on the hair shaft close to the scalp (**Figure 13-25**). The nits appear as small white, iridescent shells on the hair. After hatching, the lice

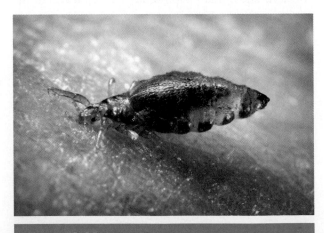

Figure 13-24

Louse.

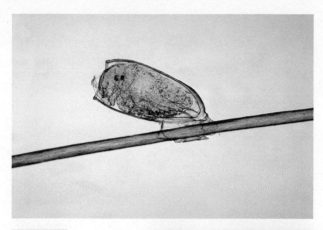

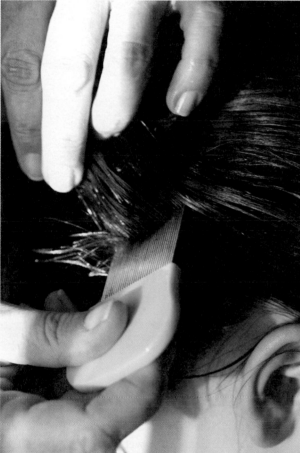

Figure 13-25

Nits.

bite and suck the blood. The site of the bite develops a highly pruritic macule or papule. Pediculosis is easily transmitted through close contact. Several topical treatments are available, but multiple applications are usually needed to successfully eradicate the infestation. Clothing, linens, and other fabrics will likely require treatment as well.

Traumatic Integumentary Disorders

Traumatic integumentary disorders can result from a wide range of injuries. Skin trauma can result in multiple skin conditions depending on the nature of these injuries (**Figure 13-26**). These injuries may be mild or life threatening depending on the location and extent of the injury. Regardless of the nature or extent of the injury, all traumatic skin conditions increase the risk for infection because of the break in the first line of defense (see Chapter 2). There are numerous traumatic skin conditions (e.g., lacerations and abrasions), but this section will focus on burns.

Burns

A burn is a skin injury that can result from a thermal (heat) or a nonthermal source. These sources may include dry heat (e.g., fire), wet heat (e.g., steam or hot liquids), radiation, friction, heated objects, natural or artificial UV light, electricity, and chemicals (e.g., acids, alkaline, and paint thinner). This injury triggers the inflammatory reaction and results in tissue destruction. The severity of the condition varies depending on location, extent, and nature of the injury. Severity is described, in part, in terms of levels (**Figure 13-27**):

- First-degree burns affect only the epidermis. These burns cause pain, erythema, and edema.

- Second-degree (partial thickness) burns affect the epidermis and dermis. These burns cause pain, erythema, edema, and blistering.

- Third-degree (full thickness) burns extend into deeper tissues. These burns cause white or blackened, charred skin that may be numb.

Complication development is usually related to burn severity. Burns may result in several complications, including:

- Local infection (particularly *Staphylococcus* infection)

- Sepsis

- Hypovolemia (burns can damage blood vessels and plasma proteins, causing fluid shifts; see Chapter 6)

- Shock (may result from sepsis or hypovolemia)

- Hypothermia (heat is lost through large injuries)

- Respiratory problems (inhaling hot air or smoke can burn airways, causing inflammation)

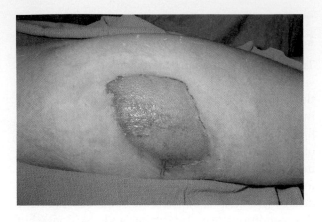

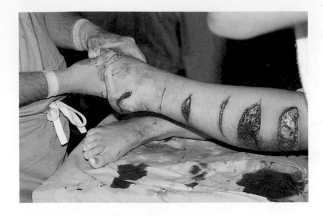

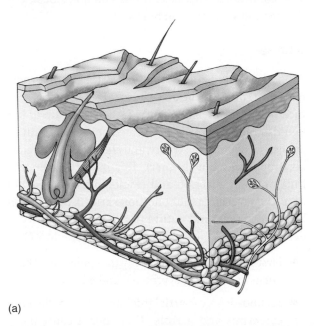

(a)

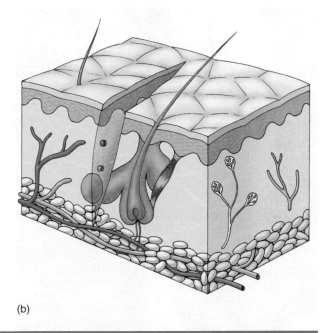

(b)

Figure 13-26

Types of wounds. (a) Abrasion. (b) Laceration.

■ Scarring

■ Contractures

Diagnostic procedures consist of a history, physical examination (including determining the total body surface area affected), chest X-ray, endoscopy (insertion of a flexible tube with a camera into the trachea and upper airways), complete blood count, and blood chemistry. Burn treatment is complex and varies depending on location and severity. Strategies for minor burns may include:

■ Remove the source of the burn.

■ If the skin is unbroken, run cool water over the area of the burn or soak it in a cool water bath (not ice water). Keep the area submerged for at least 5 minutes. A clean, cold, wet bandage or towel will also help reduce pain.

■ After flushing or soaking, cover the burn with a dry, sterile bandage or clean dressing.

■ Protect the burn from pressure and friction.

■ Administer analgesics and nonsteroidal anti-inflammatory drugs to relieve pain and swelling.

■ Apply moisturizing lotion once the skin has cooled.

■ If a second-degree burn covers an area more than 2–3 inches in diameter, or if it is located on the hands, feet, face, groin, buttocks, or a major joint, treat the burn as a major burn.

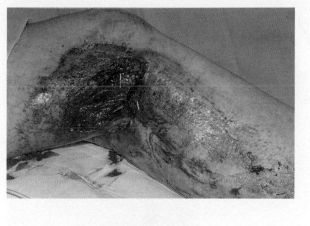

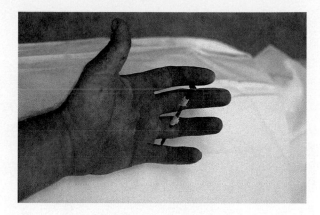

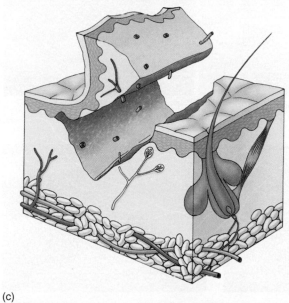

(c)

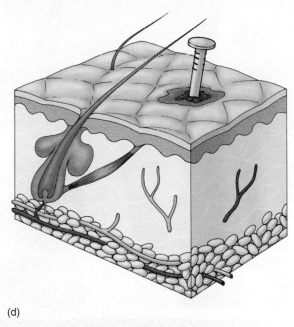

(d)

Figure 13-26 *(Continued)*

(c) Avulsion. (d) Penetrating wound.

For major burns, strategies include:

- Remove the source of the burn.

- If someone is on fire, have the person stop, drop, and roll. Wrap the person in thick material to smother the flames (e.g., a wool or cotton coat, rug, or blanket). Douse the person with water.

- Do not remove burned clothing that is stuck to the skin. The clothing may be soaked and then removed, and surgical removal may be necessary in severe cases.

- Ensure the person is breathing. Initiate rescue breathing and cardiopulmonary resuscitation if necessary. Continue to monitor respiratory sta-

tus because it can become impaired as edema worsens.

- Maintain respiratory status (e.g., endotracheal intubation with mechanical ventilation, oxygen therapy).

- Cover the burn area with a dry sterile bandage or clean cloth. Do not apply any ointments. Avoid rupturing blisters.

- If fingers or toes are involved, separate them with dry, sterile, nonadhesive dressings.

- Elevate the affected body part above the level of the heart.

- Protect the burn area from pressure and friction.

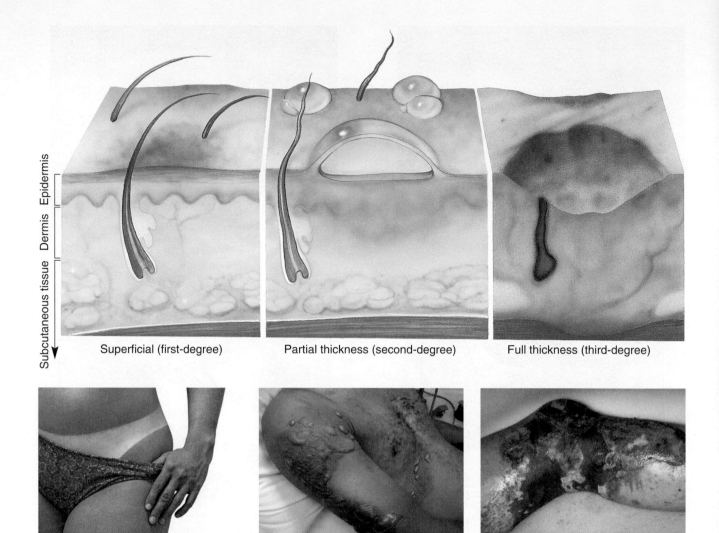

Epidermis

Dermis

Subcutaneous tissue

Superficial (first-degree) | Partial thickness (second-degree) | Full thickness (third-degree)

Figure 13-27

Burn classification.

LEARNING POINTS

There are several actions that should be avoided with burns.

- Do *not* apply ointment, butter, ice, medications, cream, oil spray, or any household remedy to a severe burn.
- Do *not* breathe, blow, or cough on the burn.
- Do *not* disturb blistered or necrotic skin.
- Do *not* remove clothing that is stuck to the skin.
- Do *not* give the person anything by mouth if there is a severe burn (surgery may be necessary).
- Do *not* immerse a severe burn in cold water because it can cause shock.
- Do *not* place a pillow under the person's head if there is an airway burn because it can close the airway.

- Take steps to prevent shock. Place the individual in Trendelenburg position and cover the person with a coat or blanket. However, do not place the person in this position if a head, neck, back, or leg injury is suspected or if it makes the person uncomfortable.

- Monitor vital signs for signs of shock (e.g., tachycardia and hypotension).

- Administer intravenous fluids (may include colloids or crystalloids) using specific formulas

- Administer oral, intravenous, or topical analgesics, sedatives, or antibiotics to reduce pain and to prevent infection.

- Implement reverse isolation (e.g., gowning and limiting visitors).

- Apply meticulous wound care to limit risk for infection and to promote healing.

- Apply protective dressings.

- Graft skin to promote tissue regeneration, prevent scarring, and aid the healing process.

- Perform surgery as necessary to close the wound, remove the dead tissue, or treat related complications (e.g., scarring and contractures).

- Conduct physical therapy to reduce effects of scar tissue.

- Increase dietary intake of protein and carbohydrates to promote healing and support the person's increased metabolic needs.

Chronic Integumentary Disorders

Numerous chronic conditions can affect the integumentary system. These conditions can vary in severity. Although most are not life threatening, many can cause significant impact on an individual's appearance.

Acne Vulgaris

Acne vulgaris is a skin condition commonly affecting adolescents, but it can occur at any age. Acne vulgaris occurs when the skin's pores become clogged with oil, debris, or bacteria. The pore can become inflamed, developing a pustule, nodule, or cyst. The clogged pore may become raised with a white top (called a whitehead), or the pore may become dark (called a blackhead) (**Figure 13-28**). If an infected pore ruptures, the material inside, including oil and bacteria, can spread to the surrounding area and cause an inflammatory reaction. Acne vulgaris commonly appears on the face

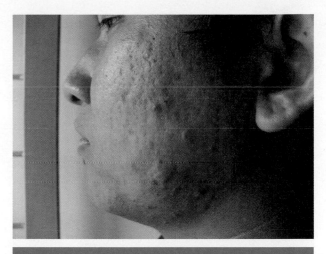

Figure 13-28

Acne vulgaris.

and shoulders, but it may also occur on the trunk, arms, legs, and buttocks. Acne vulgaris varies widely in severity. Severe cases can result in significant scarring. Risk factors for acne vulgaris include:

- Family history

- Hormonal changes (e.g., changes that occur with menstrual periods, pregnancy, birth control pill use, and stress)

- Using oily cosmetic and hair products

- Certain medications (e.g., corticosteroids, testosterone, estrogen, and phenytoin)

- High levels of humidity and sweating

Diagnostic procedures for acne vulgaris include a history and physical examination. Treatment varies depending on the severity, but these strategies often include:

- Clean skin gently with a mild, nondrying soap to remove all dirt or makeup once or twice a day, including after exercising; however, avoid excessive or repeated skin washing.

- Shampoo hair daily, especially if it is oily.

- Comb or pull hair back to keep the hair away from the face, but avoid tight headbands.

- Avoid squeezing, scratching, picking, or rubbing acne because it can lead to skin infections and scarring.

- Avoid touching affected areas.

MYTH BUSTERS

There are a couple of myths in regards to acne that warrant clearing up (no pun intended).

MYTH 1: **Eating greasy foods and chocolate worsens acne.**

Contrary to popular belief, greasy foods and chocolate have little effect on acne. Studies are ongoing to determine whether other dietary factors—including high-starch foods (such as bread, bagels and chips), which increase blood sugar—may play a role in acne.

MYTH 2: **Acne is a result of the skin being dirty.**

Acne is not caused by dirt. In fact, scrubbing the skin too hard or cleansing with harsh soaps or chemicals irritates the skin and can make acne worse. Simple cleansing of the skin to remove excess oil and dead skin cells is all that is required.

- Avoid oily cosmetics or creams; use water-based or noncomedogenic formulas.
- Use over-the-counter or prescription acne products containing benzoyl peroxide, sulfur, resorcinol, or salicylic acid.
- Administer oral or topical antibiotics (e.g., erythromycin).
- Apply retinoic acid cream or gel (e.g., Retin-A).
- Administer oral isotretinoin (Accutane).
- Administer oral contraceptives.
- Use alternative therapies including tea tree oil, zinc, guggul, and brewer's yeast.
- Apply photodynamic therapy (laser procedure).
- Apply chemical skin peels.
- Use microdermabrasion.
- Use dermabrasion.
- Use soft-tissue fillers (e.g., collagen and fat).
- Limit sun exposure.

Rosacea

Rosacea is a chronic inflammatory skin condition that typically affects the face. Rosacea is poorly understood, but it is prevalent in persons who are fair skinned, bruise easily, and women. Rosacea may present as erythema, prominent spiderlike blood vessels (telangi-

ectasia), swelling, or acnelike eruptions (**Figure 13-29**). Additional manifestations may include a thickening of the skin on the nose (rhinophyma), a burning or stinging sensation, and red, watery eyes. If left untreated, rosacea is progressive, but most people with rosacea experience remissions and exacerbations. Exacerbation triggers are specific to the individual. Triggers may include sun exposure, sweating, stress, spicy food, alcohol, hot beverages, wind, hot baths, and cold weather. Diagnostic procedures for rosacea include a history and physical examination. There is no known cure for rosacea. Treatment strategies center on identifying and avoiding possible triggers and thus reducing exacerbations. These strategies may include:

- Avoiding excessive scrubbing when cleaning
- Avoiding sun exposure (e.g., wearing protective clothing, limiting exposure time especially between 10:00 a.m. and 4:00 p.m.) and using sunscreen that protects against both UVA and UVB rays every day

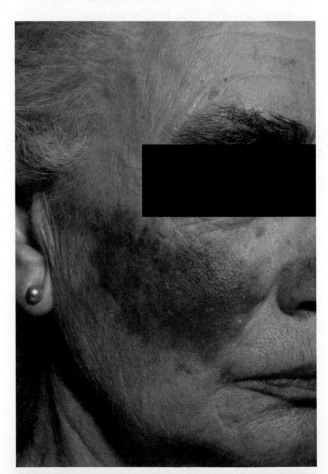

Figure 13-29

Rosacea

- Avoiding prolonged physical exertion in hot weather
- Managing stress (e.g., through deep breathing and yoga)
- Limiting spicy foods, alcohol, and hot beverages
- Avoiding any other triggers
- Using topical or oral antibiotics to control skin eruptions
- Applying retinoic acid cream or gel (e.g., Retin-A)
- Taking oral isotretinoin (Accutane)
- Performing laser surgery to help reduce the redness
- Performing surgical reduction of enlarged nose tissue
- Applying green- or yellow-tinted prefoundation creams and powders to reduce the appearance of redness

Integumentary Cancers

Skin cancer is an abnormal growth of skin cells. According to the Centers for Disease Control and Prevention (CDC) (2006), skin cancer is the most frequently occurring cancer. Prevalence rates are highest in males, African Americans, those with fair complexion, and those with a family history. The overall 5-year survival rate is approximately 38%. UV exposure, natural or artificial, is by far the most significant risk factor. For this reason, most skin cancers occur on areas that have the most sun exposure (e.g., the arms and neck). There are three major types of skin cancer—basal cell carcinoma, squamous cell carcinoma, and melanoma. Basal cell carcinoma, the most common, develops from abnormal growth of the cells in the lowest layer of the epidermis. Squamous cell carcinoma involves changes in the squamous cells, found in the middle layer of the epidermis. Melanoma develops in the melanocytes; it is the least common type but the most serious. Basal and squamous cell carcinomas rarely metastasize, but melanomas often metastasize to other areas.

Skin cancers can vary widely in appearance; they can be small, shiny, waxy, scaly, rough, firm, red, crusty, bleeding, and so on (**Figure 13-30**). Therefore, any suspicious skin lesion should be examined. Suspicious features may include:

- Asymmetry—part of the lesion is different from the other parts

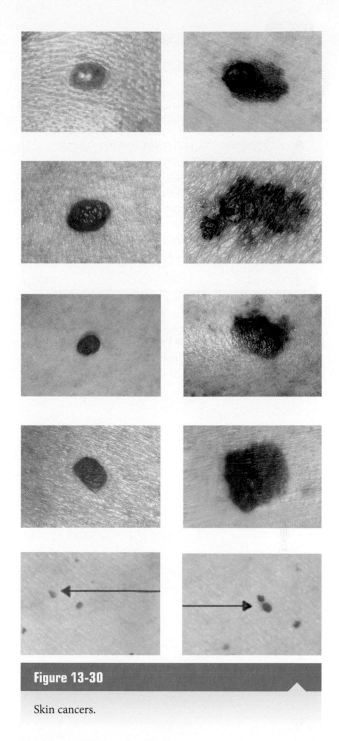

Figure 13-30

Skin cancers.

- Borders that are irregular
- Color that varies from one area to another with shades of tan, brown, or black (sometimes white, red, or blue)
- Diameter that is usually (but not always) larger than 6 mm in size
- Any skin growth that bleeds or will not heal
- Any skin growth that changes in appearance over time

LEARNING POINTS

All skin lesions, such as moles, should be monitored for any suspicious changes. These changes can be identified as easy as A, B, C, and D.

A = Asymmetry—part of the lesion is different from the other.

B = Borders—irregular.

C = Color—varies from one area to another with shades of tan, brown, or black (sometimes white, red, or blue).

D = Diameter—usually (but not always) larger than 6 mm in size (the diameter of a pencil eraser).

Most skin cancers can be prevented by limiting or avoiding exposure to UV light (e.g., by using sunscreen and wearing protective clothing). Early detection is crucial to positive outcomes. Diagnostic procedures for skin cancer typically include a history, physical examination, and biopsy. With early detection, even the most aggressive forms can be successfully treated. Removal of the cancerous growths offers the best prognosis. Treatment strategies may include:

- Cryosurgery
- Excisional surgery
- Laser therapy
- Mohs' surgery (the skin growth is removed layer by layer, examining each layer under the microscope, until no abnormal cells remain)
- Curettage and electrodesiccation (involves scraping layers of cancer cells away using a circular blade [curet] and then using an electric needle to destroy any remaining cancer cells)
- Radiation therapy
- Chemotherapy

Chapter Summary

The integumentary system plays a vital role in homeostasis and well-being by protecting the body from invasions, maintaining water balance, sensing changes in the environment, and regulating body temperature. Conditions affecting this system can cause issues with any or all of these functions. Some of these conditions can be prevented by limiting UV light exposure by using sunscreen that protects against UVA and UVB rays, wearing protective clothing, and limiting time outdoors especially between 10:00 a.m. and 4:00 p.m., when those rays are the most intense. Early diagnosis and treatment of other conditions can improve prognosis.

References

Centers for Disease Control and Prevention. (2006). Retrieved from http://www.cdc.gov/cancer/skin/basic_info/index.htm

Chiras, D. (2008). *Human biology* (6th ed.). Sudbury, MA: Jones and Bartlett.

Elling, B., Elling, K., & Rothenberg, M. (2004). *Anatomy and physiology.* Sudbury, MA: Jones and Bartlett.

Gould, B. (2006). *Pathophysiology for the health professions* (3rd ed.). Philadelphia, PA: Elsevier.

Professional guide to pathophysiology (2nd ed.). (2007). Philadelphia, PA: Lippincott Williams & Wilkins.

Resources

www.cancer.gov

www.cancer.org

www.cdc.gov

www.nayoclinic.com

www.medlineplus.gov

www.nih.gov

www.who.int

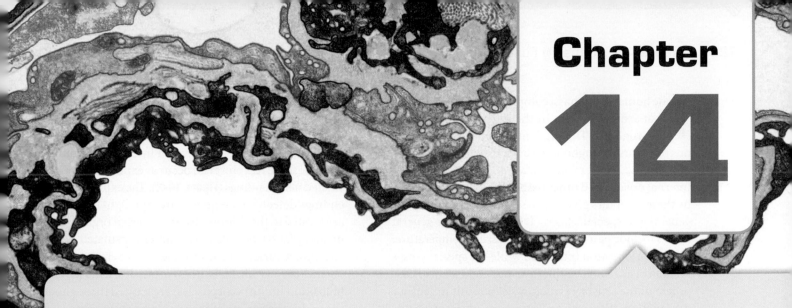

Sensory Function

- Discuss normal sensory anatomy and physiology.
- Compare and contrast congenital sensory disorders.
- Describe and discuss sensory conditions associated with aging.
- Compare and contrast infectious and inflammatory sensory disorders.
- Describe and discuss traumatic sensory disorders.
- Describe and discuss chronic sensory disorders.
- Describe and discuss sensory cancers.
- Describe and discuss miscellaneous sensory conditions.

KEY TERMS

amblyopia	ear	nystagmus	retina
anotia	eustachian tube	open-angle (chronic) glaucoma	retinal detachment
anterior chamber	external ear canal	optic nerve	rod
aqueous humor	eye	organ of Corti	saccule
atresia	glaucoma	ossicle	sclera
auricle	incus	otitis externa	secondary glaucoma
cataract	inner ear	otitis media	semicircular canal
choroid	intractable pain	otosclerosis	somatic pain
ciliary body	iris	outer ear	stapes
closed-angle (acute) glaucoma	keratitis	oval window	strabismus
cochlea	lacrimal duct	pain	tinnitus
cone	lacrimal gland	pain threshold	tympanic membrane
congenital cataract	lens	pain tolerance	utricle
congenital glaucoma	macular degeneration	phantom pain	vertigo
congenital hearing loss	malleus	posterior chamber	vestibular apparatus
conjunctiva	Meniere's disease	presbycusis	vestibule
conjunctivitis	microtia	presbyopia	visceral pain
cornea	middle ear	pupil	vitreous humor
diplopia	neuropathic pain	referred pain	

The human body has a complex surveillance system that senses changes in the internal and external environment. This vigilant system utilizes numerous receptors throughout the body to detect even subtle alterations. These receptors are located in the skin, internal organs, and other tissue. The stimuli perceived by these receptors give rise to sensations including the general and special senses (**Table 14-1**). These general senses include pain, light touch, pressure, temperature, and proprioception (position) while the special senses include taste, smell, sight, hearing, and balance. Disorders of the sensory structures can result in sensory dysfunction. These disorders can result from a wide range of causes including congenital defects, advancing age, infections, and cancers.

Anatomy and Physiology

The ability to sense changes in an ever-changing internal and external environment allows the body to respond and function. Sensations are detected by receptors, which then convert the stimuli into nerve impulses. These impulses travel to the brain by cranial or spinal nerves to be processed and appreciated (**Figure 14-1**). The human body contains five types of receptors for the general and special senses—mechanoreceptors (activated by mechanical stimuli such as touch or pressure), chemoreceptors (activated by chemicals in the blood, food, or air), thermoreceptors (activated by heat or cold), photoreceptors (activated by light), and nociceptors (activated by painful stimuli). General sense receptors can occur as exposed or encapsulated nerve endings (**Figure 14-2**). The exposed nerve endings detect pain, temperature, and light touch and are located in the skin, bones, and internal organs. One or more layers of cells surround encapsulated nerve endings. A variety of encapsulated nerve endings (e.g., Pacini's corpuscles, Meissner's corpuscles, Krause's end bulbs, and Ruffini's corpuscles) are located throughout the body for a variety of senses. Many of these sensory receptors (especially pain, temperature, and pressure) will stop generating impulses after an extended exposure to stimuli through adaptation.

Pain is associated with many conditions and, therefore, warrants further discussion. Pain is a protective mechanism, warning one's body when something is wrong. In addition, pain is the most common reason that people seek medical attention and can be used to aid diagnosis. Pain is a subjective feeling, and the perception of pain (**pain threshold**) can be influenced by affective (emotional), behavior, cognitive (beliefs and attitudes), sensory (perceptual), and physiologic factors. Unrelieved pain can delay healing, stimulate the

---

Table 14-1 Summary of the General and Special Senses

Sense	Stimulus	Receptor
General senses	Pain	Naked nerve endings
	Light touch	Merkel's discs; naked nerve endings around hair follicles; Meissner's corpuscles; Ruffini's corpuscles; Krause's end-bulbs
	Pressure	Pacinian corpuscles
	Temperature	Naked nerve endings
	Proprioception	Golgi tendon organs; muscle spindles; receptors similar to Meissner's corpuscles in joints
Special senses	Taste	Taste buds
	Smell	Olfactory epithelium
	Sight	Retina
	Hearing	Organ of Corti
	Balance	Crista ampularis in the semicircular canals; maculae in utricle and saccule

Source: Chiras, D. (2008). *Human biology* (6th ed.). Sudbury, MA: Jones & Bartlett Learning.

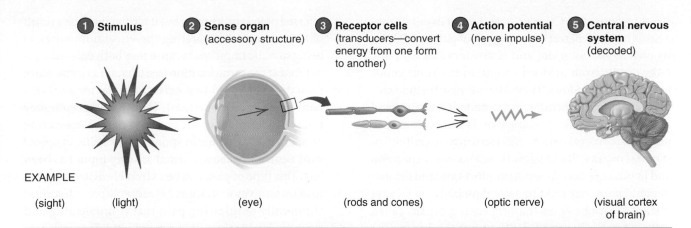

1 **Stimulus**

2 **Sense organ** (accessory structure)

3 **Receptor cells** (transducers—convert energy from one form to another)

4 **Action potential** (nerve impulse)

5 **Central nervous system** (decoded)

EXAMPLE

(sight)   (light)   (eye)   (rods and cones)   (optic nerve)   (visual cortex of brain)

Figure 14-1

The general sensory pathway.

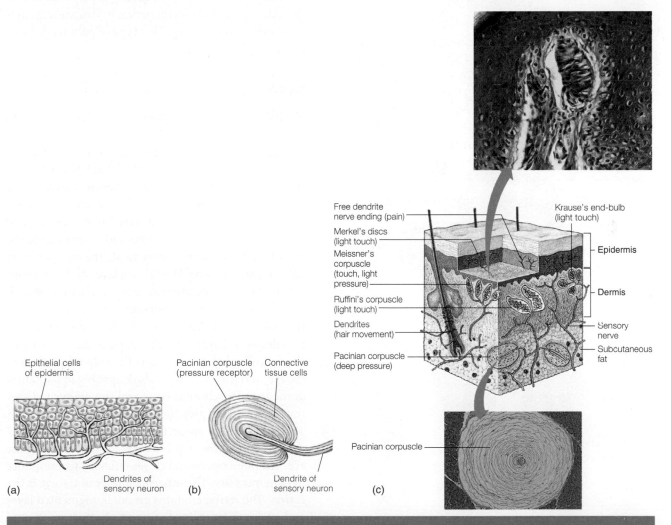

Free dendrite nerve ending (pain)

Merkel's discs (light touch)

Meissner's corpuscle (touch, light pressure)

Ruffini's corpuscle (light touch)

Dendrites (hair movement)

Pacinian corpuscle (deep pressure)

Krause's end-bulb (light touch)

Epidermis

Dermis

Sensory nerve

Subcutaneous fat

Epithelial cells of epidermis

Pacinian corpuscle (pressure receptor)   Connective tissue cells

Pacinian corpuscle

(a)   Dendrites of sensory neuron

(b)   Dendrite of sensory neuron

(c)

Figure 14-2

General sense receptors are either (a) exposed nerve endings or (b) encapsulated nerve endings. (c) The skin houses many of the receptors for the general senses. The Pacinian corpuscle, often located in the dermis of the skin, detects pressure. Meissner's corpuscle, found just beneath the epidermis, detects light touch.

stress response (see Chapter 2), and result in **pain toler-ance**. The body perceives two types of pain, each with its own cause, location, and characteristics. **Somatic pain** results from noxious stimuli to the skin, joints, muscles, and tendons. These stimuli may include cutting, crushing, pinching, extreme temperature, and irritating chemicals. Somatic pain is generally easy to pinpoint. **Visceral pain** results from noxious stimuli to internal organs. These stimuli may include expansion and hypoxia. Visceral pain is usually vague and diffuse. Visceral pain may even be sensed on body surfaces at distant locations from the originating organ, called **referred pain** (**Figure 14-3**). The exact mechanism for

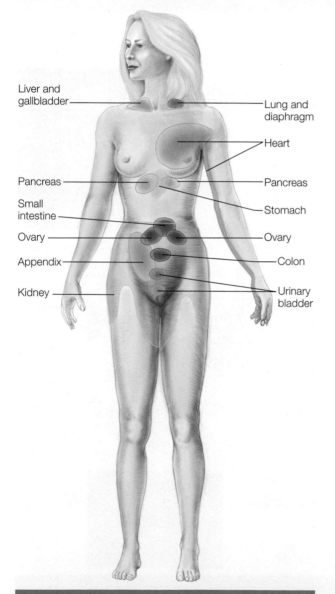

referred pain is unknown, but it is thought to be a result of the brain misinterpreting the visceral impulses as being somatic impulses because they both enter the spinal cord at the same location (see Chapter 11). **Phantom pain** describes pain that exists after the removal of a body part (e.g., amputation). The affected person may feel the discomfort of the removed part. The severing of neurons may result in spontaneous firing of spinal cord neurons because normal sensory input has been lost. This type of pain can be extremely distressing but usually resolves with time. **Intractable pain** describes chronically progressing pain that is unrelenting and severely debilitating. This type of pain does not usually respond well to typical pharmacologic pain treatments (e.g., analgesics and narcotics). Intractable pain is common with severe injuries, especially crushing injuries. **Neuropathic pain** describes pain that results from damage to peripheral nerves by disease (e.g., diabetes mellitus) or injury. This type of pain tends to be chronic and intractable.

Eyes

The human **eye** is a remarkable organ that allows us to perceive the environment in which we live. The human eyes are globe-shaped organs located in orbits in the anterior skull. The eye consists of three distinct layers (**Figure 14-4; Table 14-2**). The outermost layer of the eye is comprised of a durable, fibrous material called the **sclera** (white area) and a clear lens on the anterior side called the **cornea**. Tendons and muscles attach to the sclera to control eye movement. The cornea allows light to enter the eye. The middle layer of the eye consists of the **choroid**, which contains melanin to absorb stray light. The anterior portion of the choroid forms the **ciliary body**. The ciliary body contains smooth muscle fibers that control the shape of the lens to focus on incoming light. The **iris** is the colored portion of the eye, and the **pupil** is the dark opening in the center of the iris. The choroid layer and the pigmented section of the retina give the pupil its black appearance. The iris contains smooth muscle fibers that control the diameter of the pupil to regulate light entering the eye. The pupil opens and closes reflexively in response to light intensity. The innermost layer of the eye is the **retina**. The retina contains an outer, pigmented layer and an inner layer consisting of photoreceptors and nerve cells (**Figure 14-5**). The retina is weakly attached to the choroid, making it vulnerable to damage. The retina contains two types of photoreceptors—rods and cones. Each eye contains nearly 150 million **rods** that are sensitive to low light and function at night. How-

Figure 14-3

Referred pain. Visceral pain is often felt on the body surface at the points indicated by the colored areas.

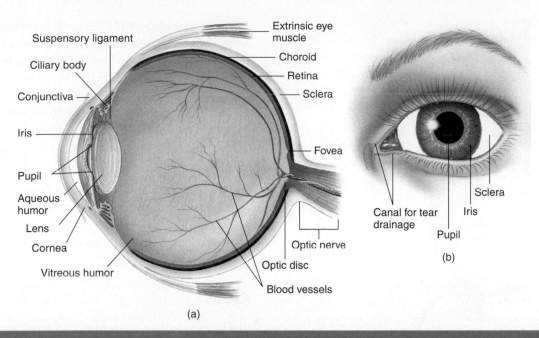

(a)

(b)

Figure 14-4

Anatomy of the eye.

Table 14-2 Structures and Functions of the Eye

Structure		Function
Wall		
Outer layer	Sclera	Provides insertion for extrinsic eye muscles
	Cornea	Allows light to enter; bends incoming light
Middle layer	Choroid	Absorbs stray light; provides nutrients to eye structures
	Ciliary body	Regulates lens, allowing it to focus images
	Iris	Regulates amount of light entering the eye
Inner layer	Retina	Responds to light, converting light to nerve impulses
Accessory structures and components	Lens	Focuses images on the retina
	Vitreous humor	Holds retina and lens in place
	Aqueous humor	Supplies nutrients to structures in contact with the anterior cavity of the eye
	Optic nerve	Transmits impulses from the retina to the brain

Source: Chiras, D. (2008). *Human biology* (6th ed.). Sudbury, MA: Jones & Bartlett Learning.

ever, each eye only contains about 6 million **cones** that can only operate in bright light and are responsible for visual acuity and color vision. The axons of the ganglion cells come together at the back of the eye to form the **optic nerve**. This area contains no photoreceptors and is insensitive to light. Visual images are cast upside down onto the retina, and impulses are transmitted to

the visual cortex in the brain. The retina processes some of the image, and then the brain processes the rest.

The **lens** is a transparent, flexible structure that lies behind the iris. Smooth muscles attached to the lens alter its shape to focus on objects. The lens separates the eye interior into two cavities—the anterior and posterior chambers. The **anterior chamber** is in front of the lens, while the **posterior chamber** is behind the lens. The anterior chamber contains watery liquid called **aqueous humor** that provides nutrients to the cornea and lens and carries away cellular waste products. A clear, gelatinous material called **vitreous humor** fills the posterior chamber. Pressures of these liquids give the eye its shape.

The inner surface of the eyelid and the exposed surface of the eye are covered by a fragile membrane called the **conjunctiva** and kept moist by the **lacrimal glands**. Blinking cleans the eye by sweeping the fluid across the eye. Tears drain on the inner side of the eye through two **lacrimal ducts**.

Ears

The human **ear** serves to detect and process sound as well as detect body position and maintain balance. The human ear has three separate divisions—outer, middle, and inner ear (**Figure 14-6; Table 14-3**). The **outer ear** consists of the auricle (or pinna), ear lobe,

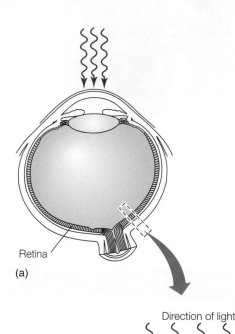

Retina

(a)

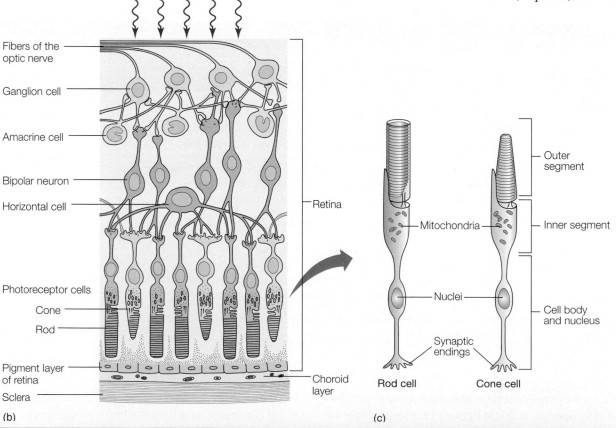

Direction of light

Fibers of the optic nerve

Ganglion cell

Amacrine cell

Bipolar neuron

Horizontal cell

Photoreceptor cells
Cone
Rod

Pigment layer of retina

Sclera

(b)

Retina

Choroid layer

Outer segment

Inner segment

Mitochondria

Nuclei

Cell body and nucleus

Synaptic endings

Rod cell   Cone cell

(c)

Figure 14-5

The retina. (a) Cross section through the wall of the eye, showing (b) arrangement of the cellular components of the retina. (c) The structure of the rods and cones.

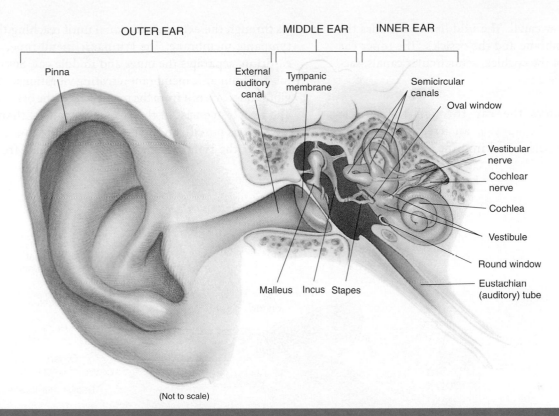

OUTER EAR   MIDDLE EAR   INNER EAR

Pinna

External auditory canal

Tympanic membrane

Semicircular canals

Oval window

Vestibular nerve

Cochlear nerve

Cochlea

Vestibule

Round window

Eustachian (auditory) tube

Malleus   Incus   Stapes

(Not to scale)

Figure 14-6

The structure of the ear.

Table 14-3 Structures and Functions of the Ear

Part	Structure	Function
Outer ear	Auricle	Funnels sound waves into external auditory canal
	Ear lobe	
	External auditory canal	Directs sound waves to the eardrum
Middle ear	Tympanic membrane or eardrum	Vibrates when struck by sound waves
	Ossicles	Transmit sound to the cochlea in the inner ear
Inner ear	Cochlea	Converts fluid waves to nerve impulses
	Semicircular canals	Detect head movement
	Saccule and utricle	Detect head movement and linear acceleration

Source: Chiras, D. (2008). *Human biology* (6th ed.). Sudbury, MA: Jones & Bartlett Learning.

and external ear canal. The **middle ear** includes the tympanic membrane and the ossicles. The **inner ear** is comprised of the cochlea, semicircular canals, saccule, and utricle.

Sound enters the ear through the auricle (**Figure 14-7**). The **auricle**, an irregularly shaped cartilage, channels sound into the ear. Sound trav-els through the **external ear canal** until reaching the tympanic membrane. The **tympanic membrane**, or eardrum, separates the outer and middle ear. Sound hits the tympanic membrane, creating vibrations. The vibrations transmit from the membrane to the ossicles. The **ossicles** consist of three bones—malleus (hammer), incus (anvil), and stapes (stirrup). The **malleus** lies near the tympanic membrane. Vibrations from

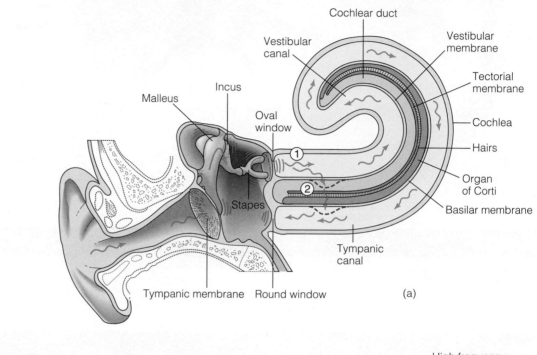

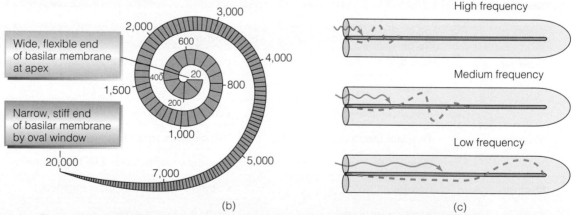

The numbers indicate the frequencies with which different regions of the basilar membrane maximally vibrate.

Figure 14-7

Transmission of sound through the ear. The cochlea is unwound here to simplify matters. (a) Vibrations are transmitted from the stirrup (stapes) to the oval window. Fluid pressure waves are established in the vestibular canal and pass to the tympanic canal, causing the basilar membrane to vibrate. (b) A representation of the basilar membrane, showing the points along its length where the various wavelengths of sound are perceived. Notice that the basilar membrane is narrowest at the base of the cochlea at the oval window end and widest at the apex. (c) High-frequency sounds set the basilar membrane near the base of the cochlea into motion. Hair cells send impulses to the brain, which interprets the signals as a high-pitch sound. Low-frequency sounds stimulate the basilar membrane where it is widest and most flexible.

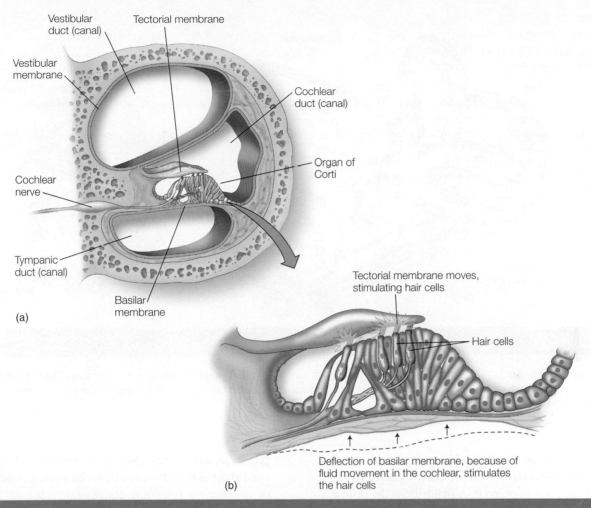

Vestibular duct (canal)

Tectorial membrane

Vestibular membrane

Cochlear duct (canal)

Cochlear nerve

Organ of Corti

Tympanic duct (canal)

Basilar membrane

(a)

Tectorial membrane moves, stimulating hair cells

Hair cells

Deflection of basilar membrane, because of fluid movement in the cochlear, stimulates the hair cells

(b)

Figure 14-8

Cross section of the cochlea. (a) Notice the three fluid-filled canals and the central position of the organ of Corti. (b) Hair cells of the organ of Corti are embedded in the overlying tectorial membrane. When the basilar membrane vibrates, the hair cells are stimulated.

the membranes cause the malleus to rock back and forth. This rocking causes the incus to vibrate, which, in turn, causes the stapes to move in and out against the oval window. The oval window is the opening to the inner ear covered with a membrane. The vibrations created by the tympanic membrane amplify as they are transmitted through the structures to the inner ear. Movement of the oval window causes fluid within the cochlea to vibrate, creating waves. The cochlea is a spiral-shaped structure that houses the organ of Corti (Figure 14-8). The organ of Corti contains hearing receptors, the hair cells. Vibrations at the organ of Corti stimulate hair movement. Dendrites wrap the bases of these hair cells. Hair movement causes the dendrites to form nerve impulses that travel to the brain via the vestibulocochlear nerve, cranial nerve VIII (see Chapter 11).

The inner ear also holds the vestibular apparatus (Figure 14-9). The vestibular apparatus includes two parts—the semicircular canals and vestibule. The semicircular canals are three ringlike, fluid-filled structures that house receptors for body position and movement. The fluid in the semicircular canals works much like a carpenter's level. Movement of the head causes the fluid in the semicircular canal to move. Fluid movement stimulates dendrites to send impulses to the brain to report this movement. The vestibule is a bony chamber positioned between the cochlea and semicircular canals. The vestibule houses receptors that respond to body position and movement. The vestibule contains the utricle and saccule that have receptor organs. Nerve impulses generated in the vestibular apparatus travel to a cluster of nerve cell bodies in the brain stem. At the brain stem, these impulses combine

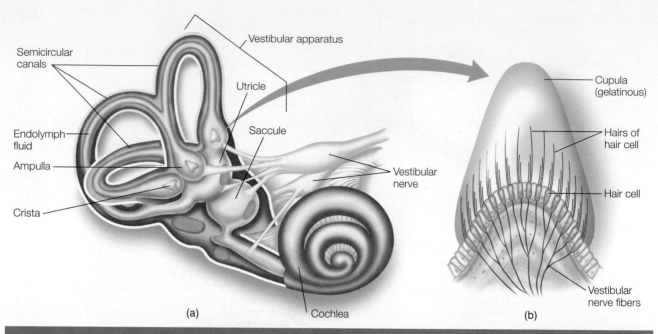

(a)

(b)

Figure 14-9

Vestibular apparatus. (a) This illustration shows the location of the cristae in the ampullae of the semicircular canals. The semicircular canals are filled with endolymph. (b) When the head spins, the endolymph is set into motion, deflecting the gelatinous cupula of the crista, thus stimulating the receptor cells.

with input from the eyes, skin, joints, and muscles. This center directs the information to many areas of the brain (see Chapter 11). A majority of the information travels a pathway to the cerebral cortex, increasing awareness of position and movement. Another pathway leads to the muscles of the limbs and torso to maintain balance and correct body position if necessary.

The middle ear also opens into the pharynx via the **eustachian tube**. The eustachian tube acts as a pressure valve. Normally, the eustachian tube remains closed, but the tube may become open with activities such as yawning and swallowing. Opening the eustachian tube allows air to flow in and out of the middle ear, equalizing the internal and external pressure on the tympanic membrane. The function of the eustachian tube is apparent when ears pop while taking off in an airplane. This popping sensation is a result of pressure being released from the eustachian tubes.

Congenital Sensory Disorders

Congenital sensory disorders vary widely in severity. Many conditions occur because of an error during embryonic development. These errors may occur randomly, due to environmental influences, or because of

genetic abnormalities. These errors may result in minor conditions with only aesthetic problems (e.g., microtia) or life-altering states (e.g., congenital cataracts). Treatment is often unnecessary, but when needed, treatment options are usually limited.

Eyes

Congenital eye conditions are rare. These conditions vary widely in severity, but vision impairment is present to some degree in most cases. These conditions seldom happen in isolation and are often associated with other disorders.

Congenital Cataracts

Congenital cataracts refer to a clouding of the lens that is present at birth. This clouding of the usually clear lens results in hazy vision. In most cases, no specific cause can be identified. However, congenital cataracts have been associated with several genetic and chromosomal conditions (e.g., Down syndrome, Patau syndrome, Lowe syndrome, and galactosemia) as well as intrauterine infection exposure (e.g., congenital rubella).

In addition to clouding of the lens, clinical manifestations usually include a failure of the affected infant

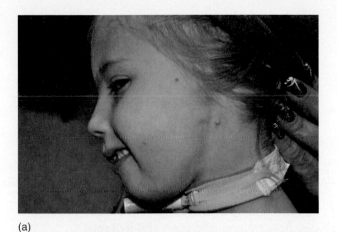

(a)

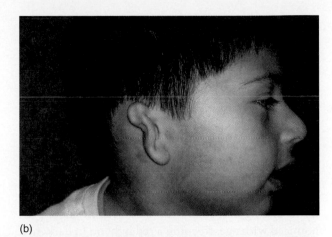

(b)

Figure 14-10

(a) Anotia. (b) Microtia.

to demonstrate visual awareness and presence of nystagmus (rapid, involuntary back-and-forth eye movement). Diagnostic procedures for congenital cataracts consist of a history and physical examination (including a thorough ophthalmology exam). Additional tests may be necessary to determine other associated conditions. In some cases, congenital cataracts are mild and do not affect vision, and these cases require no treatment. Moderate to severe cataracts that affect vision will require cataract removal surgery, followed by placement of an artificial intraocular lens. Patching to force the child to use the weaker eye may be required to prevent amblyopia (lazy eye). Treatment for any underlying disorder may also be needed.

Ears

Congenital conditions affecting the ears usually result from an absence or malformation of the external ear. These conditions may or may not affect hearing. Anotia refers to the absence of the auricle, while microtia refers to an underdeveloped, small auricle (Figure 14-10). Persons with anotia and microtia may also lack an external ear canal (atresia). These conditions are more common in males than in females and are often associated with other congenital conditions affecting the head (e.g., hemifacial microsomia, Goldenhar syndrome, and Treacher-Collins syndrome). These congenital ear conditions may be unilateral or bilateral. In addition to these structural abnormalities, congenital hearing loss can occur because of damage associated with maternal rubella and syphilis infection during pregnancy.

Sensory Conditions Associated With Aging

The way in which the body senses and responds to sensory input changes with age. In general, the senses become less acute and less able to distinguish details. These sensory changes vary in severity but can have a tremendous impact on lifestyle and quality of life. Aging increases the threshold needed to perceive sensory input, so the amount of sensory input needed to be aware of the sensation becomes greater. Physical changes in the body part related to the sensation account for most of the other sensation changes. Hearing and vision changes can be the most dramatic, but all senses can be affected by aging. Equipment such as glasses and hearing aids or changes in lifestyle can compensate for many of the sensory aging changes.

Eyes

Age-related eye changes may begin as early as 30 years of age. Some changes include less tear production as well as structural deteriorations. All of the eye structures change to some degree with aging. The cornea becomes less sensitive, so injuries may go unnoticed. By age 60, pupils decrease to about one third of the size they were at age 20. The pupil may also react more slowly in response to darkness or bright light than it did in one's youth. The lens becomes yellowed, less flexible, and slightly cloudy. The fat pads supporting the eye decrease and the eye sinks back into the skull. The eye muscles weaken, decreasing the ability to rotate the eye fully and limiting the visual field. Visual acuity also may gradually decline. Glasses or contact lenses may help correct these age-related vision changes. Nearly all persons 55 years of age or older need glasses at least part of the time. However, the severity of changes varies. Only 15–20% of elderly persons have vision deficits severe enough to impair driving ability, and only 5% become unable to read. The most common problem is difficulty focusing the eyes, a condition called **pres-byopia**. Additionally, intolerance to a glare as well as difficulty adapting to darkness and brightness may be experienced, making driving at night difficult. Inability to distinguish colors can also become more pronounced with age. Keeping a red light on in darkened rooms (such as the hallway or bathroom) may make it easier to see than using a regular night light because it produces less glare than a white light bulb.

Ears

All the ear structures thicken and change with aging, affecting balance and hearing. Hearing may decline slightly, especially with high-frequency sounds. This hearing loss accelerates in people who were exposed to excessive noise or smoking when they were younger. This age-related hearing loss is called **presbycusis**. Some hearing loss is almost inevitable. An estimated 30% of all people over 65 have significant hearing impairment. Hearing acuity (sharpness) may decline slightly beginning at about 50 years of age, possibly caused by changes in the auditory nerve. In addition, the brain may have a slight decreased ability to process or translate sounds into meaningful information. Impacted cerumen is another cause of impaired hearing and is more common with increasing age. Sensorineural hearing loss involves damage to the inner ear, auditory nerve, or the brain. This type of hearing loss may or may not respond to treatment, but hearing aids can improve function. Conductive hearing loss occurs when sound has problems transmitting through the outer and middle ear to the inner ear. Surgery or a hearing aid may be helpful for this type of hearing loss, depending on the specific cause. Persistent, abnormal ear noise (tinnitus) is another common hearing problem, especially for older adults. Tinnitus may be described as a ringing, buzzing, roaring, or humming sound. Tinnitus is usually a result of mild hearing loss.

Infectious and Inflammatory Sensory Disorders

Infectious sensory disorders can result from a wide range of causative agents. These agents often trigger the inflammatory response. These conditions may be acute or chronic and vary widely in severity. In most cases, infectious sensory disorders usually resolve with treatment.

Eyes

Eye infections can result from a variety of organisms, usually bacteria and viruses. Many of these infections are self-limited, and most respond well to treatment. However, severe or untreated infections can lead to visual impairment. These conditions can also be caused by other events that can trigger the inflammatory process (e.g., trauma, allergens, and irritants).

Conjunctivitis

Conjunctivitis refers to an infection or inflammation of the conjunctiva, the lining of the eyelids and sclera (**Figure 14-11**). Conjunctivitis may be caused by viruses (most common), bacteria (e.g., *Staphylococcus*, *Chlamydia*, and gonorrhea), allergens (e.g., pollen and dust), chemical irritants, and trauma. Each cause produces slightly different manifestations. Regardless of cause, conjunctivitis can generate blurry vision and photophobia. Viral infections normally produce a watery or mucuslike exudate. Bacterial infections usually produce a yellow-green exudate. Allergens and irritants typically produce redness, itching, and excessive tearing. Risk factors of conjunctivitis include wearing contact lenses as well as using contaminated makeup or ophthalmic medications. Bacterial and viral conjunctivitis is highly contagious through direct contact, and steps are necessary to prevent transmission (e.g., hand washing, limiting contact, proper eye hygiene, and discarding contaminated ophthalmic products).

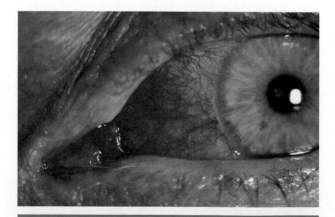

Figure 14-11

Conjunctivitis.

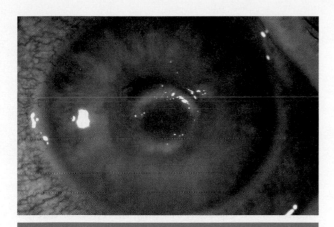

Figure 14-12

Keratitis.

Many cases of conjunctivitis will resolve without treatment. Treatment may vary depending on the underlying cause. These strategies may include ophthalmic or oral antibiotics, antihistamines, and corticosteroid agents. Because of the risk of maternal transmission of sexually transmitted infections during delivery and those infections potentially causing blindness, infants are generally treated with ophthalmic antibiotics shortly after birth. Additionally, warm moist compresses can soothe the discomfort associated with conjunctivitis.

Keratitis

Keratitis refers to an inflammation of the cornea that can be triggered by an infection or trauma (**Figure 14-12**). The HSV type 1 can be self-transmitted from the mouth and cause an ulcerated form of keratitis. Clinical manifestations reflect the inflammatory process and include severe pain, photophobia, and visual disturbances. Treatment varies depending on the underlying etiology, but strategies often include ophthalmic or oral antibiotics and corticosteroid agents.

Ears

Ear infections can result from a variety of pathogens, usually bacterial or viral. These conditions are classified based on the area of the ear infected and typically resolve with treatment.

Otitis Media

Otitis media describes an infection or inflammation of the middle ear. Otitis media is a common condition in young children. The eustachian tubes of young children are narrower, straighter, and shorter than those of adults and older children. This developmental variation in anatomy decreases the ability of fluid to drain from the middle ear adequately. In addition to these structural differences, a young child's immune system is less equipped to manage infections (see Chapter 2) than that of an adult or older child. An additional cause of fluid accumulation in the middle ear is adenoid enlargement, usually due to inflammation. Because of their close proximity to the eustachian tubes, enlargement of the adenoids can compress the tubes. Typically, otitis media begins as a viral upper respiratory infection, so otitis media is more common in the winter months than it is the rest of the year. The viral infection migrates to the middle ear, causing fluid accumulation behind the tympanic membrane. The collection of fluid provides a prime medium for secondary bacterial growth. Additional risk factors include child care in group settings, feeding infants in the supine position, environmental smoke exposure, and a history of allergic rhinitis. *Streptococcus pneumoniae* and *Haemophilus influenzae* are frequent bacterial causes of otitis media. Otitis media can lead to rupture of the tympanic membrane, scar tissue formation, and conductive hearing loss. Additionally, the infection can spread to nearby structures and cause mastoiditis, cholesteatoma (a benign epithelial cell tumor on the tympanic membrane), meningitis, and osteomylitis.

Clinical manifestations can vary depending on age and may be asymptomatic. When present, these manifestations frequently include:

- Ear pain (related to pressure in the middle ear)
- Crying or irritability
- Rubbing or pulling at the ear
- Mild hearing deficits
- Sleep disturbances
- Red, bulging tympanic membrane
- Indications of infection (e.g., fever, malaise, and chills)
- Purulent or clear exudate from the external ear canal (if the tympanic membrane ruptures)
- Nausea or vomiting
- Headache

Diagnostic procedures for otitis media consist of a history and a physical examination (including an otologic examination). The otologic examination usually includes visualization of the tympanic membrane, tympanometry (which measures tympanic membrane

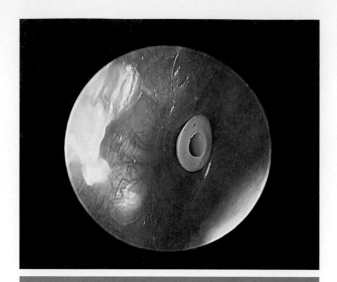

Figure 14-13

Tympanostomy tubes.

movement), and acoustic reflectometry (reflection of sound). Treatment focuses on eradicating any infection present, decreasing the amount of fluid in the middle ear, and managing pain. Strategies may include oral or otologic antibiotics and analgesics. Additionally, oral decongestant and antihistamine agents may be administered. Antipyretics may be necessary to control fever. Drainage tubes (tympanostomy tubes) can be inserted to facilitate fluid drainage for children with recurrent otitis media (**Figure 14-13**). Removal of the adenoids may also be performed with the tympanostomy tubes.

Otitis Externa

Otitis externa, or swimmer's ear, refers to an infection or inflammation of the external ear canal or auricle. Otitis externa is usually bacterial in origin (often *Pseudomonas aeruginosa*) but may also be fungal. Otitis externa generally arises from moisture in the ear that creates an environment for bacterial or fungal growth or introduction of the organisms from external sources. Risk factors include swimming in contaminated water, scratching the outside or inside of the ear, and insertion of foreign objects (e.g., cotton swabs, earphones, and ear plugs) into the ears. Most cases of otitis externa are mild and respond well to treatment, but occasionally otitis externa can lead to hearing loss, cellulitis, necrosis, osteomylitis, and meningitis. Clinical manifestations of otitis externa include ear pain that worsens with auricle movement, purulent exudate,

itching, a sensation of fullness in the ear, and hearing deficits. Diagnostic procedures typically consist of a history, physical examination (including an otologic examination), and exudate analysis (e.g., culture and sensitivity). Because of easy access of the external ear canal, treatment strategies are typically applied locally. These strategies may include otologic antibiotic, antifungal, corticosteroid, and analgesic agents. Additionally, the external ear canal may be cleaned (e.g., via lavage of warm saline). Prevention strategies include drying the ears after swimming or bathing with an alcohol-based product, avoiding insertion of foreign objects into the ear, and treating pools properly.

Traumatic Sensory Disorders

Traumatic sensory disorders can result from a wide range of injuries. These conditions can vary widely in severity. Often prognosis depends on prompt treatment.

Eyes

Eye trauma can result from numerous types of injuries. These injuries may result from direct physical trauma or chemical burns. Any of the eye structures can be involved, including the eyelid, cornea, or the entire eye globe. These conditions may vary in severity from mild (e.g., black eye) to sight threatening (e.g., corneal abrasions and closed-angle glaucoma). The eye is vulnerable to injury, and vision deficits often result. Clinical manifestations may vary depending on the nature of the injury. These manifestations may include eye pain, edema, blurry vision, diplopia (double vision), dry eyes, photophobia, floaters, pupil dilatation, and pupils that are unresponsive to light. Early diagnosis and treatment can prevent or limit the severity of visual deficits. Diagnostic procedures consist of a history and physical examination (including an ophthalmic examination often by an ophthalmologist). Treatment strategies may include:

- Flushing irritant out of the eye with sterile saline
- Avoiding rubbing the eye (can worsen the damage)
- Leaving an embedded object in the eye
- Covering the eye with a sterile dressing or cloth
- Applying eye patches to protect the eye during the healing process
- Repairing any damage surgically

CLINICAL CASE

One night B.S., a 24-year-old female, was cleaning her ears with a cotton swab as she does every night as a part of her hygiene routine. She was in a hurry to go out on a date. As she was cleaning her ears with the cotton swab, her hand slipped, and the swab went deep into her right ear. Her ear immediately began to bleed. She continued to get dressed for her date, assuming the bleeding would stop, but it did not. She decided to cancel the date and have her ear checked by a healthcare provider at the after-hours clinic.

At the clinic, the healthcare provider told B.S. that she likely perforated her tympanic membrane, and it would likely heal in a couple of weeks. The bleeding continued for the next 24 hours, so B.S. called back to the clinic. The healthcare provider at the clinic referred her to an ear, nose, and throat specialist the next day. During her visit with the ear, nose, and throat specialist, B.S. explained the incident with the cotton swab, and the specialist reminded her as she had heard many times before, "Never put anything smaller than your elbow in your ear." Upon examination, the ear, nose, and throat specialist determined that B.S. had a severe perforation of her tympanic membrane that required surgical repair with skin grafting to prevent permanent severe hearing loss.

Postsurgical repair, B.S. continues to have significant hearing loss in her right ear. The risk for graft rejection remains. Steps to protect her hearing are vital including limiting exposure to excessive noise and avoiding ototoxic medications.

Ears

Ear trauma can result from a variety of injuries to any of the internal or external ear structures. These injuries may include direct physical trauma (e.g., foreign objects and insects) and excessively loud noises (e.g., explosions and gunshots). These events can result in permanent hearing deficits. Clinical manifestations of ear trauma may include bloody or clear exudate, tinnitus, dizziness, ear pain, hearing deficits, nausea, vomiting, edema, and a sensation that an object is in the ear. Treatment strategies vary depending on the nature of the injury. These strategies may include:

- Removing the object if it is visible and easily removed
- Performing surgery to remove objects or repair the damage
- Limiting exposure to loud sounds as structures heal

Chronic Sensory Disorders

Numerous chronic conditions can affect the sensory organs. These conditions are often mild and easily managed. In some cases, these conditions can cause significant sensory deficits.

Eyes

Many chronic conditions affecting the eyes are progressive and can result in visual deficits. Most of these conditions can be prevented. With early treatment, most cases can be managed.

Glaucoma

Glaucoma refers to a group of eye conditions that lead to damage to the optic nerve. This damage is often caused by increased intraocular pressure, but it can also be caused by decreased blood flow to the optic nerve (**Figure 14-14**). Pressures inside the eye can climb because of blocked outflow of aqueous humor or increased production of aqueous humor. These increased pressures cause ischemia and degeneration of the optic nerve. Glaucoma is the second leading cause of blindness (diabetic retinopathy is number one). There are four types of glaucoma, including:

- Open-angle (chronic) glaucoma. This is the most common type. For reasons that are unclear, intraocular pressure increases gradually over an extended period. This type of glaucoma tends to run in families, and rates are six to eight times higher among African American people than among those of other races. Clinical manifestations typically include painless, insidious, bilateral changes in vision (e.g., tunnel vision, blurred vision, halos around lights, and decreased color discrimination). Because the vision changes are gradual and there are typically no other manifestations, open-angle glaucoma can often be overlooked as presbyopia.

- Closed-angle (acute) glaucoma. This type is a medical emergency, and it is a result of a sudden blockage of aqueous humor outflow. This blockage can be caused by trauma, sudden pupil dilatation (e.g., exposure to bright light after prolonged exposure to darkness), prolonged pupil dilatation (e.g., medications for eye examinations), and emotional stress. Closed-angle glaucoma is typically unilateral, but it may affect both eyes. Clinical manifestations are normally sudden in onset and worsen quickly. These manifestations may include severe

(a) Normal flow of aqueous humor

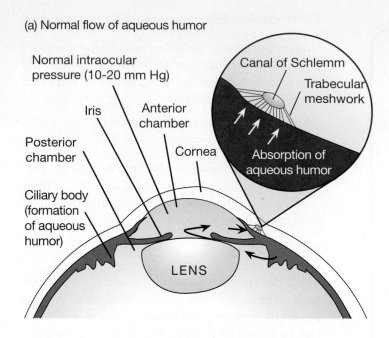

(b) Chronic (open-angle) glaucoma

Degeneration and obstruction of trabecular meshwork and canal of Schlemm decreases absorption of aqueous humor

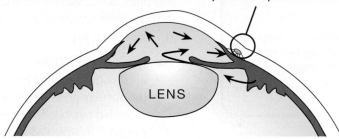

(c) Acute (narrow-or closed-angle) glaucoma

Iris in anterior position   Narrow iridoocorneal angle blocks drainage into canal of Schlemm

High intraocular pressure

LENS

Figure 14-14

Types of glaucoma.

eye pain, headache, nausea, vomiting, a nonreactive pupil, redness, haziness of the cornea, and vision changes (e.g., halos around lights).

- **Congenital glaucoma.** This type of glaucoma is present at birth. This type is a result of abnormal development of outflow channels (trabecular meshwork) of the eye. Congenital glaucoma follows an X-linked, recessive hereditary pattern. This type may go unnoticed for a few months. Clinical manifestations may include excessive lacrimation, photophobia, corneal edema, gray-white appearance to the cornea, enlarged eye globe, and vision deficits.

- **Secondary glaucoma.** This type of glaucoma is a result of certain medications (e.g., corticosteroids), eye diseases (e.g., uveitis and nearsightedness), and systemic diseases (e.g., arteriosclerosis and diabetes mellitus).

Diagnostic procedures for glaucoma consist of a history and physical examination (including an ophthalmic examination). The ophthalmic examination typically involves a gonioscopy (use of a special lens to see the outflow channels of the angle), tonometry (which measures intraocular pressure), optic nerve imaging, pupillary reflex response, retinal examination, slit lamp examination (using a microscope and light to examine the anterior eye structures), visual acuity testing, and visual field measurement. Treatment focuses on decreasing intraocular pressure. Early detection and treatment are crucial to preserve vision. Those persons at risk for glaucoma should be routinely screened (usually once a year). Treatment strategies vary depending on the type. Strategies for open-angle glaucoma may include:

- Ophthalmic medications (usually a combination of two or three types), including the following:

  - Beta blockers (to reduce aqueous humor production)
  - Alpha agonists (to reduce production of and increase drainage of aqueous humor)
  - Carbonic anhydrase inhibitors (to reduce aqueous humor production)
  - Prostaglandin-like compounds (to increase aqueous humor outflow)
  - Miotic or cholinergic agents (to increase aqueous humor outflow)
  - Epinephrine compounds (to increase aqueous humor outflow)
  - Alpha-2 adrenergic agonists (to protect the optic nerve)

- Oral medications (not generally effective when used alone), including carbonic anhydrase inhibitors
- N-methyl d-aspartate receptor antagonist (may protect the optic nerve)
- Laser surgery to open aqueous humor outflow
- Filtering surgery (to remove a small section of the trabecular meshwork)
- Drainage implants

The main strategy for treating closed-angle glaucoma is iridotomy (a surgical laser procedure to open a new channel in the iris).

The main strategy for treating congenital glaucoma is surgery to open the aqueous humor outflow channels (e.g., laser, filtering, and drainage implants).

Strategies to treat secondary glaucoma include:

- Chronic disease management
- Treating or eliminating underlying causes
- Previously discussed glaucoma pharmacologic and surgical treatments

Cataracts

A **cataract** is opacity or clouding of the lens (**Figure 14-15**). Cataracts can occur as a congenital condition (previously discussed) or develop later in life. Risk factors for adult-onset cataracts include family history, advancing age, smoking, ultraviolet (UV) light exposure (natural or artificial), metabolic conditions (e.g., diabetes mellitus), certain medications (e.g., corticosteroids), and eye injury (e.g., trauma and infection). Cataracts may affect one or both eyes and do not

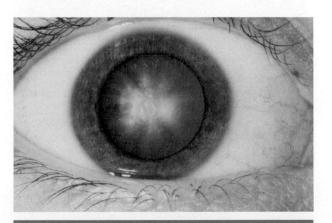

Figure 14-15

Cataracts.

necessarily affect eyes symmetrically. In addition to the cloudy appearance of the lens, clinical manifestations may include:

- Cloudy, fuzzy, foggy, or filmy vision (**Figure 14-16**)
- Color intensity loss
- Diplopia
- Impaired night vision gradually progressing to impaired day vision
- Halos around lights
- Photosensitivity
- Frequent changes in eyeglass or contact prescription

Diagnostic procedures for cataracts consist of a history and physical examination (including an ophthalmic examination). The ophthalmic examination typically involves visual acuity testing, retinal exami-

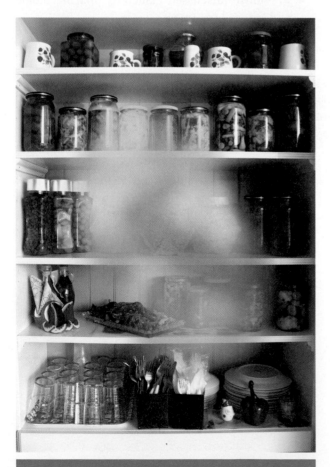

Figure 14-16

Visual changes associated with cataracts.

nation, and slit lamp examination. Surgery is the only effective treatment for cataracts. Surgical procedures may include removal of the cataract (e.g., phacoemulsification) or a lens transplant. Surgery is typically performed one eye at a time as an outpatient procedure with a local anesthetic. Recovery time is usually short, and the prognosis is good. Additional strategies may include managing or eliminating contributing factors.

Macular Degeneration

Macular degeneration refers to a deterioration of the macular area of the retina. Macular degeneration is caused by impaired blood supply to the macula that results in the cellular waste accumulation and ischemia. The most significant risk factor for this condition is advancing age. Macular degeneration has a family tendency and is most prevalent in females and Caucasians. Additional risk factors include smoking, high-fat diet, and obesity. There are two types of macular generation—dry and wet. Dry macular degeneration occurs when the blood vessels under the macula become thin and brittle. Small yellow deposits (drusen) form under the macula. These deposits increase in size and number, blurring vision and creating a dim spot in the central vision. Almost all people with macular degeneration start with the dry form. Wet macular degeneration occurs in only about 10% of people with macular degeneration. Brittle vessels break down, and new, abnormal, fragile blood vessels grow under the macula (choroidal neovascularization). These vessels leak blood and fluid, leading to macula damage. Although not as common, this form causes most of the vision loss associated with the condition. Dry macular degeneration progresses gradually (over years) in contrast to the wet form, which results in a sudden, rapid vision loss (over weeks or months).

Macular degeneration is often asymptomatic initially. The most common manifestations of the dry form are blurry vision with a loss of central vision. The most frequent manifestations of the wet form are distortion of straight lines, dark spots in central vision, and sudden loss of central vision.

Diagnostic procedures for macular degeneration consist of a history and physical examination (including an ophthalmic examination). The ophthalmic examination usually involves visual acuity using the Amsler grid, retinal examination, fluorescein angiogram (uses dye and a camera to evaluate retinal blood flow), and optical coherence tomography (noninvasive retinal imaging). No treatment exists for dry macular degeneration. However, a combination of vitamins, antioxidants, and zinc may slow the disease's progression. This combination of vitamins is often called the Age-Related Eye Disease study formula. Smokers should not use this treatment. The recommended supplements contain:

- 500 milligrams of vitamin C
- 400 international units of beta-carotene
- 80 milligrams of zinc
- 2 milligrams of copper

Although there is no cure for wet macular degeneration, treatment strategies may include:

- Laser surgery, specifically laser photocoagulation (lasers destroy the abnormal blood vessels)
- Photodynamic therapy (a light activates an injected drug to destroy leaking blood vessels)
- Antiangiogenesis or anti-vascular endothelial growth factor therapy (medications injected into the eye that slow the formation of new blood vessels in the eye)

Low-vision aids (e.g., magnifying glasses and large print) and occupational therapy can improve independence and quality of life.

Ears

Many chronic conditions affecting the ears are progressive and can result in hearing deficits. Many of these conditions are preventable. With early treatment, most cases can be managed.

Otosclerosis

Otosclerosis refers to an abnormal bone growth in the middle ear, usually involving an imbalance in bone formation and resorption. The cause of otosclerosis is unknown, but there appears to be a hereditary component. In this condition, an abnormal sponge-like bone grows in the middle ear, preventing the ear structures from vibrating in response to sound waves. As the abnormal bone grows, hearing loss progressively worsens. Nerve loss can occur in conjunction with the conductive hearing loss. According to the National Institutes of Health (2008), otosclerosis affects about 10% of Americas, usually beginning in early to mid-adulthood. Otosclerosis is most common in women and Caucasians. Pregnancy may also trigger otoscle-

rosis. Typically, otosclerosis affects both ears. Tinnitus may also be present. Diagnostic procedures consist of a history, physical examination (including a hearing test), and temporal-bone computed tomography (CT). Treatment for otosclerosis focuses on minimizing hearing loss or improving hearing. These strategies may include:

- Medications such as oral fluoride, calcium, or vitamin D may help to control the hearing loss, but the efficacy remains in question
- Hearing aids to treat the hearing loss
- Surgery to remove the stapes (stapedectomy) and replace it with a prosthesis to cure the condition
- Laser surgery to create an opening in the stapes (stapedotomy) with or without the placement of the prosthetic device

Meniere's Disease

Meniere's disease is a disorder of the inner ear that results from endolymph swelling. This swelling stretches the membranes and interferes with the hair receptors in the cochlea and vestibule. The exact cause is unknown, but Meniere's disease may be associated with head injuries, otitis media, and syphilis. Additional risk factors include allergic rhinitis, alcohol consumption, stress, fatigue, certain medications (e.g., aspirin), and respiratory infections. Clinical manifestations of Meniere's disease typically occur in waves of acute episodes that last several months followed by brief periods of relief. These attacks may be triggered by changes in barometric pressure or any of the risk factors. These manifestations include intermittent episodes of vertigo, tinnitus, unilateral hearing loss, and a sensation of fullness. Repeated episodes can lead to permanent hearing loss. Diagnostic procedures for Meniere's disease consist of a history, physical examination (including a neurologic assessment), hearing test, balance test, electrocholeography (which measures fluid accumulation in the ear), electronystagmography (balance sensors are placed in the inner ear to assess balance in relation to eye movement), caloric stimulation (instillation of warm or cold solution into the inner ear to test eye reflexes), head CT, and head magnetic resonance imaging (MRI). There is no cure for Meniere's disease. Treatment focuses on relieving inner ear pressure and relieving symptoms. Strategies may include:

- Antihistamine agents
- Benzodiazepines
- Anticholinergic agents

- Diuretics
- Antiemetic agents
- Limitation of dietary sodium intake (to promote fluid retention)
- Avoiding triggers (e.g., alcohol and stress)
- Middle ear injections of gentamicin (an ototoxic antibiotic that can reduce balance structures) or corticosteroids (can reduce swelling)
- Partial or complete surgical removal of the endolymph or inner ear
- Vestibular nerve resection
- Hearing aids
- Physical therapy to improve balance

Sensory Cancers

Any of the sensory organs can develop cancer, but it is rare. Severity varies depending on cancer type, and treatment often follows the typical cancer management regimens (e.g., chemotherapy, radiation, and surgery) (see Chapter 3). Ear cancer is extremely rare and typically involves skin cancer (see Chapter 13) of the auricle. For this reason, ear cancer will not be included in this discussion.

Eyes

Cancer of the eye is uncommon, affecting genders and ethnic groups relatively evenly. Eye cancer can affect any part of the eye from the eyelid to the intraocular structures. The most common intraocular cancers in adults are melanoma and lymphoma. The most frequent eye cancer in children is retinoblastoma. Cancer can also metastasize to the eye from other parts of the body. According to the National Cancer Institute (2008), the overall 5-year survival rate for all eye cancers is nearly 84%. Clinical manifestations of eye cancer typically include some sort of visual disturbance (e.g., losing part of the visual field and seeing flashing lights). Most cases are found during a routine ophthalmic examination (e.g., finding dark spots on the iris). Additional diagnostic procedures may include a history, ultrasound, fluorescein angiography (imaging of blood vessels in the eye using contrast dye), biopsy, and other tests to detect and evaluate metastasis (e.g., CT and MRI). Treatment varies depending on the cancer type, location, and size. Surgery is the foundation of most eye cancer treatment. Surgery may include removal of all (enucleation) or part of the eye (e.g., iridectomy and choroidectomy). Additionally, radiation may be used (e.g., teletherapy and brachytherapy). A prosthetic eye may be used if the entire eye is removed.

Miscellaneous Sensory Organ Conditions

Several sensory organ conditions that do not fall under the previously discussed categories warrant discussion.

Eyes

A few eye conditions that do not fit previously discussed categories can occur. These conditions may be manifestations of other problems or happen alone. Some of these conditions are minor, causing minimal deficits. Other conditions can cause severe visual deficits.

Strabismus

Strabismus, or cross-eyes, is a gaze deviation of one eye (**Figure 14-17**). With strabismus, the eyes do not coordinate to focus on the same object together, resulting in diplopia. This condition most often appears at birth or shortly after. In children, the brain will begin to ignore the input from one of the eyes. If the brain continues to ignore one eye, the eye will never function properly, and permanent visual deficits may result (e.g., amblyopia). A weak or hypertonic eye muscle, a short muscle, or a neurologic deficit can cause strabismus. These defects are often associated with chromosomal defects (e.g., Down syndrome), intrauterine infection exposure (e.g., congenital rubella), eye cancers (e.g., retinoblastoma), and traumatic brain injuries. Diagnostic procedures for strabismus consist of a history and physical examination (including an ophthalmic examination and a neurologic examination). Treatment focuses on strengthening the weak eye and realigning the eyes. Treatment often involves resting the normally aligned eye to strengthen the misaligned eye. Strategies usually include glasses (e.g., prism glasses), eye muscle exercises, eye patching, and surgery.

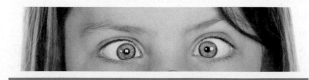

Figure 14-17

Strabismus.

Amblyopia

Amblyopia, or lazy eye, is the loss of one eye's ability to see details. Amblyopia is the most common cause of vision problems in children. Amblyopia occurs when the brain and eyes do not work together properly; the brain favors one eye. The preferred eye has normal vision, but because the brain ignores the other eye, vision does not develop normally. The normal eye attempts to compensate for the affected eye, creating a vicious cycle where the normal eye becomes stronger and the affected eye becomes weaker. The brain stops growing between 5 and 10 years of age, at which time the condition becomes permanent. Strabismus is the most frequent cause of amblyopia. Other causes include a family history, bilateral astigmatism, congenital cataracts, farsightedness, and nearsightedness. Diagnostic procedures for strabismus consist of a history and physical examination (including an ophthalmic examination). Much like with strabismus, treatment focuses on strengthening the weak eye and realigning the eyes. Treatment often involves resting the normal eye to strengthen the weaker eye. Strategies usually include wearing glasses (e.g., prism glasses), eye muscle exercises, eye patching, ophthalmic medication (atropine may be used to dilate the pupil of the normal eye to "chemically patch" it), and surgery.

Retinal Detachment

Retinal detachment is an acute condition that occurs when the retina separates from its supporting structures. This separation can happen spontaneously or because of severe nearsightedness (myoplia), trauma, diabetes mellitus, inflammation, degenerative aging changes, and scar tissue. Retinal detachment occurs when vitreous humor leaks through a retinal tear and accumulates underneath the retina. Leakage can also occur through tiny holes where the retina has thinned due to aging or other retinal disorders. Less commonly, fluid can leak directly underneath the retina, without a tear or break. As vitreous humor collects underneath it, the retina peels away from the underlying choroid. These detached areas may expand over time, like wallpaper that, once torn, slowly peels off a wall. The retina becomes ischemic and stops functioning, causing vision loss.

Retinal detachment is typically painless. Clinical manifestations of retinal detachment often include flashes of light in the peripheral visual field, blurred vision, floaters, and darkening vision (like a curtain drawing across a visual field). Diagnostic procedures consist of a history and physical examination (including an ophthalmic examination). The ophthalmic examination may involve an electroretinogram (a record of the electrical currents in the retina produced by visual stimuli), fluorescein angiography, intraocular pressure measurements, ophthalmoscopy, a refraction test, retinal photography, color discrimination, visual acuity testing, slit lamp examination, and eye ultrasound. Retinal detachment is a medical emergency requiring immediate treatment. Surgery is often the best treatment option. Surgical options include a cryopexy (intense cold application to the area with an ice probe to form scar tissue, which holds the retina to the underlying layer), laser surgery (to seal the tears or holes in the retina), pneumatic retinopexy (placing a gas bubble in the eye to help the retina float back into place), scleral buckle (indents the eye wall), and vitrectomy (removes gel or scar tissue pulling on the retina). These procedures may be performed alone or in combination with each other.

Ears

A few ear conditions that do not fit previously discussed categories can occur. These conditions may be manifestations of other problems or happen alone. Most of these conditions are mild, causing minor issues.

Tinnitus

Tinnitus describes hearing abnormal noises in the ear. This noise may be described as a ringing, buzzing, humming, whistling, roaring, or blowing. Tinnitus is a common problem, affecting approximately 50 million Americans (American Tinnitus Association, 2010). Tinnitus is not a condition itself, but, rather, it is symptom of an underlying issue. Although tinnitus can be bothersome, it does not usually warrant significant concern. Tinnitus may be associated with presbycusis, exposure to excessive noise, cerumen impaction, otosclerosis, Meniere's disease, stress, head injury, acoustic neuroma (a benign tumor on the acoustic nerve), atherosclerosis, hypertension, carotid stenosis, arteriovenous malformation, caffeine, and ototoxic medications (e.g., many antibiotics, aspirin, chemotherapies, and diuretics). Diagnostic procedures for tinnitus focus on the identification of the underlying causes. These procedures may consist of a history, physical examination (including a complete hearing test and otoscopic examination), and additional tests to identify the underlying cause. Treating the underlying cause (e.g., removing cerumen and controlling blood pressure) will resolve tinnitus in most cases. If needed, additional strategies may include:

- Tricyclic antidepressants to reduce tinnitus symptoms
- Alprazolam (Niravam, Xanax), a benzodiazepine, to reduce tinnitus symptoms
- Acamprosate (Campral), a drug used to treat alcoholism, to relieve tinnitus
- Masking tinnitus symptoms with white noise machines and hearing aids
- Avoiding things that can worsen tinnitus (e.g., caffeine, smoking, and ototoxic medications)

Vertigo

Vertigo refers to an illusion of motion. Vertigo is not the same as dizziness. Dizziness is feeling "lightheaded" or as though one might faint. People experiencing vertigo have a sensation that they or the room is spinning or moving. There are two types of vertigo—peripheral and central. Peripheral vertigo occurs when there is a problem with the vestibular labyrinth, semicircular canals, or the vestibular nerve. Certain medications (e.g., aminoglycoside antibiotics), head injuries, Meniere's disease, nerve compression, infections, and inflammation may cause this type of vertigo. Central vertigo occurs when there is a problem in the brain, particularly in the brain stem or cerebellum. Arteriosclerosis, certain medications (e.g., antiseizure agents and aspirin), alcohol, migraines, multiple sclerosis, and seizures may cause this type of vertigo. In addition to the sensation of movement, clinical manifestations may include nausea and vomiting. Diagnostic strategies for vertigo include a history, physical examination, and other tests to determine the underlying etiology (e.g., head CT and MRI). Pharmacology is the mainstay of treatment. These medications include anticholinergic agents, antihistamines (especially meclizine [Antivert]), benzodiazepines, and antiemetics. Safety precautions should also be taken to prevent injury from falls (e.g., changing positions slowly and mobility assistance).

Chapter Summary

The sensory organs work together to sense changes in the body's internal and external environment. This information is then relayed to the nervous system for interpretation and response. Disorders of these organs can significantly affect the body's sensory function and can even be life altering. Some of these conditions can be prevented by restricting noise exposure (e.g., wearing protective ear coverings and minimizing music volume) and shielding eyes (e.g., by wearing protective eye goggles and UV-protective sunglasses). Early diagnosis and treatment of other conditions can improve prognosis.

References

American Tinnitus Association. (2010). Retrieved from http://www.ata.org/for-patients/faqs

Chiras, D. (2008). *Human biology* (6th ed.). Sudbury, MA: Jones and Bartlett.

Elling, B., Elling, K., & Rothenberg, M. (2004). *Anatomy and physiology*. Sudbury, MA: Jones and Bartlett.

Gould, B. (2006). *Pathophysiology for the health professions* (3rd ed.). Philadelphia, PA: Elsevier.

National Cancer Institute. (2008). Retrieved from http://seer.cancer.gov/statfacts/html/eye.html

National Institutes of Health. (2008). Retrieved from http://www.nlm.nih.gov/medlineplus/ency/article/001036.htm

Professional guide to pathophysiology (2nd ed.). (2007). Philadelphia, PA: Lippincott Williams & Wilkins.

Resources

www.cancer.gov

www.cancer.org

www.cdc.gov

www.mayoclinic.com

www.medlineplus.gov

www.nih.gov

www.who.int

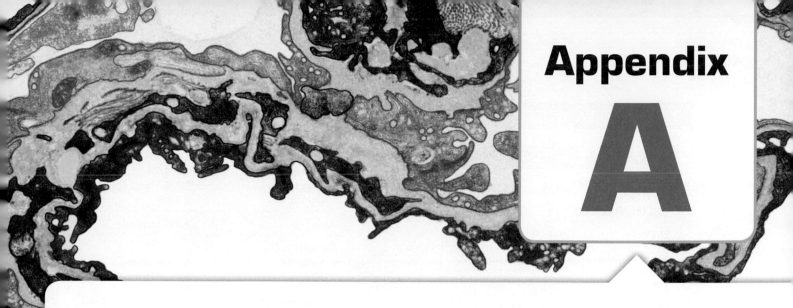

Normal Lab Values

Normal Lab Values

Cardiac Packet	
CPK-MB/CPK Relative Index	< 2.5%
CPK–Total	WM: 60–320 units/L WF: 50–200 units/L BM: 130–450 units/L BF: 60–270 units/L
Glucose	70–110 mg/dL
LDH–Total	100–190 units/L
LDH-1	14–26%
Troponin 1	Negative

CBC	
RBCs Count	M: 4.5–6.0 million/cc F: 4.0–5.5 million/cc
Hct	M: 40–50% F: 35–45%
Hgb	M: 14–18 g/dL F: 12–16 g/dL

RBC Indices
  MCV
  MCH
  MCHC
  RDW
	
	80–95 μm^3
	27–31 pg
	32–36 g/dL
	11–15%

CBC (Continued)	
WBCs Count	5000–10,000/mm^3

Granulocytes
  Neutrophils
  Eosinophils
  Basophils
	
	2500–8000/mm^3
	50–500/mm^3
	25–100/mm^3

Agranulocytes
  Lymphocytes
  Monocytes
	
	1000–4000/mm^3
	100–700/mm^3

Platelets Count	150,000–400,000/mm^3

Chem 7, Chem 12, Chem 20, Hepatic Function Panel, Renal Function Panel, Abdominal Pain Panel	
ALP	30–100 units/L
ALT (SGPT)	5–40 units/L
Amylase	50–190 units/L
AST (SGOT)	5–40 units/L

Bilirubin–Total
  Direct
  Indirect
	0.1–1.25 mg/dL
	0.1–0.3 mg/dL
	0.2–1.0 mg/dL

BUN	8–20 mg/dL
Ca^{++}–Total Ionized	9–11 mg/dL 4.25–5.25 mg/dL

Normal Lab Values *(Continued)*

Coagulation Tests

Coagulation Factors	
I (Fibrinogen)	200–400 mg/dL
II (Prothrombin)	80–120%
D-Dimer	< 250 mcg/L
FDPs	< 10 mcg/mL
Platelet Count	150,000–400,000/mm^3
PT	11–15 sec
PTT	60–80 sec
aPTT	25–40 sec
Thrombin Time	10–13 sec

CSF

Pressure	70–200 mm H$_2$O
Color	Clear
Protein	10–45 mg/dL
Glucose	45–78 mg/dL
WBCs–Total	< 5 cells/mm^3
Neutrophils	0–4%
Lymphocytes	60–80%
Monocytes	20–50%

Electrolyte Panel

Na$^+$	135–145 mEq/L
K$^+$	3.5–5 mEq/L
Cl	91–110 mEq/L
CO$_2$	20–30 mEq/L

Lipid Profile

HDL	M: > 45 mg/dL
	F: > 55 mg/dL
LDL	60–180 mg/dL
VLDL	25–50%
Total Cholesterol	< 200 mg/dL
Triglycerides	M: 40–60 mg/dL
	F: > 35–135 mg/dL

Toxicology–Toxic Levels

Drug Serum Screen

Acetaminophen	> 250 mcg/mL

Alcohol	
Intoxicated	0.1–0.4%
Stuporous	0.4–0.5%
Comatose	> 0.5%
ASA	> 300 mcg/mL
Barbitals	
Sedatives	> 10 mcg/mL
Anticonvulsant	> 40 mcg/mL
Carboxyhemoglobin	> 20%
Dilantin	> 20 mcg/mL
Lead	> 40 mcg/mL
Lithium	> 2.0 mEq/L

Drug Urine Screen

Amphetamine	> 3 mcg/mL
Diet Suppressants	
Dextroamphetamine	> 15 mcg/mL
Phenmetrazine	> 50 mcg/mL
Methamphetamine	> 40 mcg/mL
Mercury	> 100 mcg/day

Urinalysis

Volume	750–1800 cc/day
pH	4.6–8.0
Appearance	Clear
Color	Amber
Specific Gravity	1.003–1.030
Osmolality	250–1000 mOsm/L
Albumin	10–100 mg/day
Amylase	< 17 units/h
Calcium	< 250 mg/day
Creatinine	0.75–1.5 g/day
Glucose	< 500 mg/day
Potassium	25–125 mEq/day
Protein	0–8 mg/dL
Sodium	40–220 mEq/day
Urea Nitrogen	10–20 g/day
Uric Acid	250–750 mg/day

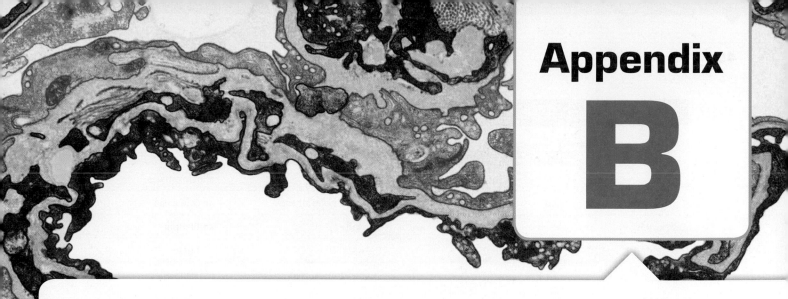

Word Roots and Combining Forms

Word Roots and Combining Forms

Root Word	Combining Form	Definition	Example
A			
abdomen	abdomin/o	abdomen	abdominocentesis
acanth		thorn	acanthosis
achilles	achill/o	Achilles' heel	achillobursitis
acid	acid/o	acid (pH)	acidosis
acoust	acoust/o	hearing	acoustics
acr	acr/o	extremity	acroarthritis
actin	actin/o	ray	actinodermatitis
acu	acul/o	needle	acupuncture
aden	aden/o	gland	adenosis
adip	adip/o	fat	adipocyte
adren	adren/o	adrenal gland	adrenomegaly
aer	aer/o	air	aerophore
agglutinat	agglutinat/o	clumping	agglutination
albin	albin/o	white	albinuria
albumin	albumin/o	protein	albuminuria
alkali	alkali/o	basic (pH)	alkalosis

Word Roots and Combining Forms *(Continued)*

Root Word	Combining Form	Definition	Example
all	all/o	other	allochromasia
alveoli	alveol/o	small hole, air sac	alveoloclasia
ambly	ambly/o	dull	amblyopia
ambul	ambul/o	walk	ambulate
ametr	ametr/o	disproportionate	ametropia
amnion	amni/o	amnion	amniocentesis
amyl	amyl/o	starch	amylorrhea
andr	andr/o	man (male)	androgenus
angi	angi/o	vessel	angioplasty
angina	angin/o	choke	anginose
aniso	anis/o	unequal	anisocytosis
ankyl	ankyl/o	stiffened, crooked	ankylosis
anus	an/o	anus	anoscope
anthrac	anthrac/o	coal	anthracosis
antr	antr/o	cavity	antroscopy
append	append/o	appendix	appendectomy
aort	aort/o	aorta	aortography
arachn	arachn/o	spider	arachroid
arteri	artcri/o	artery	arterial
arthr	arthr/o	joint	arthroscopy
atel	atel/o	imperfect, incomplete	atelectasis
ather	ather/o	fatty	atherosclerosis
atri	atri/o	atrium, chamber	atriomegaly
audi	audi/o	hear	audiology
aur	aur/o	ear	aural
axill	axill/o	armpit	axillany
B			
bacteri	bacteri/o	bacteria	bacteriuria
balan	balan/o	glans	balanitis
bas	bas/o	base (pH)	basophyl
bil	bil/i	gall, bile	biliary
bilirubin	bilirubin/o	bilirubin	hyperbilirubinism
bio	bi/o	life	biosphere

Word Roots and Combining Forms *(Continued)*

Root Word	Combining Form	Definition	Example
blephar	blephar/o	eyelid	blepharitis
bol	bol/o	cast, throw	anabolic
brachy	brachy/o	arm	brachyocephalic
bronch	bronch/o	bronchi	bronchitis
bucc	bucc/o	cheek	buccocclusion
burs	burs/o	pouch	bursitis
C			
cac	cac/o	bad, diseased	cachexia
calc	calc/i	calcium	calciuria
calcane	calcane/o	heel bone	calcaneodynia
capn	capn/i	smoke, carbon dioxide	hypercapnia
carcin	carcin/o	cancer	carcinoma
cardi	cardi/o	heart	cardioplagia
carp	carp/o	wrist	carpopedal
cata	cat/a	down, downward	catatonic
caud	caud/o	tail	caudal
caus	caus/o	heat	causalgia
cecum	cec/o	cecum	cecoileostomy
celi	celi/o	abdomen	celioma
centr	centr/i	center	centrilobular
cephal	cephal/o	head	cephalhydrocele
cerebell	cerebell/o	little brain (cerebellum)	cerebellospinal
cerebr	cerebr/o	brain (cerebrum)	cerebromalacia
cerumin	cerumin/o	wax	ceruminolysis
cervic	cervic/o	neck	cervicofacial
cheil	cheil/o	lip	cheilosis
chem	chem/o	chemical	chemotherapy
cholangi	cholangi/o	bile vessel	cholangioma
chole	chole/o	gall, bile	cholecystogram
choledoch	choledoch/o	common bile duct	choledochotomy
cholester	cholester/o	cholesterol, fat	cholesterosis
chondr	chondr/o	cartilage	chondrocarcinoma
chori	chori/o	chorion	chorioadenonia

Word Roots and Combining Forms (Continued)

Root Word	Combining Form	Definition	Example
choroid	choroid/o	choroid	choroiditis
cine	cine/o	motion	cineradiography
cinemato	cinemat/o	motion	cinematoradiograph
cirrho	cirrh/o	yellow, tawny	cirrhosis
cis	cis/o	cut	excision
cistern	cistern/o	reservoir, cavity	cisternography
clavic	clavic/o	clavicle	clavicotomy
clavicul	clavicul/o	clavicle	clavicular
cleid	cleid/o	clavicle	cleidorrhexis
clon	clon/o	turmoil	clonogenic
coagul	coagul/o	clot	coagulopathy
coccidioid	coccidioid/o	fungus	coccidioidmycosis
coccyx	coccyg/o	tail bone	coccygodynia
cochle	cochle/o	snail	cochleotopic
coit	coit/o	coming together	coitis
coll	cull/o	glutinous, jelly-like	colragenitis
colon	colon/o	colon	colonoscopy
colp	colp/o	vagina	colporrhapy
condyl	condyl/o	knuckle	condyloma
coni	coni/o	dust	coniosis
copr	copr/o	feces, excrement	coprostasis
cord	cord/o	cord	cordotomy
coria	cori/o	pupil (eye)	diplocoria
cortic	cortic/o	cortex	corticosterone
cost	cost/o	rib	costosternal
cox	cox/o	hip	coxalgia
crani	crani/o	skull	craniotomy
cretin	cretin/o	cretin	cretinism
crin	crin/o	secrete	endocrinology
crypt		hidden	cryptorchism
culd	culd/o	cul-de-sac	culdocentesis
cutane	cutan/o	skin	subcutaneous
cycl	cycl/o	ciliary body	cycloplegia

Word Roots and Combining Forms *(Continued)*

Root Word	Combining Form	Definition	Example
cyst	cyst/o	bladder	cystistaxia
cyt	cyt/o	cell	cytoplasm
D			
dacry	dacry/o	tear	dacryoma
dactyl	dactyl/o	finger, toe	dactylospasm
dem	dem/o	people	endemic
dendr	dendr/o	branched	dendritis
dent	dent/i	tooth	dentifrice
derm	derm/o	skin	dermomycosis
dermat	dermat/o	skin	dermatitis
didym	didym/o	testis	didymalgia
dilat	dilat/o	widen	dilation
dipl	dipl/o	double	diplopia
dips	dips/o	thirst	dipsomania
disk	disk/o	disk	diskectomy
diverticul	diverticul/o	diverticula	diverticulitis
dont	dont/o	tooth	oligodontia
dos	dos/i	giving	dosimeter
duoden	duoden/o	duodenum	duodenostomy
dur	dur/o	hard	duroarachnitis
E			
electr	electr/o	electricity	electrocardiogram
embol	embol/o	throwing in	embolism
emmetr	emmetr/o	ideal	emmetropia
emphys	emphys/o	inflate	emphysema
encephal	encephal/o	brain	encephalogram
enter	enter/o	intestine	enteritis
epidem	epidem/o	upon people	epidemic
epididym	epididym/o	epididymis	epididymectomy
episi	episi/o	vulva, pudenda	episiotomy
erythrocyt	erythrocyt/o	red blood cell	erythrocytosis
esophage	esophag/o	esophagus	esophagocele
esthesi	esthesi/o	feeling	anesthesia

Word Roots and Combining Forms *(Continued)*

Root Word	Combining Form	Definition	Example
F			
fasci	fasci/o	hand	fasciodis
fibr	fibr/o	fiber	fibroma
fibrin	fibrin/o	fiber	fibrinogen
fibul	fibul/o	fibula	fibular
fluor/o	fluor/o	fluorescence	fluoroscopy
foramin	foramin/o	foramen, opening	foraminoctomy
format	format/o	formation	malformation
G			
galact	galact/o	milk	galactorrhea
gangli	gangli/o	knot	ganglionectomy
gastr	gastr/o	stomach	gastritis
gen	gen/o	beginning, origin	genesis
genet	genet/o	producing	genetics
genit	genit/o	genitals	genitourinary
genital	genital/o	genitals	hypogenitalia
ger	ger/o	old age	geriatric
geront	geront/o	aged	gerontology
gigant	gigant/o	giant	gigantism
gingiv	gingiv/o	gums	gingivitis
glandul	glandul/o	little acorn, gland	glandular
glomerul	glomerul/o	little ball	glomerulitis
gloss	gloss/o	tongue	glossopharyngeal
gluc	gluc/o	glucose, sugar	glucocorticoid
glyc	glyc/o	sugar	glycogenesis
gonad	gonad/o	ovaries, testes	gonadotropin
goni	goni/o	angle	gonioscope
granul	granul/o	granular	granulocyte
gravid	gravid/o	pregnant	primigravida
gynec	gynec/o	female	gynecology
H			
halat	halat/o	breathe	inhalation
hem	hem/o	blood	hemoglobin

Word Roots and Combining Forms *(Continued)*

Root Word	Combining Form	Definition	Example
hemat	hemat/o	blood	hematocrit
hepat	hepat/o	liver	hepatoma
herni	herni/o	hernia	herniotomy
hidr	hidr/o	sweat	anhidrosis
hirsut	hirsut/o	hair	hirsutism
hist	hist/o	tissue	histology
hol	hol/o	whole	holography
humer	humer/o	humerus	humeral
hydr	hydr/o	water	hydrocele
hymen	hymen/o	hymen	hymenectomy
hypo	hypn/o	sleep	hypnosis
hyster	hyster/o	womb, uterus	hysterectomy
I			
ichthy	ichthy/o	fish (scaly)	ichthyosos
icter	icter/o	jaundice	icterogenic
ile	ile/o	ileum	ileostomy
ili	ili/o	ilium	iliosacral
immun	immun/o	safe, protect	immunotherapy
insul	insul/o	pancreatic islets	insuloma
insulin	insulin/o	insulin	insulinogenic
ion	ion/o	ion	ionoradioscope
irid	irid/o	iris	iridomalacia
ischem	ischem/o	hold back	ischemic
ischi	ischi/o	hip	ischiodynia
J			
jejun	jejun/o	jejunum	jejunotomy
K			
kary	kary/o	nucleu (cell)	karyotype
kel	kel/o	tumor	keloid
kerat	kerat/o	cornea	keratitis
ket	ket/o	ketone	ketosis
kinesi	kinesi/o	motion	bradykinesia
kinet	kinet/o	motion	kinetosis

Word Roots and Combining Forms (Continued)

Root Word	Combining Form	Definition	Example
kyph	kyph/o	hump	kyphosis
L			
labyrinth	labyrinth/o	maze	labyrinthitis
lacrim	lacrim/o	tear	lacrimotomy
lamin	lamin/o	shin plate	laminectomy
lapar	lapar/o	flank, abdomen	laparotomy
laryng	laryng/o	larynx	laryngoscope
later	later/o	side	lateroflexion
laxat	laxat/o	loosen	laxative
lei	lei/o	smooth	leiomyosarcoma
letharg	letharg/o	drowsiness	lethargy
lingu	lingu/o	tongue	nigralingua
lip	lip/o	fat	lipoatrophy
lith	lith/o	stone	lithotripsy
lob	lob/o	lobe	lobotomy
log	log/o	word, study	logomania
lord	lord/o	bending, curvature	lordosis
lumb	lumb/o	loin	lumbodynia
lymph	lymph/o	lymph, lymph gland	lymphoma
M			
mamm	mamm/o	breast	mammogram
mandibul	mandibul/o	lower jaw	mandibular
mast	mast/a	breast	mastectomy
maxill	maxill/o	upper jaw	maxillotomy
meat	meat/o	passage	meatotomy
mediastin	mediastin/o	mediastinum	mediastinits
medull	medull/o	marrow, spinal	medulloepithelioma
melan	melan/o	black	melanoma
men	men/o	month, menstruate	dysmenorrhea
mening	mening/o	membrane	meningitis
menisc	menic/o	crescent shape	menicitis
metr	metr/o	uterus	metritis
micturit	micturit/o	urinate	micturition

Word Roots and Combining Forms *(Continued)*

Root Word	Combining Form	Definition	Example
mitr	mitr/o	mitral valve	mitral
morph	morph/o	form, shape	morphology
muc	muc/o	mucous	mucositis
muscul	muscul/o	muscle	musculoskelectal
my	my/o	muscle	myoblast
myc	myc/o	fungus	mycosis
myel	myel/o	spinal cord	myeloma
myring	myring/o	membrane, mucous	myringoplasty
N			
narc	narc/o	night, sleep	narcosis
nas	nas/o	nose	nasogastric
necr	necr/o	death	necrosis
nephr	nephr/o	kidney	nephrema
neur	neur/o	nerve	neuroma
neutr	neutr/o	neither, neutral (pH)	neutrophyl
noct	noct/o	night	nocturia
nucle	nucle/o	nucleus, central	nuclear
nyct	nyct/o	night	nyctalgia
nyctal	nyctal/o	blind, night	nyctalopia
O			
ocul	ocul/o	eye	oculopupillary
olecran	olecran/o	elbow	olecranarthopathy
oment	oment/o	omentun	omentectomy
omphal	omphal/o	umbilicus	omphalitis
onc	onc/o	tumor	oncology
onych	onych/o	nail	onychitis
oophor	oophor/o	ovary	oophoritis
ophthalm	ophthalm/o	eye	ophthalmopathy
opt	opt/o	eye	optomyometer
orchi	orchi/o	testicle	orchitis
orchid	orchid/o	testicle	orchidopexy
organ	organ/o	organ	organomegaly
oscill	oscill/o	swing	oscillopsia

Word Roots and Combining Forms (Continued)

Root Word	Combining Form	Definition	Example
osm	osm/o	smell	anosmia
oste	oste/o	bone	osteorrhapy
ot	ot/o, ov/i, ov/o	ear, egg	otosclerosis, oviduct, ovoplasm
ovul	ovul/o	egg, ovum	ovulate
ox	ox/o	oxygen	anoxia
oxy	oxy/o	oxygen	oxytoxin
P			
palat	palat/o	palate	palatitis
pancreat	pancreat/o	pancreas	pancreatitis
papill	papill/o	papilla	papilledema
par	par/o	bear	paroxism
parathyr	parathyr/o	parathyroid gland	parathyroidism
patell	patell/o	patella, kneecap	patellapexy
path	path/o	disease	pathology
ped	ped/o	foot	pedal
ped	ped/i	child	pediatrics
pedicul	pedicul/o	louse	pediculosis
pen	pen/o	penis	penitis
pept	pept/o	digest	peptogenic
perine	perine/o	perineum	perineocele
phac	phac/o	lens	phacosclerosis
phag	phag/u	eat, engulf	phagocyte
phalange	phalang/o	finger, toe	phalangectomy
pharmac	pharmac/o	drug	pharmacotherapy
pharyng	pharyng/o	pharynx	pharyngitis
phe	phe/o	dusky, muzzle	pheochromocytoma
phim	phim/o	muscle	phimosis
phleb	phleb/o	vein	phlebitis
phon	phon/o	sound, voice	phonopathy
phragm	phragm/o	partition	diaphram
phragma	phragmat/o	partition	diaphragmatocele
phren	phren/o	diaphragm	phrenoplegia
physi	physi/o	nature	physiology

Word Roots and Combining Forms *(Continued)*

Root Word	Combining Form	Definition	Example
physic	physic/o	nature	physician
pin	pin/o	drink, pinlitary gland	pinocytosis
pineal	pineal/o	pineal body	pinealoma
pituitar	pituitary/o	pituitary gland	pituitarism
pleur	pleur/o	pleura	pleuritis
pneum	pneum/o	air	pneumothorax
pneumon	pneumon/o	lung	pneumonitis
poikil	poikil/o	irregular shape, passage	poikilocytosis
por	por/o	passage	poroma
porphyr	porphyry/o	porphyrin, purple	porphyrinuria
presby	presby/o	old	presbycusis
proct	proct/o	rectum, anus	proctatestomy, proctalgia
prostat	prostat/o	prostate	prostatectomy
psych	psych/o	mind	psychology
pteryg	pteryg/o	winglike	pterygomandibular
ptyal	ptyal/o	salvia	ptyalorrhea
pub	pub/o	pubis	pubovesical
pulm	pulm/o	lung	pulmometer
pulmon	pulmon/o	lung	pulmonectomy
pupill	pupill/o	pupil	pupillary
py	py/o	pus	pyorrhea
pyel	pyel/o	renal pelvis	pyelonephritis
pylor	pylor/o	pyloris	pyloroplasty
pyr	pyr/o	fire	pyrogenic
pyret	pyret/o	fever	pyretogenic
R			
rachi	rachi/o	spine	rachiomyelitis
radi	radi/o	ray, radius	radionecrosis
radiat	radiat/o	radiant	radiation
radic	radic/o	root	radicotomy
radicul	radicul/o	root	radiculitis
rect	rect/o	rectum, loosen	rectocele, relaxation
ren	ren/o	kidney	renogastric

Word Roots and Combining Forms *(Continued)*

Root Word	Combining Form	Definition	Example
reticul	reticul/o	net, network	reticulocyte
retin	retin/o	retina	retinitis
rhabd	rhabd/o	rod	rhabdomyoma
rhin	rhin/o	nose	rhinorrhagia
rhythm	rhythm/o	rhythm	arrhythmia
rhytid	rhytid/o	wrinkle	rhytidectomy
S			
sacr	sacr/o	sacrum	sacrodynia
salping	salping/o	tube	salpingoexy
sanguin	sanguin/o	blood	consanguinity
sarc	sarc/o	flesh	sarcoma
scapul	scapul/o	scapula	scapulopexy
schiz	schiz/o	split	schizophrenia
scler	scler/o	hard, fibrous	scleroderma
scoli	scoli/o	curvature	scoliosis
scot	scot/o	dark	scotoma
seb	seb/o	oil	seborrhea
senil	senile/o	old	senilism
ser	ser/o	serum	serology
sial	sial/o	saliva	sialadenitis
sid	sid/o	iron	sideropenia
sigmoid	sigmoid/o	sigmoid, colon	sigmoidoscope
sin	sin/o	curve	sinoatrial
sit	sit/o	foot	sitotherapy
somat	somat/o	body	somatotrophic
somn	somn/o	sleep	somnambulism
son	son/o	sound	sonogram
sperm	sperm/o	seed	spermolysis
spermat	spermt/o	seed	spermatocyst
sphincter	sphincter/o	closure	sphincteroplasty
sphygm	sphygm/o	pulse	sphygmomanometer
spin	spin/o	thorn, spine	spinocerebellar
spir	spir/o	breath	spirometer

Word Roots and Combining Forms *(Continued)*

Root Word	Combining Form	Definition	Example
spir	spir/o	coil	spiradenoma
splen	splen/o	spleen	splenectomy
spondyl	spondyl/o	vertebra	spondylitis
staped	staped/o	stapes, stirrup	stapedectomy
staphyl	staphyl/o	cluster, uvula	staphyloplasty
steat	steat/o	fat	steatolysis
sten	sten/o	narrowing	stenosis
stern	stern/o	sternum	sternalgia
steth	steth/o	chest	stethoscope
stigmat	stigmat/o	point	stigmatism
stomat	stomat/o	mouth, opening	stomatitis
strept	strept/o	chain	streptococcus
sympath	sympathy/o	sympathy	sympathectomy
syphil	syphil/o	syphilis	syphilopsychosis
T			
tars	tars/o	ankle bone	tarsectomy
ten	ten/o	tendon	tenorrhagia
tendin	tendin/o	tendon	tendinitis
tendon	tendon/o	tendon	tendonitis
terat	terat/o	monster	teratoma
test	test/o	testis	testalgia
thalass	thalass/o	sea	thalassemia
than	than/o	death	euthanasia
thel	thel/o	nipple	thelorrhagia
therm	therm/o	heat	hydrothermic
thromb	thromb/o	blood clot	thrombosis
thym	thym/o	thymus	thymopexy
thyr	thyr/o	thyroid	thyroptoss
tibi	tibi/o	tibia	tibial
tinnit	tinnit/o	jingling	tinnitus
toc	toc/o	birth	tocology
tom	tom/o	cut	tomography
ton	ton/o	tone, tension	tonography

Word Roots and Combining Forms *(Continued)*

Root Word	Combining Form	Definition	Example
tonsill	tonsill/o	tonsil	tonsillitis
top	top/o	place	topography
torti	torti/o	twisted	torticollis
toxic	toxic/o	poison	toxicology
trache	trache/o	trachea	tracheostomy
traumat	traumat/o	wound, injure	traumatology
trephinat	trephinat/o	bore	trephination
trich	trich/o	hair	trichomycosis
trigon	trigon/o	trigone	trigonitis
trop	trop/o	turn	neurotropism
tubercul	tubercul/o	swelling	tuberculosis
tympan	tympan/o	drum	tympanitis
U			
ul	ul/o	scar	ulectomy
ulcer	ulcer/o	surface excavation	ulcerogenic
uln	uln/o	elbow	ulnad
ungu	ungu/o	nail	ungula
ur	ur/o	urine	uremia
ureter	ureter/o	ureter	ureterolith
urethr	urethr/o	urethra	urethrocystitis
urin	urin/i	urine	uriniparous
urinat	urinat/o	urine	urination
uter	uter/o	uterus	uteralgia
uve	uve/o	uvea	uveitis
V			
vag	vag/o	vagus nerve, wandering	vagotomy
vagin	vagin/o	vagina	vaginectom
varic	varic/o	twisted vein	varicocele
vas	vas/o	vessel, duct	vasotripsy
vascul	vascul/o	small vessel	vasculopathy
vector	vector/o	carrier	vectorcardiogram
ven	ven/o	vein	venostasis
vener	vener/o	desire, love (sexual intercourse)	venereal

Word Roots and Combining Forms *(Continued)*

Root Word	Combining Form	Definition	Example
veni	veni/o	vein	venisuture
ventricul	ventricul/o	ventricle	ventriculitis
vertebr	vertebr/o	vertebra	vertebrectomy
vertig	vertig/o	dizziness, vesicle	vertigo
vesic	vesic/o	vesicle	vesicocele
vesicul	vesicul/o	vesicle	vesiculotomy
vir	vir/o	virus	viruria
viril	viril/o	masculine	virilism
viscer	viscer/o	body organs	visceroenic
vitamin	vitamin/o	vitamin	hypervitaminosis
vitre	vitre/o	vitreous humor	vitreous
vulv	vulv/o	vulva	vulvovaginitis
X			
xanth	xanth/o	yellow	xanthemia
xen	xen/o	alien, foreign	xenophobia
xiph	xiph/o	sword	xiphoid
Z			
zo	zo/o	animal	zooderma
zon	zon/o	encircling area	zonesthesia
zyg	zyg/o	joined	zygodactyly

Source: © Y.H. Hui, PhD.

Glossary

achlorhydria Decrease in stomach acid production, occasionally because of atrophic gastritis.

acne vulgaris A skin condition commonly affecting adolescents, but it can occur at any age. Acne vulgaris occurs when the skin's pores becomes clogged with oil, debris, or bacteria. The pore can become inflamed, developing a pustule, nodule, or cyst.

acquired immunity Immunity that results from subsequent exposures to an antigen because memory cells recall the antigen as foreign, and antibody production is rapid.

acromegaly Increase in bone size caused by excessive growth hormone levels in adulthood.

actin One of two types of myofilament. It is involved in muscular contractions, cellular movement, and cell shape maintenance.

action potential Creating neural charges.

active acquired immunity The process gained by actively having an antigen through invasion or vaccination. In active immunity, a person makes his or her own antibodies, and protection is usually long term.

active tuberculosis infection Phase of tuberculosis that occurs when the primary infection can no longer be controlled. During this phase, tuberculosis can spread throughout the lungs and to other organs.

active transport The movement of a substance from an area of lower concentration to an area of higher concentration, against a concentration gradient.

acute A disease that is short term, occurring and resolving quickly.

acute bronchitis An inflammation of the tracheobronchial tree or large bronchi. This inflammation is most commonly caused by a wide range of viruses. The airways become inflamed and narrowed due to the results of the inflammatory process.

acute gastritis Type of gastritis that usually develops suddenly and is likely to be accompanied by nausea and epigastric pain. It can be a mild, transient irritation, or it can be a severe ulceration with hemorrhage.

acute renal failure (ARF) A sudden loss of renal function. This loss is generally reversible and is most common in critically ill, hospitalized patients. Also called acute kidney injury.

acute respiratory distress syndrome (ARDS) A sudden failure of the respiratory system often occurring from fluid accumulation in the alveoli. ARDS has many other names, such as shock lung, wet lung, and stiff lung.

acute respiratory failure A serious, life-threatening condition that can be the result of many pulmonary disorders. The oxygen levels become dangerously low, or carbon dioxide levels become dangerously high. The low oxygen levels are unable to meet the body's metabolic needs.

acute tissue rejection The most common and treatable type of tissue rejection. This type of rejection usually occurs between 4 days and 3 months following a transplant. Acute reactions are cell mediated and result in transplant cell destruction (lyses) or necrosis.

adaptation Method by which cells attempt to prevent their own death from environmental changes. They may modify their size, numbers, or types in an attempt to manage these changes and maintain homeostasis.

Addison's disease A deficiency of adrenal cortex hormones.

adrenal gland Gland with an inner portion and outer portion that is located on a kidney.

afferent arteriole Point at which the blood enters the glomerulus.

afferent nerve A type of nerve of the peripheral nervous system. It carries impulses from the body to the brain. Also called sensory nerve.

afferent tract Fibers that carry sensory information in the form of action potentials from the periphery back to the brain. Also called ascending fibers.

afterload The pressure that the left ventricle must exert in order to get the blood out of the heart and into the aorta. The higher the afterload, the harder it is for the heart to eject the blood, thus lowering stroke volume. Both afterload and preload can affect blood pressure. As afterload and preload increase, blood pressure increases.

AIDS dementia complex Dementia that occurs in later stages of AIDS. The human immunodeficiency virus invades the brain tissue and may be exacerbated by other infections and tumors that are frequently associated with AIDS. Also called HIV-associated encephalopathy.

alarm The first stage of the general adaptation syndrome. This stage includes the generalized stimulation of the sympathetic nervous system resulting in the release of catecholamines and cortisol, or the fight-or-flight response.

albinism   A recessive condition that results in little or no melanin production.

aldosterone   A hormone secreted by the adrenal cortex that increases blood volume by increasing the reabsorption of sodium in the kidneys; sodium attracts water. Increasing water reabsorption will increase blood volume. The principal mineralcorticoid.

allele   One gene that may have many variants, which determines a characteristic.

allogenic   Type of transplant in which tissue is used from the same species of similar tissue type, but it is not identical. Most transplants use allogenic tissue.

alpha cell   One of five types of cells in the islets of Langerhans; secretes glucagon.

alveolus (plural: **alveoli**)   Hollow, saclike structures that are the final branchings of the respiratory tree and act as the primary gas exchange units of the lung.

Alzheimer's disease (AD)   The most common form of dementia. The disease causes healthy brain tissue to degenerate and atrophy.

amblyopia   The loss of one eye's ability to see details. Amblyopia is the most common cause of vision problems in children. Amblyopia occurs when the brain and eyes do not work together properly; the brain favors one eye. Also called lazy eye.

amenorrhea   The absence of menstruation.

ammonia   A metabolic waste managed by the kidneys. It is highly toxic and results from the breakdown of amio acids in the liver.

amphiarthrose   A slightly moveable joint that can be seen in the vertebral column.

ampulla   A pouch that joins the seminal vesicles to form the ejaculatory duct.

amylin   Substance that is released from the beta cells along with insulin. Amylin has a synergistic relationship with insulin to control glucose.

amyotrophic lateral sclerosis (ALS)   A disease that involves damage of the upper motor neurons of the cerebral cortex and lower motor neurons of the brain stem and spinal cord. Also called Lou Gehrig's disease after the famous baseball player who died of it.

anaphase   Phase of mitosis in which chromosomes separate and move to opposite poles.

anaphylactic shock   Type of distributive shock that is a consequence of an allergic reaction. The allergic reaction leads to a cascade of events similar to that of septic shock, except the mediators differ. Additionally, bronchospasms and laryngeal edema that can impair the patient's respiratory status occur.

anaplasia   The loss of differentiation that occurs with cancer.

anasarca   Edema that is generalized throughout the body.

anemia   A common acquired or inherited disorder of the erythrocytes that impairs the oxygen-carrying capacity of the blood.

aneurysm   Condition in the walls of an artery caused by high pressures, plaque, and infections. These walls weaken and balloon outward.

angina   Chest pain with a cardiac origin.

anion   A negatively charged electrolyte.

anion gap   The difference between the sum of cations and anions found in plasma.

ankylosing spondylitis   A progressive inflammatory disorder affecting the sacroiliac joints, intervertebral spaces, and costovertebral joints.

ankylosis   Joint fixation and deformity.

anotia   The absence of the auricle.

anteflexed   Tilted forward.

anterior eye chamber   The cavity of the eye interior that is in front of the lens.

antibody-producing cell   Type of B cell that produces millions of antibody molecules during its 24-hour life span.

antidiuretic hormone (ADH)   Hormone secreted by the posterior pituitary gland that increases water reabsorption in the kidney, which, in turn, increases blood volume and blood pressure. Antidiuretic hormone is a vasoconstrictor.

antigen   A foreign agent.

aorta   The largest artery in the body that originates from the left ventricle.

aortic valve   A three-leaflet valve that guides the passage of blood from the left ventricle to the aorta and prevents the backward flow of blood.

apocrine gland   Gland that opens into hair follicles in the axillae, scalp, face, and external genitalia.

apoptosis   Mechanism of programmed cell death that occurs because of morphologic changes.

appendicitis   An inflammation of the vermiform appendix. The inflammation can be life threatening and is most often caused by an infection.

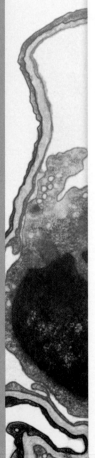

appendicular skeleton One of two divisions of the human skeleton. It consists of bones that form the arms, shoulders, pelvis, and legs.

appendix A small, wormlike structure attached to the cecum with seemingly no function but plenty of potential to cause harm if it becomes inflamed.

aqueous humor Watery liquid in the anterior chamber of the eye that provides nutrients to the cornea and lens and carries away cellular waste products.

arachnoid layer The middle layer of the meninges, named for its spider web–like vascular system.

areola An area of pigmentation surrounding the nipple.

areolar gland Gland that produces secretions that protect and lubricate the nipple and areola during breastfeeding.

arrhythmia Deviations from normal electric conduction in the heart. Arrhythmias vary in severity and are classified according to their origins. Also called dysrhythmia.

arterial blood gas (ABG) The long-standing, principal diagnostic tool for evaluating acid–base balance.

arteriole Small blood vessel that branches off arteries that are near the heart.

artery A blood vessel that carries blood away from the heart.

ascending fibers Fibers that carry sensory information in the form of action potentials from the periphery back to the brain. The ascending fibers have a variety of tracts that communicate specific sensory input. Also called afferent tracts.

ascending testicle A testicle that has returned to the lower abdomen and cannot easily be guided back into the scrotum. Also called an acquired undescended testicle.

ascites Fluid that accumulates in the peritoneal cavity.

aspiration The entrance of food into the trachea and lungs.

aspiration pneumonia Type of pneumonia that frequently occurs when the gag reflex is impaired because of a brain injury or anesthesia. Aspiration pneumonia can also occur because of impaired lower esophageal sphincter closure secondary to nasogastric tube placement or disease (e.g., gastroesophageal reflux disease).

asthma A chronic pulmonary disease that produces intermittent, reversible airway obstruction. Asthma is characterized by acute airway inflammation, bronchoconstriction, bronchospasm, bronchiole edema, and mucus production. Asthma is the most common chronic illness in children.

atelectasis Incomplete alveolar expansion or collapse of the alveoli. It occurs when the walls of the alveoli stick together.

atherosclerosis A chronic inflammatory disease characterized by thickening and hardening of the arterial wall. Lesions (or plaques) comprised of lipids develop on the vessel wall and calcify over time. Development of these lesions causes vessel obstruction, platelet aggregation, and vasoconstriction.

atopic eczema A chronic inflammatory skin condition triggered by an allergen.

atresia Lack of an external ear canal.

atrial natriuretic peptide A hormone that is released when the atria of the myocardium is overstretched, indicating increased fluid volume.

atrioventricular (AV) node Area of the heart located between atria and ventricles that receives impulses from the sinoatrial node. The impulses are delayed or move slowly through the atrioventicular node to allow for complete ventricular filling. This area can initiate impulses if the sinoatrial node begins failing.

atrophic gastritis Stomach condition caused by shrinkage and inflammation of the stomach lining.

atrophy State that occurs because of decreased work demands on a cell. When cellular work demands decrease, the cells decrease in size and number.

aura An unusual sensation (e.g., smells, tastes, or visual hallucinations) just prior to an impending seizure. Some people with focal seizures, especially complex focal seizures, may experience auras. These auras are actually simple focal seizures in which the person maintains consciousness.

auricle The irregularly shaped cartilage that channels sound into the ear.

autoimmune Type of reaction in which the body's normal defenses become self-destructive— recognizing self as foreign.

autologous Type of transplant in which the host and the donor are the same person, such as when someone donates his or her own blood prior to a scheduled surgery and then receives it during the surgery.

automaticity A process whereby cardiac cells generate an impulse to contract even with no external nerve stimulus.

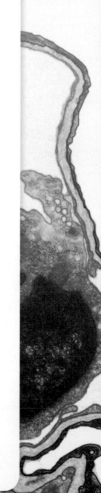

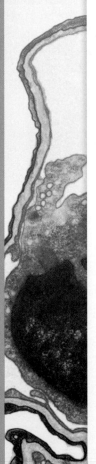

automatism Strange, repetitious behavior exhibited by a person having a complex focal seizure.

autonomic hyperreflexia A massive sympathetic response that can cause headaches, hypertension, tachycardia, seizures, stroke, and death; most commonly associated with spinal cord injuries above the sixth thoracic vertebra.

autonomic nervous system System that controls smooth muscles and is responsible for the fight-or-flight response.

autoregulation A mechanism to maintain tissue perfusion in which the blood vessels dilate to increase blood flow and constrict if the intracranial pressure is increased.

autosomal dominant Type of disorder in which a single gene mutation is passed from an affected parent to an offspring regardless of sex. Autosomal dominant disorders occur with homozygous and heterozygous allele pairs.

autosomal recessive Type of disorder in which single gene mutations are passed from an affected parent to an offspring regardless of sex, but they occur only in homozygous allele pairs.

autosome A paired set of chromosomes in DNA.

axial skeleton One of two divisions of the human skeleton. It forms the long axis of the body and includes the skull, vertebral column, and rib cage.

axon A projection of a neuron that makes connections with nearby cells. Axons transmit impulses away from the cell body.

azotemia A buildup of waste products.

B cell A cell that is a major part of the body's third line of defense. B cells mature in the bone marrow where they differentiate into memory cells or immunoglobulin-secreting (antibody) cells. B cells eliminate bacteria, neutralize bacterial toxins, prevent viral reinfection, and produce immediate inflammatory response. Each B cell has receptor sites for a specific antigen, and when it encounters the antigen, the B cell activates and multiplies into either an antibody-producing cell or a memory cell.

bacterial pneumonia A form of pneumonia that is more severe than viral pneumonia and can result from viral pneumonia.

baroreceptor Receptor in the carotid artery that detects the pressure in the heart and arteries.

Bartholin's gland Gland that lies just within the labia minor and provides lubrication during sexual intercourse.

basal ganglion (plural: ganglia) A key structure deep within the cerebrum, diencephalon, and midbrain. The basal ganglia play a pivotal role in coordination, motor movement, and posture.

base excess/deficit The concentration of buffer, in particular bicarbonate. Positive values indicate an excess of base or a deficit of acid. Negative values indicate a deficit of base or an excess of acid.

basilar skull fracture A skull fracture located at the base of the skull and usually accompanied by cerebrospinal fluid leakage.

benign Near-normal, differentiated condition of a cell or tumor, which causes fewer problems than an abnormal cell or tumor. Benign cells are usually encapsulated and are unable to metastasize.

benign prostatic hyperplasia (BPH) A common, nonmalignant enlargement of the prostate gland that occurs as men age.

beta cell One of five types of cells in the islets of Langerhans; secretes insulin.

bicarbonate-carbonic acid system A buffer mechanism that is the largest system in the extracellular fluid. Carbonic acid and bicarbonate (base) are the key players in this system.

bile A green or yellowish liquid that contains water, bile salts (formed from cholesterol), conjugated bilirubin, cholesterol, and electrolytes (including bicarbonate).

birthmark A skin anomaly that is present at birth or shortly after.

bladder A reservoir where urine is held until excretion.

bladder cancer Any cancer that forms in the tissue of the bladder.

blue bloaters Nickname given to those patients with chronic bronchitis, who are unable to increase ventilatory effort to maintain adequate gas exchange. These patients eventually develop cyanosis and edema.

bone A specialized form of connective tissue. It is a living, metabolically active tissue that is the site of fat and mineral storage (especially calcium) as well as hematopoiesis.

bone marrow Soft, fatty tissue found inside of bones.

Bowman's capsule A double membrane chamber that surrounds the glomerulus.

brain Organ located within the skull that contains billions of neurons.

brain stem Part of the central nervous system that includes the pons, cerebellum, and medulla. It connects the brain to the spinal cord. The brain stem is crucial for many basic body functions, and injury to the brain stem can easily result in death.

breast cancer Cancer of the breast; the most common malignancy in women, and the second leading cause of cancer death in women.

bronchiole Part of the lung that controls airflow.

bronchiolitis A common viral infection of the bronchioles most frequently caused by the respiratory syncytial virus. The infection most often occurs in children under 1 year of age, and incidence increases in the fall and winter months.

bronchopneumonia The most frequent type of pneumonia. It is generally a patchy pneumonia throughout several lobes.

bronchus (plural: **bronchi**) Large tube leading from the trachea to the lungs that carries air to and from the lungs.

bundle branches Specialized cardiac muscle cells that branch off the bundle of His to conduct electrical impulses through the ventricles.

bundle of His Collection of specialized cardiac muscle cells that conduct electrical impulses from the atrioventricular (AV) node.

burn A skin injury that can result from a thermal or a nonthermal source. These sources may include dry heat, wet heat, radiation, friction, heated objects, natural or artificial UV light, electricity, and chemicals.

café au lait spot Common type of birthmark that is the color of coffee with milk.

calcitonin Hormone secreted by the thyroid that regulates serum calcium levels. It alters serum calcium levels by inhibiting osteoclast activity and stimulating osteoblast activity.

calcium The most abundant mineral in the body. It is necessary for bone and teeth formation, muscle contractility, coagulation, and other body processes.

callus A mass of cells and fibers that bridges broken bone ends together inside and outside.

calyx (plural: **calyces**) Tube through which urine drains from the renal pyramid of the medulla to the renal pelvis for excretion through the ureters.

cancer The disease state associated with uncontrolled cellular growth. Key features include rapid, uncontrolled proliferation and a loss of differentiation.

candidiasis A yeast infection caused by the common fungus *Candida albicans*.

capillary A branch of an arteriole. It has thin walls to allow oxygen and nutrients to pass out of the capillaries into the cells. Additionally, carbon dioxide and waste products are passed from the cells into the capillaries.

carbuncle A cluster of boils.

carcinogenesis The process by which cancer develops. It occurs in three phases: initiation, promotion, and progression.

cardiac muscle Type of muscle that comprises the heart and is under involuntary control.

cardiac output The amount of blood the heart pumps in one minute. Cardiac output is determined by stroke volume and heart rate (CO = SV × HR, where CO is cardiac output, SV is stroke volume, and HR is heart rate).

cardiac tamponade Condition that results when the fluid accumulates in the pericardial cavity to the point that it compresses the heart. This compression prevents the heart from filling during diastole, resulting in decreased cardiac output.

cardiogenic shock Type of shock in which the left ventricle cannot maintain adequate cardiac output. Compensatory mechanisms of heart failure are triggered; however, these mechanisms increase cardiac workload and oxygen consumption, resulting in decreased contractility. Consequently, tissue and organ perfusion decrease, leading to multisystem organ failure.

cardiomyopathy A group of conditions affecting the myocardium. Cardiomyopathies are classified into three groups: dilated, hypertrophic, and restrictive.

cartilage A shiny connective tissue that is tough and flexible. Several types of cartilage can be found throughout the body in the ears, nose, bones, and joints.

caseous necrosis Type of necrosis that occurs when the necrotic cells disintegrate, but the cellular debris remains for months or years.

cataract Opacity or clouding of the lens.

cation A positively charged electrolyte.

cauda equina Individual nerve roots of the spinal cord at the vertebral canal.

cauda equina syndrome Injury to the nerve roots in the area of the cauda equina.

cecum A pouch at the end of the small intestine.

celiac disease An inherited, autoimmune, malabsorption disorder. Also called celiac sprue.

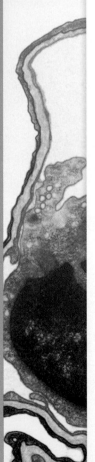

cell membrane The semipermeable boundary containing the cell and its components.

cellulitis An infection deep in the dermis and subcutaneous tissue. Cellulitis usually results from a direct invasion through a break in the skin, especially those breaks where contamination is likely.

central nervous system (CNS) System made up of the brain and spinal cord.

cerebellum Part of the brain stem that communicates with other regions of the brain to coordinate the synergistic motion of muscle movement and balance as well as cognition.

cerebral aneurysm A localized outpouching of a cerebral artery. This weakening of the artery may occur as a congenital defect or develop later in life.

cerebral contusion A bruising of the brain with rupture of small blood vessels and edema. Most contusions result from a blunt blow to the head that causes the brain to make a sudden impact with the skull.

cerebral palsy (CP) A group of nonprogressive disorders that appear in infancy or early childhood and permanently affect motor movement and muscle coordination. In addition to motor dysfunction, other cerebral functioning may be affected.

cerebral vascular accident (CVA) An interruption of cerebral blood supply. A CVA is an infarction of the brain, so it is often referred to as a brain attack. Also called a stroke.

cerebrospinal fluid (CSF) A plasmalike liquid that fills the space between the arachnoid and the pia mater layers to provide additional cushion and support to the central nervous system.

cerebrum The largest region of the brain; it controls the higher thought processes.

cervical cancer Cancer of the cervix. The Pap smear can now detect precancerous changes. Procedures can be performed to remove these precancerous cells, limiting the likelihood of these changes progressing to permanent malignant changes.

cervix The narrow opening from the uterus to the vagina.

chancre An infected, ulcerative lesion often associated with sexually transmitted infections such as syphilis.

chemoreceptor A receptor that detects chemical changes in the blood.

chlamydia One of the most prevalent sexually transmitted infections. Caused by *Chlamydia trachomatis*.

chloride A mineral electrolyte and the major extracellular anion. Chloride assists in fluid distribution by attaching to sodium or water.

cholecystitis Inflammation or infection in the biliary system caused by calculi.

cholelithiasis Gallstones; a common condition that affects both genders and all ethnic groups relatively equally.

chondrosarcoma A slow-growing tumor that begins in cartilage cells that are commonly found on the ends of bones.

chordee A downward curvature of the penis.

chorea Uncontrolled, rapid, jerky movements.

choroid The part of the middle layer of the eye that contains melanin to absorb stray light.

chromosome A nucleotide in DNA.

chronic State that occurs when an acute disease does not resolve in a short period of time. A chronic disease often has fewer notable signs than an acute disease, and it occurs over a longer period of time. Chronic diseases might not ever resolve but may become manageable.

chronic bronchitis An obstructive respiratory disorder characterized by inflammation of the bronchi, a productive cough, and excessive mucus production. Chronic bronchitis differs from acute bronchitis in that the chronic type is not necessarily caused by an infection, and symptoms persist longer.

chronic gastritis Type of gastritis that develops gradually and is likely to be accompanied by a dull epigastric pain and a sensation of fullness after minimal intake. It can be asymptomatic.

chronic obstructive pulmonary disease (COPD) A group of chronic respiratory disorders characterized by irreversible, progressive tissue degeneration and airway obstruction.

chronic overdistention Condition caused by a perceived inability to interrrupt work to void. This chronic avoidance of emptying the bladder results in detrusor muscle areflexia and overflow incontinence. Also called nurse's bladder and teacher's bladder.

chronic renal failure (CRF) A gradual loss of renal function that is irreversible.

chronic tissue rejection Type of tissue rejection that occurs from about 4 months to years after the transplant. This reaction is mostly likely due to an antibody-mediated immune response. Antibodies and complements deposit in the transplanted tissue vessel walls, resulting in decreased blood flow and ischemia.

chronotropic The rate of contraction.

Chvostek's sign An indicator of hypocalcemia in which a spasm or brief contraction of the corner of the mouth, nose, eye, and muscles in the cheek result from tapping the facial nerve in front of the ear.

chyme A mixture of food that has been chemically digested and churned in the stomach.

ciliary body The part of the middle layer of the eye that contains smooth muscle fibers that control the shape of the lens to focus on incoming light.

cilium (plural: cilia) Organelle that moves in a wavelike motion to propel the mucus and trapped particles upwards to the mouth where they can be expectorated.

cirrhosis Chronic, progressive, irreversible, diffuse damage to the liver resulting in decreased liver function.

cleft lip Congenital defect that results from failure of the maxillary processes and nasal elevations or upper lip to fuse during development. It may occur with a cleft palate. A cleft lip and palate can affect the appearance of one's face and may lead to problems with feeding, speech, ear infections, and hearing problems.

cleft palate An opening between the oral cavity and the nasal cavity. It may occur with a cleft lip. A cleft lip and palate can affect the appearance of one's face and may lead to problems with feeding, speech, ear infections, and hearing problems.

clitoris Part of the vulva formed by the connection of the two labia minor. The clitoris is sensitive to stimulation and becomes filled with blood during sexual arousal. The clitoris contains two corpora cavernosa, similar to the penis.

closed-angle (acute) glaucoma Type of glaucoma that is a result of a sudden blockage of aqueous humor outflow and is a medical emergency.

closed fracture Type of fracture in which the skin is intact.

coagulative necrosis Type of necrosis that usually results as an interruption in blood flow.

cochlea A spiral-shaped structure in the inner ear that houses the organ of Corti.

colon Part of the lower gastrointestinal tract that makes up most of the large intestine. The colon has three relatively straight sections (ascending, transverse, and descending). The colon absorbs 90% of the water and electrolytes that enter.

colorectal cancer Cancer of the colon and/or rectum.

comminuted fracture A fracture with multiple fracture lines and bone pieces.

comminuted skull fracture A skull fracture with several fracture lines.

communicating hydrocephalus Cerebrospinal accumulation that occurs when the fluid is not properly absorbed by the bloodstream.

community-acquired pneumonia Pneumonia that is acquired outside the hospital or healthcare setting.

compact bone The hard outer surface of a bone.

compartment syndrome A serious condition that results from pressure increases in a compartment, usually the muscle fascia in the case of fractures. The pressure impinges on the nerves and blood vessels contained within the compartment, potentially compromising the distal extremity.

compensatory mechanism Physiologic response to homeostatic imbalance in attempt to maintain normalcy.

complete fracture Type of fracture in which the bone is broken into two or more separate pieces.

complication A new problem that arises as a result of a disease.

compound skull fracture A skull fracture where brain tissue is exposed.

compression fracture A fracture in which the bone is crushed or collapses into small pieces.

concussion A momentary interruption of brain function. Concussions usually result from a mild blow to the head that causes sudden movement of the brain, disrupting neurologic functioning. Concussions may or may not lead to a loss of consciousness. Amnesia, confusion, sleep disturbances, and headaches may follow a concussion for weeks or months.

conductivity The ability cells to conduct electrical impulses.

condyloma acuminatum (plural: condylomata acuminata) Benign genital wart caused by a group of viruses called the human papillomaviruses.

cone A photoreceptor in the eye that operates in bright light and is responsible for visual acuity and color vision. There are about 6 million cones in the human eye.

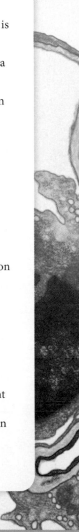

congenital Conditions involving defects or damage to a developing fetus.

congenital cataract A clouding of the lens that is present at birth. This clouding of the usually clear lens results in hazy vision.

congenital glaucoma Type of glaucoma that is present at birth. This type is a result of abnormal development of outflow channels (trabecular meshwork) of the eye.

congenital hearing loss Loss of hearing that can occur because of damage associated with maternal rubella and syphilis infection during pregnancy.

conjunctiva A fragile membrane that covers the inner surface of the eyelid and the exposed surface of the eye.

conjunctivitis An infection or inflammation of the conjunctiva, the lining of the eyelids and sclera.

constipation A change in bowel pattern characterized by infrequent passage of stool.

constrictive pericarditis Condition that results from chronic inflammation of the pericardium. The pericardium becomes thick and fibrous and adheres to the heart. The loss of elasticity restricts cardiac filling, which causes systemic congestion and decreases cardiac output.

contact dermatitis An acute inflammatory reaction triggered by direct exposure to an irritant or allergen-producing substance.

convalescence The stage of recovery following a disease that may last for days or months.

cornea A clear lens on the anterior side of the outermost layer of the eye that allows light to enter the eye.

coronary artery disease (CAD) Disease that occurs when atherosclerosis develops in the arteries supplying the myocardium. Blood flow temporarily diminishes in the coronary arteries, causing subsequent oxygen reduction to the cardiac muscle.

cortex The outer portion of an adrenal gland that is regulated by negative feedback involving the hypothalamus and adrenocorticotropic hormones.

cortisol The principal glucocorticoid, which increases serum glucose levels.

countercoup The second area of damage in a traumatic brain injury. Where the brain first impacts with the skull is the coup; then the brain rebounds and impacts with the opposite side of the skull, which is the countercoup.

coup The initial area the brain impacts with the skull in a traumatic brain injury.

Cowper's glands Two pea-sized glands adjacent to the urethra that secrete another alkaline fluid into the urethra to neutralize acidity caused by urine transportation. The Cowper's glands' secretions can sometimes be seen at the meatus before ejaculation. This secretion aids in lubrication of the penis during sexual intercourse and may contain some sperm left over from a previous ejaculation.

cranial nerves Set of nerves through which the brain accomplishes a variety of physiologically vital functions and cognitive activities. Twelve pairs branch directly from the base of the brain.

crenation Shrinkage of a cell as a result of too much water moving out of the cell.

crepitus A grating sound.

Creutzfeldt-Jakob disease (CJD) A rare, but rapidly progressive form of dementia caused by an infectious prion.

Crohn's disease An insidious, slow-developing, progressive condition that often develops in adolescence. Crohn's disease is characterized by patchy areas of inflammation involving the full thickness of the intestinal wall and ulcerations.

cryptorchidism A congenital condition in which one or both testes do not descend from the abdomen to the scrotum prior to birth.

curative A goal of treatment aimed at eradicating disease.

Curling's ulcer Stress ulcer associated with a burn.

Cushing's reflex A mechanism to maintain tissue perfusion in which a complex cascade of events results in increased blood pressure.

Cushing's syndrome Excessive cortisol levels that result from the increased corticotropin levels.

Cushing's triad Increased blood pressure, bradycardia, and changes in respiratory pattern that result from unresolved vasoconstriction, increased cardiac contractility, and increased cardiac output.

Cushing's ulcer Stress ulcer associated with a head injury.

cystic fibrosis A common inherited respiratory disorder that presents at birth. This life-threatening condition causes severe lung damage and nutrition deficits.

cystitis Inflammation of the bladder.

cystocele Condition that occurs when the bladder protrudes into the anterior wall of the vagina.

cytoplasm A colorless, viscous liquid inside the cell that contains water, nutrients, ions, dissolved gases, and waste products where the cellular work takes place.

cytotoxic cell Type of T cell that destroys cells infected with viruses by releasing lymphokines that destroy cell walls. Also called killer cell and effector cell.

deamination The process of stripping amino groups from molecules.

defecation The expulsion of the feces from the rectum.

dehydration Fluid deficit.

delta cell One of five types of cells in the islets of Langerhans; secretes somatostatin.

dementia A group of conditions in which cortical function is decreased, impairing cognitive skills and motor coordination. Issues with memory are common with dementia and include short-term memory losses as well as confusion of historical events.

dendrite A projection of a neuron that makes connections with nearby cells. Dendrites transmit impulses toward the cell body.

depolarization An increase in electrical charge through the exchange of ions across the cell membrane caused by the rapid inflow of positively charged sodium ions.

depressed fracture Type of fracture that occurs in the skull when the broken piece is forced inward on the brain.

depressed skull fracture A skull fracture in which bone fragments are displaced into the brain.

dermatome The area of the skin innervated by a given pair of spinal sensory nerves. Each spinal nerve, with the exception of the first cervical vertebra, has a specific body surface area to which it obtains sensory information.

dermis The middle layer of the skin, which is comprised of dense, irregular connective tissue and little fat tissue. The dermis includes nerves, hair follicles, smooth muscle, glands, blood vessels, and lymphatic vessels.

descending fibers Fibers that carry motor impulses in the form of action potentials from the brain to the fibers of the peripheral nervous system. Also called efferent tracts.

detrusor hyperreflexia Increased contractile activity of the detrusor muscle of the bladder, resulting in urinary incontinence.

diabetes insipidus Excessive fluid excretion in the kidneys caused by deficient antidiuretic hormone levels.

diabetes mellitus (DM) A group of conditions characterized by hyperglycemia (high serum glucose levels) resulting from defects in insulin production, insulin action, or both.

diabetic ketoacidosis A pH imbalance characterized by increased ketones in the urine caused by insufficient insulin; if cells are starved for energy, the body may begin to break down fat-producing toxic acids (ketones).

diaphragm A dome-shaped muscle that separates the thoracic and abdominal cavities and aids in respirations.

diaphysis The body of a bone.

diarrhea A change in bowel pattern characterized by an increased frequency, amount, and water content of the stool.

diastole The bottom number in a blood pressure reading, which indicates rest or relaxation by the ventricles.

diastolic dysfunction Type of heart failure characterized by decreased ventricular filling resulting from abnormal myocardial relaxation and increased left ventricular pressure. This type of heart failure is caused by conditions that stiffen the myocardium, such as coronary artery disease, hypertrophic and restrictive cardiomyopathy, and pericardial disease.

diencephalon Part of the brain that includes the thalamus and hypothalamus.

differentiation A process by which cells become specialized in terms of cell type, function, structure, and cell cycle. This process does not begin until approximately 15–60 days after the sperm and ova unite.

diffusion The movement of solutes (particles dissolved in a solvent) from an area of higher concentration to lower concentration.

dilated cardiomyopathy Type of cardiomyopathy that affects systolic function. It is the most common type of cardiomyopathy.

diplopia Double vision.

disease The state when a bodily function is no longer occurring normally. Diseases range from merely

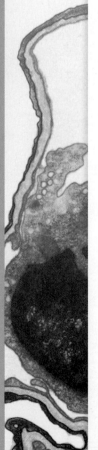

causing temporary stress to causing life-changing complications.

dislocation The separation of two bones where they meet at a joint.

dissecting aneurysm A false aneurysm in which weakening occurs in the inner layers of a blood vessel.

disseminated intravascular coagulation (DIC) A life-threatening disorder that occurs as a complication of other diseases and conditions. Clotting factors become abnormally active, often because of an inappropriate immune reaction. Hypercoagulation is followed by hemorrhaging as the clotting factors are completely utilized.

distributive shock Type of shock in which vasodilatation causes hypovolemia.

diverticular disease Conditions related to the development of diverticula.

diverticulitis A state in which diverticula have become inflamed, usually because of retained fecal matter. Diverticulitis can result in potentially fatal obstructions, infection, abscess, perforation, peritonitis, hemorrhage, and shock.

diverticulosis Asymptomatic diverticular disease. Usually there are multiple diverticula present.

diverticulum (plural: diverticula) Outwardly bulging pouch of the intestinal wall that occurs when mucosa sections or large intestine submucosa layers herniate through a weakened muscular layer.

DNA Deoxyribonucleic acid. A double-stranded chain of nucleotides called chromosomes.

dominant More powerful. In genetics, the dominant allele is more likely to be expressed in the offspring than the recessive one.

dorsal root Root formed from about 6–8 dorsal rootlets. The roots combine to form the spinal nerve.

dromotropic The rate of electrical conduction.

drug-induced asthma A type of asthma that is frequently caused by aspirin and can be fatal. Reactions can be delayed up to 12 hours after drug ingestion.

dry gangrene Type of gangrene that occurs when bacterial presence is minimal, and the skin has a dry, dark brown, or black appearance.

duodenal ulcer Type of ulcer that is commonly associated with excessive acid or *H. pylori* infections. Manifestations typically include epigastric pain that is relieved in the presence of food.

dura mater The tough outer layer of the central nervous system.

dwarfism Short stature caused by deficient levels of growth hormone, somatotropin, or somatotropin-releasing hormone.

dyslipidemia A raised level of lipids in the blood. These lipids include cholesterol and triglycerides, which are necessary for cellular membrane formation. Also called hyperlipidemia.

dysmenorrhea Painful menstruation to the extent that it impairs usual daily activities.

dysphagia Difficulty swallowing.

dysplasia The final cellular adaptation, in which cells mutate into cells of a different size, shape, and appearance.

dysrhythmia Deviations from normal electric conduction in the heart. Dysrhythmias vary in severity and are classified according to their origins. Also called arrythmia.

ear Organ that detects and processes sound and detects body position and maintains balance.

eccrine gland Gland that secretes sweat through skin pores in response to the sympathetic nervous system. Also called merocrine gland.

eclampsia An acute and life-threatening complication of pregnancy, characterized by tonic-clonic seizures, usually occurring in a patient who had developed preeclampsia.

ectopic pregnancy Pregnancy in which the zygote does not reach the uterus and implants outside the uterus.

ectopic testes Undescended testes that deviate from the path of descent.

edema Excess fluid in the interstitial space. Edema is a problem of fluid distribution, not necessarily of fluid overload.

effector cell One of two major types of T cells that work to destroy antigens. Also called killer cell.

efferent arteriole Point at which blood exits the glomerulus.

efferent nerve A type of nerve that carries impulses from the brain to the corresponding muscle receptor, resulting in muscle contraction and movement. Also called motor nerve.

efferent tracts Tracts that carry motor impulses in the form of action potentials from the brain to the fibers of the peripheral nervous system. Also called descending fibers.

ejaculation Propulsion of sperm-containing fluid.

ejaculatory duct Canal in the male reproductive tract formed by union of the vas deferens and the duct from the seminal vesicle

electrolyte A chemical that is a charged conductor when it is dissolved in water.

embolus A portion or all of a thrombus that breaks loose and travels through the circulatory system until it embeds in a smaller vessel. Any other traveling bodies (e.g., air, fat, tissue, bacteria, amniotic fluid, tumor cells, and foreign substances) can become emboli as well.

emesis The involuntary or voluntary forceful ejection of chyme from the stomach up through the esophagus and out the mouth. It is a common event that can result from a wide range of conditions. Also called vomiting.

emphysema An obstructive respiratory disorder that results in the destruction of the alveolar walls leading to large, permanently inflated alveoli.

encephalitis An inflammation of the brain and spinal cord, usually resulting from an infection.

end-stage renal disease The final phase of chronic renal failure, which is marked by 90% of nephron destruction and a drop in GFR to 10 mL/min (normal is 125 mL/min). The kidneys lose their ability to maintain any sense of homeostasis. Waste products, fluid, and electrolytes accumulate significantly.

endocardium The inner epithelial layer of the heart that makes up the valves.

endocytosis The act of bringing a substance into a cell.

endometrial cancer Cancer of the uterus, a common malignancy in women.

endometriosis Condition in which the endometrium begins growing in areas outside the uterus.

endometrium The inner mucosal lining of the uterine wall that undergoes hormonal changes to facilitate and maintain pregnancy.

enuresis The involuntary urination by a child after the age of 4–5 years, when bladder control is expected.

enzyme Protein that facilitates chemical reactions in cells.

epidemic Increasing disease numbers in a group.

epidemiology Tracking patterns of diseases in a group of people. This tracking includes occurrence, incidence, prevalence, transmission, and distribution of the disease.

epidermis The outermost layer of the skin. It is comprised of squamous epithelia.

epididymis Structure in the male reproductive tract that stores sperm until ejaculation, up to 6 weeks.

epididymitis An inflammation of the epididymis, the duct connecting the testes to the vas deferens.

epidural hematoma Hematoma that results from bleeding between the dura and skull, usually caused by an arterial tear.

epiglottis Part of the respiratory system that closes the larynx when food is swallowed.

epiglottitis A life-threatening inflammation of the epiglottis, the protective cartilage lid covering the trachea opening.

epilepsy A disorder that results from spontaneous firing of abnormal neurons; it is characterized by recurrent seizures for which there is no underlying or correctable cause.

epinephrine Hormone produced by the medulla during times of stress. With norepinephrine, it mediates the fight-or-flight response of the sympathetic nervous system.

epiphysis The growth plates at either end of a bone.

epispadias The urethral meatus occurring on the dorsal surface of the penis instead of the end.

epithalamus Dorsal posterior segment of the diencephalon, which includes the habenula, the stria medullaris, and the pineal body.

epsilon cell One of five types of cells in the islets of Langerhans; secretes ghrelin.

erectile dysfunction (ED) The inability to attain or maintain a penile erection sufficient to complete sexual intercourse. Also called impotence.

erythrocyte Red blood cell.

erythropoietin Hormone produced by the kidney that promotes the formation of red blood cells in the bone marrow.

esophageal cancer Cancer of the esophagus; usually a squamous cell carcinoma.

esophagus Part of the upper gastrointestinal system that has muscular rings to move the food toward the stomach.

essential hypertension Type of hypertension in which there is no identifiable cause, which occurs in 90–95% of hypertension cases in adults. This type of hypertension tends to develop gradually over many years. Also called primary hypertension.

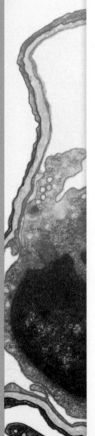

etiology The cause of a disease.

eustachian tube A pressure valve for the tympanic membrane.

Ewing's sarcoma An aggressive tumor in which the origin is unknown. Ewing's sarcoma may begin in nerve tissue within the bone.

exacerbation Disease state that occurs when the manifestations increase after a period of remission.

excitability The ability of the cells to respond to electrical impulses.

exercise-induced asthma Common type of asthma that usually occurs 10–15 minutes after activity ends. Symptoms can linger for an hour with exercise-induced asthma.

exhaustion The third stage of the general adaptation syndrome. This stage is initiated if the stressor is prolonged or overwhelms the body. During the exhaustion phase, the body becomes depleted and damage may appear as homeostasis can no longer be maintained. As the body's defenses are utilized, disease or death results.

exocytosis The release of materials from a cell, usually with the assistance of a vesicle.

exophthalmos Protruding eyes with decreased blinking and movement.

expiration Exhalation. One of two phases of breathing.

expiratory reserve volume The amount of air beyond tidal volume that can be exhaled forcefully, which is beyond the normal passive exhalation.

exsanguination The spillage of blood out of the circulatory system as the result of a ruptured aneurysm.

external ear canal Part of the ear through which sound travels until reaching the tympanic membrane.

extracellular fluid Fluid found outside the cells.

extrinsic asthma A result of increased IgE synthesis and airway inflammation, resulting in mast cell destruction and inflammatory mediator release. Extrinsic triggers include allergens such as food, pollen, dust, and medications. It usually presents in childhood or adolescence.

eye Globe-shaped organs located in orbits in the anterior skull that allow the brain to perceive the environment.

facilitated diffusion The movement of substances from an area of lower concentration to an area of higher concentration with the assistance of a carrier molecule.

fallopian tubes Two cylinders that extend from the fundus of the uterus to near the ovaries.

fascia Fibrous connective tissue that surrounds muscles. This fascia may also surround muscle groups.

fat embolism Condition that occurs when fatty marrow enters the bloodstream after a fracture to one of the long bones. The emboli can travel to vital organs such as the lungs, brain, or heart.

fat necrosis Type of necrosis that occurs when lipase enzymes break down intracellular triglycerides into free fatty acids.

fatty streaks Early stages of atherosclerosis. These streaks are made up of macrophages, and cholesterol accumulates within the macrophages.

feces Mixture of the undigested or unabsorbed remnants in the colon, along with bacteria (one third of the feces). Feces also introduce mucus (approximately 300 mL daily) to aid in bowel movements, even in times of decreased dietary intake.

fibrocystic breast disease The presence of numerous benign nodules in the breast.

fibromyalgia A syndrome predominately characterized by widespread muscular pains and fatigue. Fibromyalgia affects muscles, tendons, and surrounding tissue, but it does not affect the joints.

fibrous plaque Lesion of atherosclerosis. A pearly, white area within an artery that causes the intimal surface to bulge into the lumen. It is composed of lipid, cell debris, smooth muscle cells, collagen, and, in older persons, calcium.

first line of defense Part of the immune system that includes physical and chemical barriers that indiscriminately protect against all invaders (nonspecific immunity). The most prominent barriers in this first line are the skin and mucous membranes.

flat bone Strong, flat plate of bone that provides protection to the body's vital organs and a base for muscular attachment. Anterior and posterior surfaces of flat bones are formed from compact bone to provide strength, and the center consists of spongy bone and varying amounts of bone marrow.

flexor reflex A withdrawal reflex in response to touching an unpleasant stimulus. The flexor reflex causes the muscles of a limb to withdrawal the limb from the source of the stimulus without any conscious action.

fluid deficit Condition that occurs when total body fluid levels are not sufficient to meet the body's needs.

fluid excess Condition that occurs when total body fluid levels are greater than the body's needs.

fluid volume deficit Fluid deficit of the intravascular compartment. Also called hypovolemia.

fluid volume excess Excess fluid in the intravascular compartment. Also called hypervolemia

focal seizure One of two categories of seizure; occurs in just one part of the brain. Also called partial seizure.

follicle One of several functional units of the thyroid gland. These follicles produce thyroxine (T_4), triiodothyronine (T_3), and thyrocalcitonin (calcitonin).

folliculitis Infections involving the hair follicles. Folliculitis is characterized by tender, swollen areas that form around hair follicles, often on the neck, breasts, buttocks, and face.

foramen magnum The large and only opening in the skull.

forced expiratory volume in one second The amount of air that can be forcibly exhaled from the lungs in the first second of a forced exhalation.

forced vital capacity The amount of air that can be forcibly exhaled from the lungs after a forced inspiration.

foreskin A sheath of loose skin that covers the glans penis at birth. The foreskin is often surgically removed for hygienic, cultural, or religious reasons.

fracture A break in the rigid structure of the bone.

frank blood Blood that is bright red.

free radicals Injurious, unstable agents that can cause cell death.

frontal lobe Lobe of the brain that facilitates voluntary motor activity and plays a role in personality traits.

fully compensated A pH level that has returned to normal.

functional incontinence Type of incontinence that occurs in many older adults, especially people in nursing homes, because a physical or mental impairment prevents them from making it to the toilet in time.

furuncle An infection that begins in the hair follicles and then spreads into the surrounding dermis. A furuncle lesion starts as a firm, red, painful nodule that develops into a large, painful mass, which frequently drains large amounts of purulent exudate. Also called boil.

fusiform aneurysm An aneurysm that occurs around the entire circumference of a blood vessel. One of two major types of true aneurysm.

gallbladder A small, saclike organ located on the under surface of the liver that is a reservoir for bile. In addition to storing the bile, the gallbladder concentrates the bile by removing water.

gangrene A form of coagulative necrosis that has a combination of impaired blood flow and bacterial invasion.

gas gangrene Type of gangrene that develops because of *Clostridium*, an anaerobic bacterium. This type of gangrene is the most serious and has the most potential for being fatal.

gastric cancer Cancer of the stomach that occurs in several forms.

gastric ulcer Type of stomach ulcer that is uncommon but deadly. Gastric ulcers typically are associated with malignancy and nonsteroidal anti-inflammatory drug use. Pain associated with gastric ulcers typically worsens with eating.

gastritis An inflammation of the mucosal lining of the stomach that can be acute or chronic.

gastroenteritis Inflammation of the stomach and intestines usually because of an infection or allergic reaction.

gastroesophageal reflux disease (GERD) A condition where chyme periodically backs up from the stomach into the esophagus. Occasionally, bile can back up into the esophagus. The presence of these gastric secretions irritates the esophageal mucosa.

gene A segment of deoxyribonucleic acid (DNA) that serves as a template of protein synthesis.

general adaptation syndrome A cluster of systemic manifestations as a result of modifying in an attempt to cope with a stressor.

generalized seizure A seizure that results from abnormal neuronal activity on both sides of the brain. A generalized seizure may cause loss of consciousness, falls, or massive muscle spasms.

genetics The study of heredity—the passage of physical, biochemical, and physiologic traits from biological parents to their children.

genital herpes A sexually transmitted infection that causes blisters on the genitals and in the reproductive tract.

gestation The support of fetal development from conception to birth by the female reproductive system.

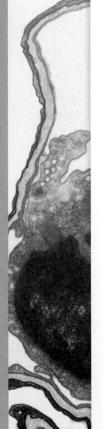

gestational diabetes A form of glucose intolerance diagnosed during pregnancy.

ghrelin Substance secreted by the epsilon cells; stimulates hunger.

gigantism Tall stature caused by excessive growth hormone levels prior to puberty.

glaucoma A group of eye conditions that lead to damage to the optic nerve. This damage is often caused by increased intraocular pressure, but it can also be caused by decreased blood flow to the optic nerve.

glomerular filtration rate (GFR) The best measure of renal functioning; it measures the speed at which blood moves through the glomerulus. GFR can be calculated using a formula that incorporates serum creatinine levels, age, gender, and ethnicity. Usual GFR is approximately 125 mL/minute.

glomerulonephritis A bilateral inflammatory disorder of the glomeruli that typically follows a streptococcal infection.

glomerulus A cluster of capillaries in the kidneys through which blood passes.

glucagon Substance secreted by alpha cells that is released when serum glucose levels fall. Glucagon stimulates the breakdown of glycogen to glucose, which raises serum glucose levels.

glucocorticoid Steroid that is secreted by the middle region of the adrenal cortex.

glucose A sugar molecule that provides energy.

goiter A visible enlargement of the thyroid gland.

gonadocorticoid Sex hormone secreted by the innermost region of the adrenal cortex.

gonorrhea Sexually transmitted infection caused by *Neisseria gonorrhoeae*. Referred to colloquially as the clap.

gout An inflammatory disease resulting from deposits of uric acid crystals in tissues and fluids within the body.

graft-versus-host rejection Type of tissue rejection in which the graft fights the host. This potentially life-threatening type of reaction occurs *only* with bone marrow transplants. The immunocompetent graft cells recognize the host cells as foreign and organize a cell-mediated attack. The host is usually immunocompromised and unable to fight the graft cells.

Graves' disease An autoimmune condition that stimulates thyroid hormone production.

greenstick fracture An incomplete fracture in which the bone is bent and only the outer curve of the bend is broken.

gross total incontinence A continuous leaking of urine, day and night, or the periodic uncontrollable leaking of large volumes of urine. In these cases, the bladder has no storage capacity.

gyrus (plural: **gyri**) A fold that increases the surface area of the cerebrum. At birth, these folds are minimal, but they increase as the brain develops into adulthood.

Hashimoto's thyroiditis The most common cause of thyroid gland failure. Also called autoimmune thyroiditis.

HCO₃ Bicarbonate. Part of the body's buffer system. It is secreted by the kidneys.

HDL High-density lipoprotein. HDL assists with removing cholesterol from the body. Also called good cholesterol.

health The absence of disease. Health can be expanded to include wellness of mind, body, and spirit. It is one's normal state.

heart failure A condition in which the heart is unable to pump an adequate amount of blood to meet metabolic needs. This pump inadequacy leads to decreased cardiac output, increased preload, and increased afterload. These three events result in decreased contractility and stroke volume. It is often referred to as congestive heart failure.

helper cell A type of regulator cell that activates, or calls up, B cells to produce antibodies.

hemangioma A vascular birthmark that appears as a bright red patch or a nodule of extra blood vessels in the skin. Also called a strawberry.

hematemesis Blood in the vomitus. Blood in the vomitus has a characteristic brown, granular appearance like coffee grounds.

hematocrit A laboratory expression of how much of the blood volume is being occupied by the erythrocytes.

hematoma A collection of blood in the tissue that develops from ruptured blood vessels. Hematomas can develop immediately or slowly and are classified by their location.

hematopoiesis The process of blood formation; it occurs primarily in the bone marrow.

hemoglobin Part of an erythrocyte. It binds to oxygen, giving blood its red color.

hemoglobin buffer system Buffer mechanism in the erythrocytes that works by binding to or releasing hydrogen and carbon dioxide.

hemoglobin S An abnormal type of hemoglobin that distorts the shape of erythrocytes, especially when there is low oxygen. These fragile, sickle-shaped cells deliver less oxygen to the body's tissues. These cells also can clog more easily in small blood vessels and break into pieces that disrupt blood flow.

hemolysis Excessive destruction of erythrocytes that causes hemolytic anemia.

hemophilia A An X-linked recessive bleeding disorder. Hemophilia A is a deficit or abnormality of clotting factor VIII. Also called classic hemophilia.

hemorrhagic stroke The most deadly kind of stroke. Occurs when blood vessels rupture inside the brain.

hepatic artery Part of the liver's dual blood supply; it carries oxygenated blood from the general circulation to the liver at a rate of approximately 300 mL per minute to nourish the liver.

hepatitis An inflammation of the liver that can be caused by infections (usually viral), alcohol, medications, or autoimmune disease.

hepatobiliary system The liver, gallbladder, and pancreas, collectively. They are called a system because of their close proximity to each other and their complementary functions.

herniated intervertebral disk A state in which the nucleus pulposus protrudes through the annulus fibrosus. Also called slipped disk and ruptured disk.

herniation The displacement of brain tissue.

herpes simplex type 1 A viral infection typically affecting the lips, mouth, and face. The common infection usually begins in childhood. Also called cold sore.

herpes simplex virus (HSV) One of a family of more than 70 herpes viruses; the cause of genital herpes.

herpes zoster A viral infection caused by the varicella-zoster virus. The condition appears in adulthood years after a primary infection of varicella (chickenpox) in childhood. The virus lies dormant on a cranial nerve or a spinal nerve dermatome until it is activated years later. The virus affects this nerve only. Also called shingles.

heterozygous Allele pair in which one is dominant and the other is recessive for a particular gene.

hiatal hernia Condition that occurs when a section of the stomach protrudes upward through an opening in the diaphragm toward the lung.

homeostasis Equilibrium, balance, consistency, or stability. It is a self-regulating, give-and-take system that responds to minor changes in the body through compensation mechanisms. Compensation mechanisms attempt to counteract those changes and return the body to its normal state.

homozygous Identical allele pair for a particular gene.

host-versus-graft rejection Most common type of tissue rejection. The host fights the graft.

human papillomavirus (HPV) Benign warts that cause genital warts. There are more than 70 different types of HPV, several of which can cause genital warts. In addition to genital warts, HPVs can lead to the development of reproductive (e.g., cervical and penile) and anal cancers.

Huntington's disease (HD) A condition caused by a genetically programmed degeneration of neurons in the brain. It is an autosomal dominant disorder involving a defect on chromosome 4. Also called Huntington's chorea.

hyaline cartilage The type of cartilage most associated with bone, often found in joints.

hydrocele Fluid accumulation between the layers of the tinica vaginalis or along the spermatic cord.

hydrocephalus A condition in which excess CSF accumulates within the skull, which dilates the ventricles and compresses the brain and blood vessels. The pressure from the excess CSF thins the cortex, causing severe brain damage.

hydronephrosis An abnormal dilation of the renal pelvis and the calyces of one or both kidneys that occurs secondary to a disease.

hymen A thin connective tissue that covers the external vaginal opening to some degree.

hyperacute tissue rejection Type of tissue rejection in which tissue rejections occur immediately to 3 days after the transplant. Hyperacute reactions occur due to a complement response in which the recipient has antibodies against the donor. This complement response triggers a systemic inflammatory reaction. The response is so quick that often the tissue has not had a chance to establish vascularization; as a result, the tissue becomes permanently necrotic.

hypercalcemia Condition that occurs when ionizing calcium levels climb above 5 mEq/L. Hypercalcemia results from excessive intake of ionizing calcium or release of ionizing calcium from the bone as well as inadequate excretion.

hyperchloremia An excess amount of chloride in the blood (> 108 mE/L). It is usually a result of an underlying condition and without its own clinical manifestations.

hyperglycemia An excess amount of glucose in the blood (> 180 mg/dL). It can be a result of an underlying conditions (e.g., diabetes mellitus) or medications (e.g., corticosteroid agents).

hyperkalemia Serum potassium levels greater than 5 mEq/L. Hyperkalemia is unusual in the healthy individual and may be a medical emergency.

hypermagnesemia Condition that occurs when magnesium levels increase above 2.5 mEq/L. Hypermagnesemia is rare and usually results from renal failure as well as excessive laxative or antacid use.

hypernatremia Condition that results from high serum sodium levels (> 145 mEq/L). The excessive sodium levels generally lead to high serum osmolality (> 295 mOsm/kg) because of the imbalance between sodium and water.

hyperparathyroidism A condition of excessive parathyroid hormone production by the parathyroid glands.

hyperphosphatemia Condition that occurs when phosphorus levels climb above 4.5 mg/dL.

hyperpituitarism A condition in which the pituitary gland secretes excessive amounts of one or all of the pituitary hormones.

hyperplasia An increase in the number of cells in an organ or tissue. This increase only occurs in cells that have the ability to perform mitotic division, such as epithelial cells.

hyperprolactinemia Excessive prolactin levels that result in menstrual dysfunction and galactorrhea (inappropriate lactation).

hypersensitivity An inflated or inappropriate response to an antigen. The result is inflammation and destruction of healthy tissue. Hypersensitivity reactions may be immediate, occurring within minutes to hours of reexposure, or delayed, occurring several hours after reexposure.

hypertension A prolonged elevation in blood pressure.

hyperthyroidism Hypermetabolic state caused by excessive thyroid hormones that result from increased thyrotropin levels.

hypertonic solution An intravascular solution that has a higher concentration of solutes than those in the intravascular compartment. Hypertonic solutions cause fluid to shift from the intracellular to the intravascular space.

hypertrophic cardiomyopathy Type of cardiomyopathy that mainly affects diastolic function.

hypertrophy Condition that occurs when cells increase in size in an attempt to meet increased work demand. This change may be a result of normal or abnormal changes.

hypervolemia Excess fluid in the intravascular compartment.

hypocalcemia Condition that occurs when ionized calcium levels fall below 4 mEq/L. Hypocalcemia occurs from increased losses or decreased intake of ionized calcium.

hypochloremia Condition that occurs when chloride levels fall below 98 mEq/L. Hypochloremia rarely occurs in the absence of other electrolyte abnormalities and, therefore, does not have its own set of clinical manifestations

hypodermis The innermost layer of the skin. It is comprised of soft, fatty tissue, as well as blood vessels, nerves, and immune cells. Also called subcutaneous tissue.

hypoglycemia A low serum glucose level.

hypokalemia Condition that occurs when potassium levels drop below 3.5 mEq/L. Usually, hypokalemia results from excessive loss, inadequate intake, or increased potassium cellular uptake.

hypomagnesemia Condition that occurs when magnesium levels drop below 1.8 mEq/L.

hyponatremia Condition that results from low serum sodium levels (< 135 mEq/L). Serum osmolality levels also fall below 275 mOsm.

hypoparathyroidism A condition in which the parathyroid gland does not produce sufficient amounts of parathyroid hormone.

hypophosphatemia Condition that occurs when phosphorus levels drop below 2.5 mg/dL.

hypopituitarism A rare, complex condition in which the pituitary gland does not produce sufficient amounts of some or all of its hormones.

hypospadias Condition in which the urethral meatus is on the ventral surface of the penis instead of the end.

hypothalamic-pituitary axis Hormones produced by the anterior pituitary gland and regulated by the hypothalamus.

hypothalamus The basal portion of the diencephalon, which regulates the pituitary gland. The hypothalamus connects the nervous and endocrine systems; it regulates many bodily functions.

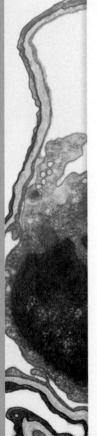

hypothyroidism A condition in which the thyroid does not produce sufficient amounts of the thyroid hormones.

hypotonic solution An intravascular solution that has a lower concentration of solutes than those in the intravascular compartment. Hypotonic solutions cause fluid to shift from the intravascular to the intracellular space.

hypovolemia Fluid deficit of the intravascular compartment.

hypovolemic shock Type of shock in which venous return reduces because of external blood volume losses. Preload drops, decreasing ventricular filling and stroke volume.

iatrogenic Caused by an unintended effect of a medical treatment.

idiopathic Unknown.

idiopathic thrombocytopenic purpura (ITP) A hypocoagulopathy state as a result of the immune system destroying its own platelets. It can be acute or chronic.

immunodeficiency A diminished or absent immune response that increases susceptibility to infections.

impacted fracture Type of fracture in which one end of the bone is forced into the adjacent bone.

impetigo A common and highly contagious skin infection. Although it can occur without an apparent break, it typically arises from a break in the skin. Impetigo spreads easily to others by direct contact with skin or contaminated objects. Lesions usually begin as a small vesicle that enlarges and ruptures, forming the characteristic honey-colored crust.

impregnation The fertilization of eggs.

incomplete fracture Type of fracture in which the bone is partially broken.

increased intracranial pressure Increased volume in the limited space of the cranial cavity. Increased intracranial pressure may occur because of a traumatic brain injury or because of other conditions that would increase the volume in the skull.

incus Bone in the ear that vibrates as a result of the malleus rocking, which, in turn, causes the stapes to move in and out against the oval window. Also called anvil.

infarction Permanent damage to tissue.

infectious mononucleosis A disease caused by the Epstein-Barr virus, a common virus of the herpes family. Most people are exposed to the virus as children, and because of the exposure, they develop immunity to the virus and do not ever develop infectious mononucleosis. Also known as mono and the kissing disease.

infectious rhinitis The common cold, a viral upper respiratory infection. The most frequent culprit is the rhinovirus, but it can be caused by many viruses.

infective endocarditis An infection of the endocardium. It was previously called bacterial endocarditis.

inferior vena cava Large vein that carries deoxygenated blood from the lower half of the body to the right atrium.

infertility A biologic inability to contribute to reproduction.

inflammatory bowel disease Chronic inflammation of the gastrointestinal tract, usually the intestines.

inflammatory response A series of reactions triggered by damage or trauma to body tissue.

influenza A viral infection that may affect the upper and lower respiratory tract. There are three strains: A, B, and C. The virus is highly adaptive and constantly mutates, preventing the development of any long-term immune defense.

initiation Phase of carcinogenesis in which the exposure of the cell to a substance or event causes DNA damage or mutation.

inner ear Division of the ear that is comprised of the cochlea, semicircular canals, saccule, and utricle.

inotropic The strength of contraction.

insidious Onset of a disease with vague symptoms.

inspiration Inhalation. One of two phases of breathing. Inspiration is an active neural process that begins with nerve impulses traveling from the brain to the diaphragm.

inspiratory reserve volume The amount of air beyond the tidal volume that can be taken in with the deepest inhalation.

insulin Hormone secreted by beta cells that is released when serum glucose levels increase. Insulin stimulates cellular uptake of glucose, which decreases serum glucose levels.

interferon A small protein that is released from cells infected by viruses. It prevents the virus from replicating and boosts the immune system.

interneuron A neuron that connects the sensory and motor neurons in the spinal cord.

interstitial A fluid compartment between the cells.

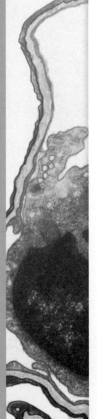

interstitial pneumonia A type of pneumonia that occurs in the areas between the alveoli. Interstitial pneumonia is routinely caused by viruses (e.g., influenza type A and B) or by uncommon bacteria (e.g., *Legionella*). Also called atypical pneumonia.

intestinal obstruction Blockage of intestinal contents in the small intestine or large intestine.

intracellular fluid Fluid found inside the cells.

intracerebral hematoma A hematoma that results from bleeding in the brain tissue. Intracerebral hematomas are caused by contusion or shearing injuries but can also result from hypertension, cerebral vascular accidents (strokes), aneurysms, or vascular abnormalities.

intractable pain Chronically progressing pain that is unrelenting and severely debilitating. This type of pain does not usually respond well to typical pharmacologic pain treatments. Intractable pain is common with severe injuries, especially crushing injuries.

intrarenal condition Cause of acute renal failure that directly damages the structures of the kidneys.

intravascular A fluid compartment inside the blood vessels.

intrinsic asthma Type of asthma that usually presents after age 35 and is not an allergic reaction. Intrinsic triggers include upper respiratory infections, air pollution, emotional stress, smoke, exercise, and cold exposure.

iris The colored portion of the eye. The iris contains smooth muscle fibers that control the diameter of the pupil to regulate light entering the eye.

irregular bone One of five types of bones found within the skeleton. Irregular bones do not fall into any other category, due to their nonuniform shape. Irregular bones primarily consist of spongy bone, with a thin outer layer of compact bone.

irritable bowel syndrome (IBS) A chronic gastrointestinal condition characterized by exacerbations associated with stress. Irritable bowel syndrome includes alterations in bowel pattern and abdominal pain not explained by structural or biochemical abnormalities.

ischemia Decreased blood flow to tissue or an organ. It essentially strangles the tissue or organ by limiting necessary nutrients and oxygen.

ischemic stroke The most common type of stroke. Caused by an interruption in blood flow, often resulting from a thrombus or emboli.

islet of Langerhans Area situated among the many small acini in the pancreas that carries out endocrine functions. The human pancreas contains approximately 1 million islets of Langerhans, and each islet of Langerhans contains five types of cells.

isotonic solution An intravascular solution that has concentrations of solutes equal to those in the intravascular compartment. Because of these solute concentrations, isotonic solutions allow fluid to move equally between compartments.

isthmus A thin band of tissue that connects the two lobes of the thyroid gland by extending across the anterior aspect of the trachea.

jaundice A yellowish discoloration of the skin and sclera caused by an excessive amount of bilirubin in the bloodstream. Can be a result of bile entering the bloodstream or erythrocyte lysis.

joint A structure that connects bones of the skeleton. Joints are classified by their degree of movement: moveable, slightly moveable, and immoveable.

joint capsule The saclike envelope enclosing the cavity of a synovial joint.

karyotype A representation of a person's individual set of chromosomes.

keratin A protein that strengthens skin.

keratitis An inflammation of the cornea that can be triggered by an infection or trauma.

killer cell A type of T cell that destroys cells infected with viruses by releasing lymphokines that destroy cell walls. Also called cytotoxic cell and effector cell.

kyphosis An increase in the curvature of the thoracic spine outward. Also called hunchback.

labia majora The two large, fatty skin folds that protect the perineum and aid in lubrication.

labia minora Two small, firm skin folds just inside the labia majora.

lacrimal duct The duct through which tears drain on the inner side of each eye.

lacrimal gland The gland that keeps the inner surface of the eyelid and the exposed surface of the eye moist.

lactation The production and secretion of milk for the feeding of offspring.

lamella (plural: **lamellae**) A thin layer of osteocytes.

large intestine Part of the lower gastrointestinal tract. It is 5 feet long in adults and contains the cecum, colon, and rectum.

laryngitis An inflammation of the larynx that is usually a result of an infection, increased upper respiratory exudate, or overuse. With laryngitis, the vocal cords become irritated and edematous because of the inflammatory process. This inflammation distorts sounds, leading to hoarseness and in some cases making the voice undetectable.

laryngotracheobronchitis A common viral infection in children 1–2 years of age. Older children and adults may also contract it. It usually begins as an upper respiratory infection with nasal congestion and cough. The larynx and surrounding area swell, leading to airway narrowing and obstruction. This swelling can lead to respiratory failure. Also called croup.

larynx The voice box. The larynx is made of cartilage and plays a central role in swallowing and talking.

latent herpes genitalis The second stage of genital herpes, which begins once the antibodies are formed.

latent syphilis The final stage of syphilis. The early latency stage begins when the secondary symptoms disappear and lasts 1–4 years. The late latency stage can last for years as the infection spreads to the brain, nervous system, heart, skin, and bones. Also called tertiary syphilis.

LDL Low-density lipoprotein. It is a major contributor of plaque formation associated with atherosclerosis. Also called bad cholesterol.

left atrium Receiving chamber on the left side of the heart. Receives blood from the pulmonary circulation, and blood leaves this chamber and travels to the left ventricle.

left-sided heart failure Type of heart failure that results from ineffective left ventricular contractility. As cardiac output falls, blood that is not being pumped out into the body backs up in the left atrium and then the pulmonary circulation.

left ventricle Pumping chamber on the left side of the heart. This chamber pumps blood to the systemic circulation.

legionnaires' disease A specific type of pneumonia that is caused by *Legionella pneumophila*. The bacteria thrive in warm, moist environments, particularly air conditioning systems and spas. Legionnaires' disease is not contagious. Most people acquire this type of pneumonia from inhaling the bacteria as they are spread by an air conditioning system or spa.

leiomyoma A uterine fibroid; a firm, rubbery growth of the myometrium.

lens A transparent, flexible structure that lies behind the iris. Smooth muscles attached to the lens alter its shape to focus on objects.

lentigo A large, pigmented spot that may appear in a sun-exposed area. Also called age spot and liver spot.

leukemia A cancer of the leukocytes. With leukemia, the bone marrow makes abnormal leukocytes. Leukemia cells do not die when they should, sometimes crowding out normal leukocytes, erythrocytes, and thrombocytes. This crowding makes it difficult for normal blood cells to do their work.

leukocyte White blood cell.

leukocytopenia Refers to decreased white blood cell levels; can indicate an immune deficiency state (e.g., bone marrow suppression).

leukocytosis Describes states of increased white blood cell levels; can indicate an active infectious process.

ligament A bundle of dense connective tissue that connects bones to bones in a joint and provide support to the joint.

linear skull fracture A simple crack in the skull.

lipid A broad group of naturally occurring molecules which includes fats, fat-soluble vitamins (such as vitamins A, D, E and K), monoglycerides, diglycerides, phospholipids, and others. The main biological functions of lipids include energy storage, as structural components of cell membranes, and as important signaling molecules.

lipid bilayer A fatty double covering that makes up the membrane of a cell. The interior surface of the bilayer is uncharged and primarily lipids. The exterior surface of the bilayer is charged and is less fatty than the interior surface.

liquefaction necrosis Type of necrosis that occurs when caustic enzymes dissolve and liquefy necrotic cells.

liver An organ that performs as many as 500 different functions. Some of the liver's primary roles are vital for homeostasis.

liver cancer Cancer of the liver. It most commonly occurs as a secondary tumor that has metastasized from the breast, lung, or other gastrointestinal structures.

lobar pneumonia Type of pneumonia that is confined to a single lobe in the lung and is described by that affected lobe (e.g., right upper lobe).

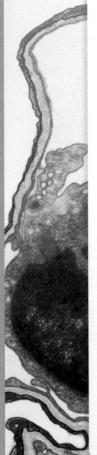

lobe Subdivision of a bodily organ or part, delineated by shape or connective tissue. Examples can be seen in the lung and brain.

local adaptation syndrome The localized version of general adaptation syndrome. In this syndrome, the body is making an attempt to limit the damage associated with the stressor by confining the stressor to one location.

long bone One of five types of bones found within the skeleton. A long bone has a body that is longer than it is wide, growth plates at either end, a hard outer surface, and an inner region that is less dense than the outer region and contains bone marrow.

longitudinal fissure The dividing point of the cerebrum into right and left hemispheres.

lordosis An exaggerated concave of the lumbar spine. Also called swayback.

lower esophageal sphincter (LES) Part of the upper gastrointestinal system that relaxes to allow the food to enter the stomach and prevents the stomach contents from refluxing into the esophagus.

lung Organ responsible for gas exchange.

lung cancer Cancer of the lung. The third most common neoplasm that can arise as a primary and secondary tumor.

lymph Fluid that drains from the lymph capillaries into larger vessels and ducts that empty into large veins at the base of the neck. The movement of lymph occurs much in the same way that blood moves through veins, with the assistance of valves and movement.

lymphatic system An extensive network of vessels and glands that returns excess fluid in body tissue to the circulatory system and works with the immune system.

lymphedema Swelling, usually in the arms and legs, because of lymph obstruction. Lymphedema can occur on its own or as a result of another disease or condition.

lysis Bursting of a cell that occurs if too much water enters the cell membrane, causing excessive swelling.

macular degeneration A deterioration of the macular area of the retina caused by impaired blood supply to the macula that results in the cellular waste accumulation and ischemia.

macular stain The most common type of vascular birthmark. These birthmarks are faint red marks often occurring on the forehead, eyelids, posterior neck, nose, upper lip, or posterior head. Also called salmon patch, angel kiss, and stork bite.

magnesium An intracellular cation that is mostly stored in the bone and muscle.

malignant State of a tumor that is usually made up of undifferentiated, nonfunctioning cells that are reproducing rapidly. Malignant tumors often penetrate surrounding tissue and spread to secondary sites.

malignant hypertension An intensified form of hypertension that may not respond well to treatment efforts.

malleus A bone that lies near the tympanic membrane. Vibrations from the membranes cause the malleus to rock back and forth. Also called hammer.

mammary glands Glands located in the breast of the male and female, but function only in females. The mammary glands produce milk when stimulated to do so.

manifestation The clinical effects or evidence of a disease. Manifestations may include both signs, what can be seen or measured, and symptoms, what the patient describes.

mastication Chewing.

mastitis An inflammation of the breast tissue that can be associated with infection and lactation.

matrix Extracellular material in which osteocytes are embedded. The matrix consists of calcium phosphate crystals that make the bones hard and strong. The matrix also contains collagen fibers that reinforce the bone, giving it flexible strength.

meatus The opening or passageway.

medulla 1. The part of the brain stem that acts as the conduction pathway for ascending and descending nerve tracts. The medulla coordinates heart rate, peripheral vascular resistance, breathing, swallowing, vomiting, coughing, and sneezing. 2. The inner portion of an adrenal gland. It is regulated by nerve impulses from the hypothalamus and produces epinephrine and norepinephrine during times of stress.

meiosis A form of cell division that occurs only in mature sperm and ova.

melanin A pigment that provides color and protection from ultraviolet rays. Disorders involving melanin result in alterations in skin coloring and can leave the skin vulnerable to the harmful effects of UV light. Melanin disorders include albinism and vitiligo.

melena Dark, tarry stool from a significant amount of bleeding high in the gastrointestinal tract.

memory cell Type of B cell that aids quick response to subsequent exposures to an antigen because memory cells recall the antigen as foreign, and antibody production is rapid.

Meniere's disease A disorder of the inner ear that results from endolymph swelling, which stretches the membranes and interferes with the hair receptors in the cochlea and vestibule.

meninges A set of three tough membranes that encase the central nervous system.

meningitis An inflammation of the meninges, usually resulting from an infection.

meningocele A rare form of spina bifida that involves a bony defect, but the meninges protrude through the vertebral opening.

menopause The complete and permanent cessation of the menstrual cycle.

menorrhagia Increased menstrual blood flow amount and duration.

menstrual cycle A series of monthly changes that begin at puberty and continue through the reproductive years.

menstruation Shedding of the endometrium. It generally occurs on a regular basis (usually every 28 days) during the reproductive years of women. Also called period.

mesentery A double-layer peritoneum containing blood vessels and nerves that supplies the intestinal wall.

metabolic acidosis Condition that results from a deficiency of bicarbonate or an excess of hydrogen.

metabolic alkalosis Condition that results from an excess of bicarbonate or a deficiency of hydrogen.

metabolic syndrome A cluster of risk factors occurring together—hyperglycemia, high blood pressure, hypercholesterolemia, and increased waist circumference. Metabolic syndrome increases the risk of cardiovascular disease, diabetes mellitus, and stroke.

metaphase Phase of mitosis in which the spindle fibers attach to centromeres and chromosomes align.

metaplasia The process of one adult cell being replaced by another cell type.

metrorrhagia Vaginal bleeding between menstrual periods in premenopausal women.

microtia An underdeveloped, small auricle.

micturition Urination.

midbrain The smallest region of the brain, and it acts as a sort of relay station for auditory and visual information. The midbrain controls the visual and auditory systems as well as eye movement.

middle ear Division of the ear that includes the tympanic membrane and the ossicles.

mineralocorticoid Steroid produced by the outermost region of the adrenal cortex.

minute respiratory volume The amount inhaled and exhaled in 1 minute. It is determined by the tidal volume multiplied by the respirations per minute.

mitosis The most common form of cell division, where the cell divides into two separate cells. In mitosis, the division of one cell results in two genetically identical and equal daughter cells. This process occurs in four phases: prophase, metaphase, anaphase, and telophase.

mitral valve A bicuspid valve that guides the passage of blood from the left atria to the left ventricle and prevents the backward flow of blood

mixed dysfunction A categorization of heart failure that is a combination of systolic and diastolic dysfunction.

mixed incontinence Type of incontinence that occurs when symptoms of more than one type of urinary incontinence are experienced.

mole A brown nevus. Moles can be tan, brown, or black; can be flat or raised; and may have hair growth.

Mongolian spot Type of birthmark that is a flat, bluish-gray area often found on the lower back or buttocks. These birthmarks are most common on those with darker complexions.

Monro-Kellie hypothesis A supposition that states that the cranial cavity cannot be compressed, and the volume inside the cavity is fixed (normal intracranial pressure is 60–200 mm H_2O or 4–15 mm Hg). The skull and its components create a state of volume equilibrium, such that any increase in volume of one component must be compensated by a decrease in volume of another.

mons pubis The pad of fat over the symphysis pubis that becomes covered with hair after puberty.

motor nerve A type of nerve that carries impulses from the brain to the corresponding muscle receptor, resulting in muscle contraction and movement. Also called efferent nerve.

mucosa The innermost of four layers of the walls of the gastrointestinal tract. The mucosa produces mucus.

mucus A thick, sticky substance produced by the goblet cells in the epithelial lining of the nose, trachea, and bronchi.

multifactorial disorder A result of an interaction between genes and environmental factors. Such a disorder does not follow a clear-cut pattern of inheritance. Multifactorial disorders may be present at birth, as with cleft lip or palate, or they may be expressed later in life, as with hypertension.

multiple myeloma A cancer of the plasma cells that most often affects older adults. Multiple myeloma is characterized by excessive numbers of abnormal plasma cells in the bone marrow crowding out the blood-forming cells and causing Bence Jones proteins to be excreted in the urine.

multiple sclerosis (MS) A debilitating autoimmune condition that involves a progressive and irreversible demyelination of brain, spinal cord, and cranial nerves neurons. This damage occurs in diffuse patches throughout the nervous system and slows or stops nerve impulses.

muscle fiber Muscle cell that is a cylinder with multiple nuclei.

muscle layer One of four layers of the walls of the gastrointestinal tract. It includes circular and longitudinal smooth muscle layers. This layer contracts in a wavelike motion to propel food through the gastrointestinal tract.

muscular dystrophy (MD) A group of inherited disorders characterized by degeneration of skeletal muscle. Muscles become weaker as damage worsens. There are nine different forms of muscular dystrophy.

myasthenia gravis An autoimmune condition in which acetylcholine receptors are impaired or destroyed by IgG autoantibodies, leading to a disruption of normal communication between the nerve and muscle at the neuromuscular junction.

myasthenic crisis A potentially life-threatening complication of myasthenia gravis that occurs when the muscles become too weak to maintain adequate ventilation.

myelin sheath Covering that surrounds axons to increase the rate of impulse transmission.

myelomeningocele The most severe form of spina bifida. In this form, the spinal canal remains open along several vertebrae in the lower or middle back. Also called open spina bifida.

myocardial infarction (MI) Death of the myocardium from sudden blockage of coronary artery blood flow. Other names for a myocardial infarction include heart attack and acute coronary syndrome.

myocarditis An inflammation of the myocardium. This is an uncommon condition, in which there is a period of at least several weeks (in some cases a decade) between exposure of the causative agent and the development of symptoms.

myocardium The middle layer of the heart; the muscle portion of the organ.

myofibril A threadlike structure that extends the entire length of the muscle fiber.

myofilament Protein fibers found in muscle fibers.

myometrium The middle layer of the uterine wall, made up of smooth muscle and a vascular system. During pregnancy, the vascular system radically increases to support the fetus.

myosin One of two types of myofilament. It is the darker and thicker of the two. Myosin myofilaments are fibrous globulins that work with actin to form actomyosin.

myxedema Advanced hypothyroidism. The condition is rare, but when it occurs, it can be life threatening. Clinical manifestations include marked hypotension, respiratory depression, hypothermia, lethargy, and coma.

nausea A subjective urge to vomit that may precede vomiting.

necrosis A cell's inability to survive due to the extent of damage.

necrotizing fasciitis A rare, serious infection that can aggressively destroy skin, fat, muscle, and other tissue. One out of four people with this infection will die because of it. Also called flesh-eating bacteria.

negative feedback system One of two types of feedback systems that maintains homeostasis (the other is a positive feedback system). The negative feedback system is the most common type and works to maintain a deficit in the system. Examples of negative feedback systems include temperature and glucose regulation.

neoplasm A cellular growth that is no longer responding to normal regulator processes, usually because of a mutation. Also called a tumor.

nephritic syndrome Inflammatory injury to the glomeruli that can occur because of antibodies interacting with normally occurring antigens in the glomeruli.

nephron One of 1–2 million microscopic filtering units in the kidney. Each is similar to a long-stemmed funnel and has multiple sections, and each section is responsible for excreting or reabsorbing specific substances.

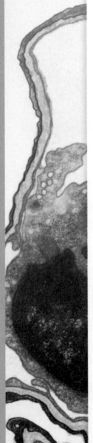

nephrotic syndrome Condition that results from antibody-antigen complexes lodging in the glomerular membrane, triggering the complement system.

nerve Part of the peripheral nervous system that consists of bundles of nerve fibers, and each fiber is part of the neuron.

neurogenic bladder All bladder dysfunction caused by an interruption of normal bladder nerve innervation.

neurogenic shock Type of distributive shock in which a loss of sympathetic tone in vascular smooth muscle and autonomic function lead to massive vasodilatation. Blood pools in the venous system, leading to decreased venous return, cardiac output, and hypotension.

neuroglia Type of cells that provide several important supportive roles in the nervous system. Neuroglia cells scaffold neural tissue as well as isolate and protect neuron cell membranes. Additionally, neuroglia cells regulate interstitial fluid, defend the neuron against pathogens, and assist with neural repair.

neuromelanin A specialized, dark pigment found in the brain.

neuron The fundamental unit of the nervous system. Neurons generate bioelectric impulses and transmit them from one area of the body to another.

neuropathic pain Pain that results from damage to peripheral nerves by disease or injury. This type of pain tends to be chronic and intractable.

neurotransmitter Chemical that is released from the presynaptic terminal and crosses the synaptic cleft in one direction to stimulate an electrical reaction in nearby neurons.

neutropenia An insufficient number of circulating neutrophils (fewer than 1,500 cells/μL; the normal range is 2,000–7,500 cells/μL). With fewer of these first responders, the body is poorly equipped to fight infections. The degree to which the body can fight infections, especially bacterial infections, is related to the severity of the neutropenia.

neutrophil An infection-fighting agent. Usually the first to arrive on the scene of an infection, neutrophils are attracted by various chemicals released by infected tissue. Neutrophils escape from the capillary wall and migrate to the site of infection. Once they get to the site, neutrophils phagocytize microorganisms, preventing the infection from spreading.

nipple Part of the breast surrounded by the areola.

nocturnal asthma Type of asthma that usually occurs between 3:00 and 7:00 a.m. and is thought to be related to circadian rhythms. At night, cortisol and epinephrine levels decrease, while histamine levels increase.

nocturnal enuresis Bed-wetting.

node of Ranvier Node that separates Schwann cells.

non–small cell carcinoma An aggressive type of lung cancer. It is the most common type of malignant lung cancer. It has several subgroups—squamous cell carcinoma, adenocarcinoma, and bronchioalveolar carcinoma. It is often referred to as bronchogenic carcinoma.

noncommunicating hydrocephalus Type of hydrocephalus that occurs when the cerebrospinal fluid flow is disrupted or not properly absorbed by the bloodstream. Also called obstructive hydrocephalus.

nonvolatile acid An acid produced from sources other than carbon dioxide, and is not excreted by the lungs.

norepinephrine Hormone produced by the medulla during times of stress. With epinephrine, it mediates the fight-or-flight response of the sympathetic nervous system.

nosocomial pneumonia Pneumonia that develops more than 48 hours after a hospital admission.

nucleotide Molecules that join together to form RNA and DNA.

nucleus The control center of the cell, which contains all the genetic information (DNA) for the cell and is surrounded by a double membrane. The nucleus regulates cell growth, metabolism, and reproduction.

nystagmus Rapid, involuntary back-and-forth eye movement.

oblique fracture A fracture at an angle to the bone shaft.

obstructive hydrocephalus A type of hydrocephalus that occurs when cerebrospinal fluid flow is disrupted or not properly absorbed by the bloodstream. Also called obstructive hydrocephalus.

occipital lobe Lobe of the brain that processes visual information.

occult blood Blood that occurs in small amounts and is not usually apparent.

occupational asthma A type of asthma that is caused by a reaction to substances encountered at work. Symptoms develop over time, worsening with each exposure and improving when one is away from work.

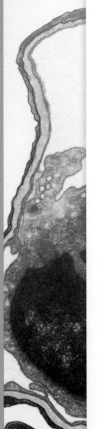

oligomenorrhea Infrequent menstruation; a long menstrual cycle.

oncogene Gene that activates cell division and influences embryonic development.

oogenesis The generation of eggs.

open-angle (chronic) glaucoma Type of glaucoma in which intraocular pressure increases gradually over an extended period. This is the most common type.

open fracture Type of fracture in which the skin is broken. The bone fragments or edges may be angled and protrude out of the skin. Open fractures have more damage to soft tissue and are at risk for infection.

opportunistic infection An infection caused by pathogens that do not normally cause disease in healthy individuals.

optic nerve The nerve formed at the back of the eye by axons of the ganglion cells coming together. This area contains no photoreceptors and is insensitive to light.

oral cancer Cancer anywhere in the mouth. Most are squamous cell carcinomas of the tongue and mouth floor. Approximately 75% of cases can be attributed to smoked and smokeless tobacco.

organ of Corti Part of the cochlea that contains hearing receptors, the hair cells. Vibrations at the organ of Corti stimulate hair movement.

organelle An internal cellular structure. Organelles perform the work that maintains the cell's life.

orgasm The climax of pleasurable sensations.

osmolarity Solute concentration.

osmosis The movement of water or another solvent across the cellular membrane from an area of low solute concentration to an area of high solute concentration.

osmotic pressure The tendency of water to move by osmosis.

ossicle Part of the ear consisting of three bones—malleus, incus, and stapes.

osteoarthritis (OA) A localized joint disease characterized by deterioration of articulating cartilage and its underlying bone as well as bony overgrowth. The surface of the cartilage becomes rough and worn, interfering with joint movement. Also called the wear-and-tear arthritis and degenerative joint disease.

osteoblast Cell on the outer surface of the periosteum that aids in remodeling and repair by rebuilding new compact bone to increase bone strength.

osteoclast A cell that breaks down some spongy bone.

osteocyte Osteoblast that has become surrounded by calcified extracellular material.

osteomalacia A softening and weakening of bones in adults, usually because of an extreme and prolonged vitamin D, calcium, or phosphate deficiency.

osteomyelitis An infection of the bone tissue.

osteonecrosis Death of bone tissue due to a loss of blood supply. Also called avascular necrosis.

osteopenia Bone mass that is less than expected for age, ethnicity, or gender.

osteoporosis A condition characterized by a progressive loss of bone calcium that leaves the bones brittle.

osteosarcoma An aggressive tumor that begins in the bone cells, usually in the femur, tibia, or fibula.

otitis externa An infection or inflammation of the external ear canal or auricle. Also called swimmer's ear.

otitis media An infection or inflammation of the middle ear. Otitis media is a common condition in young children.

otosclerosis An abnormal bone growth in the middle ear, usually involving an imbalance in bone formation and resorption.

outer ear Division of the ear that consists of the auricle (or pinna), ear lobe, and external ear canal.

oval window The opening to the inner ear covered with a membrane. Movement of the oval window causes fluid within the cochlea to vibrate, creating waves.

ovarian cancer Cancer of the ovaries. There is no reliable screening test, it is difficult to treat, and it often has metastasized at the time of diagnosis. However, advances in treatment are improving the survival rates.

ovarian cyst A benign, fluid-filled sac on the ovary. Often the cyst forms in the ovulation process. Instead of the follicle releasing the egg, the fluid stays in the follicle, creating a cyst.

ovaries Paired, almond-shaped organs located on each side of the uterus.

overactive bladder Urge incontinence with no known cause.

overflow incontinence Incontinence as a result of an inability to empty the bladder.

ovulation The transportation of the eggs.

pacemaker Cells that create the rhythmic, chemical impulses that in turn cause contraction of the heart muscle. The rate at which these impulses fire controls the heart rate.

PaCO₂ The partial pressure of carbon dioxide; it indicates the adequacy of pulmonary ventilation.

Paget's disease A progressive condition characterized by abnormal bone destruction and remodeling, which results in bone deformities.

pain A subjective feeling that serves as a protective mechanism, warning the body when something is wrong. In addition, pain is the most common reason that people seek medical attention and can be used to aid diagnosis.

pain threshold The perception of pain.

pain tolerance The amount of pain that an individual can physically and emotionally withstand.

palliative A goal of treatment aimed at increasing comfort.

pancreas An organ with exocrine digestive functions and endocrine functions. The pancreas lies underneath the stomach and liver and between the two kidneys in the retroperitoneum.

pancreatic cancer An aggressive malignancy (most commonly adenocarcinoma) of the pancreas that can quickly spread to structures nearby.

pancreatic polypeptide Substance secreted by cells that is thought to regulate some of the pancreatic activities.

pancreatitis An inflammation of the pancreas that can be acute or chronic.

pancytopenia A lack of erythrocytes, leukocytes, and platelets.

pandemic An epidemic that has spread to a larger population.

papule A small, red, elevated area of the skin.

paralytic ileus A functional intestinal obstruction.

paraphimosis A condition in which the foreskin is retracted and cannot be returned over the glans penis.

parasympathetic nervous system Subdivision of the autonomic nervous system that is responsible for the rest-and-digest response.

parathyroid gland A gland located on the posterior surface of the thyroid. There are usually four; each parathyroid gland secretes the parathyroid hormone.

parathyroid hormone (PTH) A hormone that works in opposition to calcitonin to regulate serum calcium levels.

parietal lobe The lobe of the brain that receives and interprets sensory input with the exception of smell, hearing, and vision.

parietal peritoneum layer The outer layer of the peritoneum that covers the abdominal wall as well as the top of the bladder and uterus.

Parkinson's disease A progressive condition involving the destruction of the substantia nigra in the brain. This destruction results in a lack of dopamine, a chemical messenger that allows smooth, coordinated muscle movement.

partial pressure of oxygen The concentration of oxygen in the blood.

partially compensated A pH level that is abnormal.

parturition The birth of the fetus.

passive acquired immunity The process gained by receiving antibodies made outside the body by another person, animal, or recombinant DNA. In passive immunity, the person is not actively producing antibodies, and protection is short lived. Examples of passive immunity include mother-to-fetus transfer through placenta or breastfeeding transference.

pathogenesis The development of a disease.

pathologic fracture A type of fracture in that results from a weakness in the bone structure secondary to conditions such as tumors or osteoporosis.

pathophysiology The study of changes in normal anatomy and physiology goes wrong.

pediculosis A lice infestation that can take three forms—*Pediculus humanus corpus* (body louse), *Pediculus pubic* (pubic louse), and *Pediculus humanus capitis* (head louse). Lice are small, brown, parasitic insects that feed off human blood and cannot survive for long without the human host.

pelvic inflammatory disease (PID) An infection of the female reproductive system.

penile cancer Cancer of the penis. The exact cause is unknown, but risk is thought to be increased by the presence of smegma, being uncircumcised, poor hygiene, phimosis, and HPV infection.

penis Part of the male external genitalia; contains erectile tissue that fills with blood during sexual arousal.

peptic ulcer disease (PUD) Erosive lesions affecting the lining of the stomach or duodenum.

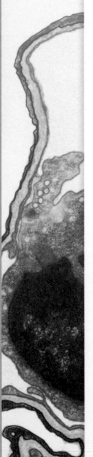

perfusion The process of delivering oxygen and nutrients with arterial blood to tissue.

pericardial effusion Fluid accumulation between the pericardium and the heart.

pericarditis An inflammation of the pericardium. The fluid may be serous, purulent, serosanguineous, or hemorrhagic. As the pericardial tissue becomes inflamed, the swollen tissue rubs together, creating friction.

pericardium Sac that encloses, protects, and supports the heart.

perimetrium The outer, serous layer of the uterine wall that covers all of the fundus, part of the corpus, but none of the cervix.

periosteum A layer of connective tissue that covers compact bone surfaces. The periosteum serves as the site of muscle attachment (via tendons).

peripheral nerve A nerve that branches from a plexus and supplies sensory and motor functions to many areas of the body.

peripheral nervous system (PNS) A division of the nervous system made up of the nerves.

peripheral vascular disease (PVD) A narrowing in the peripheral vessels. Most often this condition is caused by atherosclerosis, but it can also be caused by thrombus, inflammation (e.g., thromboangiitis obliterans), or vasospasms (e.g., Raynaud's disease and Raynaud's phenomenon).

peripheral vascular resistance (PVR) The force opposing the blood in the peripheral circulation. PVR increases as the diameter and elasticity of the blood vessels decreases.

peristalsis The wavelike contraction of the muscle layer of the gastrointestinal tract that propels food through the gastrointestinal tract.

peritoneal cavity The space between the parietal peritoneum layer and the visceral peritoneum layer that contains serous fluid to decrease friction and facilitate movement.

peritoneum The large serous membrane that lines the abdominal cavity.

peritonitis An inflammation of the peritoneum that can be life threatening.

pH A measure of hydrogen concentration in the plasma. The pH measure is a negative logarithm that reflects hydrogen concentrations; the higher the hydrogen concentration, the lower the pH number.

phagocytosis Endocytosis that involves solid particles. Also called cell eating.

phantom pain Pain that exists after the removal of a body part. The affected person may feel the discomfort of the removed part. The severing of neurons may result in spontaneous firing of spinal cord neurons because normal sensory input has been lost. This type of pain can be very distressing but usually resolves with time.

pharynx Passageway that connects the oral and nasal cavities to the larynx.

phenotype The outwardly, physical expression of genes, such as eye color.

pheochromocytoma A rare tumor of the adrenal medulla. The tumor excretes epinephrine and norepinephrine and can be life threatening because of the effects of epinephrine and norepinephrine.

phimosis Condition that occurs when the foreskin cannot be retracted from the glans penis.

phosphate buffer system Buffer mechanism that acts much like the bicarbonate-carbonic acid system. Buffering in this system primarily takes place in the kidneys by moving hydrogen.

phosphorus Phosphate. It is found in the bones and, in smaller quantities, in the bloodstream.

pia mater The innermost layer of the meninges; it rests directly on the brain and spinal cord.

pigmented birthmark A birthmark made of a cluster of pigment cells, which cause color in skin. These birthmarks can be many different colors, from tan to brown, gray to black, or even blue.

pink puffers Nickname given to those patients with emphysema, who often hyperventilate, creating a pink appearance to their skin.

pinocytosis Endocytosis that involves a liquid. Also called cell drinking.

pituitary gland Pea-sized gland located at the base of the brain. The pituitary gland can be divided into two parts—the anterior and posterior pituitary gland. The pituitary gland is often referred to as the master gland. Despite its size, the pituitary gland secretes several hormones that influence many different body functions.

placenta A vascular organ that develops during pregnancy to nourish the fetus through the umbilical cord.

plasma Liquid portion of the blood primarily comprised of protein.

plasma membrane The semipermeable boundary of a cell containing the cell and its components. Also called cell membrane.

plasmin An enzyme that dissolves clots once healing has occurred.

pleural effusion The accumulation of excess fluid in the pleural cavity that can compress the lung and limit expansion during inhalation.

pleurisy Inflammation of the pleural membranes, which leads to swollen and irregular tissue. This inflammation is often associated with pneumonia and creates friction in the pleural membranes.

plexus An organized collaboration of several intersected nerves.

***pneumocystis carinii* pneumonia** A specific type of pneumonia that is caused by a yeastlike fungus, *Pneumocystosis jiroveci*. This type of pneumonia occurs as an opportunistic infection and can be fatal to the immune compromised (e.g., children or those with AIDS or cancer).

pneumonia An inflammatory process caused by numerous infectious agents (e.g., bacteria, viruses, and fungi) and injurious agents or events (e.g., aspiration and smoke). *Streptococcus pneumonia* is responsible for 75% of all cases of pneumonia.

pneumothorax Air in the pleural cavity. The presence of atmospheric air in the pleural cavity and the separation to pleural membranes can lead to atelectasis. The pressure can cause a partial or complete collapse of a lung.

polycystic kidney disease (PKD) An inherited disorder characterized by numerous grape-like clusters of fluid-filled cysts in both kidneys.

polycystic ovary syndrome A condition in which the ovary enlarges and contains numerous cysts.

polydipsia Excessive thirst.

polymenorrhea Frequent menstruation due to a short menstrual cycle.

polyphagia An increase in hunger sensation.

polyuria An increase in the amount of water that is excreted.

pons The part of the brain stem that contains nerves that regulate sleep and breathing.

port-wine stain Vascular birthmark that looks like wine was spilled on an area of the body. These birthmarks most often occur on the face, neck, arms, and legs.

portal hypertension Increase in vessel pressures sin the hepatic artery and the portal vein. This increased pressure is often associated with liver disease.

portal vein Part of the liver's dual blood supply; it carries partially deoxygenated blood from the stomach, pancreas, and spleen, as well as from the small and large intestines to the liver at a rate of approximately 1,000 mL per minute so that the liver can process nutrients and digestion byproducts.

positive feedback system One of two types of feedback systems that maintains homeostasis (the other is a negative feedback system). The positive feedback system works to increase an output in the system. An example of a positive feedback system include a blood clot.

posterior eye chamber The cavity of the eye interior that is behind the lens.

postictal period The time period following a generalized seizure, during which the individual may be confused, fatigued, and fall into a deep sleep.

postrenal condition Cause of acute renal failure that interferes with the urine excretion.

postsynaptic cell membrane The membrane that receives and responds to a signal (binds neurotransmitter) from the presynaptic cell.

potassium The primary intracellular cation. Potassium plays a crucial role in electrical conduction, acid–base balance, and metabolism (carbohydrate, protein, and glucose).

PP cell One of five types of cells in the islets of Langerhans; secretes a pancreatic polypeptide.

predisposing factor Tendency that puts an individual at risk for developing certain diseases.

pregnancy-induced hypertension (PIH) Hypertension that occurs for the first time during pregnancy. It occurs in 5–8% of all pregnancies.

preload The amount of blood returning to the heart, which the heart has to manage. Both afterload and preload can affect blood pressure. As afterload and preload increase, blood pressure increases.

premenstrual dysphoric syndrome A severe form of premenstrual syndrome (PMS) that is characterized by severe depression, tension, and irritability.

premenstrual syndrome (PMS) A group of physical and emotional symptoms that affect many women for reasons not fully understood.

prerenal condition Cause of acute renal failure that disrupts blood flow on its way to the kidneys.

presbycusis Age-related hearing loss.

presbyopia Difficulty focusing the eyes resulting from age-related changes.

presynaptic terminal Terminal bouton or some similar structure. It is a specialized area within the axon of the presynaptic cell that contains neurotransmitters enclosed in small membrane-bound spheres.

priapism A prolonged, painful erection.

primary immune deficit Type of immunodeficiency that involves basic developmental failures, many resulting from genetic or congenital abnormalities (e.g., hypogammaglobulinemia).

primary herpes genitalis The first stage of genital herpes. Usually occurs within 2–10 days of exposure and is characterized by blister or open lesions, fever, headache, muscle aches, swollen lymph nodes in the groin area, painful urination, and vaginal discharge.

primary hypertension Type of hypertension in which there is no identifiable cause. It occurs in 90–95% of hypertension cases in adults and tends to develop gradually over many years. Also called essential hypertension.

primary syphilis The first stage of syphilis. Painless chancres (usually one) form at the site of infection about 2–3 weeks after initial infection.

primary TB infection One of two stages of tuberculosis pathogenesis. In this stage, infection occurs when the bacillus first enters the body.

prion An abnormal protein particle that causes proteins to fold abnormally, especially in nervous tissue.

prodrome In herpes simplex virus, a tingling or burning sensation at the site just before a lesion appears.

prognosis An individual's likelihood of surviving, making a full recovery, or regaining normal functioning after developing a disease.

programmed cell death The process of eliminating unwanted cells.

progression Phase of carcinogenesis in which the tumor invades, metastasizes, and becomes drug resistant. It is the final phase of carcinogenesis, and it is irreversible.

progressive stage of shock State of shock that begins when the compensatory mechanisms fail to maintain cardiac output. Tissues become hypoxic, cells switch to anaerobic metabolism, lactic acid builds up, and metabolic acidosis develops.

prolactin A hormone from the anterior pituitary gland that prompts milk production.

proliferation The regulated process by which cells divide and reproduce.

promotion Phase of carcinogenesis in which the mutated cells are exposed to factors that promote growth. It may occur just after initiation or years later, and it can be reversible if the promoting factors are removed.

prophase Phase of mitosis in which the chromosomes condense and the nuclear membrane disintegrates.

prophylactic Goal of treatment aimed at preventing disease.

prostate cancer Cancer of the prostate. It is the most common cancer among men. The slow-growing tumor is often confined to the prostate, improving the prognosis.

prostate gland A chestnut-shaped gland at the base of the urethra that produces fluid that mixes with the sperm and secretions of the seminal vesicles. This prostate fluid further deceases acidity, increases sperm motility, and prolongs sperm life.

prostatitis Inflammation of the prostate that can be acute or chronic.

protein buffer system The most abundant buffering system. Proteins can act as an acid or base by binding to or releasing hydrogen. Proteins exist in intracellular and extracellular fluid but are the most abundant inside the cell.

protoplasm A colorless, viscous liquid containing water, nutrients, ions, dissolved gases, and waste products where the cellular work takes place. Also called cytoplasm.

psoriasis A common chronic inflammatory condition that affects the life cycle of the skin cells.

pulmonary artery Vessel that carries deoxygenated blood from the right ventricle to the lungs for oxygenation.

pulmonary circulation The portion of the cardiovascular system that carries oxygen-depleted blood away from the heart, to the lungs, and returns oxygenated blood back to the heart.

pulmonary vein Vessel that carries oxygenated blood from the lungs to the left atrium.

pulmonic valve A three-leaflet valve that guides the passage of blood from the right ventricle to the pulmonary artery and prevents the backward flow of blood.

pulse pressure The difference between the systolic and diastolic blood pressures.

pupil The dark opening in the center of the iris that opens and closes reflexively in response to light intensity.

Purkinje network of fibers Area of specialized cells in the heart that receives impulses from the bundle branches and stimulates ventricular contraction.

pus Yellowish-white wound drainage.

pyelonephritis An infection that has reached one or both kidneys.

pyloric sphincter A muscular ring through which chyme passes as it leaves the stomach in small, varying amounts. The pyloric sphincter prevents reflux of bile from the small intestines into the stomach.

pyloric stenosis A narrowing and obstruction of the pyloric sphincter.

pyrogen A molecule released by macrophages that have been exposed by bacteria.

Raynaud's disease A condition that is result of vasospasms of arteries—most often of the hands—that occurs because of sympathetic stimulation.

recessive Less influential. In genetics, the recessive allele is less likely to be expressed in the offspring than the dominant one.

rectocele Condition that occurs when the rectum protrudes through the posterior wall of the vagina.

rectum A reservoir to store feces.

recurrent herpes genitalis The fourth stage of genital herpes; characterized by the reactivation of the virus and clinical manifestations.

red marrow Bone marrow that serves as the blood-cell factory (hematopoiesis). As humans age, this red marrow is slowly replaced by fat, creating yellow marrow.

reduce A fracture treatment in which the broken bone fragments are brought together to promote healing. This reduction can be accomplished by manual manipulation or surgery.

referred pain Pain at distant locations from the originating organ.

reflex incontinence Urinary incontinence caused by trauma or damage to the nervous system.

regulator cell One of two major types of T cells that work to destroy antigens. Regulator cells include helper T cells and suppressor T cells.

regurgitation Insufficiency or incompetence. In the heart, it occurs when the valve leaflets do not completely close. Incompetent valves allow blood to flow in both directions.

remission Disease state that occurs when the manifestations subside.

renal artery The artery that supplies each kidney with blood.

renal capsule Connective tissue that surrounds the kidneys.

renal cell carcinoma The most frequently occurring kidney cancer in adults. Most common in those 50–70 years of age.

renal cortex The area immediately beneath the renal capsule that contains the functional units of the kidney.

renal failure The kidneys' inability to function adequately. Renal failure is classified as either acute or chronic.

renal hilum The opening in the kidney that the renal artery and nerves enter and the renal vein and ureter exit.

renal impairment Reduced renal reserve; the first phase of chronic renal failure. About 60% of nephrons are lost.

renal insufficiency The second phase of chronic renal failure. Waste products begin to accumulate as renal function declines and 75% of the nephrons are lost.

renal pelvis Funnel-like area in the center of the kidney in which urine drains.

renal sinus A cavity into which the renal hilum opens.

renin-angiotensin-aldosterone A vital control and compensatory mechanism that is activated when renal blood flow is decreased, often in hypotensive states. When blood flow is decreased to the kidneys, renin is released from the kidneys, which, in turn, activates angiotension I to convert to angiotension II (a vasoconstrictor) and stimulates aldosterone secretion. In hypotensive states, this mechanism raises blood pressure and maintains vital organs. In chronic disease states such as hypertension, this mechanism is inappropriately activated because of vasoconstriction to the kidneys, further contributing to the hypertension.

repolarization **1.** The recovery of the ventricles, represented by T waves. Repolarization of the atria does not appear on an electrocardiogram because it is hidden by the other more prominent waveforms. **2.** Restoration of the resting potential of the cell membrane.

residual volume Volume of air left in the lungs after maximum exhalation.

resistance The second stage of the general adaptation syndrome. In this stage, the body chooses the most effective and advantageous defense. Cortisol levels and the sympathetic nervous system return

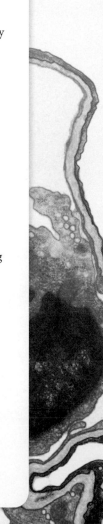

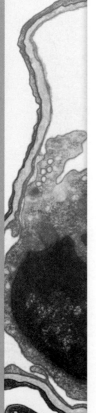

to normal, causing the fight-or-flight symptoms to disappear. The body will either adapt or alter in an attempt to limit problems or become desensitized to the stressor.

respiratory acidosis Condition that results from carbon dioxide retention, increasing carbonic acid and, in turn, decreasing pH level.

respiratory alkalosis Condition that results from excess exhalation of carbon dioxide that leads to carbonic acid deficits and pH increases.

resting potential A slight charge that the plasma side of the neuron membrane has at rest because of the sodium ions concentrated on the outside of the cell.

restrictive cardiomyopathy Type of cardiomyopathy that is characterized by rigidity of the ventricles leading to diastolic dysfunction.

retching A strong, unproductive effort to vomit.

retention An inability to empty the bladder.

reticular activation system Specialized nerve fibers through which the reticular formation sends impulses to the cerebral cortex. The reticular formation and reticular activation system are responsible for alertness during the day and can prevent sleeping at night.

reticular formation A region of the brain stem in which most of the branches of the many nerve fibers passing through the brain stem terminate. The reticular formation acts like a gatekeeper, receiving all incoming and outgoing information. The reticular formation sends impulses to the cerebral cortex through specialized nerve fibers.

retina The innermost layer of the eye. The retina contains an outer, pigmented layer and an inner layer consisting of photoreceptors and nerve cells. The retina is weakly attached to the choroid, making it vulnerable to damage.

retinal detachment An acute condition that occurs when the retina separates from its supporting structures.

retractile testicle A testicle that moves back and forth between the scrotum and the lower abdomen. Such a testicle is easily returned to the scrotum through gentle manipulation.

retroflexed Tilted backward. Often used in reference to the uterus.

rheumatoid arthritis (RA) A systemic, autoimmune condition involving multiple joints. In RA, the inflammatory process primarily affects the synovial membrane, but it can also affect other organs.

rickets A softening and weakening of bones in children, usually because of an extreme and prolonged vitamin D, calcium, or phosphate deficiency.

right atrium Receiving chamber on the right side of the heart. Receives blood from the peripheral circulation, and blood leaves this chamber and travels to the right ventricle.

right-sided heart failure Type of heart failure that results from an ineffective right ventricular contractility. As a result, blood does not move appropriately out of the right ventricle. Blood backs up into the right atrium and then to the peripheral circulation, causing increased pressures in the capillary bed.

right ventricle Pumping chamber of the left side of the heart. Pumps blood to the pulmonary circulation.

rod A photoreceptor in the eye that is sensitive to low light and that functions at night. There are nearly 150 million in the human eye.

rootlet A small nerve along the dorsal and ventral surfaces of the spinal cord from which spinal nerves arise.

rosacea A chronic inflammatory skin condition that typically affects the face. Rosacea is poorly understood, but it is prevalent in persons who are fair skinned, bruise easily, and women. Rosacea may present as erythema, prominent spiderlike blood vessels (telangiectasia), swelling, or acnelike eruptions

rugae Wrinkles in the stomach that unfold as the stomach fills.

saccular aneurysm A bulge on the side of a blood vessel. One of two major types of true aneurysm.

saccule A bed of sensory cells situated in the inner ear. It translates head movements into neural impulses which the brain can interpret.

sarcomere Repeated structural unit into which myofilaments are organized.

scabies A result of a mite infestation. The female mites burrow into the epidermis, laying eggs over a period of several weeks. The larvae hatch from the eggs and then migrate to the skin's surface. The larvae burrow in search of nutrients and mature to repeat the cycle. The burrowing and fecal matter left by the mites triggers the inflammatory process, leading to erythema and pruritus.

Schwann cell A cell that produces the myelin sheath.

sciatica A radiating, aching pain, sometimes with tingling and numbness, that starts in the buttock and extends down the back or side of one leg.

sclera White, fibrous material of the outermost layer of the eye.

scoliosis A lateral deviation of the spine. This lateral curvature may affect the thoracic or lumbar area or both. Scoliosis may also include a rotation of the vertebrae on their axis.

scrotum A sac of skin just below the penis that contains the testes, epididymis, and lower spermatic cords.

sebaceous gland A gland that produces sebum.

sebum Secretion of the sebaceous gland that moisturizes and protects the skin.

second line of defense Part of the immune system that responds to antigen invasions that occur as the result of tiny breaks in the skin or in the lining of the respiratory, digestive, or genitourinary tracts.

secondary glaucoma Type of glaucoma that is a result of certain medications, eye diseases, and systemic diseases.

secondary hypertension A type of hypertension that tends to appear suddenly and cause higher blood pressure than primary hypertension does.

secondary immunodeficiency An acquired immunodeficiency that involves a loss of immune function because of a specific cause (e.g., infection, splenectomy, malnutrition, hepatic disease, drug therapy, or stress).

secondary syphilis Stage of syphilis that occurs about 2–8 weeks after the first chancres form. About 33% of those who do not have their primary syphilis treated will develop this second stage. A generalized brown-red rash that does not itch characterizes this stage.

secondary tuberculosis infection Occurs when the primary TB infection can no longer be controlled, and the TB spreads throughout the lungs and other organs.

seizure A transient physical or behavior alteration that results from an abnormal electrical activity in the brain.

selectively permeable Condition that allows a cell to maintain internal balance or homeostasis.

semen Fluid made up of ejaculatory fluid and sperm. It flows from the ejaculatory duct to the urethra, where it is released from the penis during sexual intercourse.

semicircular canal A ringlike, fluid-filled structure that houses receptors for body position and movement. Movement of the head causes the fluid in the semicircular canal to move. Fluid movement stimulates dendrites to send impulses to the brain to report this movement. There are three semicircular canals in each human ear.

seminal vesicles A pair of pouches that secrete an alkaline ejaculatory fluid containing sugar, protein, and prostaglandins. The seminal vesicles join with the ampulla to form the ejaculatory duct.

sensory nerve A type of nerve of the peripheral nervous system. It carries impulses from the body to the brain. Also called afferent nerve.

septic shock Type of distributive shock in which a bacterium's endotoxins activate an immune reaction. Inflammatory mediators are triggered, increasing capillary permeability and fluid shifts from the vascular compartment to the tissue. Falling cardiac output leads to multisystem organ failure.

serosa The outermost of the four layers of the walls of the gastrointestinal tract.

sesamoid bone One of five types of bones found within the skeleton. Sesamoid bones are usually short or irregular bones embedded in a tendon. Sesamoid bones are usually present in a tendon where it passes over a joint and serves to protect the tendon.

severe acute respiratory syndrome (SARS) A rapidly spreading respiratory illness that presents similarly to atypical pneumonia. Prevalence rates are higher in Asian countries. SARS is caused by a coronavirus, SARS-CoV. Transmission occurs through inhalation of respiratory droplets or close contact or oral–fecal contact. SARS has high mortality and morbidity rates.

sex-linked Type of genetic disorder that is caused by genes located on the sex chromosomes.

sexually transmitted infection (STI) Any of a broad range infections that can be contracted through sexual contact. Sometimes referred to as sexually transmitted disease (STD).

shedding herpes genitalis The third stage of herpes, wherein the virus is reactivated but produces no symptoms.

shock A clinical syndrome resulting from inadequate tissue and organ perfusion because of decreased blood volume or circulatory stagnation.

short bone One of five types of bones found within the skeleton. Short bones are approximately as wide as they are long, and their primary function is providing support and stability with little movement. Short bones contain only a thin layer of compact bone along with spongy bone and relatively large amounts of bone marrow.

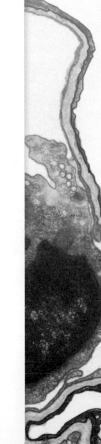

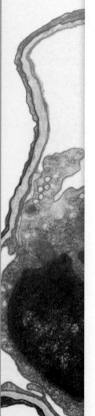

simple fracture A fracture with a single break in the bone and bone ends that maintain their alignment and position.

sinoatrial (SA) node Area of the heart where the conduction pathway originates. All impulses originating in the sinoatrial node travel through the right and left atrium, resulting in atrial contraction. The sinoatrial node automatically generates impulses ranging from 60 to 100 beats per minute (sinus rhythm).

sinusitis An inflammation of the sinus cavities most often caused by a viral infection.

skeletal muscle Muscle that connects to bone. The most frequently occurring muscle type, making up approximately 40% of the body's weight.

skeleton The 206 bones of varying shapes and sizes in the human body. The skeleton provides support and protection for vital organs such as the heart, lungs, and brain.

Skene's gland Gland in the mucosal lining of the vagina that secretes a protective, lubricating fluid during sexual intercourse.

skin Outer covering of the body comprised of three layers—endodermis, dermis, and epidermis.

skin cancer An abnormal growth of skin cells.

skin tag A benign, soft brown or flesh-colored growth, usually on the neck.

small cell carcinoma A type of lung cancer that occurs almost exclusively in heavy smokers and is less frequent than non–small cell cancers. Also called oat cell carcinoma.

small intestine The longest section of the gastrointestinal tract (approximately 20 feet long in adults). This length allows for adequate nutrient absorption as the small intestine continues the digestion process. In the small intestine, the enzymes that have been secreted into the gastrointestinal tract break the large food molecules into smaller molecules that are then absorbed.

smegma An oily secretion produced by the glans that can combine with dead skin to form a cheesy substance. If the smegma is not regularly removed from under the foreskin, the penis can become irritated and infected.

smooth muscle Type of muscle that lines walls of hollow organs and tubes and is found in the eyes, skin, and glands. Smooth muscles are involuntary.

sodium The most significant cation. Sodium is the most prevalent electrolyte of extracellular fluid, and its primary function is to control serum osmolality and water balance.

somatic pain One of two types of pain the body perceives. It results from noxious stimuli to the skin, joints, muscles, and tendons. These stimuli may include cutting, crushing, pinching, extreme temperature, and irritating chemicals. Somatic pain is generally easy to pinpoint.

somatostatin Hormone secreted by delta cells that regulates insulin and glucagon.

spermatic cord A cordlike structure, consisting of the vas deferens and its accompanying arteries, veins, nerves, and lymphatic vessels, that passes from the abdominal cavity through the inguinal canal down into the scrotum to the back of the testicle.

spermatocele A sperm-containing cyst that develops between the testes and the epididymis.

spermatogenesis The generation of sperm.

spina bifida A neural tube defect that can vary in severity from mild to debilitating. Neural tube development begins early in pregnancy, starting at the cervical area and progressing toward the lumbar area, and the neural tube usually closes by the 4th week of gestation. In spina bifida, the posterior spinous processes on the vertebra fail to fuse. This opening permits the meninges and spinal cord to herniate, resulting in neurologic impairment.

spina bifida occulta The mildest form of spina bifida. It results in a small gap in one or more of the vertebrae. The spinal nerves and meninges do not usually protrude through the opening, so most children with this form have no clinical manifestations and experience no neurologic deficits.

spinal cord A long, thin, tubular bundle of nervous tissue that exits the skull through the large and only opening in the skull, called the foramen magnum.

spinal cord injury (SCI) Injury that occurs directly to the spinal cord or indirectly to surrounding bones, tissues, or blood vessels.

spinal reflex arc The process that creates an unconscious response to stimuli.

spinal shock A temporary suppression of neurologic function because of spinal cord compression. In spinal shock, neurologic function gradually returns.

spiral fracture A fracture that twists around the bone shaft.

spongy bone The inner region of a bone that is less dense than the outer region.

spontaneous pneumothorax Type of pneumothorax that develops when air enters the pleural cavity from an opening in the internal airways.

sprain An injury to a ligament that often involves stretching or tearing of the ligament.

stable angina pectoris Type of cardiac chest pain that is a result of ischemia that is initiated by increased demand (activity) and relieved with the reduction of that demand (rest).

stapes One of the three ossicles in the middle ear. Also called stirrup.

status asthmaticus A life-threatening, prolonged asthma attack that does not respond to usual treatment.

status epilepticus Seizures that last longer than 20 minutes or subsequent seizures before the individual has fully regained consciousness.

stenosis A narrowing of a tubular structure, such as the heart valves. When the heart valves are stenosed, blood moving through the valves is reduced, causing blood to back up in the chamber just before the valve.

stomach An expandable food and liquid reservoir. When empty, the stomach wall shrinks, forming wrinkles called rugae. As the stomach fills, the rugae unfold and the wall stretches to accommodate up to 2 to 4 liters.

strabismus A gaze deviation of one eye. With strabismus, the eyes do not coordinate to focus on the same object together, resulting in diplopia. Also called cross-eyes.

strain An injury to a muscle or tendon that often involves stretching or tearing of the muscle or tendon.

stress fracture Type of fracture that occurs from repeated excessive stress. Also called fatigue fracture.

stress incontinence Loss of urine from pressure exerted on the bladder by coughing, sneezing, laughing, exercising, or lifting something heavy. Stress incontinence occurs when the sphincter muscle of the bladder weakens.

stress ulcer Type of peptic ulcer disease that develops because of a major physiologic stressor on the body.

stroke volume The amount of blood ejected from the heart with each contraction. In addition to afterload, stroke volume is affected by preload.

subarachnoid hemorrhage A hemorrhage that results from bleeding in the space between the arachnoid and pia. The primary clinical presentation is a severe headache with a sudden onset that is worse near the back of the head.

subdural hematoma A hematoma that develops between the dura and arachnoid, frequently caused by a small venous tear. Because it is a result of a venous tear, a subdural hematoma generally develops slowly.

submucosa layer One of four layers of the walls of the gastrointestinal tract. It is comprised of connective tissue that includes blood vessels, nerves, lymphatics, and secretory glands.

substantia nigra A brain structure located in the mesencephalon (midbrain) that plays an important role in reward, addiction, and movement. *Substantia nigra* is Latin for "black substance'" as parts of the substantia nigra appear darker than neighboring areas due to high levels of neuromelanin. Parkinson's disease is caused by the death of dopaminergic neurons in the substantia nigra pars compacta.

subthalamus Part of the thalamus that participates in motor activities.

sulcus (plural: sulci) The grooves in between the gyri of the brain.

superior vena cava Large vein that carries deoxygenated blood from the upper half of the body to the right atrium.

suppressor cell A type of regulator cell that turns antibody production off.

surfactant A substance on the surface of the alveoli. Surfactant is a lipoprotein produced by alveoli cells and has a detergent-like quality. Surfactant is a watery substance that produces surface tension on the alveoli, which enhances pulmonary compliance and prevents the alveoli from collapsing.

suture An immoveable joint in the skull.

sympathetic nervous system (SNS) Subdivision of the autonomic nervous system. It is responsible for the fight-or-flight response.

synapse The gap between the neurons. This gap includes the presynaptic terminal, the synaptic cleft (space between neurons), and a postsynaptic cell membrane.

synaptic cleft Space between neurons.

synarthrose An immoveable joint.

syndrome A group of signs and symptoms that occur together.

syndrome of inappropriate antidiuretic hormone (SIADH) Condition of increased renal water retention caused by excessive antidiuretic levels.

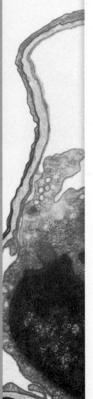

syngenic Type of transplant in which tissue from the identical twin of the host is used.

synovial fluid A transparent viscous fluid secreted by the synovial membrane that lubricates cartilage in the synovial joints.

synovial joint A freely moveable joint; it is the most common type of joint. Synovial joints contain cartilage that is lubricated by a transparent viscous fluid secreted by the synovial membrane.

syphilis An ulcerative sexually transmitted infection caused by *Treponema pallidum*, a spiral-shaped (spirochete) bacterium that requires a warm, moist environment to survive.

systemic circulation The part of the cardiovascular system that carries oxygenated blood away from the heart to the body, and returns deoxygenated blood back to the heart.

systemic lupus erythematosus (SLE) A chronic, autoimmune, inflammatory disorder that can affect any connective tissue. It is thought that B cells are activated for unknown reasons to produce autoantibodies and autoantigens that combine to form immune complexes.

systole The top number in a blood pressure reading, which indicates work by the ventricles.

systolic dysfunction Type of heart failure characterized by decreased cardiac output due to decreased contractility.

T cell A cell that is a major part of the body's third line of defense. It is produced in the bone marrow and matures in the thymus, which is why it is called a T cell. Two major types of T cells work to destroy antigens—regulator cells and effector cells.

T$_3$ Triiodothyronine; a hormone produced by the follicles of the thyroid gland to regulate cellular metabolism and growth and development.

T$_4$ Thyroxine; a hormone produced by the follicles of the thyroid gland to regulate cellular metabolism and growth and development.

telophase Phase of mitosis in which chromosomes arrive at each pole and new membranes are formed.

temporal lobe The lobe of the brain that plays an essential role in hearing and memory.

tendon Specialized tough cord or band of dense connective tissue that is a continuous extension of the periosteum.

tension pneumothorax The most serious type of pneumothorax; it occurs when the pressure in the pleural space is greater than the atmospheric pressure. This increased pressure is due to trapped air in the pleural space or entering air from a positive-pressure mechanical ventilator.

teratogen A birth defect–causing agent.

terminal bouton Miniscule bulge into which several small fibers terminate. These terminal boutons communicate with neurons, muscle fibers, or glands.

tertiary syphilis The final stage of syphilis. Also called latent syphilis. The early latency stage begins when the secondary symptoms disappear and lasts 1–4 years. The late latency stage can last for years as the infection spreads to the brain, nervous system, heart, skin, and bones.

testes Gonads; organs that produce sperm and the sex hormones.

testicular cancer Cancer of the testicles. Testicular cancer can occur as a slow-growing or fast-growing tumor. Risk for developing testicular cancer is thought to be increased by family history, infection, trauma, and cryptorchidism. Testicular cancer usually affects one testicle, but can affect both.

testicular torsion An abnormal rotation of the testis on the spermatic cord.

testosterone Hormone that gives males their classic secondary sex characteristics and sex drive. Testosterone also regulates metabolism and protein anabolism, inhibits pituitary secretion of the gonadotropins, and promotes potassium excretion and renal sodium reabsorption.

thalamus Part of the diencephalon that receives and relays most of the sensory input, affects mood, and initiates body movements (especially those associated with fear or anger).

third line of defense The body's specific immune system that includes T cells and B cells.

third spacing Significant fluid increases in compartments where fluid does not normally collect (e.g., peritoneum). Fluid is not easily exchanged among the other extracellular fluids.

thirst mechanism Part of the hypothalamus that causes an increase in oral intake.

thromboangiitis obliterans An inflammatory condition of the arteries. Also known as Buerger's disease.

thrombocyte A blood platelet.

thrombocytopenia Describes decreased platelet levels; increases the risk of bleeding and infection.

thrombocytosis Refers to increased platelet levels; increases the risk of thrombus formation.

thromboplastin A factor in blood clotting, which is stimulated by the release thromboplastin from damaged cells lining blood vessels.

thrombotic thrombocytopenic purpura (TTP) A coagulation disorder that is a result of a deficiency of an enzyme necessary for cleaving von Willebrand's factor.

thrombus A blood clot that consists of platelets, fibrin, and red and white blood cells. These clots can form anywhere in the circulatory system.

thyroid gland A gland located at the base of the neck below the larynx that consists of two lobes, one on either side of the trachea.

thyroid-stimulating hormone (TSH) Hormone produced by the pituitary gland that promotes the thyroid to produce T_3 and T_4.

thyrotoxicosis Thyroid crisis—a sudden worsening of hyperthyroidism symptoms that may occur with infection or stress. Fever, decreased mental alertness, and abdominal pain may occur. Thyrotoxicosis is a medical emergency.

tidal volume The amount of air involved in one normal inhalation and exhalation.

tinea A parasite that causes several types of superficial fungal infections described by the area of the body affected. Tinea corporis, or ringworm, is an infection of the body. Tinea pedis, or athlete's foot, involves the feet, especially the toes. Tinea unguium is an infection of the nails, typically the toenails.

tinnitus Persistent, abnormal noises in the ear. This noise may be described as a ringing, buzzing, humming, whistling, roaring, or blowing.

TNM staging Method of expressing the extent of cancer by evaluating the tumor size, nodal involvement, and metastatic progress.

tonicity The osmotic pressure of two solutions separated by a semipermeable membrane.

tophus (plural: tophi) A large, hard nodule comprised of uric acid crystals deposited in soft tissue, usually in cooler areas of the body.

trachea The windpipe; carries air from the oral and nasal cavities to the lungs.

transcellular A third compartment of fluid, in addition to the interstitial and intravascular compartments.

transient incontinence Urinary incontinence resulting from a temporary condition.

transient ischemic attack (TIA) A temporary episode of cerebral ischemia that results in symptoms of neurologic deficits. Transient ischemic attacks are often called ministrokes because these neurologic deficits mimic a cerebral vascular accident or stroke except that these deficits resolve within 24 hours (1–2 hours in most cases).

transverse fracture A fracture straight across the bone shaft.

traumatic brain injury (TBI) Injury that is usually caused by a sudden and violent blow or jolt to the head (called a closed injury) or a penetrating (known as an open injury) head injury that disrupts the normal brain function.

traumatic pneumothorax Type of pneumothorax that is caused by any blunt or penetrating injury to the chest. These injuries can inadvertently occur during certain medical procedures.

trichomoniasis Infection caused by *Trichomonas vaginalis*, a one-celled anaerobic organism. This extracellular parasite can burrow under the mucosal lining. It is colloquially referred to as the trick.

tricuspid valve A three-leaflet valve that guides the passage of blood from the right atria to the right ventricle and prevents the backward flow of blood

Trousseau's sign An indicator of hypocalcemia in which a strategically placed blood pressure cuff elicits a carpal spasm.

tuberculosis (TB) A potentially serious infectious disease that is increasing globally after a former decline.

tumor A cellular growth that is no longer responding to normal regulator processes. Also called a neoplasm.

tumor grading system The degree of differentiation of a malignancy. The grading system determines the degree of differentiation on a scale of 1 to 4 in order of clinical severity, with grade 1 cancers being well differentiated and less likely to cause problems and grade 4 cancers being undifferentiated, meaning they are highly likely to cause problems because they do not resemble any characteristics of the original tissue.

tunica adventitia The outer layer of the blood vessels, which consists of elastic and fibrous connective tissue.

tunica intima The smooth, thin, inner layer of the blood vessels.

tunica media The middle layer of the blood vessels, which is comprised of elastic tissue and smooth muscle that is responsible for the vessel's ability to constrict and dilate.

tympanic membrane Part of the ear that separates the outer ear and the middle ear. Sound hits the tympanic membrane, creating vibrations. Also called eardrum.

type 1 diabetes Type of diabetes mellitus that develops when the body's immune system destroys pancreatic beta cells. To survive, people with type 1 diabetes must have insulin delivered by injection or a pump. This form of diabetes usually strikes children and young adults, although disease onset can occur at any age. Previously called insulin-dependent diabetes and juvenile-onset diabetes.

type 2 diabetes Type of diabetes that usually begins as insulin resistance, a disorder in which the cells do not use insulin properly. As the need for insulin rises, the pancreas gradually loses its ability do produce it. It was previously called non–insulin-dependent diabetes and adult-onset diabetes.

type I hypersensitivity IgE-mediated type of hypersensitivity, in which allergens activate T cells, which bind to mast cells. Repeated exposure to relatively large doses of the allergens is usually necessary to cause this response.

type II hypersensitivity Tissue-specific type of hypersensitivity, which generally involves the destruction of a target cell by an antibody-directed, cell-surface antigen. IgG or IgM reacts with an antigen on the cell, activating the complement system. The effects of type II reactions include cell lysis and phagocytosis.

type III hypersensitivity Immune complex mediated type of hypersensitivity, in which circulating antigen-antibody complexes accumulate and are deposited in the tissue. This accumulation triggers the complement system causing local inflammation and increased vascular permeability, so more complexes accumulate.

type IV hypersensitivity Cell-mediated type of hypersensitivity, which involves a delayed processing of the antigen by the macrophages. Once processed, the antigen is presented to the T cells, resulting in the release of lymphokines that cause inflammation and antigen destruction.

type A influenza The most common type of influenza virus. It includes several subtypes, including H1N1. Type A influenza is usually responsible for the most serious epidemics and global pandemics.

type B influenza Type of influenza virus that can also cause regional epidemics, but the disease it produces is generally milder than that caused by type A.

type C influenza Type of influenza virus that causes sporadic cases and minor, local outbreaks. Type C has never been connected with a large epidemic.

ulcerative colitis A progressive condition of the rectum and colon mucosa that usually develops in the second or third decade of life. Inflammation causes epithelium loss, surface erosion, and ulceration.

uncompensated A pH level that is still normal.

unstable angina A change in cardiac chest pain; the pain becomes unpredictable, occurs at rest, or increases in frequency or intensity. It is considered a preinfarction state.

urea One of the three most significant metabolic wastes managed by the kidneys.

uremia Waste accumulation due to renal impairment.

ureter Part of the urinary system that transports the urine using peristaltic actions to the bladder for storage.

urethra Tube that empties the urinary bladder.

urge incontinence A sudden, intense urge to urinate, followed by an involuntary loss of urine.

uric acid A metabolism byproduct managed by the kidneys that is a results of the breakdown of nucleotides, the building blocks of DNA.

urinary incontinence Involuntary loss of urine.

urinary tract infection (UTI) Infection of the urinary tract that often ascends from the urinary meatus. Typically caused by *Escherichia coli* and more frequent in females.

urination The voluntary contraction of the bladder and relaxation of the external sphincter, forcing urine out through the urethra.

urolithiasis The presence of renal calculi.

urticaria Raised erythematous skin lesions that are a result of a type I hypersensitivity reaction. Also called hives.

uterine prolapse The descent of the uterus or cervix into the vagina.

uterus A hollow, pear-shaped organ held in place by the broad, round, and uterosacral ligaments.

utricle A division of the inner ear that detects motion and position.

vagina A hollow, tunnel-like structure that extends from the cervix to the external genitalia.

varicocele A dilated vein in the spermatic cord.

varicose vein A dilated, tortuous, engorged vein that develops because of improper venous valve function. The most common location is the legs, but varicose veins can be found in the esophagus (esophageal varices) and the rectum (hemorrhoids). Also called varicosity.

vas deferens Part of the male duct system that carries sperm out of the testes.

vascular birthmark Birthmark that consists of blood vessels that have not formed correctly; therefore, these birthmarks are generally red.

vein A blood vessel that carries blood back to the heart.

ventilation The transportation of air from the atmosphere to the lungs and out again.

ventilation/perfusion ratio A measurement used to assess the efficacy and adequacy of ventilation and perfusion. Also called VQ ratio.

ventral root A root formed from about 6–8 ventral rootlets. The roots combine to form the spinal nerve.

ventricle A hollow area. In the brain, ventricles are interconnected, and cerebrospinal fluid fills and flows freely between them. In the heart, they are pumping chambers.

venule A blood vessel that is larger than a capillary. Venules merge together to form veins.

verruca (plural: verrucae) A viral infection caused by a number of the human papillomaviruses. Verrucae can develop at any age and often resolve spontaneously. They can be transmitted through direct skin contact between people or within the same person.

vertebral canal Part of the central nervous system through which the spinal cord extends to the second lumbar vertebra.

vertigo An illusion of motion. People experiencing vertigo have a sensation that they or the room is spinning or moving.

vesicle A blister.

vestibular apparatus Part of the inner ear that includes the semicircular canals and the vestibule.

vestibule **1.** A bony chamber positioned between the cochlea and semicircular canals. The vestibule houses receptors that respond to body position and movement. **2.** The area of the vagina that contains the urethral and vaginal opening.

viral pneumonia A form of pneumonia that is usually mild and heals without intervention, but it can lead to a virulent bacterial pneumonia.

visceral pain One of two types of pain the body perceives. It results from noxious stimuli to internal organs and may include expansion and hypoxia. Visceral pain is usually vague and diffuse. Visceral pain may even be sensed on body surfaces at distant locations from the originating organ.

visceral peritoneum layer The inner layer of the peritoneum that encases the abdominal organs.

vital capacity The sum of the tidal volume and reserves in the lungs.

vitiligo A rare condition characterized by small patchy areas of hypopigmentation. Vitiligo occurs when the cells that produce melanin die or no longer form melanin, causing slowly enlarging white patches of irregular shapes on the skin.

vitreous humor A clear, gelatinous material that fills the posterior chamber.

vomiting The involuntary or voluntary forceful ejection of chyme from the stomach up through the esophagus and out of the mouth. It is a common event that often results from a wide range of conditions. Also called emesis.

von Willebrand's disease A common bleeding disorder caused by a defect or deficiency of a blood clotting protein, called von Willebrand factor.

vulva The structures of external female genitalia. These structures include the mons pubis, the labia majora, the labia minora, the clitoris, and the vestibule.

water intoxication Fluid excess that occurs in the intracellular space.

welt A raised erythematous skin lesion.

wet gangrene Type of gangrene that occurs with liquefaction necrosis. Extensive damage from bacteria and white blood cells produce a liquid wound.

white matter Bundles of myelinated nerves.

Wilms' tumor A rare kidney cancer that primarily affects children. Also called nephroblastoma.

yellow marrow Bone marrow that begins to form during adolescence and is present in most bones by adulthood. Yellow marrow can be reactivated to produce blood cells under certain circumstances.

zygote A fertilized egg.

Index

D

deaminiation process, 182
decerebrate response, 343*f*
decorticate response, 343*f*
decubitus ulcers, 408
deep vein thrombosis (DVT), 95*f*
defecation, 256
dehydration, 156
delta cells, 295
dementia, 356–359
dendrites, 315–316
deoxyribonucleic acid (DNA), 2, 16*f*, 22, 182, 355
depolarization, 74, 157, 316
depressed fractures, 338, 379
dermatitis, 409, 410
dermatome, 325
dermis, 402
descending fibers, 324
detrusor hyperreflexia, 184
detrusor muscle areflexia, 184
diabetes insipidus, 156, 158, 298
diabetes mellitus, 300–304
  diagnosis, 302*t*
  fluid deficit in, 156
  gestational, 303
  metabolic syndrome, 303–304
  pancreatitis in, 270
  type 1, 302
  type 2, 302–303
diabetic ketoacidosis, 160, 301
diaphoresis, 156
diaphragm, 118–119
diaphyses, 365
diarrhea, 272–273, 281
diastole, 75
diastolic dysfunction, 104
DIC (disseminated intravascular coagulation), 65–66, 67*f*, 271
diencephalon, 317, 318–320
dietary cholesterol, 88–89
differentiation, 8–11, 16–17
diffusion, 5–6
digestion, 251–253
dilated cardiomyopathy, 81–83, Error! No page number
diminution (immunodeficiency) malfunction, 41
diplopia, 440, 446
dislocation, 380–382

dissecting aneurysm, 85, 88*f*
disseminated intravascular coagulation (DIC), 65–66, 67*f*, 271
distributive shock, 108
diverticula, 283–285
diverticular disease, 283–285
diverticulitis, 274, 284–285
diverticulosis, 284
dizziness, 448
DNA (deoxyribonucleic acid), 2, 16*f*, 22, 182, 355
dopamine, 352–353
dorsal root, 325
dorsal root ganglion, 329*f*
Down syndrome, 27–28
dromotropic effect, 75
drug-induced asthma, 134
dry gangrene, 14–15
dry macular degeneration, 444–445
duodenal ulcers, 263
dura mater, 314
DVT (deep vein thrombosis), 95*f*
dwarfism, 298
dyslipidemia, 85–90
dysmenorrhea, 224
dysphagia, 258, 259*f*
dysplasia, 11, 12, 244
dysrhythmias, 74, 84–85, 86*f*–87*f*
dysuria, 189

E

ear(s)
  anatomy and physiology, 432–436
    age-related changes, 438
  disorders. *See also specific disorder*
    chronic, 445–446
    congenital, 437
    infectious/inflammatory, 439–440
    miscellaneous, 447–448
    traumatic, 441
ear drum, 433–434
ear lobe, 432–433
ear trauma, 441
EBV (Epstein-Barr virus), 56, 237
eccrine glands, 402–403
eclampsia, 99
ectopic pregnancy, 212
ectopic testes, 218–219

extracellular fluid
  bicarbonate-carbonic acid system, 167
  sodium, 157
  third spacing, 152
extrinsic asthma, 133
eye(s), 406
  anatomy and physiology, 430–432
    age-related changes, 437–438
  disorders. *See also specific disorder*
    cancer, 446
    chronic, 441–445
    congenital, 436–437
    infectious/inflammatory, 438–439
    miscellaneous, 446–447
    traumatic, 440
eye cancer, 446
eye trauma, 440

F

facilitated diffusion, 6, 7*f*
factor VIII concentrates, 65
fallopian tubes, 209, 212
familial dyslipidemia, 88
farsightedness, 406
fascia, 374–375, 379
fat embolism, 379
fat necrosis, 13–14
fatty acid derivatives, 293
fatty streaks, 91
feces. *See* stools
female reproductive system
  anatomy and physiology, 209–216, 210*f*, 211*f. See also specific organs*
  disorders, 223–230. *See also specific disorder*
    cancer, 243–245
    infectious, 231–232
    infertility, 226–227, 228–229
    menstrual, 223–225
    ovarian, 228–229, 245
    pelvic support, 225–226
    uterine, 226–228
fertilization, 214
fever, 36
fibrocystic breast disease, 229
fibroids, 227–228
fibromyalgia, 397
fibrous plaque, 91

fight-or-flight response, 32, 297, 326–328
first line of defense, 34
first-degree burns, 417, 420*f*
flaccid paralysis, 354
flat bones, 366
flesh-eating bacteria, 414
flexor reflex, 325
flora, 403
flu (influenza), 126–128
fluid balance, 152, 152–157
fluid deficit, 156–157
fluid excess, 154–156
fluid movement, 152–154
focal seizures, 349–350
focal vitiligo, 407
follicles, 211–212
follicle-stimulating hormone (FSH), 209, 211–212, 214
folliculitis, 413
foramen magnum, 321
forced expiratory volume in one second, 120
forced vital capacity, 120
foreskin, 206, 219–220
fracture(s), 377–380
  reduction, 379–380
  skull, 338–339
fragile X syndrome, 26, 27*f*
freckles, 406
free radicals, 15
frontal lobe, 318, 321*f*
FSH (follicle-stimulating hormone), 209, 211–212, 214
full thickness burns, 417, 420*f*
fulminant hepatitis, 265
functional blindness, 406
functional incontinence, 184
furuncles, 413
fusiform aneurysm, 85, 88*f*

G

galactosemia, 436
gallbladder, 194, 255, 263–265
gallstones (cholelithiasis), 194, 263–265
gangrene, 14–15
gas exchange, respiratory, 71*f*, 112–118, 136
gas gangrene, 15
gastric cancer, 286

Photo Credits

Half Title Page, Title Page, Chapter Openers, © Science Photo Library/age fotostock

Learning Points icon, © Jubal Harshaw/Shutterstock.com

Myth Busters icon, Courtesy of National Cancer Institute

Case Study icon, © Science Photo Library/age fotostock

Chapter Summary icon, © Photocrea Michael Bednarek/ShutterStock, Inc.

Page xvi, Source: AAOS. (2006). *Paramedic: Pathophysiology.* Sudbury, MA: Jones & Bartlett Learning.

Chapter 1

1-1A, Mycoplasma photo courtesy of Tim Pietzcker, Universitat Ulm; 1-1B, Yeast photo courtesy of Fred Winston, Harvard Medical School; 1-1C, Fibroblast photo courtesy of Junzo Desaki, Ehime University School of Medicine; 1-1D, Nerve cell photo courtesy of Gerald J. Obermair and Bernhard E. Flucher, Innsbruck Medical University; 1-1E, Plant cell photo courtesy of Ming H. Chen, University of Alberta; 1-2, Source: Lewin, B., Cassimeris, L., Lingappa, V., & Plopper, G. (2007). *Cells.* Sudbury, MA: Jones & Bartlett Learning; 1-3, Photo reproduced from *The Journal of Cell Biology*, 1988, vol. 107, pp. 101–114, by copyright permission of The Rockefeller University Press; 1-4, Source: AAOS. (2004). *Paramedic: Anatomy & Physiology.* Sudbury, MA: Jones & Bartlett Learning; 1-5 through 1-8, Source: Chiras, D. (2008). *Human Biology* (6th ed.). Sudbury, MA: Jones & Bartlett Learning; 1-9, Source: AAOS. (2004). *Paramedic: Anatomy & Physiology.* Sudbury, MA: Jones & Bartlett Learning; 1-10, 1-12, Source: Lewin, B., Cassimeris, L., Lingappa, V., & Plopper, G. (2007). *Cells.* Sudbury, MA: Jones & Bartlett Learning; 1-13, © University of Alabama at Birmingham Department of Pathology PEIR Digital Library (http://peir.net); 1-14, Gibson, M. S., Puckett, M. L., & Shelly, M. E. (2004). Renal tuberculosis. *Radiographics, 24*(1), 251–256. Courtesy of Dr. Michael S. Gibson; 1-15, © Dr. E. Walker/Photo Researchers, Inc.; 1-16, © CNRI/Photo Researchers, Inc.; 1-17, © SPL/Photo Researchers, Inc.; 1-18, © Stevie Grand/SPL/Photo Researchers, Inc.; 1-19, E. Schröpfer, S. Rauthe, and T. Meyer. (2008). "Diagnosis and misdiagnosis of necrotizing soft tissue infections: three case reports." *Cases Journal,* 1, 252; 1-24, © 2005 Terese Winslow, U.S. Govt. has certain rights; 1-25, Courtesy of Rick Guidotti, Positive Exposure/National Marfan Foundation; 1-26, © SPL/Photo Researchers, Inc.; 1-27, Courtesy of Nikki Deal; 1-28, Courtesy of Leonard V. Crowley, MD, Century College; 1-29, Courtesy of Sarah Coulter-Danner; 1-30, © Wellcome Images/Custom Medical Stock Photo; 1-31, Courtesy of www.dermnet.com

Chapter 2

2-4, 2-5, Source: Chiras, D. (2008). *Human Biology* (6th ed.). Sudbury, MA: Jones & Bartlett Learning; 2-6, Source: Adapted from Gould, B. (2010). *Pathophysiology for the Health Professions* (4th ed.). Philadelphia, PA: Elsevier; 2-7, 2-8, Source: Pommerville, J. C. (2011). *Alcamo's Fundamentals of Microbiology* (9th ed.). Sudbury, MA: Jones & Bartlett Learning.

Chapter 3

3-2, © SPL/Photo Researchers, Inc.; 3-3, Source: Dean, L., "Mutations and blood clots: How point mutations in clotting factor genes conspire to increase the risk of thrombosis." In L. Dean, J. McEntyre (Eds.), *Coffee Break: Tutorials for NCBI Tools* [Internet]. Retrieved from http://www.ncbi.nlm.nih.gov/books/NBK2318; 3-4, Source: Chiras, D. (2008). *Human Biology* (6th ed.). Sudbury, MA: Jones & Bartlett Learning; 3-6, © Dr. E. Walker/Science Photo Library/Custom Medical Stock Photo; 3-8, © Joaquin Carrillo Farga/Photo Researchers, Inc.; 3-9, © Michael Abbey/Photo Researchers, Inc.; 3-10, © Stanley Fleger/Visuals Unlimited

Chapter 4

4-1, 4-2, Source: AAOS. (2004). *Paramedic: Anatomy & Physiology.* Sudbury, MA: Jones & Bartlett Learning; 4-3, © SIU/Visuals Unlimited, Inc.; 4-4, © Phil Degginger/Alamy Images; 4-5 through 4-8, Source: Chiras, D. (2008). *Human Biology* (6th ed.). Sudbury, MA: Jones & Bartlett Learning; 4-9, Source: AAOS. (2004). *Paramedic: Anatomy & Physiology.* Sudbury, MA: Jones & Bartlett Learning; 4-10A, © Cabisco/Visuals Unlimited; 4-10B, © Ed Reschke/Peter Arnold, Inc.; 4-10C (top), © John D. Cunningham/Visuals Unlimited; 4-10C (bottom), © Cabisco/Visuals Unlimited; 4-11, Source: Chiras, D. (2008). *Human Biology* (6th ed.). Sudbury, MA: Jones & Bartlett Learning; 4-12, Source: AAOS. (2004). *Paramedic: Anatomy & Physiology.* Sudbury, MA: Jones & Bartlett Learning; 4-13, © Dr. E. Walker/Photo Researchers, Inc.; 4-15 (rhythm strips), Source: *Arrhythmia Recognition: The Art of Interpretation*, courtesy of Tomas B. Garcia, MD; 4-16, © CNRI/Photo Researchers, Inc.; 4-21, © Medicimage/Visuals Unlimited, Inc.; 4-22, © Medical-on-Line/Alamy Images; 4-26, © Keith/Custom Medical Stock Photo; 4-27, © Fred Marsik/Visuals Unlimited; 4-29, National Heart, Lung and Blood Institute (www.nhlbi.nih.gov); 4-30A, © SIU/Visuals Unlimited, Inc.; 4-30B, © Dr. Gladden Willis/Visuals Unlimited, Inc.

Chapter 5

5-1, Source: Chiras, D. (2008). *Human Biology* (6th ed.). Sudbury, MA: Jones & Bartlett Learning; 5-2, © David M. Phillips/Photo Researchers, Inc.; 5-3, © Chet Childs/Custom Medical Stock Photo; 5-4, © David M. Martin, MD/Photo Researchers, Inc.; 5-5, © David M. Phillips/Visuals Unlimited; 5-6, Source: Chiras, D. (2008). *Human Biology* (6th ed.). Sudbury, MA: Jones & Bartlett Learning; 5-7, Source: AAOS. (2004). *Paramedic: Anatomy & Physiology.* Sudbury, MA: Jones & Bartlett Learning; 5-8, Source: Chiras, D. (2008). *Human Biology* (6th ed.). Sudbury, MA: Jones & Bartlett Learning; 5-10, 5-11, © SIU/Visuals Unlimited; 5-16, Courtesy of Hugh Dainer, MD, PhD; 5-17, Source: Madara, M., & Pomarico-Denino, V. (2008). *Quick Look Nursing: Pathophysiology* (2nd ed.). Sudbury, MA: Jones & Bartlett Learning; 5-18, Courtesy of Benjamin J. Marais; 5-19, © Phototake, Inc./Alamy Images; 5-20, 5-21, National Heart, Lung and Blood Institute (www.nhbli.nih.gov); 5-24, Source: Madara, M., & Pomarico-Denino, V. (2008). *Quick Look Nursing: Pathophysiology* (2nd ed.). Sudbury, MA: Jones & Bartlett Learning; 5-25A, © University of Alabama at Birmingham Department of Pathology PEIR Digital Library (http://peir.net); 5-25B, Courtesy of National Cancer Institute; 5-27, Courtesy of Michael-Joseph F. Agbayani; 5-30,

Source: Madara, M., & Pomarico-Denino, V. (2008). *Quick Look Nursing: Pathophysiology* (2nd ed.). Sudbury, MA: Jones & Bartlett Learning.

Chapter 6

6-3, Courtesy of Mariana Ruiz Villarreal; 6-4, © Jones and Bartlett Publishers. Photographed by Kimberly Potvin; 6-5, 6-6, Source: Baumberger-Henry, M. (2008). *Quick Look Nursing: Fluids and Electrolytes* (2nd ed.). Sudbury, MA: Jones and Bartlett Learning; 6-7, 6-8, © Jones & Bartlett Learning. Photographed by Carolyn Arcabascio; 6-9, Source: Clark, R. K. (2005). *Anatomy and Physiology: Understanding the Human Body*. Sudbury, MA: Jones & Bartlett Learning; 6-12, Source: Baumberger-Henry, M. (2008). *Quick Look Nursing: Fluids and Electrolytes* (2nd ed.). Sudbury, MA: Jones and Bartlett Learning.

Chapter 7

7-1, Source: Chiras, D. (2008). *Human Biology* (6th ed.). Sudbury, MA: Jones & Bartlett Learning; 7-2, Source: Madara, M., & Pomarico-Denino, V. (2008). *Quick Look Nursing: Pathophysiology* (2nd ed.). Sudbury, MA: Jones & Bartlett Learning; 7-3, Courtesy of Kenjiro Kimura, MD, PhD; 7-4, 7-5, Source: AAOS. (2004). *Paramedic: Anatomy & Physiology*. Sudbury, MA: Jones & Bartlett Learning; 7-6, © Custom Medical Stock Photo; 7-7, From the University of Alabama at Birmingham Department of Pathology PEIR Digital Library © (http://peir.net); 7-8, Source: Madara, M., & Pomarico-Denino, V. (2008). *Quick Look Nursing: Pathophysiology* (2nd ed.). Sudbury, MA: Jones & Bartlett Learning; 7-9, © Eskimo71/Dreamstime.com; 7-10, © CNRI/Photo Researchers, Inc.; 7-11, © Dr. Gladden Willis/Visuals Unlimited, Inc.; 7-12, Source: AAOS. (2004). *Paramedic: Anatomy & Physiology*. Sudbury, MA: Jones & Bartlett Learning.

Chapter 8

8-1, 8-2, Source: Chiras, D. (2008). *Human Biology* (6th ed.). Sudbury, MA: Jones & Bartlett Learning; 8-3A, Daniel Sabraus/Photo Researchers, Inc., 8-3B, © Jones & Bartlett Learning; 8-3C, © John Henderson/Alamy Images; 8-4, Source: AAOS. (2004). *Paramedic: Anatomy & Physiology*. Sudbury, MA: Jones & Bartlett Learning; 8-5, Source: Greenberg, S. (2007). *Exploring the Dimensions of Human Sexuality* (3rd ed.). Sudbury, MA: Jones & Bartlett Learning; 8-6, 8-7, Source: AAOS. (2004). *Paramedic: Anatomy & Physiology*. Sudbury, MA: Jones & Bartlett Learning; 8-8, Source: Chiras, D. (2008). *Human Biology* (6th ed.). Sudbury, MA: Jones & Bartlett Learning; 8-9, 8-10, Source: AAOS. (2004). *Paramedic: Anatomy & Physiology*. Sudbury, MA: Jones & Bartlett Learning; 8-12, Source: Greenberg, S. (2007). *Exploring the Dimensions of Human Sexuality* (3rd ed.). Sudbury, MA: Jones & Bartlett Learning; 8-13A, © Daniel Sabraus/Photo Researchers, Inc.; 8-13B, © Ansell Horn/Phototake; 8-13C, © Marilyn Schrut/Phototake; 8-14, 8-15, © Wellcome Images/Custom Medical Stock Photo; 8-18, © SPL/Photo Researchers, Inc.; 8-22, © Dr. P. Marazzi/Science Photo Library; 8-24, © University of Alabama at Birmingham Department of Pathology PEIR Digital Library (http://peir.net); 8-26, Courtesy of Sarah Coulter-Danner; 8-27, 8-28, Courtesy of CDC (20088-29, Courtesy of Joe Miller/CDC; 8-30, Courtesy of Bill Schwartz/CDC; 8-31,

Courtesy of Dr. Gavin Hart and Dr. N.J. Fiumara/CDC; 8-32, Courtesy of J. Pledger, BSS/VD/CDC; 8-33, 8-34, Courtesy of CDC (2008); 8-35, Courtesy of Susan Lindsley/CDC; 8-36, Source: Greenberg, S. (2007). *Exploring the Dimensions of Human Sexuality* (3rd ed.). Sudbury, MA: Jones & Bartlett Learning; 8-37, Courtesy of CDC (2008); 8-38, Courtesy of Susan Lindsley/CDC; 8-39, Courtesy of Joe Millar/CDC; 8-40, Courtesy of CDC (2008), 8-41, Courtesy of CDC/ Susan Lindsley and William R. Smart; 8-42, Adapted from: Gould, B. (2006). *Pathophysiology for the Health Professions* (3rd ed.). Philadelphia, PA: Elsevier.

Chapter 9

9-1, 9-2, Source: Chiras, D. (2008). *Human Biology* (6th ed.). Sudbury, MA: Jones & Bartlett Learning; 9-3C, © Donna Beer Stolz, PhD, Center for Biologic Imaging, University of Pittsburgh Medical School; 9-4, 9-5, Source: Chiras, D. (2008). *Human Biology* (6th ed.). Sudbury, MA: Jones & Bartlett Learning; 9-6, © David M. Martin, MD/Photo Researchers, Inc.; 9-7, Donna Beer Stolz, PhD, Center for Biologic Imaging, University of Pittsburgh Medical School; 9-8, Courtesy of Leonard V. Crowley, MD, Century College; 9-11, © CNRI/Photo Researchers, Inc.; 9-12, © Scott Camazine/Alamy Images; 9-13, Source: Madara, M., & Pomarico-Denino, V. (2008). *Quick Look Nursing: Pathophysiology* (2nd ed.). Sudbury, MA: Jones & Bartlett Learning; 9-14, © Phototake Inc./Alamy Images; 9-15, Source: Madara, M., & Pomarico-Denino, V. (2008). *Quick Look Nursing: Pathophysiology* (2nd ed.). Sudbury, MA: Jones & Bartlett Learning; 9-21, Courtesy of Leonard V. Crowley, MD, Century College; 9-23, Biophoto Associates/Photo Researchers, Inc.; 9-24A, © Michael English, MD/Custom Medical Stock Photo; 9-24B, © G-I Associates/Custom Medical Stock Photo; 9-25, Courtesy of CDC/Sol Silverman, Jr., D.D.S., University of California, San Francisco; 9-26, © Medimage/Science Photo Library

Chapter 10

10-1, Source: Chiras, D. (2008). *Human Biology* (6th ed.). Sudbury, MA: Jones & Bartlett Learning; 10-2, Source: AAOS. (2004). *Paramedic: Anatomy & Physiology*. Sudbury, MA: Jones & Bartlett Learning; 10-3, Source: Chiras, D. (2008). *Human Biology* (6th ed.). Sudbury, MA: Jones & Bartlett Learning; 10-4, Source: AAOS. (2004). *Paramedic: Anatomy & Physiology*. Sudbury, MA: Jones & Bartlett Learning; 10-4C, © John D. Cunningham/Visuals Unlimited; 10-5, Source: AAOS. (2004). *Paramedic: Anatomy & Physiology*. Sudbury, MA: Jones & Bartlett Learning; 10-6A, © Marion Bull/Alamy Images; 10-6B, © AP Photos; 10-7, Courtesy of Tanya Angus and Karen Strutynsky (www.tanyaangus.com); 10-9A, © Science Photo Library; 10-9B, © Science Photo Library/Custom Medical Stock Photo

Chapter 11

11-1, Source: AAOS. (2004). *Paramedic: Anatomy & Physiology*. Sudbury, MA: Jones & Bartlett Learning; 11-2, © David M. Phillips/Visuals Unlimited; 11-3, © C. Raines/Visuals Unlimited; 11-4A, © Science VU/ER Lewish/Visuals Unlimited; 11-4B, © T. Reese, DW Fawcett/Visuals Unlimited; 11-5, Source: Chiras, D. (2008). *Human Biology* (6th ed.). Sudbury, MA: Jones & Bartlett Learning; 11-7, Source: AAOS. (2004). *Paramedic: Anatomy & Physiology*.

Sudbury, MA: Jones & Bartlett Learning; 11-8, From the University of Alabama at Birmingham Department of Pathology PEIR Digital Library © (http://peir.net); 11-9, Courtesy of Marcus Raichle, MD, Mallinckrodt Institute of Radiology, Washington University in St. Louis School of Medicine; 11-10, Source: AAOS. (2004). *Paramedic: Anatomy & Physiology.* Sudbury, MA: Jones & Bartlett Learning; 11-11, Source: Chiras, D. (2008). *Human Biology* (6th ed.). Sudbury, MA: Jones & Bartlett Learning; 11-12, © AbleStock; 11-13, 11-14, Source: AAOS. (2004). *Paramedic: Anatomy & Physiology.* Sudbury, MA: Jones & Bartlett Learning; 11-15, Source: Chiras, D. (2008). *Human Biology* (6th ed.). Sudbury, MA: Jones & Bartlett Learning; 11-17, 11-18, Source: AAOS. (2004). *Paramedic: Anatomy & Physiology.* Sudbury, MA: Jones & Bartlett Learning; 11-20, © SIU/ Visuals Unlimited; 11-22, © Medicimage/Visuals Unlimited, Inc.; 11-26, 11-29, Source: Madara, M. & Pomarico-Denino, V. (2008). *Quick Look Nursing: Pathophysiology* (2nd ed.). Sudbury, MA: Jones & Bartlett Learning; 11-31, Courtesy of Dr. Jason W. Schroeder, MD; 11-33, © BSIP/age fotostock; 11-34, © Medical Body Scans/Photo Researchers, Inc.; 11-41, © Biophoto Associates/Photo Researchers, Inc.; 11-42, © Peter Arnold, Inc./Alamy Images; 11-43, © BSIP/ Photo Researchers, Inc.; 11-44, © Biophoto Associates/Photo Researchers, Inc.

Chapter 12

12-1, Source: Chiras, D. (2008). *Human Biology* (6th ed.). Sudbury, MA: Jones & Bartlett Learning; 12-2, Source: AAOS. (2004). *Paramedic: Anatomy & Physiology.* Sudbury, MA: Jones & Bartlett Learning; 12-3, Source: Chiras, D. (2008). *Human Biology* (6th ed.). Sudbury, MA: Jones & Bartlett Learning; 12-4, Source: AAOS. (2004). *Paramedic: Anatomy & Physiology.* Sudbury, MA: Jones & Bartlett Learning; 12-5A, © R. Calentine/Visuals Unlimited; 12-5B, © John D. Cunningham/Visuals Unlimited; 12-5C, © R. Kessel/Visuals Unlimited; 12-6, 12-7, Source: Chiras, D. (2008). *Human Biology* (6th ed.). Sudbury, MA: Jones & Bartlett Learning; 12-8, Source: Chiras, D. (2008). *Human Biology* (6th ed.). Sudbury, MA: Jones & Bartlett Learning; 12-9, Source: AAOS. (2004). *Paramedic: Anatomy & Physiology.* Sudbury, MA: Jones & Bartlett Learning; 12-11, © Don W. Fawcett/Visuals Unlimited; 12-12, © Ed Reschke/Peter Arnold, Inc.; 12-13, Source: Chiras, D. (2008). *Human Biology* (7th ed.). Sudbury, MA: Jones & Bartlett Learning; 12-14, Source: AAOS. (2004). *Paramedic: Anatomy & Physiology.* Sudbury, MA: Jones & Bartlett Learning; 12-17A, © Carolina K. Smith, MD/ShutterStock, Inc.; 12-17B, © Andres Rodriguez/ShutterStock, Inc.; 12-18, Source: AAOS. (2004). *Paramedic: Anatomy & Physiology.* Sudbury, MA: Jones & Bartlett Learning; 12-19, AAOS. (2011). *Advanced Emergency Care Transportation of the Sick and Injured.* Sudbury, MA: Jones & Bartlett Learning; 12-20, © Robert O. Brown Photography/ShutterStock, Inc.; 12-21, Source: AAOS. (2004). *Paramedic: Anatomy & Physiology.* Sudbury, MA: Jones & Bartlett Learning; 12-25, Courtesy of Steven Goldstein, MD; 12-26A, © Photo Insolite Realite/Photo Researchers, Inc.; 12-26B, © Professor Pietro M. Motta/Photo Reseachers, Inc.; 12-27A, © picsbyst/ShutterStock, Inc.; 12-27B, © Medical Body Scans/Photo

Researchers, Inc.; 12-29; Courtesy of Paul Cunningham, MD and Sherri Rudinski. Accessed from MedPix™ (www .rad.usuhs.edu/medpix); 12-30, © Medical-on-Line/Alamy Images; 12-31, © Dr. P. Marazzi/Photo Researchers, Inc.; 12-34, © Scott Camazine/Photo Researchers, Inc.; 12-37, © CNRI/Photo Researchers, Inc.

Chapter 13

13-1, © Donna Beer Stolz, Ph.D., Center for Biologic Imaging, University of Pittsburgh Medical School; 13-2, Source: AAOS. (2004). *Paramedic: Anatomy & Physiology.* Sudbury, MA: Jones & Bartlett Learning; 13-3, © Dr P. Marazzi/Photo Researchers, Inc.; 13-4, © Julie DeGuia/ShutterStock, Inc.; 13-5, © guentermanaus/ShutterStock, Inc.; 13-6, Courtesy of Marnie Pasciuto-Wood; 13-7, Courtesy of Wassa Catlow, 13-8, Courtesy of Cassandra Hartley; 13-9, © Nadine Mitchell/Dreamstime.com; 13-10, Courtesy of Dean Ducas; 13-11, © Patrick G/age fotostock; 13-12, © Dr. Zara/age fotostock; 13-13, Courtesy of Paul Matthews; 13-14, © Wellcome Images/Custom Medical Stock Photo; 13-15, © CDC/Susan Lindsley; 13-17, © Cavallini James/age fotostock; 13-18, © CDC/Allen W. Mathies, MD/California Emergency Preparedness Office (Calif/EPO), Immunization Branch; 13-19,   © Dr. Ken Greer/Visuals Unlimited, Inc.; 13-20, © CDC/Dr. Dancewiez; 13-21, © Phototake Inc./Alamy Images; 13-22, 13-23, © Centers for Disease Control; 13-24, Courtesy of James Gathany/Frank Collins, PhD/CDC; 13-25A, © CDC/Dr. Dennis D. Juranek; 13-25B, © jader alto/age fotostock, 13-26A-D © English/Custom Medical Stock Photography; 13-27D; © Amy Walters/ShutterStock, Inc.; 13-27E, Courtesy of Rhonda Beck; 13-27F, © John Radcliffe Hospital/Photo Researchers, Inc.; 13-28, © Arthur Ng Heng Kui/ShutterStock, Inc.; 13-29, © Dr. Zara/age fotostock; 13-30, Courtesy of The Skin Cancer Foundation [www .skincancer.org]

Chapter 14

14-1, Source: AAOS. (2004). *Paramedic: Anatomy & Physiology.* Sudbury, MA: Jones & Bartlett Learning; 14-2A, © Astrid & Hans-Frieder Michler/Photo Researchers, Inc.; 14-2B, © Cabisco/Visuals Unlimited; 14-3, 14-4, Source: Chiras, D. (2008). *Human Biology* (6th ed.). Sudbury, MA: Jones & Bartlett Learning; 14-5, Source: Chiras, D. (2008). *Human Biology* (6th ed.). Sudbury, MA: Jones & Bartlett Learning; 14-6, 14-7, Source: AAOS. (2004). *Paramedic: Anatomy & Physiology.* Sudbury, MA: Jones & Bartlett Learning; 14-8, 14-9, Source: Chiras, D. (2008). *Human Biology* (6th ed.). Sudbury, MA: Jones & Bartlett Learning; 14-10, Courtesy of Dr. Arturo Bonilla, Microtia-Congenital Ear Deformity Institute (http://microtia.org); 14-11, Courtesy of John T. Halgren, MD, University of Nebraska Medical Center; 14-12, Courtesy of Christopher J. Rapuano, MD; Cornea Service, Wills Eye, Professor, Jefferson Medical College of Thomas Jefferson University, Philadelphia, PA; 14-13, Courtesy of Andrew Heaford and Richard Smith, University of Iowa; 14-15, Courtesy of the National Eye Institute/NIH; 14-16, Modified from photo © Effrosyni Labropoulou/Dreamstime.com; 14-17, © Justin Paget/ShutterStock, Inc.

Prefixes and Suffixes

Prefixes

a-	without
adeno-	gland
an-	no, not, or without
ana-	without
anti-	against
bi-	two
brady-	slow
cryo-	use of liquid nitrogen to freeze
de-	to come down
dis-	to free of, separate from, or undo
dys-	difficult; bad or faulty
electro-	electricity
endo-	internal; within or inside
epi-	over, upon, above
eu-	good or well-being
ex-	outward
hemi-	half
hemo-	blood
histo-	tissue
hydro-	water
hyper-	over, excessive
hypo-	under, decreased
inter-	between
intra-	within
mal-	bad
mano-	pressure
mito-	threads
mono-	one
oligo-	scant or scanty
pan-	entire
per-	through
peri-	around
photo-	light
poly-	much, many, excessive
post-	after
pre-	before
proto-	first or to create
quadri-	four

sub-	below, under, or beneath
supra-	above
syn-	together
tachy-	fast
tri-	three

Suffixes

-ac	pertaining to
-ad	toward
-al	pertaining to
-algia	pain
-ant	the thing of which
-ar	pertaining to
-arche	beginning
-ary	pertaining to
-asthenia	exhaustion
-atic	pertaining to
-blast	developing or immature cell
-cele	hernia, herniation
-centesis	puncture
-clasia	artificial breaking to provide movement
-crine	secrete
-cusis	hearing
-cyst	fluid-filled sac or bladder
-cyte	cell
-desis	binding or stabilizing
-drome	course or set
-dynia	pain
-ectasis	dilation
-ectomy	removal, excision
-edema	abnormal accumulation of fluid in intercellular body spaces
-elastic	elastic
-emia	condition of blood
-gen	beginning or producing
-genic	originating within
-gram	picture or record
-graph	record, diagram